Handbook of Experimental Pharmacology

Continuation of Handbuch der experimentellen Pharmakologie

Vol. 67/II

Antibiotics

Containing the Beta-Lactam Structure

Part II

Contributors

P. Actor · M. C. Browning · N. H. Georgopapadakou · J. R. E. Hoover
K. C. Kwan · A. K. Miller · J. D. Rogers · R. B. Sykes · B. M. Tune
J. V. Uri

Editors

A. L. Demain and N. A. Solomon

Springer-Verlag Berlin Heidelberg New York Tokyo 1983

Professor Dr. ARNOLD L. DEMAIN
Ms. NADINE A. SOLOMON
Fermentation Microbiology Laboratory
Department of Nutrition and Food Science
Massachusetts Institute of Technology
Cambridge, MA 02139/USA

With 46 Figures

ISBN-13:978-3-642-68903-1 e-ISBN-13:978-3-642-68901-7
DOI: 10.1007/978-3-642-68901-7

Library of Congress Cataloging in Publication Data. Main entry under title: Antibiotics containing the beta-lactam structure. (Handbook of experimental pharmacology; v. 67, pt. 1–) Includes index. 1. Antibiotics–Synthesis. 2. Beta-lactamases. 3. Fungi–Genetics. [DNLM: 1. Antibiotics–Pharmacodynamics. 2. Beta-lactamases–Pharmacodynamics. W1 HA51L v. 67/QV 350 A62935] QP905.H3 vol. 67, pt. 1, etc. 615'.1s 82-19689 [QD375] [547.7'6]

Softcover reprint of the hardcover 1st edition 1983

Product Liability: The publisher can give no guarantee for information about drug dosage and application thereof contained in this book. In every individual case the respective user must check its accuracy by consulting other pharmaceutical literature.

2122/3130-543210

Preface

It is quite amazing that the oldest group of medically useful antibiotics, the β-lactams, are still providing basic microbiologists, biochemists, and clinicians with surprises over 50 years after Fleming's discovery of penicillin production by *Penicillium*. By the end of the 1950s, the future of the penicillins seemed doubtful as resistant strains of *Staphylococcus aureus* began to increase in hospital populations. However, the development of semisynthetic penicillins provided new structures with resistance to penicillinase and with broad-spectrum activity. In the 1960s, the discovery of cephalosporin C production by *Cephalosporium* and its conversion to valuable broad-spectrum antibiotics by semisynthetic means excited the world of chemotherapy. In the early 1970s, the 40-year-old notion that β-lactams were produced only by fungi was destroyed by the discovery of cephamycin production by *Streptomyces*. Again this basic discovery was exploited by the development of the semisynthetic cefoxitin, which has even broader activity than earlier β-lactams. Later in the 1970s came the discoveries of nocardicins from *Nocardia*, clavulanic acid from *Streptomyces*, and the carbapenems from *Streptomyces*. Now in the 1980s we learn that β-lactams are produced even by unicellular bacteria and that semisynthetic derivatives of these monobactams may find their way into medicine. Indeed, the future of the prolific β-lactam family seems brighter with each passing decade.

Considering the level of excitement in this area, we felt that this would be the right time for the leaders in the field to survey past and present research, development, and clinical applications of β-lactams and prospects for future progress. We were pleasantly surprised that so many busy people agreed to give up their time to contribute to this project. The result is this volume in two parts describing all aspects of β-lactam antibiotics.

Cambridge

ARNOLD L. DEMAIN
NADINE A. SOLOMON

List of Contributors

Dr. P. Actor, Smith Kline & French Laboratories, 1500 Spring Garden Street, P.O. Box 7929, Philadelphia, PA 19101/USA

Dr. M. C. Browning, Stanford University School of Medicine, Division of Nephrology, Department of Pediatrics, Stanford, CA 94305/USA

Dr. N. H. Georgopapadakou, The Squibb Institute for Medical Research, E. R. Squibb & Sons, Inc., P.O. Box 4000, Princeton, NJ 08540/USA

Dr. J. R. E. Hoover, Chemistry Research, Smith Kline & French Laboratories, 1500 Spring Garden Street, P.O. Box 7929, Philadelphia, PA 19101/USA

Dr. K. C. Kwan, Biopharmaceutics, Merck Institute for Therapeutic Research, West Point, PA 19486/USA

Dr. A. K. Miller, 104B Duncan Hill, Westfield, NJ 07090/USA

Dr. J. D. Rogers, Merck Sharp & Dohme Research Laboratories, West Point, PA 19486/USA

Dr. R. B. Sykes, The Squibb Institute for Medical Research, E. R. Squibb & Sons, Inc., P.O. Box 4000, Princeton, NJ 08540/USA

Dr. B. M. Tune, Stanford University School of Medicine, Division of Nephrology, Department of Pediatrics, Stanford, CA 94305/USA

Dr. J. V. Uri, Clinical Investigation, Smith Kline & French Laboratories, 1500 Spring Garden Street, P.O. Box 7929, Philadelphia, PA 19101/USA

Contents

CHAPTER 12

Bacterial Enzymes Interacting with β-Lactam Antibiotics
N. H. GEORGOPAPADAKOU and R. B. SYKES. With 10 Figures

CHAPTER 13

In Vitro and In Vivo Laboratory Evaluation of β-Lactam Antibiotics

A. K. MILLER

CHAPTER 14

β-Lactam Antibiotics: Structure–Activity Relationships. J. R. E. HOOVER
With 8 Figures

CHAPTER 15

Pharmacokinetics of β-Lactam Antibiotics. K. C. KWAN and J. D. ROGERS
With 28 Figures

CHAPTER 17

Therapeutic Application of β-Lactam Antibiotics. J. V. Uri and P. Actor

Contents of Companion Volume 67, Part I

CHAPTER 12

Bacterial Enzymes Interacting with *β*-Lactam Antibiotics

N. H. GEORGOPAPADAKOU and R. B. SYKES

A. Introduction

Development of β-lactam antibiotics over the past 40 years represents an unparalleled effort in the history of antimicrobial chemotherapy. The continual emergence of new compounds, natural, semisynthetic, and synthetic, is a tribute to the research programs being carried out around the world. Alongside the intensive search for new and improved β-lactam antibiotics has been the study of enzymes that interact with these molecules.

Early studies were conducted on the penicillin-hydrolyzing enzymes (β-lactamases), initially detected by ABRAHAM and CHAIN in 1940. These enzymes, responsible for the penicillin resistance among staphylococci in the 1940s and 1950s, have since proved to be a major source of resistance in gram-negative organisms. Throughout the 40-year history of β-lactam antibiotics, β-lactamases have continually asserted their presence. They have proved to be extremely important as antibiotic resistance agents and, as such, have given impetus to antibiotic development programs. Other enzymes implicated in the hydrolysis of penicillins and cephalosporins are the acylases and esterases. Although of little importance as antibiotic-resistance agents, these enzymes have played a significant part in the production of semisynthetic β-lactam antibiotics.

The second group of enzymes interacting with β-lactam antibiotics have the opposite physiological role to the β-lactamases, i.e., they are inactivated by these compounds. The effects of penicillin on cell-wall structure and morphology were shown soon after its introduction, and by the late 1950s penicillin was reported to be a specific inhibitor of bacterial cell-wall synthesis. During the following decade, the structure of the bacterial cell wall and the mechanism of its synthesis were elucidated. Following on from these studies in the 1970s came the isolation and identification of the two types of bacterial enzymes sensitive to penicillin, peptidoglycan transpeptidase and DD-carboxypeptidase.

Abbreviations

6-APA, 6-Aminopenicillanic acid; pCMB, p-chloromercuribenzoate; Diac-L-Lys-D-Ala-D-Ala, α,ε-diacetyl-L-lysyl-D-alanyl-D-alanine; Diac-L-Lys-D-Ala-D-Lac, α,ε-diacetal-L-lysyl-D-alanyl-D-lactate; DFP, diisopropylfluorophosphate; DTNB, 5,5′-dithiobis (2-nitrobenzoic acid); pI, isoelectric point; MSF, methanesulfonyl fluoride; MIC, minimum inhibitory concentration; NEM, *N*-ethylmaleimide; PBP, penicillin-binding protein; PSE, penicillin-sensitive enzyme; SDS, sodium dodecylsulfate; UDP-MurNac-L-Ala-D-Glu-meso-Dap-D-Ala-D-Ala, UDP-*N*-acetylmuramyl-L-alanyl-γ-D-glutamyl-meso-2,6-diaminopimelyl-D-alanyl-D-alanine

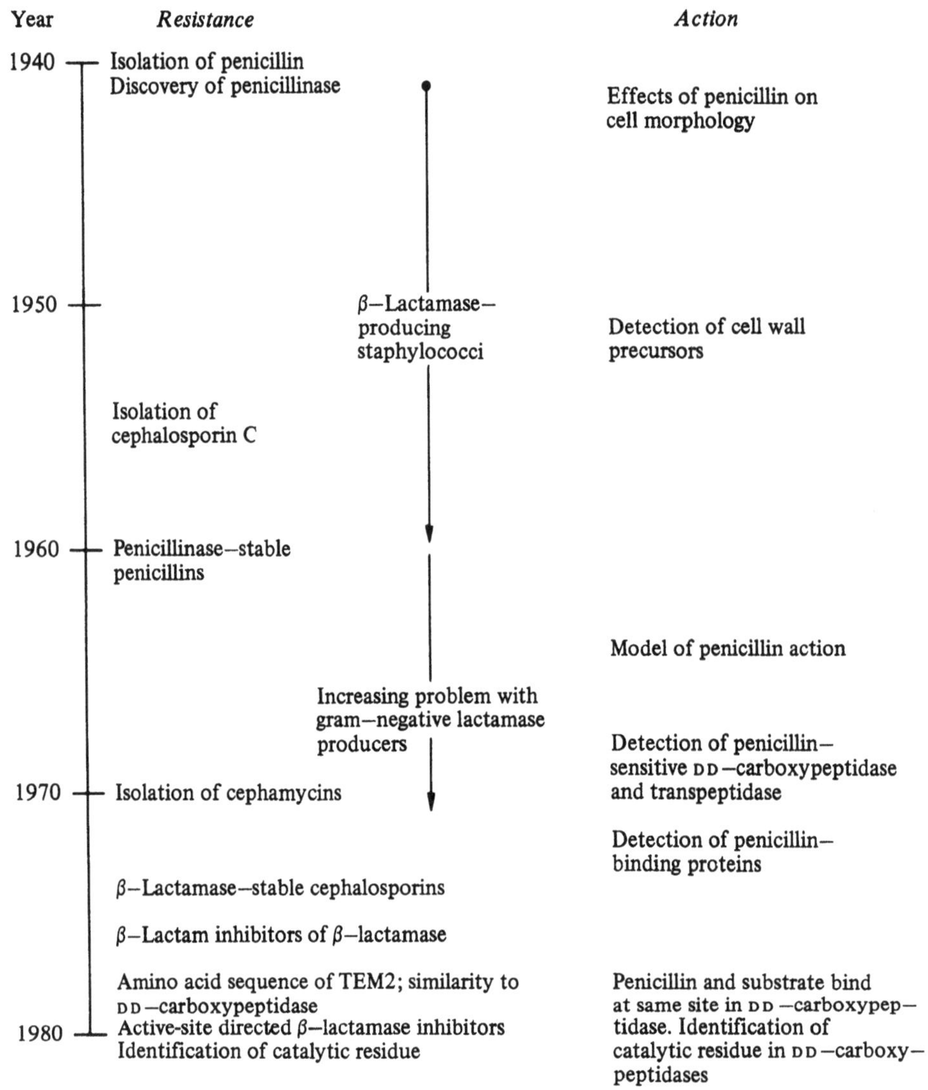

Fig. 1. Landmarks in β-lactam resistance and β-lactam action

However, the action of penicillin proved to be more complex than earlier studies had suggested. Since the early 1970s, reports have appeared describing the existence of several proteins in microbial membranes capable of covalently binding penicillin and performing important physiological functions. The presence of multiple targets for penicillin is now widely accepted. It is also established that penicillin-binding proteins (PBPs) and penicillin targets are different in different bacteria, and that these targets may respond differently to various β-lactam antibiotics.

Initially studied as two separate entities, those enzymes hydrolyzing β-lactams and those that are inactivated by β-lactams have been recently found to possess several common features. Thus, the distinction between the two groups of enzymes might be less sharp than was originally thought. β-Lactamase activity has been detected in some penicillin-sensitive enzymes (PSEs), and some β-lactams do inactivate β-lactamases. Most remarkably, the amino acid sequence at the active site of some penicillin-sensitive enzymes appears to be homologous to that of conventional β-lactamases.

The chronological sequence of developments in the area of β-lactamases and β-lactam action is shown in Fig. 1.

I. Classification of β-Lactam Antibiotics

β-Lactam antibiotics represent the largest group of commercially available antimicrobial agents. In addition, there is a large number of compounds at various stages of development.

Between 1940 and 1970 all known antimicrobially active β-lactam-containing compounds were divided into two chemical types, penicillins and cephalosporins. The penicillins (*1*) contain a β-lactam ring fused to a thiazolidine ring, whereas the cephalosporins (*2*) have the β-lactam fused to a dihydrothiazine ring. These are referred to as the classic β-lactams.

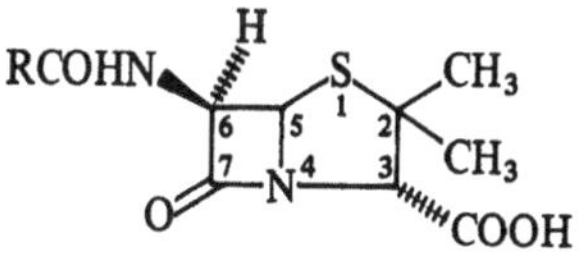

(*1*)

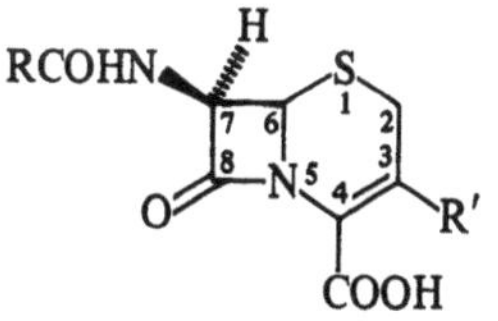

(*2*)

The discovery of the 7α-methoxy cephalosporins in 1971 (NAGARAJAN et al. 1971) provided the first new, naturally occurring β-lactam nucleus since the isolation of cephalosporin C. Although often referred to colloquially as cephamycins, they are fundamentally ceph-3-ems with a methoxy group in place of hydrogen at the 7α-position of the cephalosporin nucleus (*2*).

The first reported nonclassic β-lactam containing compounds were the amidino penicillins (*3*), e.g., mecillinam (LUND and TYBRING 1972), produced semisynthetically from 6-aminopenicillanic acid (6-APA). Another group of nonclassic semisynthetic molecules are the oxacephalosporins (*4*), e.g., moxalactam (YOSHIDA et al. 1978). All other nonclassic β-lactams presently undergoing clinical trial have been isolated from natural sources. Clavulanic acid (*5*) (HOWARTH et al. 1976; READING and COLE 1977), the first of such compounds to be isolated, has oxygen in place of sulfur in the five-membered ring. The carbapenems (*6*) include the olivanic acids (BROWN et al. 1977), thienamycins (ALBERS-SCHONBERG et al. 1978), epithienamycins (STAPLEY et al. 1977), and PS compounds (OKAMURA et al. 1978). The only active monocyclic β-lactams so far reported are the nocardicins (*7*) (AOKI et al. 1976) and the monobactams (SYKES et al. 1982).

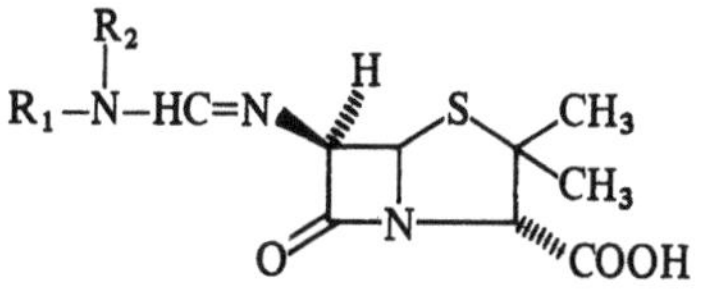

(*3*)

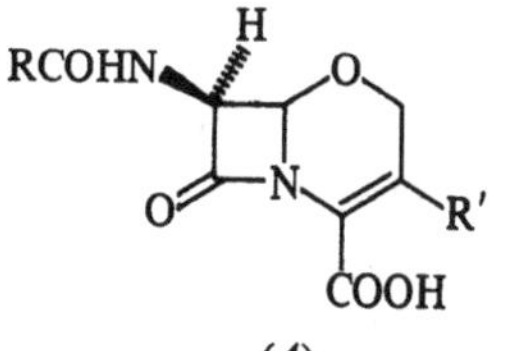

(*4*)

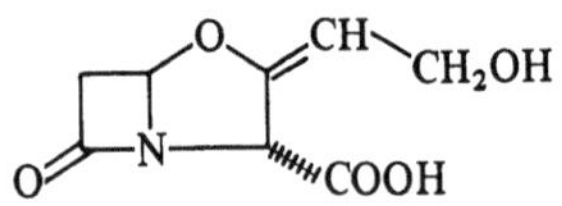

(5)

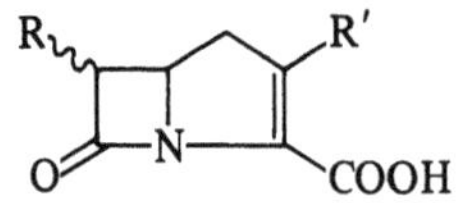

(6)

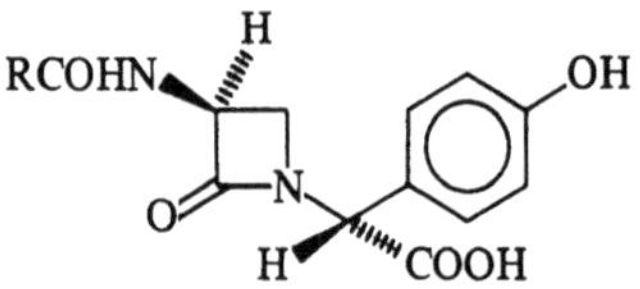

(7)

With the exception of thienamycin (*8*), side-chain substituents on the β-lactam ring of naturally occurring β-lactam antibiotics are in the β configuration. In thienamycin, the side chain is α. As will be discussed, the stereochemistry of the attachment of the side chain is of utmost importance to enzyme–β-lactam interactions.

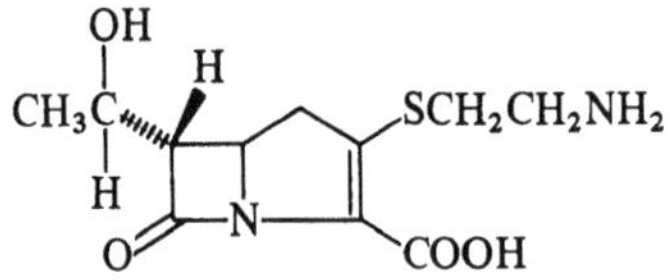

(8)

Significant discoveries in the field of β-lactam research are shown in the β-lactam calendar (Fig. 2).

II. Mode of Action of β-Lactam Antibiotics

1. Structure and Synthesis of Peptidoglycan

To understand how β-lactam antibiotics interact with their targets, it is necessary briefly to review the structure and biosynthesis of peptidoglycan. This netlike macromolecule surrounds, in one or more layers, the bacterial cytoplasmic membrane and is responsible, at least in gram-positive bacteria, for the shape and integrity of the cell. As its name implies, peptidoglycan consists of polysaccharide (glycan) strands cross-linked through short peptides. The glycan moiety consists of alternating *N*-acetylglucosamine and *N*-acetylmuramic acid residues and is relatively uniform in bacteria. In contrast, the peptide moiety, which consists of D- and L-amino acids, is variable, especially in the diamino acid cross-linking adjacent peptide strands directly or via an interpeptide bridge (Fig. 3). This structural diversity is limited to Gram-positive bacteria and is thought to be the result of the constant interaction of the cell wall with the outside environment. The peptidoglycan of gram-negative bacteria appears to have identical peptide strands linked directly via meso-diaminopimelic acid; that is, there is no interpeptide bridge (SCHLEIFER and KANDLER 1972). External to the peptidoglycan, gram-negative bacteria have an outer membrane containing a highly variable lipopolysaccharide structure which again may be the result of the constant interaction of the outer cell surface with the external environment.

In gram-positive bacteria, peptidoglycan is attached covalently to teichoic acids, which are heteropolymers made up of sugar and amino acid units and may play a role in bacterial adherence (OFEK and BEACHEY 1980). The linkage is a phosphodiester bond between *N*-acetylmuramic acid of peptidoglycan and *N*-acetylglucosamine of teichoic acid, the phosphate being derived from UDP-*N*-acetylglucosamine (COLEY et al. 1978).

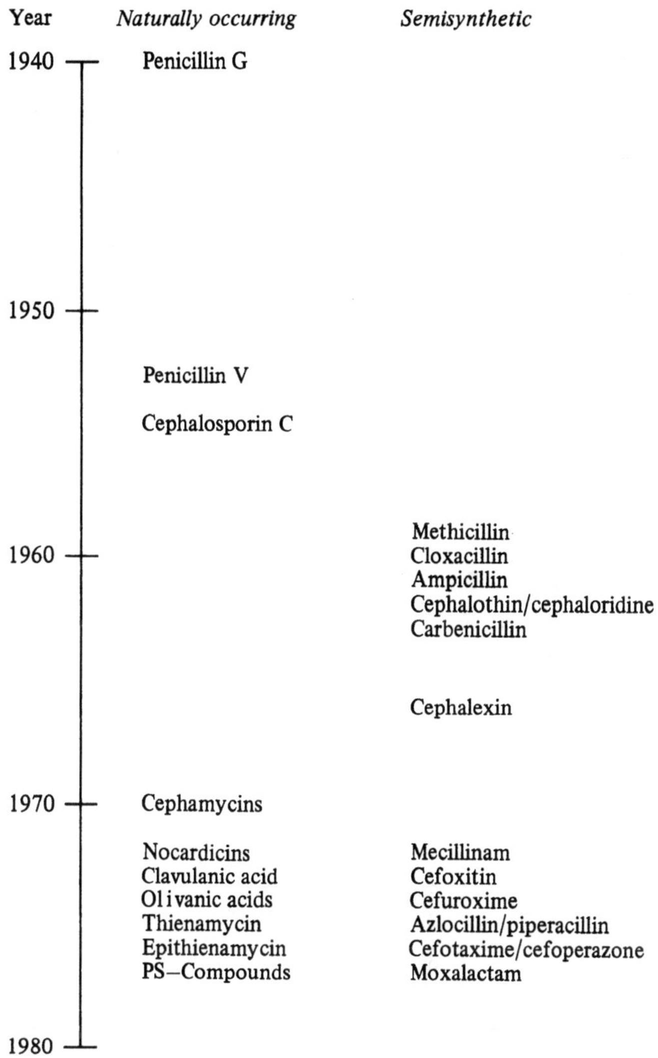

Fig. 2. β-Lactam calendar

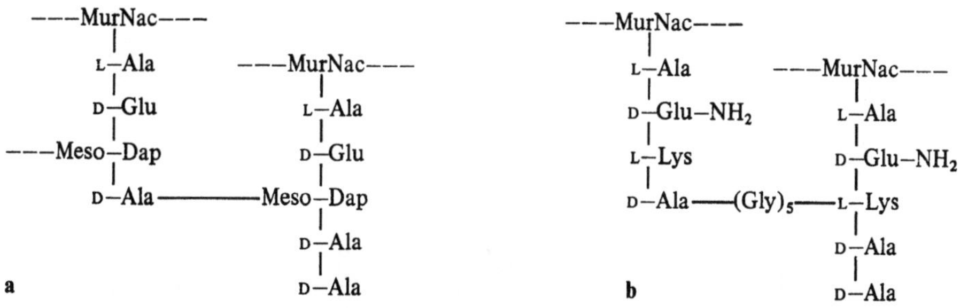

Fig. 3. Major peptidoglycan types of clinically important bacteria: **a** Gram-negative bacteria (e.g., *E. coli*) and bacilli (e.g., *B. subtilis*); **b** staphylococci (e.g., *S. aureus*) and streptococci (e.g., *S. faecalis*)

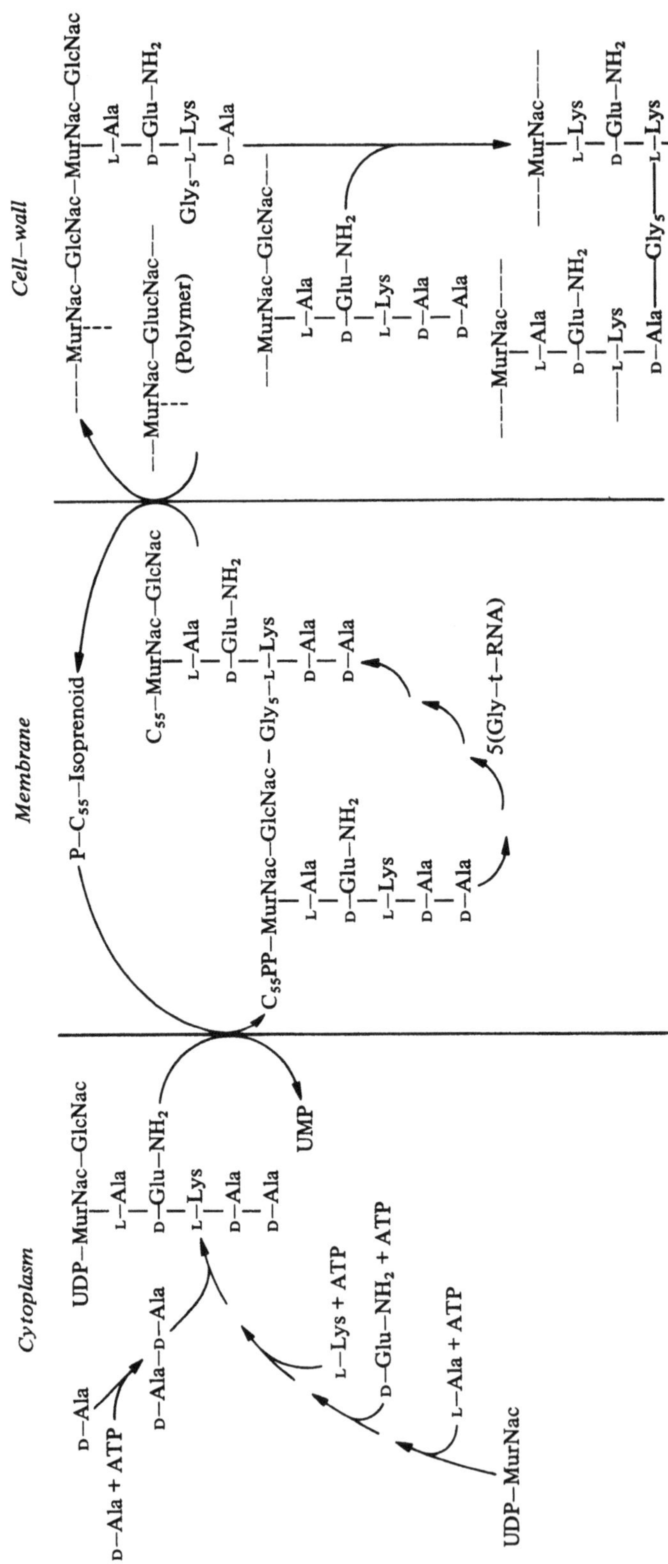

Fig. 4. Major steps in peptidoglycan biosynthesis in *S. aureus*

In gram-negative bacteria peptidoglycan is covalently attached to a major outer membrane lipoprotein (Braun's lipoprotein), of molecular weight 7,500 in *Escherichia coli*, which in effect anchors the outer membrane to the peptidoglycan (BRAUN and REHN 1969). Thus, *Salmonella typhimurium* mutants lacking the ability to cross-link Braun's lipoprotein to peptidoglycan fail to invaginate during cell division, and therefore form a defective septum (FUNG et al. 1978). The lipoprotein-peptidoglycan linkage is between the ε-amino group of lysine at the lipoprotein C-terminus and the carboxyl group of every tenth diaminopimelic acid in the peptidoglycan peptide strand. The reaction probably involves concomitant release of the penultimate D-alanine in the peptide strand (BRAUN et al. 1974).

The biosynthesis of peptidoglycan is topologically divided into three stages (Fig. 4): (1) occurring in the cytoplasm, synthesis of UDP-*N*-acetylmuramic acid pentapeptide; (2) occurring in the membrane, transfer of phospho-*N*-acetylmuramic acid, addition of *N*-acetylglucosamine and species-specific modifications (e.g., successive additions of five glycines to the ε-amino group of the lysine residue of the pentapeptide in *Staphylococcus aureus*); (3) occurring outside the membrane, transfer of new units to growing peptidoglycan and cross-linking of adjacent peptide strands.

It is the last transpeptidation reaction which has been considered to be the site of action of penicillin and other β-lactam antibiotics. Interestingly enough, in most organisms the *N*-acetylmuramyl-pentapeptide does not accumulate as a result of the action of penicillin, because it regulates its own synthesis (LUGTENBERG et al. 1972). Thus, *S. aureus*, the organism in which accumulation of cell-wall precursors was first observed (PARK 1952), may constitute an exception rather than the rule. The degree of peptidoglycan cross-linking varies among bacteria, from 30% in *Lactobacillus acidophilus* to 90% in *S. aureus* (GHUYSEN and SHOCKMAN 1973).

The molecular geometry of peptidoglycan and the enzymology of its biosynthesis during cell expansion and division is uncertain. Teleologically, one would expect different enzymes (i.e. transpeptidases) for cylindrical and hemispherical growth, septum formation, and peptidoglycan repair. Insertion of new cell-wall appears to be localized (DANEO-MOORE et al. 1975; POOLEY et al. 1978), but some turnover (two- or even three-dimensional) probably does occur as a result of autolytic activity associated with cell-wall remodelling (WESTON et al. 1977). Autolytic activity may also be responsible for cell-wall separation at the end of septation (SHOCKMAN et al. 1974; FEIN and ROGERS 1976) and, at least in some organisms, for the lytic effect of β-lactam antibiotics (ROGERS and FORSBERG 1975; TOMASZ and WAKS 1975). Cell-wall biosynthesis is integrated with cell growth (DNA replication, membrane assembly and division, but the coupling mechanisms are largely unknown.

2. The Tipper and Strominger Hypothesis for Penicillin Action

In 1965, TIPPER and STROMINGER proposed that penicillin acts as a steric analog of the terminal D-Ala-D-Ala portion of the pentapeptide chain in the nascent peptidoglycan (Fig. 5). A covalent penicilloyl-enzyme adduct is formed, which is stable to subsequent hydrolysis, and thereby transpeptidase is inactivated. It was postulated that transpeptidation also proceeds through an acyl enzyme intermediate

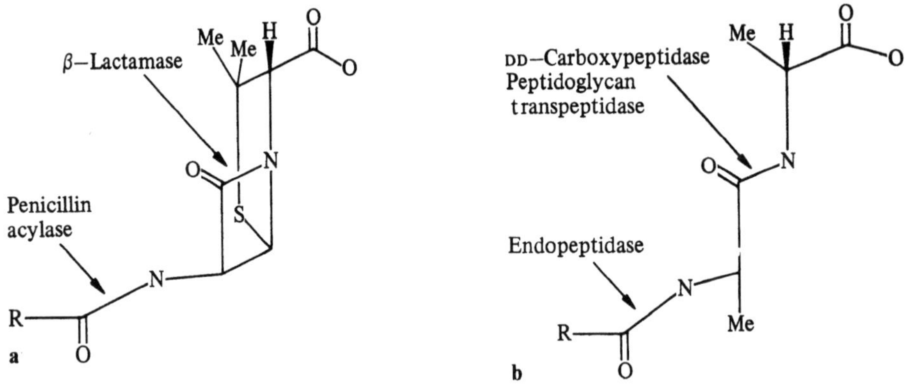

Fig. 5 a, b. Schematic presentation of penicillin (**a**) and the acyl D-Ala-D-Ala end of the peptide strand in the nascent peptidoglycan (**b**). Corresponding sites of enzymatic attack in the two molecules are indicated by *arrows*. Hydrogens are omitted for the sake of clarity, except where necessary to indicate stereochemistry. (After TIPPER and STROMINGER 1965)

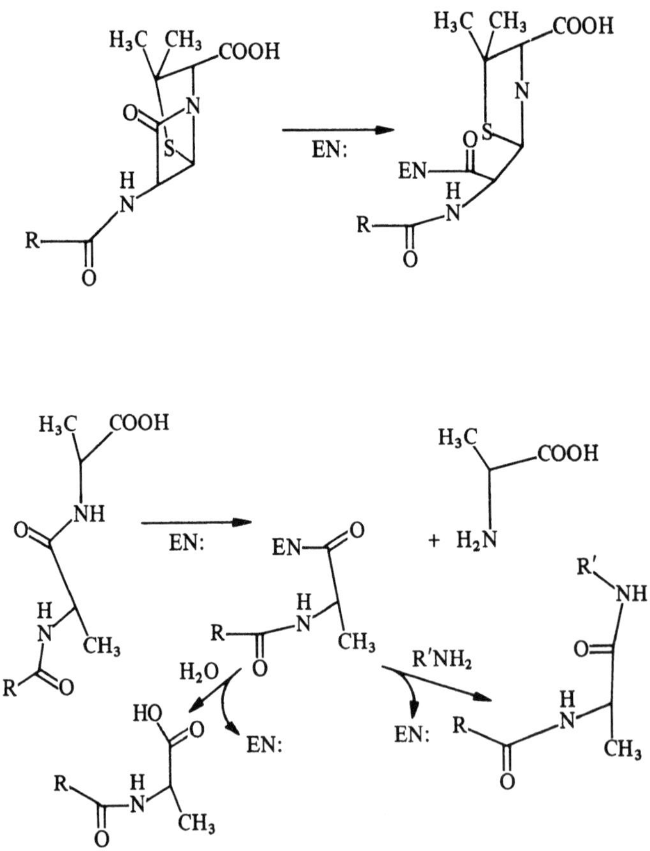

Fig. 6. Transpeptidase reaction and inactivation by penicillin. *R′* represents the peptide acceptor. The carboxypeptidase reaction is also included

which is then transferred to an amino acid acceptor of an adjacent peptide strand (Fig. 6).

The model predicted that:

1. Peptidoglycan enzymes, other than transpeptidase, cleaving the peptide bond in R-D-Ala-D-Ala (where R is a diamino acid residue) at the end of the peptidoglycan should also bind penicillin.
2. Penicilinases have evolved from peptidoglycan enzymes acting on the peptide bond in R-D-Ala-D-Ala. That is, there may be a continuum from cell-wall-synthesizing enzymes to β-lactam-inactivating enzymes.
3. A penicilloyl enzyme is also formed during penicillin hydrolysis by β-lactamases.
4. Enzymes binding to the R-D-Ala-D-Ala portion at the end of the peptidoglycan strands but not cleaving the peptide bond in R-D-Ala$\downarrow$D-Ala would be insensitive to penicillin.
5. Peptidoglycan enzymes acting on the peptide bond in R-D-Ala$\downarrow$D-Ala might have given rise to enzymes hydrolyzing the penicillin side chain.

The above model has since been refined (penicillin is now believed to act as a steric analog (LEE 1971; BOYD 1977) or a K_{cat} inhibitor (RANDO 1975) but otherwise is basically correct, and all of its predictions have been experimentally realized:

1. DD-carboxypeptidases, bacterial enzymes hydrolyzing the peptide bond in R-D-Ala$\downarrow$D-Ala are inhibited to various degrees by penicillin.
2. DD-carboxypeptidases exist which possess transpeptidase activity as well as weak but measurable penicillinase activity (TAMURA et al. 1976; KOZARICH and STROMINGER 1978).
3. Acyl enzyme intermediate has been recently trapped with β-lactamase (FISHER et al. 1980).
4. Neither the lipoprotein-peptidoglycan cross-linking enzyme (BRAUN et al. 1974) nor LD-carboxypeptidase (IZAKI et al. 1968) are penicillin-sensitive enzymes.

Although the putative acyl-enzyme intermediate of the peptidoglycan transpeptidase reaction has never been isolated, that of the analogous DD-carboxypeptidase reaction has (RASMUSSEN and STROMINGER 1978).

There still remain, however, some unanswered questions as to the degree of steric similarity of penicillin to the D-Ala-D-Ala portion of the pentapeptide and the extent to which they bind at the same site. Epipenicillin [6-α-penicillin], whose configuration more closely approximates the DD-dipeptide, is a less potent antibiotic than penicillin (SAWAI et al. 1970). 6-Methylpenicillins, which are also better analogs of the substrate than is penicillin, are less potent antibiotics (HO et al. 1972); however, some but not all 7-methoxy cephalosporins *are* potent inhibitors (GEORGOPAPADAKOU et al. 1979; HO et al. 1973; CURTIS et al. 1979b).

III. Classification of Enzymes Interacting with β-Lactam Antibiotics

1. Enzymes Acting on Peptidoglycan

There are two types of enzymes known to be inhibited by β-lactam antibiotics: DD-*carboxypeptidases* and *peptidoglycan transpeptidases*. Some DD-carboxypeptidases are referred to as DD-carboxypeptidases-transpeptidases to indicate the fact that

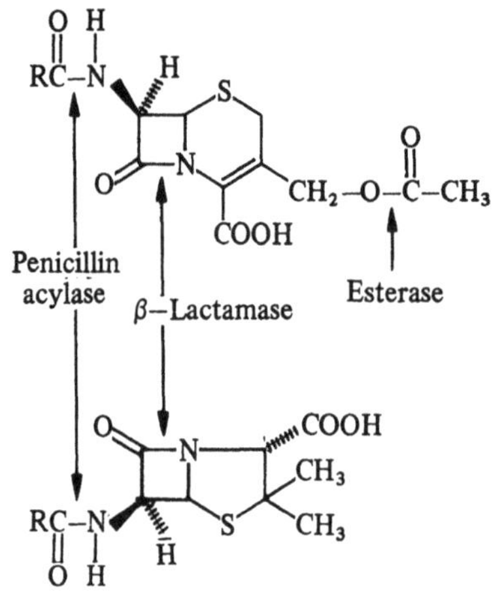

Fig. 7. Interaction of penicillins and cephalosporins with hydrolyzing enzymes

they can also catalyze transfer reactions in vitro (Sect. C.I.2). Both DD-carboxypeptidases and peptidoglycan transpeptidases almost certainly proceed through similar mechanisms, involving formation of an acyl-enzyme intermediate followed by transfer to an amino acid acceptor (transpeptidase) or to water (carboxypeptidase). Both enzymes are usually membrane bound (carboxypeptidase can be soluble too; Sect. C.I.2) and they both bind penicillin covalently.

Peptidoglycan transpeptidase is known to perform an important physiological function and has been considered the classic target for penicillin and other β-lactam antibiotics. The physiological role of DD-carboxypeptidase is less clear. It is obviously essential in organisms where tetrapeptides instead of pentapeptides are involved in cross-linking, as in *Gaffkya homari* (HAMMES and KANDLER 1976). It is also possible that it regulates the degree of cross-linking by competing with transpeptidase for peptide strands. DD-carboxypeptidase, although often the major PBP, is seldom a lethal target for penicillin.

2. Enzymes Degrading β-Lactam Antibiotics

Although β-lactam antibiotics provide a substrate for a number of hydrolytic enzymes, by far the most important are the β-lactamases. These enzymes hydrolyze the cyclic amide bond of susceptible β-lactam antibiotics to give antibiotically inactive products (Fig. 7). In the case of penicillins, the products of hydrolysis are penicilloates which are stable and easily detectable. With cephalosporins, the corresponding cephalosporoates are usually unstable, the resulting fragmentation pattern being dependent on the nature of the C-3 substituent (NEWTON et al. 1967). Thus the detection of cephalosporin hydrolysis products is often complicated.

A second type of enzymatic degradation of β-lactam antibiotics involves removal of acyl side chains by amino acid acylases (often referred to as penicillin acylases or amidases) (Fig. 7). Penicillin acylases are widely distributed among bacteria and fungi (COLE 1969a). They are enzymes of rather low substrate specificity, hydrolyzing side chains from both penicillins and cephalosporins with pH optima around 8.0 (COLE 1969a). Recently, the deacylation of the carbapenem PS-5 (*9*) to NS-5 (*10*) by both L- and D-amino acid acylases from animal and microbial sources has been reported (FUKUGAWA et al. 1980). Although removal of acyl side chains from β-lactam antibiotics usually leads to compounds with markedly reduced antibacterial activity, loss of the acyl side chain from certain naturally occurring carbapenems leads to increased antibacterial activity. In addition to hydrolyzing the side chains from β-lactam antibiotics, acylases can hydrolyze various acylamino acids, amides and esters (COLE 1969b).

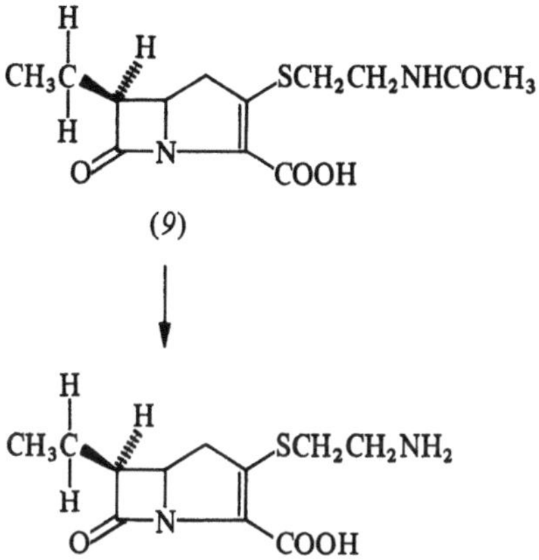

(*10*)

Acylases are usually assayed with penicillin as substrate (COLE et al. 1975). Recently, a colorimetric assay employing phenylacetyl aminobenzoic acid has been reported (SZEWCZUK et al. 1980).

Acylases are of minor, if any, importance in antibiotic resistance but are commercially exploited in the enzymatic cleavage of penicillins and cephalosporins in the production of semisynthetic derivatives. Unfortunately, no acylase is known to remove the D-α-aminoadipoyl side chain from naturally occurring cephalosporin C (*11*), a reaction which would greatly facilitate production of semisynthetic cephalosporins.

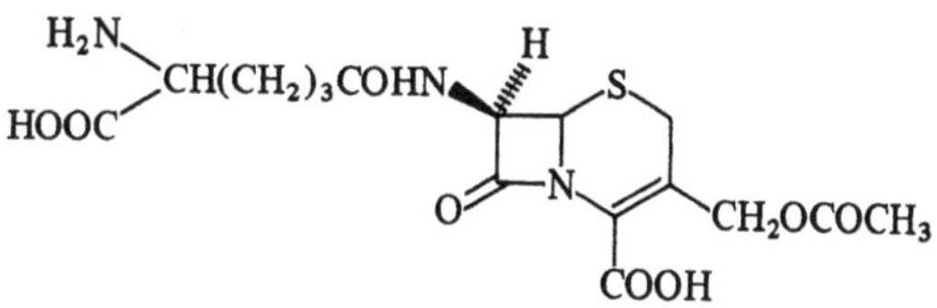

(*11*)

A third enzymatic degradation involves removal by esterases of the acetyl group of cephalosporins containing an acetoxymethyl group at C-3, e.g., cephalothin (Fig. 7). Such a cleavage produces compounds of reduced antimicrobial activity. A recent report (NISHIURA et al. 1978) describes the microbial degradation of cephalothin to deacetyl cephalothin by a strain of *E. coli*. The presence of esterases in mammalian tissue are exploited for cleaving microbiologically inactive penicillin esters (pro-drugs), such as talampicillin (*12*) to release the active compounds, in this case ampicillin. Esterases are also used commercially for cleaving the acetoxymethyl group of cephalosporin C in the production of semisynthetic cephalosporins.

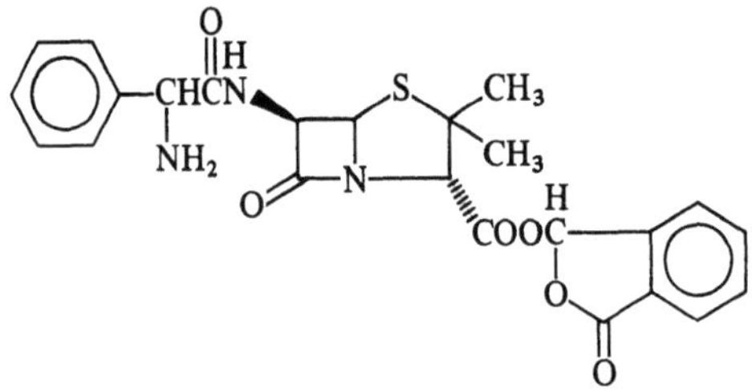

(*12*)

Enzymes specifically interacting with the thienamycin class of compounds (carbapenems) have recently been isolated from mammalian kidney (KAHAN and KROPP 1980).

B. Bacterial Proteins Binding β-Lactam Antibiotics

I. General

All bacteria examined to date contain several proteins which specifically and covalently bind penicillin (PBPs). In retrospect, the finding of multiple PBPs in bacteria (BLUMBERG and STROMINGER 1974) is not unexpected. Cell-wall biosynthesis may involve several reactions that proceed through cleavage of the peptide bond in the D-Ala-D-Ala portion of the nascent peptidoglycan. For example, cylindrical and hemispherical growth or septation could involve different transpeptidases, each subject to specific spatial and temporal controls. Generation of tetrapeptides for subsequent transpeptidation (HAMMES and KANDLER 1976) or regulation of the degree of cross-linking would also involve different DD-carboxypeptidases. According to the Tipper and Strominger hypothesis, all these enzymes could covalently bind penicillin and, if the complexes are stable enough, would be detected as PBPs. Indeed, both DD-carboxypeptidase and transpeptidase are penicillin sensitive and bind penicillin covalently. Presumably, other proteins which bind penicillin are penicillin-sensitive enzymes and the failure to detect enzyme activity (CHASE et al. 1977; KLEPPE and STROMINGER 1979) is due to low amounts of enzyme, inactivation during isolation, low turnover numbers or inappropriate assay conditions.

On sodium dodecylsulfate (SDS)–polyacrylamide gels, PBPs have molecular weights (MW) usually ranging from 40,000 to 120,000 and are numbered in order of decreasing molecular weight. They are present in amounts ranging from a few molecules to a couple of thousand molecules per cell (SPRATT 1977a). Perhaps it is not accidental that the targets of penicillin and other β-lactam antibiotics have been found to be relatively minor PBPs (BUCHANAN and STROMINGER 1976; REYNOLDS et al. 1978; SUZUKI et al. 1978). Accessibility of PBPs to and affinity for β-lactam antibiotics are also important factors in the overall inhibitory effect of these compounds.

Binding to PBPs is usually determined by measuring competition with ^{14}C-penicillin G binding. Typically, whole cells or bacterial membranes are incubated for 10 min at 30 °C with a nonradioactive β-lactam antibiotic. Then ^{14}C-penicillin G is added and the incubation is continued for another 10 min. Proteins are solubilized with detergent and fractionated on SDS-polyarylamide gels (LAEMMLI 1970). Fluorography of the gels (BONNER and LASKEY 1974) followed by microdensitometry of the fluorogram permits quantitative determination of protein-bound radioactivity. The PBP methodology is thoroughly discussed by SPRATT (1977a).

In a variation of the above procedure, membranes are solubilized with nonionic detergent prior to the binding assay (GEORGOPAPADAKOU and LIU 1980a). In another variation, applicable whenever β-lactamases are suspected to be present, membranes are preincubated for 10 min with clavulanic acid (2 μg/ml) prior to the binding assay (GEORGOPAPADAKOU and LIU 1979, unpublished work).

The PBP binding assay is convenient and, in the case of membranes, permits determination of binding under conditions where permeability barriers and β-lactamases are largely absent. An inherent limitation of this type of assay is that binding to proteins other than PBPs cannot be examined. Penicillin G, traditionally considered the prototype of β-lactam antibiotics, may not adequately represent all of them (YANO et al. 1979; NISHIDA et al. 1977). Thus, it may often be prudent to examine the binding directly, using radiolabeled β-lactam antibiotics. PBP binding results, done mostly with nonradiolabeled compounds and ^{14}C-penicillin G, have been correlated with MICs and morphological changes. The correlations rest on several important assumptions: (a) that neither bound antibiotic nor bound penicillin G are released during the assay; (b) that the PBP amount is limiting for cell growth [although it is conceivable that an essential PBP, like a nonessential one (e.g., PBP 5/6 in *E. coli*), might be present in excess]; (c) that penicillin G binding is a necessary and sufficient condition for enzymatic activity [although in the case of PBP 5/6 of *E. coli* enzymatic activity can be lost without the concomitant loss of penicillin binding ability] (CURTIS and STROMINGER 1978); (d) that image density in the x-ray film after fluorography is linearly correlated with radioactivity. This last point is a purely technical one which, however, should be borne in mind since there can be a hundred-fold difference between amounts of individual PBPs in an organism.

Most PBPs have no demonstrable enzymatic activity, but they nevertheless seem to perform important physiological functions. Thus far, such functions have been assigned to individual PBPs only in *E. coli* (SPRATT 1977a; SUZUKI et al. 1978) and related bacteria (CURTIS et al. 1979a). There, binding of β-lactam antibiotics to individual PBPs has been associated with distinct morphological changes and essential PBPs, associated with elongation, cell shape or septation, have been identified.

The picture is less clear with bacteria which have different PBP patterns (Fig. 8), and in which binding of penicillin to individual PBPs is not associated with morphological changes. The situation is even more complicated by the presence of enzyme multiplicity revealed by microbiological and physiological studies. That is, more than one protein may be responsible for a single physiological function. As a result, deletion of an essential PBP may result in compensatory increases in other PBPs (TAMAKI et al. 1977; GILES and REYNOLDS 1979).

The spatial and temporal distribution of PBPs in the cell is largely unknown. Minor PBPs associated with localized functions (e.g., septum formation) are ex-

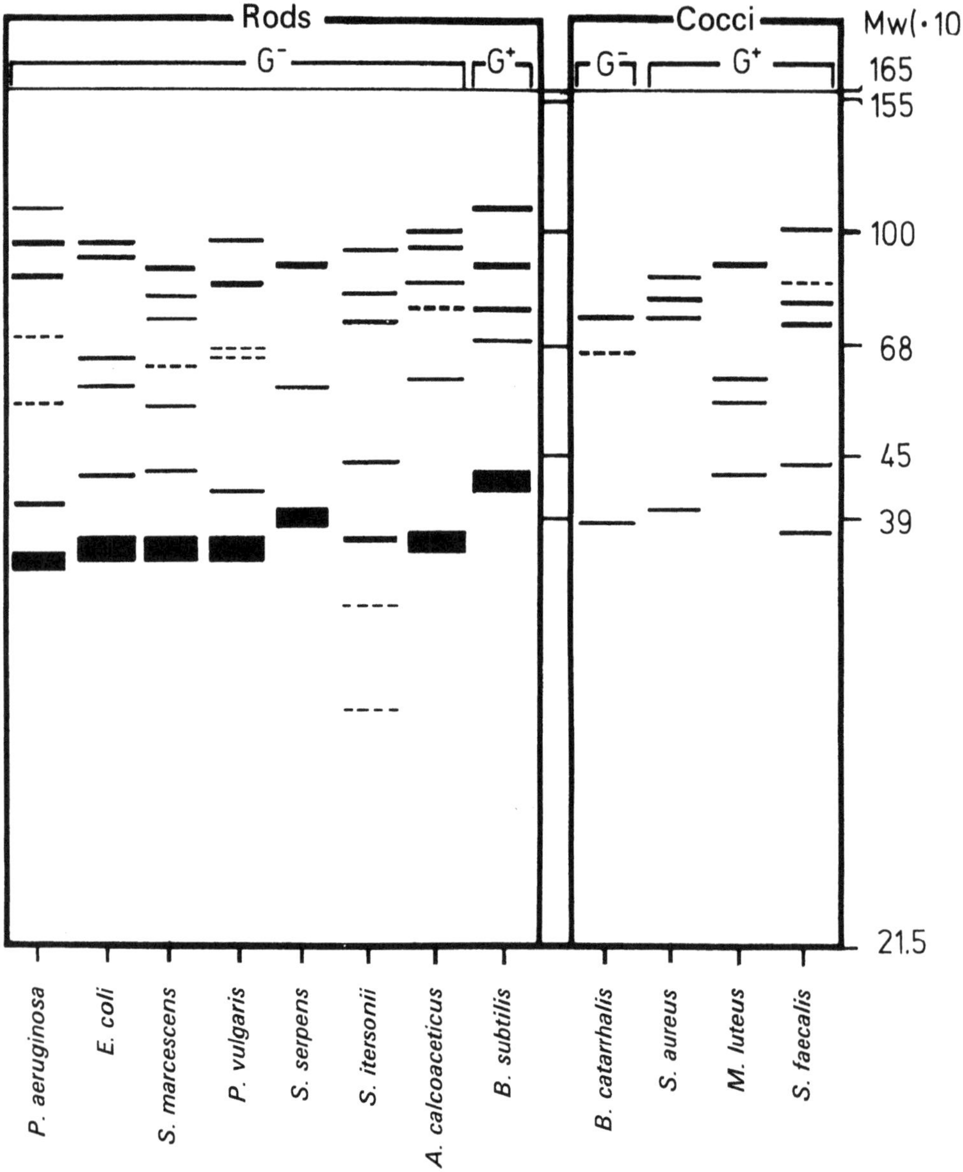

Fig. 8. Schematic drawing of PBPs from representative bacteria based on fluorograms of SDS gels of solubilized membranes that had been incubated with ^{14}C-penicillin G. Individual PBPs are represented by *lines* whose relative thickness indicates relative abundance. Very minor PBPs are indicated by *broken lines*. Lines are drawn according to the molecular weight of PBPs and the mobilities of molecular weight markers in each gel

pected to be concentrated in specific regions in the cytoplasmic membrane, becoming major PBPs in those regions. But evidence to support this suggestion is lacking (GOODELL and SCHWARTZ 1977). Also, activity of cell-wall synthesizing enzymes varies throughout growth (GLASER and LINDSAY 1977, MIRELMAN et al. 1978) which is consistent with the notion that cell-wall biosynthesis is a discontinuous process (ROGERS 1970). But PBP patterns have not yet been followed during synchronous growth and division.

PBPs must have common features in the structure and function as evidenced by their ability to bind penicillin (TIPPER and STROMINGER 1965). However, differences between PBPs exist and PBP patterns (relative amounts, molecular weights, sensitivity to β-lactam antibiotics, ability to release bound penicillin) appear to parallel taxonomic/evolutionary lines (COCKS and WILSON 1972; FOX et al. 1980) and, possibly, the structural diversity of peptidoglycan. Since the most variable amino acid in peptidoglycan is the one corresponding to the side chain of penicillin, it is not surprising that PBP affinity of β-lactam antibiotics is different in different organisms.

II. Penicillin-Binding Proteins in Gram-Negative Bacteria

Although PBP patterns in gram-negative bacteria are diverse, those of enterobacteria are remarkably similar. Unfortunately, as most studies have involved enterobacteria, a false impression has been created of the universality of the enterobacterial PBP pattern (CURTIS et al. 1979a). Perhaps the only universal feature of PBPs is a 35,000- to 40,000-dalton protein, present in varying amounts, which is moderately sensitive to β-lactam antibiotics and has weak but measurable β-lactamase activity. In *E. coli* and related enterobacteria it is the major PBP and has DD-carboxypeptidase activity.

1. Escherichia coli

Seven PBPs (molecular weights: 40,00–90,000) are consistently found in *E. coli* (SPRATT and PARDEE 1975). They are coded by separate genes which appear to be dispersed on the *E. coli* chromosome (SUZUKI et al. 1978; TAMAKI et al. 1980). Their properties are outlined in Table 1. Two additional PBPs, of molecular weights 35,000 and 30,000, are occasionally found. All PBPs are located in the cytoplasmic membrane and, with the exception of the 49,000-dalton protein (PBP 4), are rendered soluble only after treatment with detergents. Physiological studies have indicated that the 91,000-, 66,000-, and 60,000-dalton proteins are involved respectively in elongation, shape, and septation (SPRATT 1975). Microbiological studies, involving *E. coli* mutants with individual PBPs altered, have confirmed the above

Table 1. Properties of *E. coli* PBPs (SPRATT, 1977)

Mobility in SDS-PAGE	Protein	MW	Copies/cell	Function
	1a, 1b	91,000	230	Elongation (transpeptidase)
	2	66,000	20	Shape
	3	60,000	50	Septation
	4	49,000	110	Carboxypeptidase IB
	5	42,000	800	Carboxypeptidase IA
	6	40,000	570	Carboxypeptidase IA

assignment of physiological functions and have established these three proteins as the killing sites for β-lactam antibiotics in *E. coli* (SUZUKI et al. 1978).

Depending on their PBP binding profile, different β-lactam antibiotics or different concentrations of the same β-lactam antibiotic may cause different morphological changes. For example, penicillin G causes formation of filaments at low concentrations but lysis at higher concentrations corresponding to binding to PBP 3 and 1 respectively. The properties of *E. coli* PBPs have been the subject of several recent reviews (SPRATT 1978; MATSUHASHI et al. 1979; SPRATT 1979).

Binding of β-lactam antibiotics to PBP 1 (molecular weight: 91,000) is thought to be responsible for the lytic effect of these compounds, although the exact mechanism of the process is unknown. PBP 1 is the in vivo transpeptidase (SUZUKI et al. 1978). It has been resolved into two genetically distinct components (SPRATT et al. 1977) with identical enzymatic and physiological functions but different heat stabilities and affinities toward β-lactam antibiotics (NAKAGAWA et al. 1979) (Table 1). PBP 1 a is heat labile and highly sensitive to β-lactam antibiotics. PBP 1 b, which is composed of at least three genetically indistinguishable proteins, is relatively heat stable and only moderately sensitive to β-lactam antibiotics. *E. coli* mutants lacking PBP 1 a have no phenotypic defect (SPRATT et al. 1977) while mutants lacking PBP 1 b are hypersensitive to β-lactam antibiotics (SUZUKI et al. 1978) reflecting the compensatory role of PBP 1 a. PBP 1 b has been recently purified and shown to possess transpeptidase and transglycosylase activity (SUZUKI et al. 1980).

Binding of β-lactam antibiotics to PBP 2 (molecular weight: 66,000) results in giant round cells which eventually lyse (MELCHIOR et al. 1973; SPRATT 1977 b), a process possibly involving two stages and mediated by cyclic AMP (cAMP) (YAMASAKI et al. 1976). PBP 2 is a very minor protein, accounting for less than 1% of the total PBP content of *E. coli* (SPRATT 1977 a). It is very sensitive to mecillinam (binds at less than 0.1 µg/ml), to some penicillins, and to a lesser degree to thienamycin and clavulanic acid, but is generally resistant to cephalosporins. Its enzymatic function is unknown, although it appears to release bound penicillin in the presence of hydroxylamine (0.2 *M*), a process thought to be enzymatic (BLUMBERG et al. 1974; Nishino et al. 1977). Furthermore, the serine reagent diisopropylfluorophosphate inhibits binding of penicillin to this protein suggesting that, like DD-carboxypeptidase, it might be a serine enzyme (GEORGOPAPADAKOU and LIU, unpublished work).

Binding of β-lactam antibiotics to PBP 3 (molecular weight: 60,000) results in filamentous cells (SPRATT 1975). PBP 3 is sensitive to both penicillins and cephalosporins. In contrast to PBP 1 b and 2, it appears to tolerate structural changes in the periphery of β-lactam antibiotics. For example, it is equally sensitive to CP-35,587 (*13*) (a tetrazolyl derivative of amoxycillin) and amoxycillin (Table 2), ac-

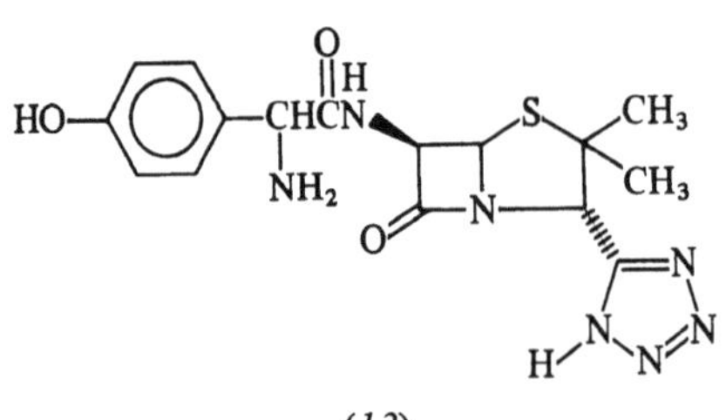

(*13*)

Table 2. Binding of amoxicillin and CP35587 to *E. coli* PBPs

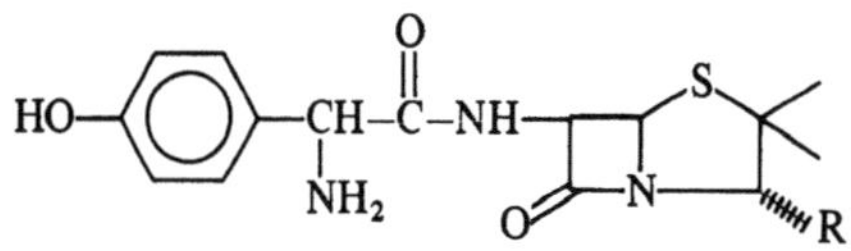

	R	μg/ml to completely inhibit pen G binding				
		PBP1	PBP2	PBP3	PBP4	PBP5/6
Amoxicillin	—COOH	10	2.0	2.0	0.1	>30
CP35587	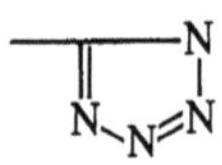	>30	≧10	2.0	30	>30

counting for the typical cephalosporin-like effects of the former compound (PRESSLITZ 1978). PBP 3 could be a transpeptidase, responsible for formation of cross wall during division, but such enzymatic activity has not yet been demonstrated. As with PBP 2, the only enzymatic activity shown is the release of bound penicillin in the presence of hydroxylamine (GEORGOPAPADAKOU and LIU 1980a).

Binding of β-lactam antibiotics to PBP 4 (molecular weight: 49,000) results in no morphological change and mutants lacking this protein grow normally. Like PBP 1a, PBP 4 is generally sensitive to β-lactam antibiotics. It possesses both DD-carboxypeptidase and "natural model" transpeptidase activities (NGUYEN-DISTECHE et al. 1974a, b; POLLOCK et al. 1974), the latter being of no demonstratable physiological significance. *E. coli* mutants lacking both PBP 1a and 1b are not viable (SUZUKI et al. 1978), suggesting that PBP 4 cannot function as a peptidoglycan transpeptidase.

Binding of β-lactam antibiotics to PBP 5/6 results in no detectable morphological change and mutants lacking 95% of PBP 5 grow normally (MATSUHASHI et al. 1978). PBP 5/6 (molecular weight: 40,000) is composed of two proteins which account for over 80% of the total PBP content in *E. coli* (SPRATT 1977a). PBP 5 is DD-carboxypeptidase 1A (SPRATT and STROMINGER 1976). This protein possesses DD-carboxypeptidase, endopeptidase and weak penicillinase activity but no natural model transpeptidase activity (NGUYEN-DISTECHE et al. 1974a, b; POLLOCK et al. 1974). Interestingly enough, mutants lacking completely PBP 5/6 are hypersensitive to β-lactam antibiotics (TAMAKI et al. 1978), possibly indicating that PBP 4 is compensating for the loss of PBP 5/6 and that DD-carboxypeptidase has an important physiological role.

2. Other Enterobacteria

As already pointed out, most enterobacteria such as *Enterobacter*, *Klebsiella*, and *Salmonella* have PBP patterns very similar to that of *E. coli* (CURTIS et al. 1979a; GEORGOPAPADAKOU and LIU 1980a) (Table 3). In these organisms the PBP numbering system used is identical to the one in *E. coli*.

Table 3. Penicillin-binding proteins in gram-negative bacteria

Organism	Spratt No.	PBP[a]-MW ($\times 10^3$)	Reference[b]
Escherichia coli	1a	1–96	SPRATT (1977a)
	1b	2–91	
	2	3–66	
	3	4–60	
	4	5–45	
	5/6	6–38	
Enterobacter cloacae	1b	1–89	
	2	2–66	
	3	3–58	
	4	4–49	
	5/6	5–41	
Enterobacter faecalis	1a	1–108	
	1b	2–100	
	1c	3–87	
	2	4–66	
	3	5–60	
	4	6–44	
	5/6	7–37	
Klebsiella pneumoniae	1a	1–98	
	1b	2–93	
	2	(3–68)	
	3	(4–62)	
	5/6	5–36	
Proteus mirabilis	1a	1–103	
	1b	2–83	

Organism	Spratt No.	PBP[a]-MW ($\times 10^3$)	Reference[b]
Pseudomonas aeruginosa	1a	1–118	NOGUCHI et al. (1979)
	1b	2–98	
	1c	3–86	
	2	(4–71)	
	3	(5–58)	
	4	6–41	
	5/6	7–35	
Pseudomonas fluorescens	1b	1–92	
	1c	2–81	
	3	(3–62)	
	4a	4–46	
	4b	5–43	
	5/6	6–36	
Spirillum itersonii		1–93	
		2–81	
		3–68	
		4–47	
		5–37	
		(6–30)	
		(7–27)	
Spirillum serpens		1–80	
		2–58	
		3–39[c]	
		4–28	
		5–25	

	2	(3–68)	
	3	(4–63)	
	4	5–45	
	5/6	6–36	
Proteus vulgaris	1a	1–103	
	1b	2–83	
	2	(3–66)	
	3	(4–62)	
	4a	(5–51)	
	4b	(6–45)	
	5/6	7–36	
Salmonella typhimurium	1a	1–108	SHEPHERD et al. (1977)
	1b	2–103	
	2	3–62	
	3	4–56	
	4	5–42	
	5/6	6–35	
Serratia marcescens	1a	1–95	
	1b	2–87	
	1c	3–78	
	2	(4–65)	
	3	5–60	
	4	6–50	
	5/6	7–36	
		(8–34)	
Acinetobacter calcoaceticus		1–102	
		2–94	
		(3–83)	
		(4–78)	
		5–62	
		6–36	
Branhamella catarrhalis		1–77[d]	
		2–68	
		3–39	
Caulobacter crescentus		1–132	KOYASU et al. (1980)
		2–98	
		3–77	
		4–64	
		5–50	
Haemophilus influenzae		1–90	MAKOVER et al. (1980)
		2–84	
		3–75	
		4–68	
		5–64	
		6–48	
		7–27	

[a] Major PBPs are underlined. Very minor PBPs ($\leqslant 1\%$ of total PBPs) are enclosed in parentheses
[b] Unless indicated otherwise, data are from GEORGOPAPADAKOU and LIU 1980a
[c] Major PBPs in whole cells but not solubilized membranes; partially soluble (i.e., found mostly in the supernatant after sonication and centrifugation), especially the 47,000-dalton PBP
[d] Although the major PBP, it is less than 5% of the 40,000-dalton (major) PBP of *E. coli*

PBP 1 (molecular weight: 90,000–110,000) is composed of two proteins, one highly sensitive to β-lactam antibiotics, the other moderately so. PBP 2 (molecular weight: 62,000–66,000) is sensitive to mecillinam but insensitive to most other β-lactam antibiotics. PBP 3 (molecular weight: 56,000–62,000) is sensitive to both penicillins and cephalosporins. PBP 4 (molecular weight: 45,000–49,000) sometimes solubilized during membrane isolation as in *Klebsiella pneumoniae*, is generally sensitive to β-lactam antibiotics and, in the case of *S. typhimurium*, has been shown to possess DD-carboxypeptidase and natural model transpeptidase activities (SHEPHERD et al. 1977). PBP 5/6 (molecular weight: 36,000–40,000), the major PBP, is moderately sensitive to β-lactam antibiotics and possesses DD-carboxypeptidase and weak penicillinase activity (MARTIN et al. 1975; SCHILF et al. 1978; SHEPHERD et al. 1977; GEORGOPAPADAKOU and LIU 1980a).

The PBP patterns of *Proteus* and *Serratia* differ somewhat from those of the rest of enterobacteria (Table 3). Significantly, it has been suggested that both genera are taxonomically and evolutionarily distant from the rest of enterobacteria (GRIMONT and GRIMONT 1978). *Proteus* PBPs are almost identical from species to species (OHYA et al. 1979) and can be correlated fairly easily with those of *E. coli*. *Serratia* PBPs are generally resistant to β-lactam antibiotics (GEORGOPAPADAKOU and LIU, unpublished work) which might account to some extent for the resistance of these organisms to most β-lactam antibiotics. In both *Proteus* and *Serratia*, the major PBP is a 36,000-dalton protein with weak penicillinase activity (SCHILF et al. 1978; GEORGOPAPADAKOU and LIU, unpublished work).

3. Pseudomonads

Pseudomonas aeruginosa has a PBP pattern very similar to that of *E. coli* except that PBP 1 appears to consist of three proteins with molecular weights 118,000, 98,000, and 86,000 (Table 3). The 118,000-dalton protein is not present in all *P. aeruginosa* strains examined, leading to the suggestion that the 98,000-dalton and 86,000-dalton proteins correspond, respectively, to PBPs 1 b and 1 a of *E. coli* (NOGUCHI et al. 1979). It is possible that the 98,000- and 118,000-dalton proteins in *P. aeruginosa* correspond to PBPs 1 b and 1 a of *E. coli* and that the 86,000-dalton protein has no *E. coli* counterpart. Curiously, mecillinam appears to inhibit penicillin binding to the 86,000-dalton protein at concentrations less than 10 μg/ml (GEORGOPAPADAKOU and LIU, unpublished work).

Binding of β-lactam antibiotics to *P. aeruginosa* PBPs results in morphological changes similar to those observed in *E. coli*, although the concentration range over which these occur may differ as a result of differences in permeability (NIKAIDO and NAKAE 1979), β-lactamases (OHMORI et al. 1977) and PBP affinity (CURTIS et al. 1979b). α-Sulfocephalosporins constitute an important exception in that PBP 3 of *P. aeruginosa* is very sensitive to them while PBP 3 of *E. coli* is resistant. Consequently, these compounds induce filamentation and lysis in *P. aeruginosa* but only lysis in *E. coli* (CURTIS et al. 1980).

Pseudomonas fluorescens has a PBP pattern almost identical to that of *P. aeruginosa*. The absence of PBPs 1 a, 2, and 3 (Table 3) is probably artifactual (all three are very minor PBPs in *P. aeruginosa*). In both *P. fluorescens* and *P. aeruginosa* a 35,000-dalton protein is the major PBP and, as in enterobacteria, is moderately sensitive to β-lactam antibiotics and has weak penicillinase activity (GEORGOPAPADAKOU and LIU, unpublished work).

4. Other Bacteria

Branhamella catarrhalis and *Neisseria gonorrhoeae* have somewhat similar PBP patterns but different from those of enterobacteria. The 80,000- and 40,000-dalton PBPs of *B. catarrhalis* (Table 3) could correspond to PBPs 1 and 4 of *N. gonorrhoeae* observed in all strains examined (NOLAN and HILDEBRANDT 1979). The 40,000-dalton protein of *B. catarrhalis* spontaneously releases penicillin with a half-life of less than 10 min at 30 °C (GEORGOPAPADAKOU and LIU, unpublished work), a property suggesting correspondence to PBP 5/6 (DD-carboxypeptidase 1A) of *E. coli*.

Acinetobacter calcoaceticus also has a PBP pattern different from that of enterobacteria, the only common feature being a major 36,000-dalton PBP which, like PBP 5/6 of *E. coli*, spontaneously releases bound penicillin with a half-life of less than 20 min at 30 °C.

Caulobacter crescentus possesses at least five PBPs (molecular weights: 50,000–132,000) which, with the exception of the 50,000-dalton protein, are located in the cytoplasmic membrane. The 50,000-dalton PBP is located in the outer membrane (KOYASU et al. 1980).

Spirillum itersonii and *Spirillum serpens* possess seven (molecular weights: 27,000–93,000) and five (molecular weights: 25,000–80,000) PBPs, respectively. The 37,000- and 47,000-dalton proteins of *S. itersonii* appear to be water soluble while the rest are membrane bound (GEORGOPAPADAKOU and LIU 1980a).

Haemophilus influenzae possess eight PBPs (molecular weights: 27,000–90,000), the 84,000- and 75,000-dalton proteins corresponding, on the basis of sensitivity of β-lactam antibiotics, to PBPs 1a and 2 of *E. coli* (MAKOVER et al. 1980).

III. Penicillin-Binding Proteins in Gram-Positive Bacteria

The PBP patterns of gram-positive bacteria exhibit a diversity similar to that observed in gram-negative bacteria although they tend to remain similar within a genus, e.g. in *Bacillus* (Table 4). As in gram-negative bacteria, there is a 35,000–45,000-dalton protein which is present in varying amounts and is usually, but not always, (see Sect. B.III.3) moderately sensitive to β-lactam antibiotics. It possesses weak penicillinase activity and, in the cases examined, DD-carboxypeptidase activity.

1. Bacilli

Bacillus subtilis possesses six PBPs (BLUMBERG and STROMINGER 1972a) (molecular weights: 44,000–115,000), the 44,000-dalton protein (PBP 6) being the major PBP (accounts for 70% of the total PBP content) and possesses DD-carboxypeptidase activity (Sect. C.I.1.c). Mutant studies have suggested that the 98,000 dalton protein (PBP 2), a minor PBP, to be the killing site for penicillin and other β-lactam antibiotics (BUCHANAN and STROMINGER 1976). Recent physiological studies have supported this suggestion (HORIKAWA and OGAWARA 1980), but have provided no

Table 4. Penicillin-binding proteins in gram-positive bacteria

Organism	PBP[a]-MW ($\times 10^3$)	Reference[b]
Bacillus cereus	1–122 2–96 3–50	SUGINAKA et al. (1972)
Bacillus licheniformis	1–123 2–89 3–83 4–46	CHASE et al. (1978)
Bacillus megaterium	1–123 2–94 3–83 4–70 5–45	CHASE et al. (1977)
Bacillus stearothermophilus	1–105 2–78 3–76 4–45	YOCUM et al. (1974)
Bacillus subtilis	1–115 2–90 3–85 4–78 (5–71) 6–44	BLUMBERG and STROMINGER (1972a)
Nocardia lurida	1–87 2–75 3–62 4–49 5–47 6–44	
Nocardia rhodochrous	1–127 2–103 3–98 (4–55) 5–52	
Streptomyces cacaoi	1–105 2–91 3–64 4–55 5–50 6–47	OGAWARA and HORIKAWA (1980)
Streptomyces griseus	1–33[c] 2–28	
Streptomyces R61	(1–97) 2–90 (3–79) (4–51) (5–47) 6–41 7–26	
Micrococcus luteus	1–90 2–62 3–58 4–46	
Stapylococcus aureus	1–92 2–83 3–75 (4–53) 5–42	SUGINAKA et al. (1972)
Staphylococcus epidermidis	1–100 2–93 3–87 4–76 5–39	
Streptococcus faecalis	1–105 2–86 3–79 4–74 5–42 6–35	COYETTE et al. (1978)
Streptococcus lactis	1–91 (2–83) 3–81 4–78 5–39	
Streptococcus pneumoniae	1–100 2–95 3–80 4–78 5–52	WILLIAMSON et al. (1980)

[a] Major PBPs are underlined. Very minor PBPs ($\ll$ 1% of total PBPs) are enclosed in parentheses

[b] Unless indicated otherwise, data are from GEORGOPAPADAKOU and LIU 1980a

[c] About one-fifth of regular amount of protein was applied on slab gel (about 20 μg) Therefore, only major PBPs could be detected

[d] Present in solubilized membranes but not whole cells

clue as to the enzymatic activity of the protein. It has been speculated that the 98,000-dalton PBP is a peptidoglycan transpeptidase. The only other PBP with enzymatic activity is the 78,000-dalton protein (PBP 4), which has weak penicillinase activity (GEORGOPAPADAKOU and LIU 1980a; KLEPPE and STROMINGER 1979).

Bacillus stearothermophilus has a PBP pattern (molecular weights: 45,000–105,000) similar to that of *B. subtilis* (YOCUM et al. 1974), one difference being the absence of the 98,000-dalton protein (PBP 2 of *B. subtilis*). It is quite possible that this protein is also present in *B. stearothermophilus* but in amounts below the detection limit of the PBP assay. The 45,000-dalton protein (PBP 4) is a DD-carboxypeptidase and will be discussed in Sect. C.I.2.c).

In *Bacillus megaterium* five PBPs have been observed (molecular weights: 41,000–120,000), the 120,000-dalton protein (PBP1) accounting for 30% of the total PBP content (CHASE et al. 1977). Although the molecular weights of individual PBPs roughly correspond to those in *B. subtilis*, relative amounts and affinities for β-lactam antibiotics are different (CHASE et al. 1977; GEORGOPAPADAKOU and LIU, unpublished work). Most importantly, physiological studies have suggested that the killing site for penicillin is the 120,000-dalton protein (PBP 1). Consistent with the above suggestion, recent mutant studies have shown β-lactam resistance to be associated with a 10-fold decrease in the 120,000-dalton protein (PBP 1) and a concomitant 1.5-fold increase in the 83,000-dalton protein (PBP 3) (GILES and REYNOLDS 1979). It is possible that the 94,000-dalton protein (PBP 2) is also a killing site in *B. megaterium* but the highly β-lactam-sensitive PBP 1 dominates the resistance pattern. The 120,000-dalton protein (PBP 1) which has been purified to virtual homogeneity shows no enzymatic activity (CHASE 1980). In membranes plus cell-wall preparations, PBP 1 has been associated with transpeptidase activity (SHEPHERD et al. 1977). However, penicillin release from PBP1 after penicillin treatment is slower than recovery of transpeptidase activity indicating the possible presence of multiple transpeptidases.

In *Bacillus cereus* three PBPs (molecular weights: 50,000–122,000) have been observed, those equivalent to the 78,000- and 85,000-dalton *B. subtilis* PBPs being apparently missing (SUGINAKA et al. 1971). The 50,000-dalton protein (PBP 3) could be, by analogy to *B. subtilis*, a DD-carboxypeptidase. No attempt has been made to study enzymatic activity of individual PBPs or to determine the killing site of penicillin in this organism.

In *Bacillus licheniformis* four PBPs (molecular weights: 56,000–123,000) have been observed, the one equivalent to the 78,000-dalton *B. subtilis* PBP apparently missing (CHASE et al. 1978). The 46,000-dalton protein (PBP 4) is probably a DD-carboxypeptidase and the 123,000-dalton protein (PBP 1) a peptidoglycan transpeptidase, although enzymatic studies have not been performed. As in other bacilli, the 123,000-dalton PBP spontaneously releases bound penicillin (CHASE et al. 1978).

2. Micrococci

In *S. aureus* four PBPs (molecular weights: 42,000–92,000) have been observed, the 42,000-dalton protein (PBP 5) being a DD-carboxypeptidase (SUGINAKA et al. 1972; KOZARICH and STROMINGER 1978). This protein has weak penicillinase and transpeptidase activities, although it is not a peptidoglycan transpeptidase (KOZARICH and STROMINGER 1978). Physiological studies here suggested that the 87,000-dalton (PBP 1) and 75,000-dalton (PBP 3) proteins are the killing sites for β-lactam antibiotics in this organism (GEORGOPAPADAKOU and LIU 1980b).

In *Staphylococcus epidermidis* five PBPs have been observed (molecular weights: 39,000–100,000), the "extra" (relative to *S. aureus* PBPs) PBP being a 100,000-dalton protein while the rest are similar to those of *S. aureus* (GEORGOPAPADAKOU and LIU 1980a).

In *Micrococcus luteus* four PBPs (molecular weights: 46,000–90,000) have been observed, the PBP pattern differing markedly from that of staphylococci. No attempt has been made to study enzymatic activities or to determine killing sites for penicillin (GEORGOPAPADAKOU and LIU 1980a).

3. Streptococci

In *Streptococcus faecalis* five PBPs (molecular weights: 42,000–105,000 have been observed, the 42,000-dalton protein (PBP 5) being a DD-carboxypeptidase with penicillinase and transpeptidase activities (COYETTE et al. 1978) (Sect. C.I.2.c). Physiological studies, using a series of structurally related penicillins, have suggested the 42,000-dalton PBP to be the killing site for β-lactam antibiotics (COYETTE et al. 1978). However, this protein is sensitive to 0.1 µg/ml cefoxitin while the organism is not sensitive up to 100 µg/ml which argues against the above suggestion. Recent physiological studies with several structurally diverse β-lactam antibiotics have suggested that the killing sites are the 105,000-dalton (PBP 1) and 79,000-dalton (PBP 3) proteins (GEORGOPAPADAKOU and LIU 1980b).

In *Streptococcus lactis* five PBPs (molecular weights: 39,000–91,000) have been observed, the PBP pattern being somewhat different from that of *S. faecalis*. The 39,000-dalton protein (PBP 5) possesses weak penicillinase activity. This protein might be a DD-carboxypeptidase, although its high sensitivity to cephalothin (it binds at less than 0.1 mg/ml) would argue against this (GEORGOPAPADAKOU and LIU 1980a). The killing site for penicillin in this organism has not yet been determined.

In *Streptococcus pneumoniae* five PBPs (molecular weights: 52,000–100,000) have been observed (WILLIAMSON et al. 1980). Studies with penicillin-resistant clinical isolates suggested PBPs 1 and 2 to be the killing sites for β-lactam antibiotics (HACKENBECK et al. 1980). No enzymatic studies have been performed with individual PBPs.

4. Actinomycetes

In *Streptomyces cacaoi* six PBPs (molecular weights: 47,000–105,000) have been observed. The killing site for β-lactam antibiotics has been suggested to be the 91,000-dalton protein (PBP 2) (OGAWARA and HORIKAWA 1980).

In *Streptomyces* R61, six PBPs (molecular weights: 26,000–97,000) have been observed (GEORGOPAPADAKOU and LIU 1980a). The 40,000-dalton (PBP 5) and 26,000-dalton (PBP 6) proteins are, respectively, soluble and membrane-bound DD-carboxypeptidase (GHUYSEN et al. 1979). The former enzyme has been extensively studied by GHUYSEN (GHUYSEN 1977) as the model for the interactions of β-lactam antibiotics with their targets. It possesses transpeptidase and weak penicillinase activities (fragments penicillin; Sect. E.III.2).

In *Nocardia lurida* six PBPs (molecular weights: 44,000–87,000) have been observed as in *Nocardia rhodochrous* (molecular weights: 52,000–127,000) (GEORGOPAPADAKOU and LIU 1980a). No further studies with these two organisms have been done.

C. Enzymes Inhibited by β-Lactam Antibiotics

As already stated, DD-carboxypeptidase and peptidoglycan transpeptidase are the two main types of bacterial enzymes which are inhibited by β-lactam antibiotics. Endopeptidase, formally a reversal of transpeptidation and present sometimes as a secondary activity of DD-carboxypeptidases, is a third type of enzyme (Fig. 9). Both DD-carboxypeptidase and peptidoglycan transpeptidase are present in all species of bacteria examined thus far and both are PBPs. When assayed in vitro, there appears to be some spill-over of enzymatic activity between the two enzymes. That is, most DD-carboxypeptidases are capable of both hydrolysis and transpeptidation under certain conditions and have been called DD-carboxypeptidases-transpeptidases. Although this may have important mechanistic and evolutionary implications, the physiological role of each enzyme is specific. DD-carboxypeptidases possessing transpeptidase activity (such as PBP 4 of *E. coli*) do not compensate for the lack of the peptidoglycan transpeptidase [PBPs 1a and 1b of *E. coli* (SUZUKI et al. 1978)].

DD-Carboxypeptidases (molecular weight: 25,000–50,000) from a variety of species have been isolated and studied extensively. In contrast, peptidoglycan transpeptidases (molecular weight: 90,000–100,000) have only recently been isolated and their properties are largely unknown. Therefore, most of the discussion that follows relates to DD-carboxypeptidases with (e.g., *Streptomyces* R 61 DD-carboxypeptidase) or without (e.g., *B. subtilis* DD-carboxypeptidase) in vitro transpeptidase activity.

I. DD-Carboxypeptidases

With a notable exception (FRERE et al. 1978), all DD-carboxypeptidases studied thus far are readily inhibited by penicillin, 7α-methoxy cephalosporins and, to a lesser degreee, by nonmethoxylated cephalosporins. Some are excreted into the growth medium (e.g., *Streptomyces* R 61 DD-carboxypeptidase) or are found in the soluble fraction upon rupture of cells (e.g., *E. coli* DD-carboxypeptidase 1B). The majority, however, are membrane-bound and can be solubilized only by treatment with detergents.

DD-Carboxypeptidases are present in varying amounts, tending to be more abundant in cylindrical than spherical bacteria (GEORGOPAPADAKOU and LIU 1980a). They act on the peptide bond between the two terminal D-alanine residues

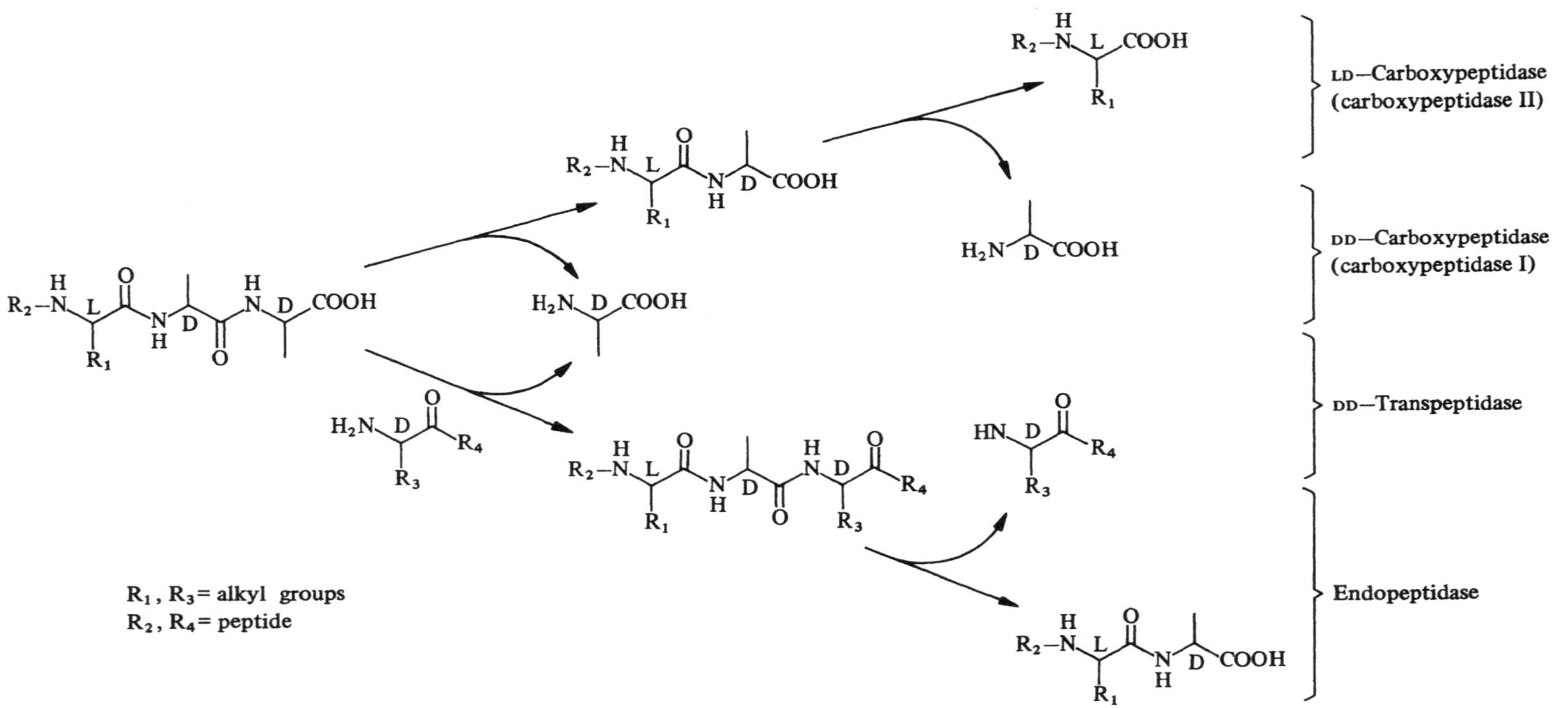

Fig. 9. Enzymes acting on UDP-MurNAc-pentapeptide

of UDP-*N*-acetylmuramyl-L-alanyl-γ-D-glutamyl-meso-2,6-diaminopimelyl-D-alanyl-D-alanine (UDP-MurNAc-L-Ala-D-Glu-meso-Dap-D-Ala-D-Ala; UDP-MurNAc-pentapeptide) and the related synthetic substrate diacetyl-L-lysyl-D-alanyl-D-alanine (Diac-L-Lys-D-Ala-D-Ala) (PERKINS et al. 1973). The general mechanism of the reactions catalyzed by DD-carboxypeptidase is shown in Fig. 9. Typically, the enzyme is incubated at 30 °C for 30 min with UDP-MurNAc-L-Ala-D-Glu-meso-Dap-^{14}C-D-Ala-^{14}C-D-Ala or ^{14}C-Diac-Lys-D-Ala-D-Ala. The hydrolysis product, ^{14}C-D-Ala or ^{14}C-Diac-L-Lys-D-Ala is subsequently separated from the substrate by high-voltage electrophoresis and quantitated by liquid scintillation counting (PERKINS et al. 1973; TAMURA et al. 1976). Both substrates bind to DD-carboxypeptidase poorly, with typical K_m values of $10^{-2}M$ (formation of acyl-enzyme intermediate is rate-determining and therefore K_m includes the acylation constant). However, they are turned over at rates ranging from 10 min^{-1} for the *B. subtilis* enzyme to 3,300 min^{-1} for the *Streptomyces* R 61 enzyme. Obviously, the in vivo activity of DD-carboxypeptidase would be a function of both enzyme amount present and molar activity.

Like most peptidases, DD-carboxypeptidases also possess esterase activity, hydrolyzing the depsipeptide analog of the synthetic substrate, diacetyl-L-lysine-D-alanyl-D-lactate (Diac-L-Lys-D-Ala-D-Lac) (RASMUSSEN and STROMINGER 1978). The K_m of this depsipeptide is substantially lower than that of the corresponding peptide reflecting a higher acylation rate (RASMUSSEN and STROMINGER 1978). It should be noted that the low K_i values of penicillin ($10^{-9}M$ in the case of *Streptomyces* R 61 DD-carboxypeptidase) have been attributed to a fast acylation step, the initial (reversible) binding having an equilibrium constant comparable to the K_m for the substrate (FRERE et al. 1975).

In addition to peptidase and esterase activities, DD-carboxypeptidases possess endopeptidase, transpeptidase and penicillinase activities, all five activities most likely occurring at the same active site. Endopeptidase activity involves cleavage of the peptide bond between D-alanine and meso-diaminopimelic acid in the disaccharide-tetrapeptide dimer (Fig. 9). The similarity of the endopeptidase to DD-carboxypeptidase reaction is evident since α to the susceptible peptide bond is a free carboxyl group on the D-symmetric center of diaminopimelic acid (R_4=OH in Fig. 9).

Depending on the nature of nucleophilic acceptor, DD-carboxypeptidase-associated transpeptidase activity can be divided into two types: (1) acceptor is hydroxylamine, glycine or another amino acid and probably binds at the donor site (transpeptidation is reversed hydrolysis); (2) acceptor is Gly-L-Ala or another peptide and binds at a site topologically distinct from the donor site (natural model transpeptidation). While the first type of activity is not uncommon for peptidases (FRUTON 1971) the second type is unique for DD-carboxypeptidases. In the absence of a readily accessible peptidoglycan transpeptidase, the natural model transpeptidation may be a plausible model for the interaction of β-lactam antibiotics with their enzyme targets.

Depending on the type of cleavage, DD-carboxypeptidase-associated penicillinase activity can be divided into two types: (1) exclusive cleavage at the amide bond of the β-lactam (only product is penicilloic acid); (2) additional cleavage at the C_5–C_6 of the β-lactam (products are, wholly or in part, phenylglycine and

Table 5. Properties of DD-carboxypeptidases

Source	MW ($\times 10^3$)	Active residue	Peptidase activity			Transpeptidase activity	Interaction with penicillin G		References
			Substrate[b]	K_m m*M*	V_{max} µmol/mg/min	Acceptor	I_{50} M	$t_{1/2}$ of Release (min)	
E. coli – membrane	40(38)[a]	ser, cys	UDPMAGDAA	4.2	1	NH_2OH, Gly	2.2×10^{-4}	5	TAMURA *et al.* (1976), CURTIS and STROMINGER (1978), NGUYEN-DIESTECHE *et al.* (1974a), GEORGOPAPADAKOU and LIU unpublished work
			UDPMAGLAA	5.6	0.26				
			DLAA	14.3	0.30				
– cytoplasm	49(45)		UDPMAGDAA	1.0	3.9	AGDAA[b]	3×10^{-7}	90	
S. typhimurium – membrane			UDPMAGDAA			AGDAA		5	SHEPHERD *et al.* (1977)
– cytoplasm			AGDAA			AGDAA		90	
P. mirabilis – membrane			UDPMAGDAA				7×10^{-7}	5	SCHILF and MARTIN (1980)
– cytoplasm			UDPMAGDAA				4×10^{-9}	90	
N. gonorrheae – membrane			UDPMAGDAA	0.18			2×10^{-8}		DAVIS *et al.* (1978)
B. stearothermophilus – membrane	46(45)	ser	UDPMAGDAA	1.4		NH_2OH, Gly, Ala	1.9×10^{-7}	10	NISHINO *et al.* (1977), YOCUM *et al.* (1974), YOCUM *et al.* (1979), HAMMARSTROM and STROMINGER (1975)
			DLAA						
B. subtilis – membrane	50(44)	ser	UDPMAGDAA	0.67		NH_2OH	2×10^{-5}		UMBREIT and STROMINGER (1973), BLUMBERG and STROMINGER (1972), YOCUM *et al.* (1979)
			DLAA	0.55	0.0016	NH_2OH		200	

B. megaterium – membrane	45(39)		UDPMAGDAA						MARQUET *et al.* (1976)
			AGDAA				1×10^{-5}		
			DLAA	1.7	0.024				
B. coagulans – membrane	29	cys	UDPMAGDAA	4.8	0.015				MCARTHUR and REYNOLDS (1979a, b, 1980)
			AGDAA	10	0.013				
S. aureus – membrane	42	ser	DLAA	100	0.24	NH_2OH, Gly	2×10^{-5}	< 1	KOZARICH and STROMINGER (1978)
S. faecalis – membrane	43(42)	ser, cys	DLAA			NH_2OH, Gly, Ala		260	COYETTE *et al.* (1977), GEORGOPAPADAKOU and LIU unpublished work
Streptomyces R61 – exocellular	38	ser, Arg	UDPMAGDAA			Gly, Ala, Meso-Dap, Gly-Gly-ε-Gly-α-Ac-L-Lys, Gly-L-Ala	1.5×10^{-9}	80	GHUYSEN (1977), GEORGOPAPADAKOU *et al.* (1981a)
			DLAA						
– membrane	26		UDPMAGDAA			AGDAA		100	GHUYSEN *et al.* (1979)
			AGDAA						
Streptomyces R 39 – exocellular	57	ser	UDPMAGDAA			Gly, Ala, Meso-Dap	1×10^{-11}	4100	GHUYSEN (1977) GHUYSEN *et al.* (1980)
			DLAA						
Streptomyces albus G – exocellular	18		UDPMAGDAA						GHUYSEN *et al.* (1979)
			DLAA						
Streptomyces sp. – membrane	22		UDPMAGDAA			AGDAA			GHUYSEN *et al.* (1979)
			AGDAA						

[a] Numbers in parentheses refer to corresponding molecular weights given in Tables 3 and 4

[b] Abbreviations: AGDAA, L-Ala-D-Glu-Meso-Dap-D-Ala-D-Ala; DLAA, Diac-L-Lys-D-Ala-D-Ala; UDPMAGDAA, UPDMurNAc-L-Ala-D-Glu-Meso-Dap-D-Ala-D-Ala; UDPMAGLAA, UPDMurNAc-L-Ala-D-Glu-L-Lys-D-Ala-D-Ala

penicillamine). The first type of activity is associated with fast release of hydrolysis products (typical half-life: 5 min) while the second type with slow release (typical half-life: 2 h). The interaction of DD-carboxypeptidases with β-lactam antibiotics will be further discussed in Sect. E.

Some of the properties of different DD-carboxypeptidases are outlined in Table 5.

1. DD-Carboxypeptidases in Gram-Negative Bacteria

DD-Carboxypeptidases have been studied in *E. coli*, *S. typhimurium*, *Proteus mirabilis*, and *N. gonorrhoeae*. *E. coli* contains two DD-carboxypeptidases (PBP 4 and 5/6) both of which have been purified by conventional methods and designated, respectively, I A and I B (TAMURA et al. 1976). DD-Carboxypeptidase I A has been also purified by affinity column chromatography on ampicillin-Sepharose (GORECKI et al. 1975). A third DD-carboxypeptidase, I C, is the soluble fraction of I B and has properties identical to those of I B (TAMURA et al. 1976); therefore, it will not be further discussed.

Carboxypeptidase I A of *E. coli* is moderately sensitive to penicillin which releases as penicilloic acid with a half-life of 5 min at 37 °C (TAMURA et al. 1976). In addition to carboxypeptidase activity (substrates: UDP-MurNAc-L-Ala-γ-D-Glu-meso-Dap-D-Ala-D-Ala, UDP-MurNAc-L-Ala-γ-D-Glu-L-Lys-D-Ala-D-Ala, Diac-L-Lys-D-Ala-D-Ala), the enzyme exhibits endopeptidase activity (substrate: UDP-MurNAc-L-Ala-γ-D-Glu-Meso-Dap-D-Ala-Meso-Dap-γ-D-Glu-L-Ala-UDP-MurNAc) and transpeptidase activity, the acceptor being simple amino compounds such as hydroxylamine and glycine (TAMURA et al. 1976). Carboxypeptidase and penicillinase activities are inhibited by sulfhydryl reagents such as *p*-chloromercuribenzoate (pCMB) ($I_{50} = 0.1$ m*M*) (CURTIS and STROMINGER 1978). However, the binding of penicillin is not inhibited by these reagents suggesting that the sulfhydryl group is involved only in the deacylation step. Predictably, an acyl-enzyme intermediate has been trapped (substrate: Diac-L-Lys-D-Ala-D-Ala) in the presence of *p*-chloromercuribenzoate (CURTIS and STROMINGER 1978). Carboxypeptidase activity is also inhibited by 10 m*M* diisopropylfluorophosphate (DFP) which appears to bind covalently to the enzyme. Radioactivity from ^{14}C-DFP remained protein-bound after SDS-polyacrylamide gel electrophoresis (GEORGOPAPADAKOU and LIU, unpublished work). Possibly, the enzyme is a serine protease. The enzyme is also inhibited by EDTA and divalent cations (both at 10 m*M*) (TAMURA et al. 1976). Mutants lacking carboxypeptidase I A have been obtained by mutagenesis (MATSUHASHI et al. 1978). Interestingly, they retained the ability to bind penicillin G, as suggested by the detection of PBP 5/6 (MATSUHASHI et al. 1979).

Carboxypeptidase I B of *E. coli* is highly sensitive to penicillin which releases slowly (half-life: 90 min at 37 °C), probably as penicilloic acid. In addition to carboxypeptidase activity (substrate: UDP-MurNAc-L-Ala-γ-D-Glu-meso-Dap-D-Ala-D-Ala) the enzyme also has natural model transeptidase activity (substrate: L-Ala-γ-D-Glu-meso-Dap-D-Ala-D-Ala), forming cross-linked tetrapeptide dimers (NGUYEN-DISTECHE et al. 1974a). *p*-Chloromercuribenzoate (2 m*M*) does not inhibit peptidase activity suggesting that a sulfhydryl group is not involved. DFP (10 m*M*) inhibits binding of penicillin indicating that this enzyme too might be a serine peptidase (GEORGOPAPADAKOU and LIU, unpublished work). Contrary to carboxypeptidase I A, carboxypeptidase I B is activated by EDTA and divalent cations (TAMURA et al. 1976).

In *S. typhimurium* two DD-carboxypeptidases have been found (PBPs 4 and 5) which appear to be homologous to those of *E. coli* (SHEPHERD et al. 1977). Both PBPs 5 and 4 release bound penicillin, with half-lives of 5 and 90 min at 37 °C, respectively. Both enzymes catalyze the synthesis of a cross-linked dimer from L-Ala-D-Glu-meso-Dap-D-Ala-D-Ala (natural model transpeptidation), PBP 5 with a lower efficiency than PBP 4.

In *P. mirabilis*, two DD-carboxypeptidases have been found (45K and 36K PBPs) one, highly sensitive to penicillin, in the bacterial form and another, moderately sensitive to penicillin, in the bacterial L-form (MARTIN et al. 1975). Both enzymes release bound penicillin, the one in the L-form as penicilloic acid and at a rate faster than the bacterial one (SCHILF et al. 1978). Thus, the two enzymes could be homologous to carboxypeptidase I A (L-form enzyme) and I B (bacterial enzyme). Indeed, this has been recently verified (SCHILF and MARTIN 1980).

In *N. gonorrhoeae* one DD-carboxypeptidase has been found and purified by conventional methods. It acts on UDP-MurNAc-L-Ala-D-Glu-meso-Dap-D-Ala-D-Ala (K_m: 0.2 m*M*) and is highly sensitive to β-lactam antibiotics including mecillinam (DAVIS et al. 1978).

2. DD-Carboxypeptidases in Gram-Positive Bacteria

DD-Carboxypeptidases have been isolated and studied in bacilli, streptococci, staphylococci, and streptomycetes. Perhaps the most detailed studies have been carried out with the *Streptomyces* R 61 enzyme, an exocellular enzyme highly sensitive to β-lactam antibiotics and capable of both hydrolysis and transpeptidation. The enzyme is also present in a membrane-bound form acting exclusively as a transpeptidase. This fact and the fact that the membrane-bound form releases bound penicillin exclusively as penicilloic acid suggest different conformations of the two enzyme forms. The discussion which follows is limited to the exocellular form of the enzyme.

a) Streptomyces R 61

Streptomyces R 61 DD-carboxypeptidase has been purified to homogeneity by conventional methods, and, on SDS-polyacrylamide gel electrophoresis, has a molecular weight of 38,000 (FRERE et al. 1973 a). Studies using a series of synthetic peptides have established that the binding site for the acyl donor consists of at least three subsites (Fig. 9): S_1, requiring a D-amino acid with its α-carboxyl group free; S_2, requiring a D-alanine or to some extent glycine; S_3, requiring a long-chain L-amino acid with its amino group substituted. Interestingly, while K_ms of peptide substrates are similar, V_{max}s are markedly different, suggesting that good substrates might induce a conformational change leading to catalytic activity (LEYH-BOUILLE et al. 1971; GEORGOPAPADAKOU et al. 1981 b).

In addition to the donor site, the enzyme possesses an acceptor site requiring an amino acid with a D-asymmetric center in the group involved in the peptide bond (e.g., glycine, D-alanine, meso-diaminopimelic acid) or dipeptides with N-terminal glycine (PERKINS et al. 1973). Significantly, the enzyme also catalyzes dimerization of a tetrapeptide analog of the synthetic substrate into the corresponding hexa- and heptapeptides:

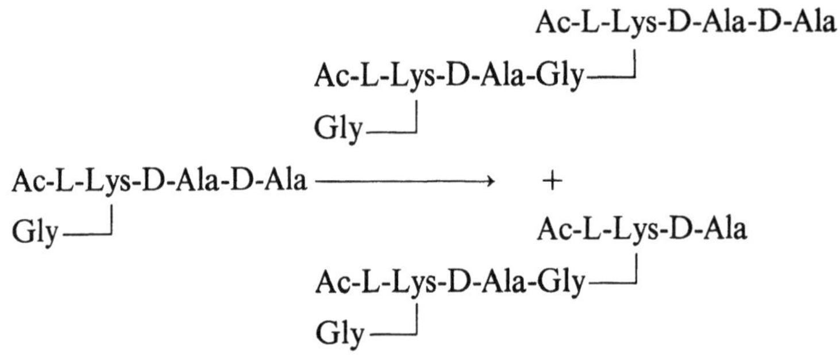

None of the good acceptors inhibits enzyme activity at the concentrations used to measure transpeptidation (1–10 m*M*), suggesting that binding occurs at a site topologically distinct from the donor site (POLLOCK et al. 1972). In both the R 61 enzyme and in other DD-carboxypeptidases acceptor concentrations have been reported as mole fractions of the acyl donor. However, the acyl donor concentrations used vary from organism to organism and even from one experiment to the next, a situation which makes interpretation of results difficult. Since transpeptidation competes with hydrolysis, in which water is the acceptor, acceptor concentrations are best stated as molar concentrations. Typically such concentrations are 1 and 10 m*M* resulting, respectively, in 10%–20% and 50%–80% transpeptidation with good amino acid acceptors (PERKINS et al. 1973; GEORGOPAPADAKOU and LIU, unpublished work). The mechanism for the transpeptidation has been suggested to be an ordered pathway in which the acceptor binds first to the enzyme (FRERE et al. 1973 b).

Peptidase activity is inhibited by the arginine-specific reagents methylglyoxal, 2,3-butanedione, and phenylglyoxal (second order rate constants: 70–120 M^{-1}) suggesting that binding of the substrate requires an arginine-carboxyl group interaction. Binding of the penicillin is also inhibited, but inhibition is less and appears to depend on the size of the α-dicarbonyl side chain (GEORGOPAPADAKOU et al. 1981 a).

Both peptidase and penicillin-binding activities are inhibited by the active-site reagents methanesulfonylfluoride (MSF) and DFP (second-order rate constants: 0.7 and 1.5 M^{-1} $\min^{-1}$). For DFP, which binds to the enzyme stoichiometrically, the inactivation rate is substantially smaller than that of classic serine proteases suggesting inefficient binding. Accordingly, a substrate-related chloromethyl ketone, Diac-L-Lys-D-Ala-CH_2Cl, which lacks the *C*-terminal group of the substrate, does not inhibit the enzyme (GEORGOPAPADAKOU, LIU, SABO, ONDETTI, unpublished work).

Interestingly, binding of α-dicarbonyls to the R 61 enzyme facilitates the subsequent binding of DFP suggesting that interaction of these compounds with the active site might induce a conformational change making the serine residue more accessible to modifying reagents (GEORGOPAPADAKOU et al. 1981 a). Conformational changes have also been postulated to occur upon binding of penicillin.

b) Other Streptomycetes

Membranes of *Streptomyces* sp. contain a 22,000-dalton protein which is predominantly a transpeptidase, catalyzing transfer reactions between Diac-L-Lys-D-Ala-D-Ala and various amino donors including dipeptides with N-terminal glycine (GHUYSEN et al. 1979). However, as far as is known, it does not catalyze natural model transpeptidations. The enzyme has been solubilized with cationic detergents and purified by conventional methods (GHUYSEN et al. 1979).

Streptomyces R 39 DD-carboxypeptidase is an exocellular enzyme of molecular weight 57 K (FRERE et al. 1974 b) which catalyzes the hydrolysis of R-D-Ala-D-Ala peptides as well as natural model transpeptidations leading to the formation of peptide dimers. The substrate requirements of its donor site appear to be more stringent than those of the R 61 enzyme. For example, glycine cannot replace D-alanine as the penultimate residue (LEYH-BOUILLE et al. 1972). Both K_m and V_{max} for different peptides are different, suggesting that conformational changes are less important in this enzyme than in R 61 DD-carboxypeptidase. Penicillin binding occurs, as in R 61, via a serine residue indicating that this enzyme is also a serine protease (GHUYSEN et al. 1980).

Streptomyces albus G DD-carboxypeptidase is an exocellular enzyme of molecular weight 18,000 which hydrolyzes R-D-Ala-D-Ala peptides but, contrary to the R 39 and R 61 enzymes, cannot catalyze even simple transpeptidations. In addition to carboxypeptidase activity, the enzyme has endopeptidase activity hydrolyzing appropriate peptide dimers. It appears to be a Zn^{2+} metalloenzyme and is relatively resistant to β-lactam antibiotics. The enzyme has also been found in a 9,000-dalton form, with identical catalytic properties and giving rise to the same peptide maps upon limited proteolysis as the 18,000-dalton form (GHUYSEN et al. 1980).

c) Bacilli

B. subtilis DD-carboxypeptidase (PBP 5) is a membrane-bound enzyme of molecular weight 50,000. It has been solubilized by nonionic detergents and purified both by conventional methods (UMBREIT and STROMINGER 1973) and by affinity chromatography on 6-APA-Sepharose (BLUMBERG and STROMINGER 1972 b). It acts on UDP-Mur-NAc-L-Ala-D-Glu-meso-Dap-D-Ala-D-Ala and Diac-L-Lys-D-Ala-D-Ala, requiring with the former substrate Zn^{2+} (10 m*M*) for activity. For either substrate the turnover number is at least two orders of magnitude smaller than with the *Streptomyces* enzymes. In addition to peptidase activity, the *B. subtilis* enzyme also has esterase activity (substrate: Diac-L-Lys-D-Ala-D-Lac) (RASMUSSEN and STROMINGER 1978) and transpeptidase activity, acceptors being simple amino compounds such as hydroxylamine (NISHINO et al. 1977).

The enzyme has an acidic pH optimum (5.5) and is inhibited by 0.1 m*M* 5,5′-dithiobis-(2-nitrobenzoic acid) (DTNB) and 10 m*M* pCMB (UMBREIT and STROMINGER 1973). With Diac-L-Lys-D-Ala-D-Lac as substrate, an acyl-enzyme has been isolated and a serine residue has been identified as the amino acid involved in the binding. The same serine residue has been shown to be involved in the binding of penicillin (YOCUM et al. 1979).

B. stearothermophilus DD-carboxypeptidase (PBP 4) has a molecular weight of 45,000 and has been purified by affinity chromatography following the procedure used for the *B. subtilis* enzyme (YOCUM et al. 1974). The properties of the two enzymes are very similar although the optimal temperatures for activity differ by over 20 °C. In addition to carboxypeptidase activity, the enzyme shows some transpeptidase activity, the amino donor being glycine or D-alanine but not meso-diaminopimelic acid (NISHINO et al. 1977).

B. megaterium DD-carboxypeptidase (PBP 5) has a molecular weight of 45,000 and has been solubilized by nonionic detergents and purified by affinity chromatography on ampicillin-Affinose (CHASE et al. 1977; CHASE 1980). The enzyme catalyzes the hydrolysis of the terminal D-alanine from UDP -MurNAc-L-Ala-D-Glu-meso-Dap-D-Ala-D-Ala or L-Ala-D-Glu-meso-Dap-D-Ala-D-Ala and simple transpeptidations with glycine or D-alanine as acceptors (CHASE et al. 1977). However, it does not catalyze model transpeptidations. The enzyme has a neutral pH optimum, is stimulated by β-mercaptoethanol and low concentrations of pCMB, and is inhibited by Cu^{2+} and Hg^{2+} (MARQUET et al. 1976).

Bacillus coagulans DD-carboxypeptidase is a membrane-bound enzyme of molecular weight 29,000 (MCARTHUR and REYNOLDS 1980). Like the DD-carboxypeptidases from other bacilli, it has been solubilized with nonionic detergents and subsequently purified to homogeneity by affinity chromatography on ampicillin-agarose (MCARTHUR and REYNOLDS 1980). A twofold increase in activity which has been observed upon solubilization is attributed to conformational changes of the enzyme (MCARTHUR and REYNOLDS 1979a). The enzyme catalyzes the hydrolysis of both UDP-MurNAc-L-Ala-D-Glu-meso-Dap-D-Ala-D-Ala and L-Ala-D-Glu-meso-Dap-D-Ala-D-Ala and simple transpeptidations with D-alanine as acceptor. It has a low pH optimum (4.9) and is inhibited by 18 m*M* DTNB but not 0.1 *M* *N*-ethylmaleimide (NEM) (MCARTHUR and REYNOLDS 1979b).

d) Micrococci

S. aureus DD-carboxypeptidase (PBP 5) is a membrane-bound enzyme of molecular weight 42,000. The enzyme has been purified to apparent homogeneity by affinity chromatography. It is moderately sensitive to penicillin which releases as penicilloic acid with a half-life at 30 °C of less than 1 min (KOZARICH and STROMINGER 1978). It catalyzes both the release of D-alanine from the synthetic substrate Diac-L-Lys-D-Ala-D-Ala and the transfer of the Diac-L-Lys-D-Ala to water or simple amino acceptors such as glycine and hydroxylamine. It does not, however, catalyze natural model transpeptidations. Acyl-enzyme complexes have been isolated by SDS-polyacrylamide gel electrophoresis both with substrate and penicillin (KOZARICH and STROMINGER 1978). Perhaps the most remarkable property of this enzyme is its ability to act both as DD-carboxypeptidase-transpeptidase and as a low efficiency β-lactamase, both peptidase and β-lactamase activities having the same V_{max} (KOZARICH and STROMINGER 1978).

e) Streptococci

S. faecalis DD-carboxypeptidase (PBP 5) is a membrane-bound enzyme of molecular weight 42,000. It has been solubilized with nonionic detergents and purified to homogeneity by affinity chromatography on ampicillin-Sepharose (COYETTE et al. 1978). The purified enzyme has properties identical to those of the membrane form. It catalyzes the hydrolysis of D-alanine from Diac-L-Lys-D-Ala-D-Ala and, under alkaline conditions, the transfer of Diac-L-Lys-D-Ala moiety to simple amino acceptors such as D-alanine, glycine and glycylglycine. It does not, however, catalyze natural model transpeptidations. The enzyme is inhibited by low concentrations of pCMB (COYETTE et al. 1980).

II. Peptidoglycan Transpeptidase

Peptidoglycan transpeptidase has been commonly studied in wall-membrane preparations (ANDERSON et al. 1966; MIRELMAN and SHARON 1972), or bacterial cells made permeable to exogenous nucleotide-sugar peptidoglycan precursors by treatment with toluene (BECK and PARK 1976) or ether (VOSBERG and HOFFMAN-BERLING 1971; MIRELMAN and NUCHAMOWITZ 1979a). Such studies usually fail to distinguish the presence of multiple transpeptidases. In addition, some transpeptidase assays are susceptible to interference from other enzymes [e.g., carboxypeptidases if the release of D-alanine is being measured (PRESSLITZ and RAY 1979)]. Nevertheless, several studies of peptidoglycan transpeptidases have been reported, the majority dealing with the effect of various β-lactam antibiotics on the enzymes. For example, *P. aeruginosa* peptidoglycan transpeptidase shows equal sensitivity to β-lactam antibiotics as the *E. coli* enzyme, indicating that the characteristic β-lactam resistance of the former organism is not due to a change in affinity of target to antibiotic (MOORE et al. 1979). Other studies have attempted, more (*E. coli*) or less (*B. megaterium*) successfully, to correlate peptidoglycan transpeptidase with specific PBPs.

A most important type of study has dealt with the question of substrate specificity of peptidoglycan transpeptidase. The obvious merit of such an approach is that it can provide a framework for the design of analogs with potential antibacterial activities. A series of UDP-MurNAc-pentapeptide analogs having the two terminal D-alanine residues replaced by other D-amino acids were biosynthesized and tested in a wall-membrane preparation from *Gaffkya homari*. Transpeptidation was affected mainly after substitution of the penultimate residue in the pentapeptide and the effect appeared in the V_{max} rather than in the K_m term (CARPENTER et al. 1976). It is tempting to speculate that, like DD-carboxypeptidases and β-lactamases, peptidoglycan transpeptidases undergo conformational change upon substrate binding, leading, in the case of good substrates, to catalytic activity. Similarly, D-norvalyl-D-alanine (D-Nva-D-Ala) was found to inhibit growth in *E. coli*, presumably by in vivo incorporation into the peptide strands of peptidoglycan (NEUHAUS et al. 1977).

Peptidoglycan transpeptidase has been recently purified from *E. coli* membranes by affinity chromatography on ampicillin-Sepharose (NAKAGAWA et al. 1979). The purified enzyme (PBP 1b) appears not to be a single protein and, in addition, may be multifunctional acting both as peptidoglycan transpeptidase and polymerase (NAKAGAWA et al. 1979; SUZUKI et al. 1980).

D. β-Lactamases

I. General

β-Lactamases are widespread in the microbial world being produced by gram-positive and gram-negative bacteria (Richmond and Sykes 1973; Sykes and Matthew 1976), blue-green algae (Kushner and Breuil 1977) and yeasts (Mehta and Nash 1978). With a few exceptions, β-lactamase activity has been detected in all bacteria tested (Sykes and Matthew 1976; Matthew and Harris 1976), the majority of *Streptomyces* strains (Ogawara 1975; Ogawara et al. 1978), and most strains of other actinomycetes (Schwartz and Schwartz 1979) including *Nocardia* (Wallace et al. 1978). Organisms other than bacteria and actinomycetes have only rarely been found to produce β-lactamases.

The majority of β-lactamases produced by gram-positive organisms are inducible and exocellular (Citri and Pollock 1966), while those produced by gram-negative organisms may be inducible or constitutive and, with few exceptions, are periplasmic (commonly referred to as cell-bound) (Richmond and Sykes 1973).

Detection of β-lactamases in gram-positive organisms is relatively easy, although induction with a β-lactamase-resistant penicillin such as cloxacillin or methicillin (0.5 μg/ml) is usually necessary for maximal enzyme production.

Among gram-negative species only in *H. influenzae* and *N. gonorrhoeae* are β-lactamases readily accessible to β-lactam substrates (Sykes and Percival 1978). In most other species, the bacterial outer membrane acts as a permeability barrier (Costerton and Cheng 1975), restricting the flow of β-lactam substrates into and products out of the cell. Such a situation makes β-lactamase detection difficult in intact cells. Thus, enzyme is usually released by disruption techniques such as osmotic shock or sonication. If an inducible β-lactamase is suspected, the organism is grown in the presence of benzylpenicillin. However, the high concentrations of inducer that are used (100–500 μg/ml) can affect outer membrane permeability leading to "pseudo-induction" (Smith 1963). Thus, induction can only be demonstrated satisfactorily by estimating cell-free enzyme levels.

Gram-positive organisms are checked for β-lactamase production with a susceptible penicillin, usually benzylpenicillin, as substrate. Among gram-negative organisms, potential cephalosporin-hydrolyzing enzyme producers are checked with a cephalosporin as substrate, usually cephaloridine. All other gram-negative organisms are screened with ampicillin or benzylpenicillin as substrate. The methods most commonly used for detecting β-lactamases are (a) acidimetric, based on the formation of an extra carboxyl group upon β-lactam hydrolysis; (b) iodometric, based on the removal of iodine by the hydrolysis products of the β-lactam from the blue-black starch–iodine complex resulting in discoloration (Jorgensen et al. 1977; Odugbemi et al. 1977; Dale and Smith 1971; Catlin 1975); (c) microbiological, based on the loss of antibacterial activity of β-lactam antibiotics upon hydrolysis; (d) colorimetric, involving the chromogenic β-lactam nitrocefin (O'Callaghan et al. 1972), a yellow-colored cephalosporin hydrolyzed by most β-lactamases to give deep red products. It is noted that the acidimetric and microbiological methods cannot differentiate between acylase and β-lactamase activity. All four methods have been thoroughly discussed in a recent review (Sykes and Matthew 1979). Assay methods are (a) acidimetric; (b) iodometric; (c) colorimetric, all three being variations of the corresponding detection methods. In addition, there is (d) hydroxylamine-based assay, involving reaction of the residual β-lactam antibiotic with hydroxylamine and subsequent spectrophotometric determination (DALE and SMITH 1971; MAYS et al. 1975); (e) spectrophotometric (kinetic assay) based on spectral changes observed upon hydrolysis of penicillins and cephalosporins (JANSSON 1965; WALEY 1974; SAMUNI 1975).

As with most enzymes, β-lactamases are characterized on the basis of substrate and inhibition profiles, molecular weights, and isoelectric points (pIs). Substrate profiles are determined from the hydrolytic activity of a β-lactamase toward a number of β-lactam antibiotics relative to a reference compound (usually benzylpenicillin) whose rate of hydrolysis is arbitrarily taken as 100. Inhibition profiles are determined from the effect on a β-lactamase of certain semisynthetic penicillins (usually cloxacillin and methicillin) and modifying agents (usually pCMB and chloride ions). Obviously, loss of β-lactamase activity after modification of a specific residue could be due either to direct involvement of that residue in catalysis or to conformational changes. Furthermore, in order for either substrate or inhibition profile to be meaningful, β-lactamase activity must be due to a single enzyme. For example, early studies on the substrate profile of *B. cereus* β-lactamase involved a mixture of two β-lactamases and thus conclusions were invalid. Molecular weights are determined by gel filtration, equilibrium centrifugation or SDS-polyacylamide gel electrophoresis, the former two methods involving nondissociating conditions and therefore producing molecular weights that are sometimes multiples of those produced by SDS-polyacylamide gel electrophoresis. Isoelectric points are determined by analytical isoelectric focusing in polyacrylamide gels under nondenaturing conditions (VESTERBERG 1973; MATTHEW 1975). After focusing, β-lactamases are detected using the chromogenic cephalosporin nitrocefin. In contrast to preparative isoelectric focusing in density gradients, analytical isoelectric focusing does not give precise absolute pI values (LABIA and BARTHELÈMY 1977) but nevertheless is useful for comparison studies.

Research on the production and spread of β-lactamases in bacteria has been greatly aided by two breakthroughs in the field of molecular genetics: (1) the discovery of R factors (OCHIAI et al. 1959) which provided the first proof of transferable nonchromosomal replicating material from one bacterial cell to another; (2) the formulation of the concept of transposition (HEDGES et al. 1974), defined as the ability of certain pieces of genetic material ("transposons") to be translocated from one plasmid to another, or from plasmid to bacterial chromosome or to bacteriophage or vice versa.

The genes for β-lactamase are located chromosomally or extrachromosomally and may be mobilized intragenetically by a recombination transposition event and intergenetically by one of the transfer mechanism such as transformation, transduction or conjugation. β-Lactamase genes thus have the potential for a high degree of mobility, explaining in part why β-lactamases have been so successful as antibiotic resistance agents (Fig. 10).

II. β-Lactamases in Gram-Positive Bacteria

As already stated, the majority of β-lactamases in gram-positive bacteria are exocellular. They are usually obtained from the culture medium by adsorption on ion

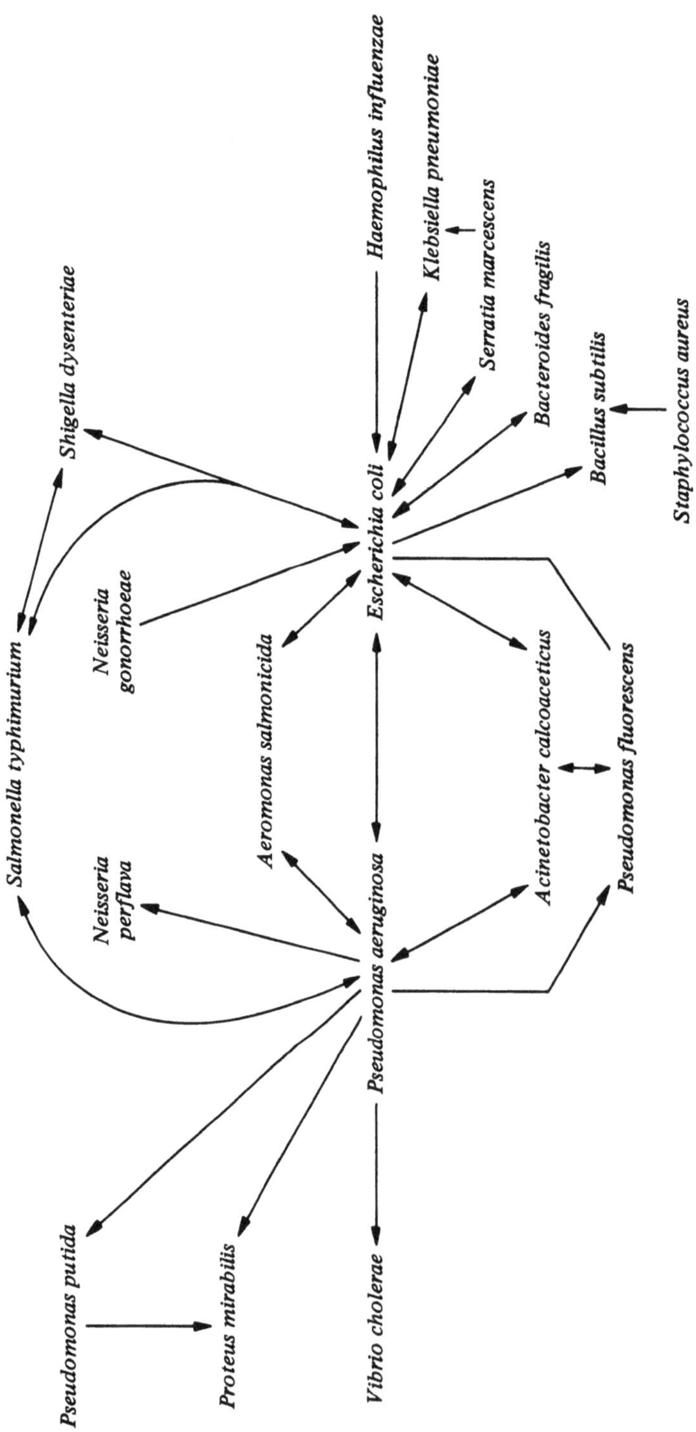

Fig. 10. Flow of plasmids between bacteria. (Adapted from Young and Mayer 1979)

Table 6. Substrate profile of staphylococcal β-lactamase

Substrate	Relative rate of hydrolysis
Penicillin G	100
Ampicillin	120
Cloxacillin	2
Cephradine	2
Cephaloridine	10

exchangers such as Amberlite (JOHNSON et al. 1973), DEAE-cellulose (JOHNSON et al. 1973) or cellulose phosphate (RICHMOND 1963). Membrane-bound β-lactamases are usually released by nonionic detergents (YAMAMOTO and LAMPEN 1976) or limited proteolysis (POLLOCK 1965).

Although *S. aureus* is the only gram-positive organism considered an important pathogen, much detailed work has been carried out with the β-lactamases from *B. cereus* and *B. licheniformis*. Only recently have β-lactamases from actinomycetes been studied in any detail.

1. Staphylococci

Since the early 1960s, it has been known that the genetic determinant for lactamase production in *S. aureus* is characteristically located extrachromosomally on a plasmid (NOVICK 1963). Transfer of this plasmid from one cell to another is mediated by transduction (HARMON and BALDWIN 1964) and is probably responsible for the spread of penicillin resistance among different staphylococcal phage types.

β-Lactamases from *S. aureus* can be serologically divided into four types, A, B, C, and D (RICHMOND 1965), the enzymes being otherwise indistinguishable. They are predominantly active against penicillins (with the exception of β-lactamase-stable penicillins, such as methicillin and the isoxazoyl penicillins), and among the cephalosporins, against cephaloridine (Table 6).

Staphylococcal β-lactamase is inducible in the majority of wild-type strains, though most studies have used a penicillinase constitutive strain (PCl) which produces large amounts of enzyme, of which 60% is exocellular and the rest membrane bound (DYKE 1979). Strains that are endemic in hospitals produce large quantities of exocellular β-lactamase but, generally, the proportion of the exocellular relative to the membrane-bound form depends on the strain studied and the conditions of growth (DYKE 1979).

It has been reported (KAMINSKI 1963) that induction of *S. aureus* β-lactamase, but not β-lactamase activity, is inhibited by micromolar concentrations of anionic detergents such as sodium dodecylsulfate. Whether this reflects inhibition of all exocellular enzymes (e.g., by perturbation of the cytoplasmic membrane) or affects specifically β-lactamase induction is unclear.

The exocellular enzyme has been purified by conventional methods (RICHMOND 1963), and its amino acid composition, molecular weight and amino acid sequence determined (AMBLER and MEADWAY 1969; AMBLER 1975). It is a single polypeptide

Table 7. Substrate profile of *Bacillus* β-lactamases

Enzyme	Substrate						Reference
	Benzyl-penicillin	Ampi-Cillin	Carben-icillin	Methi-cillin	Cepha-loridine	Cepha-lothin	
B. cereus I	100	100	22	6	1	–	SYKES and BUSH (1981)
B. cereus II	100	64	–	89	41	89	SYKES and BUSH (1981)
B. licheniformis	100	79	21	–	25	–	SYKES and BUSH (1981)

chain with a molecular weight of 29,000 and a PI of 8.9. A remarkable feature of its amino acid sequence is the extensive homology (approximately 40%) to the β-lactamases of *B. licheniformis* and *B. cereus* (AMBLER 1975; THATCHER 1975).

The enzyme is inactivated by iodine (RICHMOND 1963) and tetranitromethane (AMBLER 1975), the latter reacting preferentially with tyrosine-82. However, as in other proteins, tetranitromethane promotes intermolecular cross-linking resulting in a high-molecular-weight inactive species, which accounts for the observed inactivation, while the monomeric species has normal activity (BRISTOW and VIRDEN 1978). The enzyme is also inactivated by phenylglyoxal, a reagent normally specific for arginine residues (PAIN and VIRDEN 1979). However, the possibility of inter- and intramolecular cross-linking (involving lysine and carboxyl residues) cannot be ruled out. Recently, the enzyme has been shown to be inhibited irreversibly by phenylpropynal, activity dropping to 20% after 1 h (SCHENKEIN and PRATT 1980).

2. Bacilli

a) Aerobic

B. cereus (NRRLB-569) produces two exocellular β-lactamases, I and II (KUWABARA and ABRAHAM 1967), which are coded by separate structural genes and do not cross-react immunologically. As with most gram-positive β-lactamases, the enzymes of this strain are inducible. However, the β-lactamases of a spontaneous mutant, 569/H, are constitutive. On the basis of the coordinate regulation of β-lactamase I and II, it has been suggested that the two structural genes may lie in the same operon (POLLOCK 1971). Other *B. cereus* strains produce, in varying amounts, enzymes apparently similar to I and II of strain 569 (DAVIES et al. 1975). Most studies, and therefore the discussion that follows, deal with enzymes of *B. cereus* 569.

β-Lactamase I has been purified to homogeneity by conventional methods (KOGUT et al. 1956) and has molecular weight 30,000 daltons (DAVIES et al. 1974a). On isoelectric focusing it is resolved into three enzymes (DAVIES et al. 1974a) which differ in their N-terminal amino acid sequence but have identical specific activity (IMSANDE et al. 1970; DAVIES et al. 1974a; THATCHER 1975). Its amino acid sequence (THATCHER 1975) and substrate specificity (Table 7) is similar to those of the *S. aureus* and *B. licheniformis* enzymes. The pH optimum is between 6.0 and 7.0.

Chemical modifications involving group-specific (WALEY 1975; OGAWARA and UMEZAWA 1975) and site-specific (PATIL and DAY 1973; DURKIN et al. 1977) reagents have given equivocal results. The products of the β-lactamase reaction have been reported to reversibly inhibit the enzyme with K_is in the 10^{-2} M range (KIENER and WALEY 1978). Interestingly, boric acid, benzeneboronic acid and *m*-amino benzeneboronic acid were also reversible inhibitors with K_is in the millimolar range (KIENER and WALEY 1978). Recently, phenylpropynal has been shown to inactivate the enzyme irreversibly achieving 70% inhibition after 1 h (SCHENKEIN and PRATT 1980). Most importantly, an active site serine residue (Ser-44) has been identified (KNOTT et al. 1979) (Sect. E) which appears to be conserved in the amino acid sequences of all β-lactamases and DD-carboxypeptidases examined thus far (WAXMAN et al. 1980).

β-Lactamase II has been purified to homogeneity also by conventional methods (DAVIES et al. 1974b) and has molecular weight 22,000 daltons (KUWABARA and LLOYD 1971). It is a zinc metalloenzyme (DAVIES and ABRAHAM 1974), the presence of zinc dominating its inhibition pattern [e.g., inhibition by EDTA and *N*-ethylmaleimide (NEM) (KUWABARA and ABRAHAM 1967)]. Its amino acid sequence is not yet known, but is expected to be substantially different from that of other β-lactamases. The enzyme is active toward both penicillins and cephalosporins (NEWTON and ABRAHAM 1956) (Table 7).

The enzymes from several strains of *B. licheniformis* have been characterized by POLLOCK (1965) and his associates. There are two forms of β-lactamase, a 30,000-dalton exocellular enzyme and a larger membrane-bound form present in approximately equal amounts. The two enzymes are coded by the same gene which has been mapped by transformation analysis (SHERRATT and COLLINS 1973). However, they differ in their substrate specificities and other properties. The complete amino acid sequence of the exocellular enzyme from strain 749/C is known (AMBLER and MEADWAY 1969). The membrane-bound enzyme is a precursor of the exocellular enzyme but the exact mechanism of secretion is unknown. It had been reported that secretion involves proteolytic cleavage of an N-terminal 24-amino acid segment ending in phosphatidylserine (YAMAMOTO and LAMPEN 1976). But studies from a different laboratory with the membrane form indicated no such peptide (SIMONS et al. 1978). Furthermore, the group that had originally found a phospholipoprotein to be the membrane-bound precursor of the exocellular enzyme has since retreated from their original position (IZUI et al. 1980). Therefore, the published model for the secretion of β-lactamase in *B. licheniformis* (LAMPEN 1978) must be revised, although secretion probably does occur according to the "signal hypothesis" of BLOBEL and DOBBERSTEIN (1975). The exocellular enzyme may account for up to 30% of the total exocellular proteins in *B. licheniformis* and has been purified both by conventional methods (POLLOCK 1965) and by affinity chromatography on cephalosporin C-Sepharose (CRANE et al. 1973). Like many other β-lactamases from gram-positive bacteria, the enzyme has low activity toward cephalosporin derivatives (Table 7).

b) Anaerobic

β-Lactamases have been isolated and characterized from the anaerobic gram-positive rods *Clostridium ramosum* and *Clostridium clostridiiformis* (DEL BENE et al.

Table 8. Substrate profile of β-lactamases produced by *Clostridium* species

Organism	Relative rate of hydrolysis							Reference
	Penicillin G	Ampicillin	Carbenicillin	Cloxacillin	Cefazolin	Cephamandole	Cefoxitin	
Clostridium ramosum	100	260	<1	100	66	28	<1	DEL BENE *et al.* (1979)
Clostridium clostridiiformis	100	87	3	2	< 1	< 1	<1	DEL BENE *et al.* (1979)

Table 9. Substrate profile of β-lactamases from actinomycetes

Organism	Relative rate of hydrolysis					Reference
	Benzyl-penicillin	Ampi-cillin	Carben-icillin	Cloxa-cillin	Cepha-loridine	
Streptomyces (E750–3)	100	28	13	6	2	OGAWARA *et al.* (1978)
Nocardia	100	100	80	NT	15	WALLACE *et al.* (1978)
Micromonospora	100	190	0	0	800	SCHWARTZ and SCHWARTZ (1979)
Microbispora	100	690	200	0	1700	SCHWARTZ and SCHWARTZ (1979)

1979). The enzyme produced by *C. ramosum* has a broad substrate profile hydrolyzing both penicillins and cephalosporins (Table 8). Enzyme induction has been observed with a number of β-lactam antibiotics, resulting in a 10- to 200-fold increase in the amount of β-lactamase produced. The enzyme is inhibited by *p*-chloromercuribenzoate (*p*CMB) and cefoxitin. However, all these results are difficult to interpret as the *C. ramosum* studied has been shown to harbor the TEM-1 β-lactamase (DEL BENE et al. 1979).

The enzyme isolated from strains of *C. clostridiiformis* is highly active against penicillins but shows little if any activity against cephalosporins (Table 8). Although low levels of enzyme induction have been reported, cefoxitin was the only effective inducer. The enzyme is resistant to inhibition by *p*CMB and cefoxitin.

3. Streptomycetes

Streptomyces is one of the most abundant genera of soil microorganisms and produes a large number of antibiotics including penicillins, cephalosporins, and β-lactamase inhibitors (NAGARAJAN 1972; BROWN et al. 1977). The majority of *Streptomyces* strains studied have been shown to produce a β-lactamase predominantly active against penicillins (OGAWARA 1975) (Table 9).

The enzymes are usually exocellular, are produced constitutively (OGAWARA 1975) and are probably plasmid-mediated (OGAWARA and NOZAKI 1977). Unlike other bacterial β-lactamases, the *Streptomyces* enzymes are resistant to inactivation by iodine and *N*-bromosuccinimide (JOHNSON et al. 1973; OGAWARA 1975). The β-lactamase from *Streptomyces albus* has been purified by conventional methods (JOHNSON et al. 1973) while the enzyme from *Streptomyces cellulosae* was purified by affinity chromatography on Blue Sepharose (OGAWARA and HORIKAWA 1979).

4. Other Actinomycetes

The production of β-lactamase by actinomycetes other than streptomycetes is widespread throughout the various genera (SCHWARTZ and SCHWARTZ 1979). Unlike *Streptomyces*, these organisms tend to produce broad-spectrum β-lactamases

Table 10. Substrate profile of mycobacterial β-lactamases

Organism	Relative rate of hydrolysis				Reference
	Peni-cillin G	Ampi-cillin	Cloxa-cillin	Cepha-loridine	
Mycobacterium phlei	100	NT	NT	285	RICHMOND and SYKES (1973)
Mycobacterium smegmatis	100	68	0	77	RICHMOND and SYKES (1973)
Mycobacterium fortuitum	100	NT	0	91	RICHMOND and SYKES (1973)

NT = Not Tested

(Table 9), active against penicillins and cephalosporins. Most of the enzymes are exocellular.

Many species of mycobacteria, including pathogenic ones, produce β-lactamases which may contribute to the resistance of these organisms to β-lactam antibiotics. The enzymes have been recently reviewed by KASIC (1979). They are constitutive and intracellular, being released upon cell disruption (KASIC and PEACHAM 1968). They are generally active against both penicillins and cephalosporins (Table 10), although differences between enzymes from different species do exist. For example, the β-lactamase from *Mycobacterium tuberculosis* does not hydrolyze α-substituted penicillins and cephalosporins, such as ampicillin, while the one from *Mycobaterium smegmatis* does (KASIK and PEACHAM 1968).

III. β-Lactamases in Gram-Negative Bacteria

Since the early 1960s an overwhelming number of reports have appeared describing β-lactamases from different species of gram-negative organisms. As in gram-positive bacteria, β-lactamases are crucial factors in the resistance of gram-negative bacteria to β-lactam antibiotics. In an attempt to group the enzymes in some meaningful way, classification schemes have been proposed based mainly on biochemical and genetic data (RICHMOND and SYKES 1973; SYKES and MATTHEW 1976; SYKES and SMITH 1979). However, as new β-lactamases are discovered and once considered nonpathogenic organisms take a prominent role in clinical medicine, such schemes are subject to change.

The existence of R factors in gram-negative bacteria (Sect. D.I) complicates attempts to correlate the properties of different β-lactamases with the bacterial genus or species in which they are found. The nature of the enzyme is specified by the R factor while the amount of enzyme produced varies with the organism.

As already stated, the majority of β-lactamases in gram-negative bacteria are periplasmic, with molecular weights 25,000–30,000 (RICHMOND and SYKES 1973), although β-lactamases with molecular weights in excess of 40,000, probably dimeric, do exist (DALE and SMITH 1974, 1976). They are usually released from cells by sonication, a procedure releasing all cytoplasmic contents. An alternative method is osmotic shock (NEU and HEPPEL 1965) whereby only periplasmic proteins (less than 10% of total cell proteins) are released. The osmotic shock method releases β-lactamases of molecular weight less than 30,000 (SMITH and WYATT 1974), peptidoglycan acting apparently as a molecular sieve (BROAD and SMITH 1979). β-Lactamases of molecular weight 30,000 or more are released by spheroplasting (SMITH and WYATT 1974).

1. Anaerobic

Bacteroides fragilis is the most frequently isolated anaerobic species from clinical specimens and is involved in serious infections. The species is divided into five subspecies, *B. fragilis* being the most common clinical isolate from infections. *B. fragilis* is generally resistant to penicillin but some isolates are unusually sensitive and others highly resistant (FINEGOLD and SUTTER 1972). The subspecies are also usually penicillin resistant (JONES and FUCHS 1976; OLSSON et al. 1977).

The black-pigmented bacteroides *Bacteroides melaninogenicus* and subspecies are generally penicillin sensitive although resistant isolates have been reported (MARTIN et al. 1972; MURRAY and ROSENBLATT 1977; APPELBAUM and CHATTERTON 1978).

Most *Bacteroides* owe their resistance, at least in part, to the production of β-lactamase. From a study of over 200 clinical isolates of *B. fragilis* OLSSON et al. (1977) found 93% of strains to be β-lactamase producers. It has also been reported that the great majority of *B. fragilis* strains inhabiting the intestinal tract of humans are β-lactamase producers (OLSSON-LILJEQUIST et al. 1979). The enzymes produced by these strains are all constitutive and appear to be very closely related in terms of substrate profile, inhibition patterns and isoelectric point (Table 11).

The *B. fragilis* β-lactamase shows some specificity toward cephalosporin substrates, with the exception of cefoxitin, and is inhibited by *p*CMB, cloxacillin and cefoxitin. Thus, its substrate profile resembles that of the class I β-lactamases of RICHMOND and SYKES (1973) commonly found in *Pseudomonas*, *Enterobacter*, indole-positive PROTEUS, and *E. coli* strains. However, the inhibition patterns by both *p*CMB and cloxacillin are different.

There seems to be disagreement on whether the subspecies produce different and characteristic β-lactamases (LEUNG and WILLIAMS 1978; TALLY et al. 1977). There is little doubt that *Bacteroides* species other than *B. fragilis* produce β-lactamases, although there is some controversy as to whether such enzymes preferentially hydrolyze penicillins or cephalosporins (SALYERS et al. 1977; SHERRILL and MCCARTHY 1979) (Table 10).

The work of WÜST and WILKINS (1978) showed indirectly that β-lactamases from several *Bacteroides* species are inhibited by clavulanic acid. Although *B. fragilis* strains have been shown to harbor plasmids, none has been linked to the production of β-lactamase (DEL BENE et al. 1979).

2. Aerobic

β-Lactamases produced by this group of organisms are classified with respect to the location of their structural genes in the cell, namely chromosomal and extrachromosomal.

Table 11. Properties of β-lactamases produced by *Bacteroides* species

Organism	Relative rate of hydrolysis						Inhibition by:					References
	Benzyl-penicillin	Ampicillin	Carbenicillin	Cephaloridine	Cephalothin	Cefoxitin	*p*-Chloromercuri-benzoate	Cloxacillin	Cefoxitin	MW	Isoelectric point	
Bacteroides fragilis	5	5	5	100	90	0	5	S	S	30000	5.0	BRITZ and WILKINSON (1978); DARLAND and BIRNBAUM (1977); LEUNG and WILLIAMS (1978); OLSSON *et al.* (1977)
Bacteroides melaninogenicus, *Bacteroides oralis*	100	6	60		30		R	R	R			MURRAY and ROSENBLATT (1977); SALYERS *et al.* (1977)

S = Sensitive
R = Resistant

a) Chromosomally-Mediated β-Lactamases

The great majority of chromosomally-mediated β-lactamases, which include both constitutive and inducible enzymes, fall into the class I category of RICHMOND and SYKES (1973). These enzymes hydrolyze cephalosporins in preference to the penicillins – a number of semisynthetic penicillins being inhibitors. Organisms producing class I enzymes are widespread and of considerable clinical importance. In general, these enzymes hydrolyze susceptible cephalosporins 5–1,000 times as rapidly as benzylpenicillin and are inhibited by cloxacillin, cephamycins, and olivanic acids. They are resistant to inhibition by *p*CMB and clavulanic acid. Strains of different genera vary greatly in the amount of chromosomal β-lactamase that they produce when growing in a nutrient medium in the absence of antibiotic. Activities of enzyme range from barely detectable (i.e., less than about 0.0012 μmol/s per milligram dry weight bacteria) in species of *Haemophilus*, to 70 μmol/s per milligram in *Enterobacter cloacae* 214 (HENNESSEY 1967), and to 2,000 μmol/s per milligram in certain strains of *Klebsiella* (SAWAI et al. 1973). Chromosomally-mediated enzymes can be further divided on the basis of inducibility.

α) Inducible β-Lactamases. Inducible enzymes are found in a wide range of genera, notably: *Acinetobacter*, *Citrobacter*, *Enterobacter*, indole-positive *Proteus*, *Pseudomonas*, *Serratia* and *Yersinia*. These enzymes are often genus, species, and subspecies specific (MATTHEW and HARRIS 1976).

COUILLARD et al. (1979) examined a wide variety of enzymes from *Enterobacter*, and on the basis of isoelectric point, recorded ten enzyme types with isoelectric points between 7 and 10. Wild-type strains of *P. aeruginosa* invariably produce a chromosomally-mediated inducible β-lactamase (NORDSTRÖM and SYKES 1974). On the other hand, there is only one report of an inducible β-lactamase produced by *E. coli* (DALE 1975). Some properties of these enzymes are listed in Table 12.

Synthesis of β-lactamase can be induced in these strains either by β-lactam substrates, as would usually occur in a clinical situation (HENNESSEY 1967; SYKES and RICHMOND 1971), by β-lactamase inhibitors (HENNESSEY 1967; SABATH et al. 1965) or by compounds that are neither substrates not inhibitors (GARBER and FRIEDMAN 1970). Since induction can increase production of β-lactamase more than 100-fold (HENNESSEY 1967; NORDSTRÖM and SYKES 1974), presence of small amounts of antibiotic may give rise to bacterial populations that are resistant by virtue of increased production of chromosomal enzyme.

β) Constitutive β-Lactamases. With one exception, *E. coli* β-lactamases are noninducible, as are enzymes produced by *Shigella* and *Salmonella*. Several strains are known to produce exceptionally high levels of chromosomally-mediated enzyme. For example, the enzyme produced by *E. cloacae* P99 (FLEMING et al. 1967) is a typical *Enterobacter* enzyme on the basis of its substrate profile (Table 13) and other biochemical properties (RICHMOND and SYKES 1973). However, unlike the majority of *Enterobacter* enzymes, it is constitutive and is produced in large amounts.

The majority of *E. coli* strains produce a constitutive, chromosomally-mediated β-lactamase resembling closely the enzyme produced by strains 214T and D31 (SMITH 1963; BURMAN et al. 1968). However, the enzymes from these strains can be distinguished from each other and from the otherwise identical chromosomal

Table 12. Inducible β-lactamases

Organism	Relative rate of hydrolysis					Inhibition by:				References
	Benzyl-penicillin	Ampicillin	Carbenicillin	Cephaloridine	Cephalothin	*p*-Chloromercuri-benzoate	Cloxacillin	MW	Isoelectric point	
Acinetobacter anitratum 7844	3	1		100	60	R				Morohoshi and Saito (1977)
Chromobacter violaceum	100	4	6	310	187	R	S			Farrar and O'Dell (1976)
Citrobacter freundii GN336	100	< 5	< 5	5,500						Sawai *et al.* (1968)
Enterobacter aerogenes 58	100	0		1,100	1,000					
Enterobacter aerogenes 250	100			1,285	595		S	30,000	9.3	Letarte *et al.* (1977)
Enterobacter cloacae 214	100	10	< 5	10,000	3,000				7.5	Farrar and Krause (1970)
Escherichia coli JD41	100	40		320			S	42,000	7.6	Hennessey (1967)
Proteus vulgaris GN76	100	140		1,780						Sawai *et al.* (1968)
Proteus morganii 185	100	<10	< 5	1,000	230	R	S			Hamilton-Miller *et al.* (1965)
Proteus rettgeri 410	100	<10		3,800	2,320	R	S			Hamilton-Miller (1967)
Pseudomonas aeruginosa GN918	100	10	< 5	770	50	S	S	34,000	8.7	Yaginuma *et al.* (1973)
Pseudomonas aeruginosa NCTC8203	100	10	0	400		R	S	29,000	7.7	Sykes and Richmond (1971)
Serratia marcescens 1331E	100	0	0	2,000	2,000				8.5	Sykes and Matthew (1976)
Serratia marcescens	100	60	26	822		R	S			Farrar and Newsome (1973)
Yersinia enterocolitica W222 enzyme B	100	< 1	< 1	280	210	R	S	34,000	5.4	Cornelis and Abraham (1975)

β-lactamase of *Shigella sonnei* (SMITH et al. 1974) by starch gel electrophoresis (BOBROWSKI et al. 1976). Spontaneous *E. coli* mutants producing large amounts of a chromosomal β-lactamase have been isolated, hyperproduction being due to increased copy number of the enzyme-coding gene (NORMARK et al. 1977). Such gene amplification resulting in β-lactamase hyperproduction may be responsible for some clinical cases of ampicillin resistance (MEDEIROS and MANDEL 1979).

Most strains of *Yersinia enterocolitica* so far examined produce two distinct β-lactamases (A and B) which differ in substrate profile, sensitivity to *p*CMB, molecular weight, inducibility and isoelectric point (CORNELIS and ABRAHAM 1975) (Table 13).

In contrast to the β-lactamases produced by gram-positive organisms, only a small number of gram-negative bacteria have been reported to produce enzymes predominantly active against penicillins (penicillinases). DEBELL et al. (1978) reported an enzyme from *Vibrio parahaemolyticus* which was more active on penicillins than cephalosporins. From a survey conducted in β-lactamase producing gram-negative organisms, SYKES and MATTHEW (1976) found only one organism producing a chromosomally-mediated penicillinase.

The chromosomally-mediated broad-spectrum β-lactamases are characteristic of the genus *Klebsiella*, a group of organisms with diverse biochemical properties. The enzymes produced by these organisms are identical on the basis of substrate profile, but have different isoelectric points (MATTHEW and HARRIS 1976) (Table 13).

b) R-Factor-Mediated β-Lactamases

A study of drug resistance in strains of *Salmonella typhimurium* by ANDERSON and DATTA (1965), revealed a number of ampicillin-resistant strains capable of transferring their resistance to sensitive recipient strains. Subsequent work by DATTA and KONTOMICHALOU (1965) showed that the transfer of ampicillin resistance was associated with the production of β-lactamase. Among the organisms studied was *E. coli* strain TEM, an ampicillin-resistant strain isolated in Athens (DATTA and KONTOMICHALOU 1965). Ampicillin resistance and β-lactamase production in this strain were shown to be mediated by an R-factor which was designated TEM.

The β-lactamase associated with the TEM R-factor was subsequently isolated and purified (DATTA and RICHMOND 1966). A similar R-plasmid-mediated β-lactamase produced by strains of *P. aeruginosa* was reported by SYKES and RICHMOND (1970). Although the enzymes have identical substrate profiles and inhibition patterns, they can be distinguished by isoelectric focusing (MATTHEW et al. 1975). These enzymes, referred to as the TEM-type enzymes, occur most frequently and with the widest distribution of the R-factor-mediated enzymes.

A second R-factor-mediated β-lactamase was found by DATTA and KONTOMICHALOU (1965) in a strain of *E. coli* carrying the R-factor R 1818. The enzyme can be differentiated from the TEM-type on the basis of substrate profile; it hydrolyzes cloxacillin at a much lower rate than benzylpenicillin (Table 14). The R 1818 group of enzymes, later to be referred to as the "oxacillin-hydrolyzing enzymes," along with the TEM-type β-lactamases remained until the mid-1970s the only known R-plasmid-mediated β-lactamases in gram-negative bacteria.

Table 13. Constitutive β-lactamases

	Relative rate of hydrolysis					Inhibition by:				Reference
	Benzyl-penicillin	Ampicillin	Carbenicillin	Cephaloridine	Cephalothin	*p*-Chloromercuri-benzoate	Cloxacillin	MW	Isoelectric point	
Proteus morganii 1510	100	6	0	1,200	450	R	S	38,000	7.2	FUJII-KURIYAMA *et al.* (1977)
Enterobacter cloacae P99	100	0	0	6,600	1,300	R	S	30,000	8.5	FLEMMING *et al.* (1967)
Escherichia coli 214T	100	3	0	330	400	R	S	31,000	8.3	DALE and SMITH (1971b)
Yersinia enterocolitica W222 enzyme A	100	80	25	300	130	S	S	30,000	8.1	CORNELIS and ABRAHAM (1975)
Aeromonas liquefaciens	100	100	60	20		R	R	24,000		RICHMOND and SYKES (1973)
Aerobacter cloacae 53	100	105	10	64	15	S	R	24,000	7.5	SMITH and HAMILTON-MILLER (1963)
Klebsiella aerogenes 1082E	100	170	50	70	80	S	R	24,000	6.5	MARSHALL *et al.* (1972)
Klebsiella aerogenes 418	100	185		9		R	S	20,000		DALE and SMITH (1971)

Within the last few years, six additional plasmid-mediated β-lactamases have been recognized as distinct species in gram-negative bacteria. Two of these enzymes, SHV-1 (PITTON 1972; PETROCHEILOU et al. 1977) and HMS-1 (MATTHEW et al. 1979) are determined by plasmids carried by Enterobacteria. The other four enzymes, PSE-1, PSE-2, PSE-3 and PSE-4 are determined by plasmids which are normally *Pseudomonas*-specific (HEDGES and MATTHEW 1979).

α) TEM-Type β-Lactamases. The TEM-1 and TEM-2 β-lactamases are constitutive enzymes indistinguishable on the basis of substrate profile, inhibition pattern, molecular weight and reaction with antiserum (Table 14). However, the enzymes can be readily distinguished by differences in their isoelectric points (MATTHEW et al. 1975). Comparison of the amino acid sequence of the TEM-2 β-lactamase (AMBLER and SCOTT 1978) with the nucleotide sequence of the TEM-1 enzyme (SUTCLIFFE 1978) has revealed a single amino acid, Lys, replacing Gln at residue 14 in the TEM-2 β-lactamase.

Chemical modifications involving tetranitromethane, photooxidation and iodoacetic acid (SCOTT 1973; OGAWARA et al. 1972) have suggested the presence of a tyrosine and a histidine residue near or at the active site of the TEM enzyme. Recently, phenylpropynal has been shown to inactivate irreversibly the enzyme at 3 m*M*, achieving complete inhibition in less than 20 min (SCHENKEIN and PRATT 1980). Penicillin G protects the enzyme from inactivation, suggesting that phenylpropynal acts near or at the active site. The residue(s) modified was not identified but from spectrophotometric data it was suggested to be lysine or arginine. The enzyme is also inhibited by anionic detergents such as sodium dodecylsulfate and the anionic macrolide izumenolide (BUSH et al. 1980).

The TEM-2 β-lactamase expressed in *E. coli* W3110 carrying the R6K plasmid is being studied by x-ray crystallography (KNOX et al. 1976).

HEDGES et al. (1974) compared 29 different plasmid-mediated β-lactamases and found that the TEM-type were determined by plasmids from a wide range of compatibility groups exhibiting broad taxonomic and geographical spread. From the plasmids studied, 78% mediated the synthesis of the TEM-type β-lactamase. The authors concluded, that because this type of enzyme was so common, its structural gene must possess special properties enabling it to be translocated from one replicon to another. Later work showed that acquisition of ampicillin resistance by the R-factor was associated with an increase in plasmid molecular weight and the term transposon was proposed for such mobile R-factor antibiotic-resistance genes (HEDGES and JACOB 1974).

In studies involving 363 gram-negative plasmid-mediated β-lactamases (MATTHEW 1979) 77% were found to be of the TEM-type. Of these, the TEM-1 β-lactamase was by far the most common, representing about 90% of the TEM-type enzymes.

A disconcerting aspect of the TEM β-lactamases is their presence in strains of *Neisseria gonorrhoeae* and *Haemophilus influenzae* when these strains harbor drug resistance plasmids (SYKES et al. 1975; SYKES and PERCIVAL 1978).

β) Oxacillin-Hydrolyzing β-Lactamases. This group of R-factor-mediated β-lactamases, like the TEM-type enzymes, are synthesized constitutively. They were orig-

Table 14. Properties of plasmid-mediated β-lactamases (MATTHEW 1979)

Plasmid	β-lactamase	Relative rate of hydrolysis						Inhibition by:			MW	Isoelectric point	References
		Benzyl-penicillin	Ampicillin	Carbenicillin	Cloxacillin	Cephaloridine	Cephalothin	p-Chloromercuri-benzoate	Cloxacillin	Sodium chloride			
RGK	TEM-1	100	106	10	0	76	20	R	S	R	28,900	5.4	HEDGES et al. (1974) SUTCLIFFE (1978)
RP1	TEM-2	100	107	10	0	74	20	R	S	R	28,900	5.6	HEDGES et al. (1974) AMBLER and SCOTT (1978)
P453	SHV-1	100	212	8	< 2	56	8	R	S	R	17,000	7.6	MATTHEW et al. (1979)
P997	HMS-1	100	253	14	2	183	3	S	S	R	21,000	5.2	MATTHEW et al. (1979)
Rgn238	OXA-1	100	382	30	190	30	15	PS	R	S	23,300	7.4	HEDGES et al. (1974)
R46	OXA-2	100	179	15	200	37	25	R	R	S	44,600	7.7	HEDGES et al. (1974)
R57b	OXA-3	100	178	10	350	44	10	R	R	S	41,200	7.1	HEDGES et al. (1974)
RPL11	PSE-1	100	90	97	< 2	18	< 2	S	R		28,500	5.7	MATTHEW and SYKES (1977)
R151	PSE-2	100	267	121	371	32	< 2	S	S		12,400	6.1	MATTHEW (1978)
Rms149	PSE-3	100	101	253	3	10		R			12,000	6.9	SAWADA et al. (1974)
pMG19	PSE-4	100	88	150	< 2	40	4	R	R		32,000	5.3	HEDGES and MATTHEW (1979)

inally set apart from the TEM β-lactamases by their ability to hydrolyze isoxazolyl penicillins and methicillin (HEDGES et al. 1974). The oxacillin-hydrolyzing enzymes (oxa-enzymes) are resistant to inhibition by *p*CMB and cloxacillin but are inhibited by chloride ions (YAMAGISHI et al. 1979; DALE 1971) (Table 14). In the studies reported by MATTHEW (1979), 15% of the plasmid-mediated β-lactamases from gram-negative organisms belonged to this type of enzyme. Although the second most common group of plasmid-mediated β-lactamases, the oxacillin-hydrolyzing enzymes are relatively rare compared to the TEM enzymes.

SYKES and SMITH (1979) have suggested as a possible reason for the relative rarity of the oxacillin-hydrolyzing enzymes their lower substrate turnover relative to the TEM enzymes. On a weight basis, the TEM enzyme is about 12 times as efficient as the oxacillin-hydrolyzing enzyme mediated by R46 (DALE and SMITH 1976). Another contributing factor to the containment of this enzyme type could be limited transfer capability. To date, the oxacillin-hydrolyzing enzymes have not been shown to be mediated by transposons.

γ) SHV-1 β-Lactamase. Originally reported by PITTON in 1972, plasmid mediation of the SHV-1 enzyme has only recently been confirmed (MATTHEW et al. 1979). The enzyme has a substrate profile similar to that of the TEM β-lactamases (Table 14), with the exception of ampicillin hydrolysis. The two enzymes also differ in their ability to hydrolyze the tetrazolyl analog of amoxycillin, CP-35,587 (*13*) (PHILIPON et al. 1976).

An intriguing aspect of the purified SHV-1 enzyme has been the effect of different substrates on inhibition by *p*CMB. Hydrolysis of benzylpenicillin is unaffected by 0.5 m*M* *p*CMB whereas hydrolysis of cephaloridine is completely inhibited (MATTHEW et al. 1979). It has been suggested (MATTHEW et al. 1979) that the binding sites for the two antibiotics are different in SHV-1, an essential sulfhydryl group being present in the cephaloridine – but not in the benzylpenicillin-binding site. Alternatively, the two sites might overlap, or pCMB might bind close to the active site, thus blocking entry of certain substrates. The SHV-1 enzymes does not cross-react with other R-plasmid-mediated β-lactamase (MATTHEW 1979).

Early reports (PITTON 1972; ROUPAS and PITTON 1974) on the distribution of SHV-1 β-lactamase remarked on the high proportion of *Klebsiella* strains carrying this enzyme. Such strains have recently been implicated in serious hospital cross-infections, being resistant to a wide range of penicillins, cephalosporins and aminoglycosides (PETROCHEILOU et al. 1977). The frequency of the SHV-1 enzyme among plasmid-mediated β-lactamases, together with its taxonomic spread, suggest that its structural gene has acquired transposability. In the studies reported by MATTHEW (1979) the overall frequency of this enzyme was 4%.

δ) PSE-β-Lactamases. These enzymes are mediated by plasmids that are normally *Pseudomonas*-specific (HEDGES and MATTHEW 1979). The four PSE enzymes are distinguished by their ability to hydrolyze carbenicillin at least as fast as benzylpenicillin (Table 14). They are divided into four types on the basis of molecular weight, isoelectric point and inhibition pattern (FURTH 1975; SAWADA et al. 1974; MATTHEW and SYKES 1977). PSE-1 type β-lactamase, initially described by MATTHEW and SYKES (1977), is produced by two IncP-2 plasmids which are usually

(JACOBY and MATTHEW 1979), but not always (MEDEIROS et al. 1979) *Pseudomonas*-specific.

PSE-2 type enzyme is specified by a plasmid (R 151) which has a limited host range (BRYAN et al. 1974). PSE-3 and PSE-4 β-lactamases are determined by plasmids that are not self-transmissible by conjugation even between *Pseudomonas* strains (JACOBY and MATTHEW 1979). PSE-3 was first described by JACOBY (1977) while PSE-4 is the Dalgleish enzyme described by NEWSOME et al. (1970) and SYKES and RICHMOND (1971).

E. Interaction with the β-Lactam Nucleus

I. Components of the Interaction

1. Kinetic Parameters

The minimal scheme for the interaction of DD-carboxypeptidase-transpeptidase and β-lactamase with β-lactam antibiotics is:

$$E+B \underset{k_{-1}}{\overset{k_1}{\rightleftharpoons}} E \cdot B \overset{k_2}{\rightarrow} E-B \overset{k_3}{\rightarrow} E+P \qquad \textit{Scheme I}$$

That is, a given β-lactam antibiotic, B, reversibly binds to the enzyme, E, forming a noncovalent complex, E · B. Subsequently, it acylates the enzyme forming a covalent complex, E – B, and is finally released as inactive antibiotic, P. If k_{-1}/k_1 (K_s) and k_3 are low but k_2 is high, the antibiotic acts as inhibitor; if K_s is low but k_2 and k_3 are high, the antibiotic acts as a substrate.

Until very recently evidence for the above mechanism had come mostly from the detailed studies of Ghuysen and his co-workers with *Streptomyces* R 61 DD-carboxypeptidase (GHUYSEN et al. 1979). In that system, dissociation constants (K_s) were separated from acylation constants (k_2) by stopped-flow experiments and the individual constants for several β-lactam antibiotics were determined. The studies of FISHER et al. (1980) with *E. coli* R-TEM β-lactamase have suggested that β-lactamases may operate by a similar mechanism, including formation of an acyl-enzyme intermediate.

Structural features of the β-lactam compounds that appear to facilitate interaction are:

1. A bicyclic β-lactam nucleus, although the monocyclic β-lactam nocardicin A binds (weakly) to DD-carboxypeptidase and peptidoglycan transpeptidase (MIRELMAN and NUCHAMOWITZ 1979b; GEORGOPAPADAKOU and LIU unpublished) and is a (poor) substrate for several β-lactamases (PRATT and ANDERSON 1980)
2. An anionic group adjacent to the amino part of the amide bond in the β-lactam nucleus
3. A side chain (at C-6 in penicillins, at C-7 in cephalosporins) that can rotate freely around the amide bond (SAMUNI and MEYER 1978).

In cephalosporins, substituents at C-3 are generally tolerated by the enzymes while in penicillins they are not. For example, tetrazolyl-amoxicillin interacts poorly with PBPs and β-lactamase relative to amoxicillin (PRESSLITZ 1978; GEORGOPAPADAKOU and LIU, unpublished work).

With the possible exception of DD-carboxypeptidase from *S. albus* G, all known DD-carboxypeptidases form covalent complexes with penicillin and other β-lactam antibiotics which are subsequently broken down. The parameters of this interaction are usually reported as I_{50}s (antibiotic concentration required to inhibit activity by 50%) and half-lives of the breakdown of the complex. However, I_{50}s are not estimated under steady-state conditions, which are prerequisite for Michaelis-Menten constants such as K_i $\left(\text{defined as } \frac{K_s}{k_2} \cdot k_3\right)$. Furthermore, the breakdown rate (k_3), estimated from the half-life of the complex $[t\frac{1}{2} = -(ln0.5)/k_3]$, can be very small. In that limiting case, K_i becomes small even when the rate of formation of the complex $\left(\frac{k_2}{K_s}\right)$ is small. That is, in $K_i = \frac{K_s}{k_2} \cdot k_3$ if $k_3 \rightarrow 0$ then $K_i \rightarrow 0$.

As already stated, with *Streptomyces* R 61 DD-carboxypeptidase, the rate of formation of the enzyme-antibiotic complex can be dissected into the dissociation constant (K_s) and the acylation constant (k_2) by stopped-flow experiments (FRERE et al. 1975b; FUAD et al. 1976). The picture which has emerged is that dissociation constants are in the 0.1- to 10-m*M* range while acylation constants are in the 0.01- to 200-s^{-1} range. The 10^4 difference in acylation rates of β-lactam antibiotics of comparable chemical reactivities has been attributed to conformal changes induced by β-lactam antibiotics upon binding, which is also reflected in fluorescence quenching and circular dichroism changes (NIETO et al. 1973).

For β-lactamases, the parameters of interaction with β-lactam substrates usually reported are K_m, V_{max} and sometimes the ratio V_{max}/K_m expressing the "physiological efficiency" of the enzyme (POLLOCK 1965). In Scheme I, $K_m = \frac{k_3 K_s}{k_2 + k_3}$, k_3 also being referred to as the catalytic constant (k_{cat}). If $k_3 \gg k_2$, then $K_m = K_s$, i.e., the kinetic constant K_m becomes equal to the equilibrium constant K_s.

E. coli R-TEM β-lactamase hydrolyzes several penicillins and cephalosporins with K_m values ranging from 0.02 to 0.6 m*M* and k_3 values from 0.004 to 2000 s^{-1}, most compounds falling in the high k_3 range (FISHER et al. 1980).

Rates of formation $\left(\frac{k_2}{K_s}\right)$, reported as $\frac{k_3}{K_m}$, range from $10^8\ M^{-1}\ s^{-1}$ for penicillin to $6\ M^{-1}\ s^{-1}$ for cefoxitin. Since k_3 for the latter compound is 0.004 s^{-1} at steady state, an acyl intermediate accumulates with a half-life estimated (from k_3) to be 3 min. The relatively long half-life of the cefoxitinoyl-enzyme complex has allowed its kinetic and spectroscopic characterization and isolation. Interestingly, hydroxylamine, a better nucleophile than water, does not substantially accelerate the breakdown of the covalent complex, indicating that the cefoxitinoyl-enzyme linkage may be inaccessible (FISHER et al. 1980).

2. Conformational Changes

The general scheme for the interaction of DD-carboxypeptidase-transpeptidase and β-lactamase with β-lactam antibiotics including conformational changes is

$$\begin{array}{ccccccc} E+B & \underset{k_{-1}}{\overset{k_1}{\rightleftharpoons}} & E\cdot B & \overset{k_2}{\rightarrow} & E-B & \overset{k_3}{\rightarrow} & E+P \\ & & \downarrow\uparrow & & \downarrow\uparrow & & \\ & & E'\cdot B & \overset{k'_2}{\rightarrow} & E'-B & \overset{k'_3}{\rightarrow} & E+P'. \end{array}$$

Scheme II

That is, a given β-lactam antibiotic B alters the conformation of the enzyme upon formation of the noncovalent complex. Subsequently it acylates the enzyme and is finally released as inactive antibiotic. k'_2 and k'_3 are, respectively, the formation and breakdown rates of the conformationally altered complex, $E'-B$, and P' the breakdown product.

Conformational changes induced by the binding of penicillins have been suggested for the exocellular DD-carboxypeptidase of *Streptomyces* R61 (GHUYSEN 1977). The possible partitioning of this enzyme into two conformers will be discussed in the contect of hydrolysis products formed from penicillin (Sect. E.II).

Conformational changes might also occur during the interaction of *E. coli* R-TEM β-lactamase with cefoxitin, rendering the cefoxitinoyl-enzyme linkage inaccessible to nucleophilic attack by hydroxylamine. On the other hand, the lack of accessibility might be due to steric hindrance by the cefoxitin side chain. It is noted that clavulanic acid, which completely lacks a side chain, *is* attacked by hydroxylamine after it has formed a covalent complex with the enzyme (CHARNAS et al. 1978).

Another example of conformational changes upon binding of β-lactam antibiotics is the interaction of quinacillin with the β-lactamase from *S. aureus* PCl (VIRDEN et al. 1978). Based on kinetic evidence, a slow isomerization of the enzyme between conformational states differing in K_m and V_{max} for quinacillin has been suggested. The hydrolysis products (P and P' in Scheme II) are identical for both conformers. It is not clear whether the conformational change occurs before or after binding of quinacillin; that is, whether the enzyme occurs in two conformations both binding quinacillin, or binding of quinacillin induces a conformational change.

Perhaps the best example of β-lactam-induced conformational changes is the interaction of *B. cereus* β-lactamase I with penicillins. Some of these compounds (S-type substrates) are hydrolyzed faster than 6-APA, while others (A-type substrates) are hydrolyzed more slowly, the rate of hydrolysis depending on the structure of the side-chain (CITRI et al. 1976). The difference has been attributed to conformational changes on the enzyme upon binding to the β-lactam substrate. This has been supported by immunological studies (ZYK and CITRI 1968), chemical modification studies (CITRI and ZYK 1965) and recently by tritium exchange experiments (KIENER and WALEY 1977).

3. Nature of the Covalent Complex

As already stated, DD-carboxypeptidases, peptidoglycan transpeptidases and β-lactamases form covalent complexes with β-lactam antibiotics. The most extensive studies on the nature of the linkage have been carried out with DD-carboxypeptidases. Incubation of ^{14}C-penicillin G with *Streptomyces* R 61 DD-carboxypeptidase followed by denaturation, digestion with proteolytic enzymes, and analysis of the peptide fragments revealed that penicillin was covalently attached to a serine residue on the enzyme (FRERE et al. 1976). Similar studies with *B. subtilis* and *B. stearothermophilus* DD-carboxypeptidases (GEORGOPAPADAKOU et al. 1977; YOCUM et al. 1979) as well as the enzyme from *Streptomyces* R 39 (GHUYSEN et al. 1980) indicate that in these enzymes too, penicillin binds to a serine residue. Furthermore, the amino acid sequence of the first 40 residues from the N-terminus in the two *Bacillus* DD-carboxypeptidases are homologous with each other and with that of some β-lactamases (WAXMAN et al. 1980). Results from studies with other DD-carboxypeptidases (Sect. C) as well as with PBPs (Sect. B) are consistent with penicillin binding generally occurring at a serine residue.

Studies with *B. cereus* β-lactamase I and ^{3}H-6-β-bromopenicillanic acid (Sect. E.III.3) have shown that the compound binds to serine-44 on the enzyme. This serine residue is conserved in the amino acid sequence of several β-lactamases (AMBLER 1979) and corresponds to serine-36 in the DD-carboxypeptidases of *B. subtilis* and *B. stearothermophilus* (WAXMAN et al. 1980).

Studies with the *E. coli* R-TEM β-lactamase have suggested that β-lactam antibiotics such as cefoxitin acylate a residue, probably serine, at the active site (FISHER et al. 1980). Thus, it is tempting to speculate that the interaction of β-lactamases with β-lactam antibiotics involves formation of a covalent complex (E−B in Scheme I) with a serine residue on the enzyme.

4. Nature of Release Products

The minimal scheme for the interaction of DD-carboxypeptidase and β-lactamase with β-lactam antibiotics resulting in more than one breakdown product is

$$E+B \underset{k_{-1}}{\overset{k_1}{\rightleftharpoons}} E\cdot B \overset{k_2}{\rightarrow} E-B \begin{array}{l} \overset{k_3}{\nearrow} E+P \\ \underset{k_3'}{\searrow} E+P \end{array} \qquad \text{Scheme III}$$

The above scheme differs from Scheme II in that it postulates no conformational changes. However, it is often difficult to dissect kinetic pathways into "synchronic" components. In the absence of strong evidence for different conformational states of the enzyme, one assumes that different products are formed by the same complex, E−B. Thus, the DD-carboxypeptidases from *B. stearothermophilus* and *Streptomyces* R 61 release penicillin wholly or in part as phenylacetylglycine and *N*-formyl-D-penicillamine, the other released product being penicilloic acid (HAMMARSTROM and STROMINGER 1975; FRERE et al. 1975b). In the case of the R 61 enzyme, available evidence favors Scheme II over Scheme III; that is, each of the two products is formed by a different enzyme conformer (Sect. E.I.2).

As already discussed in Sect. C, the enterobacterial carboxypeptidase IA (PBP 5/6) releases penicillin exclusively (i.e., within the limits of detection) as penicilloic acid. Possibly, carboxypeptidase 1B (PBP 4) also releases penicillin as penicilloic acid (SCHILF and MARTIN 1980).

The high molecular weight PBPs release bound penicillin as phenylacetylglycine (and *N*-formyl-D-penicillamine), at least in the cases of *S. aureus* and *B. subtilis* (WAXMAN and STROMINGER 1979).

β-Lactamases release penicillins and cephalosporins as penicilloic acids and cephalosporoic acids respectively, the latter being further degraded nonenzymatically depending on the nature of the C-3 substituent. Interestingly, penicillin sulfoxides are fragmented by *β*-lactamases via a mechanism similar to the degradation of penicillin to phenylacetylglycine by DD-carboxypeptidases (THOMAS 1979; and personal communication), emphasizing the similarity of the microenvironment at the active site in the two types of enzymes.

II. Streptomyces R 61 DD-Carboxypeptidase

The interaction of the R 61 enzyme with penicillin G involves formation of a covalent penicilloyl-enzyme complex which is subsequently hydrolyzed with a half-life of 80 min at 37 °C (FRERE et al. 1974 a) and 200 min at 30 °C (GEORGOPAPADAKOU et al. 1982).

The mechanism for the release of penicillin G can be outlined as follows:

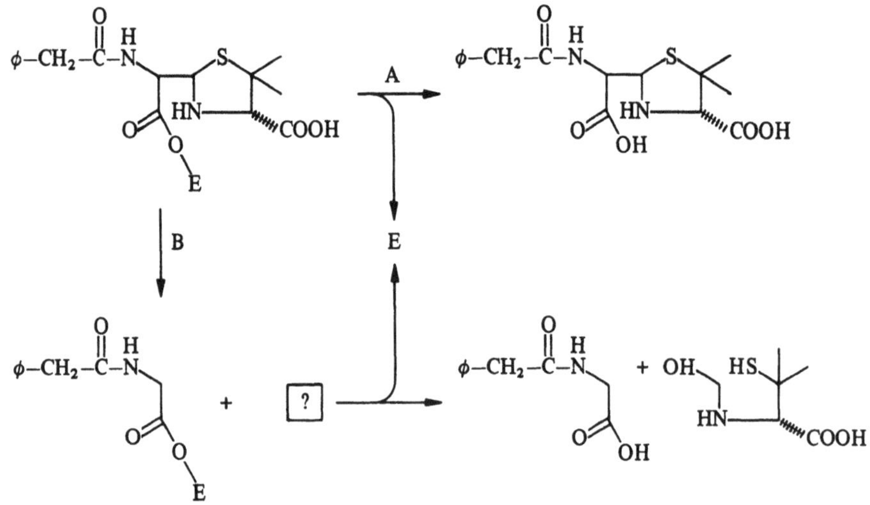

Partitioning of products between pathways A and B depends on the nature of the nucleophile acceptor. However, contrary to the *B. subtilis* enzyme, the sum of these products is independent of the nucleophilicity of the acceptor, suggesting either that the rate-determining step is other than the release of phenylacetylglycine or that the release involves conformational changes.

Penicillins such as carbenicillin, ampicillin, penicillin V (FRERE et al. 1974 a) and methylpenicillin (GEORGOPAPADAKOU et al. 1982) are released at rates similar to penicillin G. However, 6-APA, which lacks the side chain, is released an order of magnitude faster (GEORGOPAPADAKOU and LIU, unpublished work) suggesting that the side chain might be at least partially responsible for anchoring the *β*-lactam at the active site. Methoxylation at C-6 increases the rate of release by an order of magnitude, either by facilitating the secondary fragmentation or by preventing the interaction of the *β*-lactam side chain with the active site.

Cephalosporins are released by the R 61 enzyme probably without fragmentation (GHUYSEN et al. 1980). Contrary to penicillins, methoxylation at C-7 decreases the rate of release by at least two orders of magnitude (GEORGOPAPADAKOU and LIU, unpublished work), an effect similar to that observed with β-lactamases (FISHER et al. 1980).

III. β-Lactamases and β-Lactam Inhibitors

The ability of alkoxy- (e.g. methicillin) and isoxazolyl-(e.g. cloxacillin)penicillins to inhibit β-lactamases has been already discussed in the context of induction and classification of β-lactamases (Sect. D). These compounds are competitive inhibitors of some β-lactamases and act synergistically in vivo with β-lactamase-susceptible β-lactam antibiotics. However, they are of rather limited clinical use.

Since the middle 1970s, several β-lactam compounds have been reported which irreversibly inhibit β-lactamases. These are the naturally occurring clavulanic acid and carbapenems and the (semi-)synthetic penicillanic acid sulfones and halopenicillanic acids. With the exception of carbapenems, the compounds are by themselves poor antibiotics but act synergistically when combined with β-lactamase-susceptible β-lactams.

1. Clavulanic Acid

The interaction of clavulanic acid with β-lactamase has been studied in three different enzyme systems: the *E. coli* R-TEM enzyme (CHARNAS et al. 1978; FISHER et al. 1978; LABIA and PEDUZZI 1978) the *S. aureus* PCl enzyme (READING and HEPBURN 1979; CARTWRIGHT and COULSON 1979), and the *B. cereus* I enzyme (DURKIN and VISWANANTHA 1978). All three enzymes are inhibited progressively, but the rate and extent of inhibition is different with each enzyme. Substrates afford some protection against inactivation, suggesting that clavulanic acid binds at the active site.

The mechanism of inactivation has been studied most extensively with *E. coli* R-TEM β-lactamase. Incubation of this enzyme with clavulanic acid results in (a) destruction (turnover) of clavulanic acid; (b) formation of a catalytically inactive *transient* clavulanate-enzyme complex; (c) formation of a catalytically inactive *stable* clavulanate-enzyme complex. The transient complex is formed at a faster rate than the irreversibly-inactivated complex, but it decomposes to free enzyme and thus eventually all of the enzyme accumulates into the irreversibly inactivated form (FISHER et al. 1978). Isoelectric focusing of the irreversibly-inhibited enzyme shows three protein bands in addition to that corresponding to the inactive enzyme. Hydroxylamine treatment restores one-third of the catalytic activity and abolishes one of the extra protein bands (CHARNAS et al. 1978). It is possible that the band affected by hydroxylamine is a covalent clavulanate-enzyme complex involving an ester linkage with a serine residue on the enzyme. It is also possible that the other two bands represent clavulanate-enzyme complexes involving bonds resistant to hydroxylaminolysis, although it might be that they are susceptible but inaccessible to hydroxylamine.

The interaction of the R-TEM enzyme with clavulanic acid can be summarized as follows (Charnas et al. 1978):

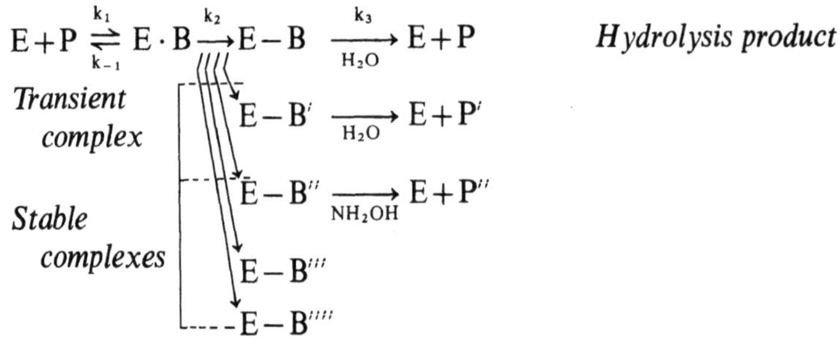

The above scheme is a variation of the general Scheme III of Sect. E.I.4.

Both transient and stable complexes show an increase in absorbance at 281 nm, which has been attributed to a secondary cleavage of the oxazolidine ring producing a β-aminoacrylate structure:

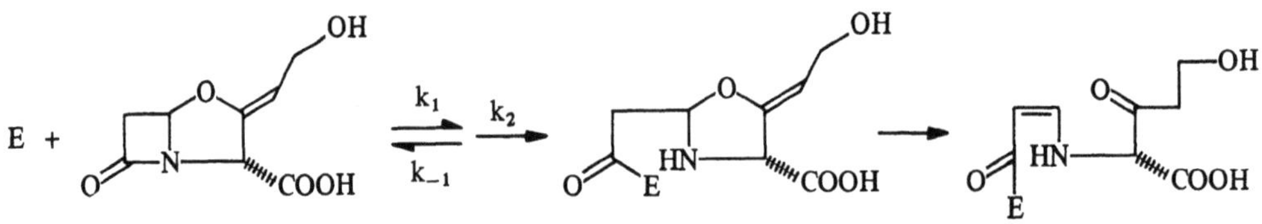

This species may subsequently react with additional groups on the enzyme resulting in different forms of inactivated enzyme revealed by isoelectric focusing (Charnas et al. 1978).

2. Penicillin Sulfones

The first such compound to be reported, as a β-lactamase inhibitor exhibiting synergy with susceptible β-lactams in a variety of bacteria, was 6-desaminopenicillanic acid sulfone (CP 45899) (*14*) (English et al. 1978). Similar to clavulanic acid, it lacks an acylamine side chain and has a weak C-5-to-sulfur bond which, like the C-5-to-oxygen bond in clavulanic acid, is the driving force for the fragmentation occurring after formation of the acyl intermediate with β-lactamases (Fisher and Knowles 1980).

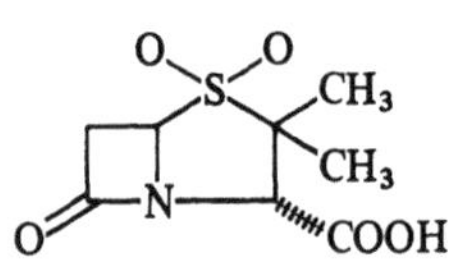

(*14*)

The mechanism of inactivation of β-lactamases by penicillin sulfones has been studied mainly with the *E. coli* R-TEM enzyme. Inactivation of this enzyme by CP 45899 results in an increase in absorbance at 280 nm, suggesting formation of a chromophore similar to that observed during inactivation by clavulanic acid. Hydroxylamine treatment partially reactivates the enzyme (by about 25%) and eliminates the chromophore (FISHER and KNOWLES 1980). A mechanistic scheme similar to that suggested for clavulanic acid has been also suggested for CP 45 899. Studies with other penicillanic acid sulfones have suggested potency to be a function of the half-life of the acyl enzyme intermediate, sulfones derived from poor substrates such as methicillin and quinacillin being more potent inactivators than those derived from good substrates such as penicillin V. Interestingly, hydroxylamine treatment does not restore any enzymatic activity after inactivation by quinacillin suggesting possible steric hindrance by the side-chain.

3. Halopenicillanic Acids

6β-Bromopenicillanic acid (*15*) is a potent inhibitor of the *B. cereus* β-lactamase I (but not β-lactamase II) and the β-lactamases from *E. coli* (R-TEM), *B. licheniformis*, and *S. aureus* (PRATT and LOOSEMORE 1978). Inhibition was shown to be progressive and irreversible with the *B. cereus* I enzyme and the *E. coli* (R-TEM) enzyme.

In studies with 6β-bromopenicillanic acid and *B. cereus* β-lactamase, the presence of benzylpenicillin significantly slowed the rate of enzyme inactivation, suggesting that the inhibitor binds at or near the enzyme active site (PRATT and LOOSEMORE 1978). As stated elsewhere (Sect. E.I.3) bromopenicillanic acid binds to a serine residue at the active site.

The inhibitory activities of 6β-bromopenicillanic acid and its iodo analog against the enzymes from *S. aureus* and *E. coli* (R-TEM) compare favorably with that of clavulanic acid, whereas the 6β-bromopenicillanic acid is less active (VON DAEHNE 1980). Predictably, 6-halopenicillin sulfones are more potent β-lactamase inhibitors than the parent penicillin sulfones (CARTWRIGHT and COULSON 1979).

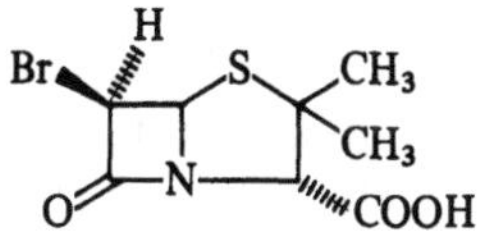

(*15*)

4. Carbapenems

a) Olivanic Acids

Olivanic acids, in addition to being broad-spectrum antibiotics, strongly inhibit β-lactamases from various bacteria. MM 4550 (*16*) is particularly active against penicillinases while MM 13902 (*17*) and MM 17880 (*18*) are particularly active against cephalosporinases such as that from *E. cloacae* (HOOD et al. 1979). With *E. coli* B 11 β-lactamase inhibition was found to be progressive and irreversible (BUTTERWORTH et al. 1979).

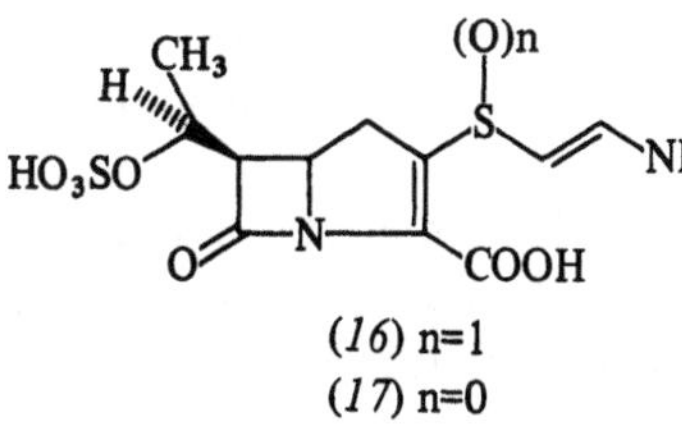

(*16*) n=1
(*17*) n=0

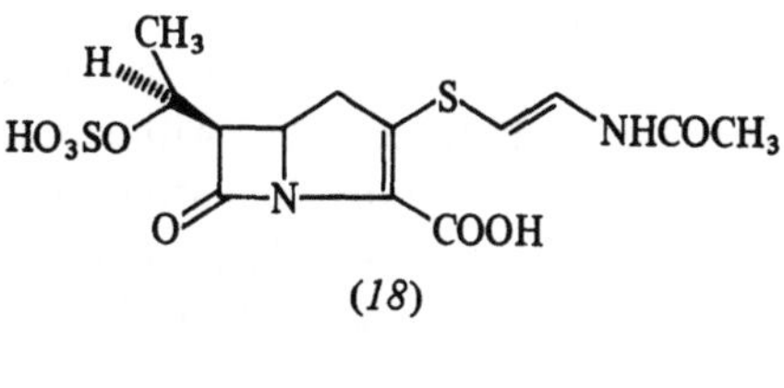

(*18*)

b) PS-5

The antibiotic PS-5 (*19*) is a potent inhibitor of several β-lactamases (OKAMURA et al. 1978). The compound is resistant to hydrolysis whereas it is susceptible to β-lactamases of *B. cereus*, *Proteus vulgaris*, *Citrobacter freundii* and *Streptomyces* species (FUKAGAWA et al. 1980a, b). Recent studies have shown the *B. licheniformis* β-lactamase to be inactivated by PS-5 according to first-order kinetics (FUKAGAWA et al. 1980a, b).

With the exception of the *B. licheniformis* enzyme, PS-5 behaves like clavulanic acid in that hydrolysis of the compound by β-lactamases is slow and the enzymes are simultaneously inactivated (FUKAGAWA et al. 1980a, b).

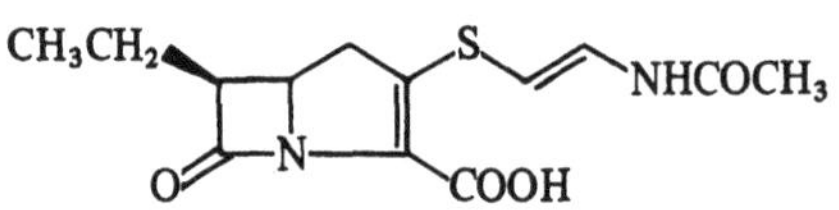

(*19*)

F. Concluding Remarks

Relying heavily on detailed studies of only a few β-lactamases and DD-carboxypeptidases we have attempted in this review to discuss the interaction of bacterial enzymes with β-lactam antibiotics and some of the properties of these enzymes. We strove to be comprehensible rather than comprehensive; excellent up-to-date reviews on specific topics exist and we have referred to them in the appropriate sections.

The single most important concept in the mode of action of β-lactam antibiotics is the TIPPER and STROMINGER (1965) hypothesis. It states that penicillin and other β-lactam antibiotics are steric analogs of the natural substrate for peptidoglycan transpeptidase(s) and their interaction with this (these) enzyme(s) parallels that of the substrate. Not surprisingly, β-lactam resistance arising from substantial changes in the target enzymes is relatively rare and occurs stepwise. Possibly, the steric similarity of β-lactams to the substrate makes decreased antibiotic affinity of the target enzyme(s) with full retention of catalytic activity toward substrate an unlikely event.

Studies with penicillin-sensitive enzymes have concentrated on DD-carboxypeptidases. These enzymes are plausible models for the interaction of penicillin with its targets but are seldom themselves the targets of penicillin action. They may be evolutionary precursors of β-lactamases as evidence for extensive homology between the two types of enzymes would suggest. In addition, most DD-carboxypeptidases possess weak penicillinase activity. The fact that peptidase activity has never been observed with β-lactamases may be due simply to limitations in detection of such activity. It is noted that membrane-bound DD-carboxypeptidases have generally low turnover numbers for the substrate. The DD-carboxypeptidase from *S. aureus* is an attractive candidate linking DD-carboxypeptidase and β-lactamases. It possesses both activities with similar V_{max}.

The effect of individual structural components of β-lactam antibiotics on the interaction with bacterial enzymes may lead to a better understanding of the nature of the interaction and to the rational design of effective inhibitors with high specificity. Such an approach has already lead to the synthesis of penicillin sulfones which inhibit β-lactamases (Sect. E.III.2). However, the different substrate profiles of various β-lactamases would argue against the feasibility of a universal β-lactamase inhibitor. Similarly, the fact that PBPs and penicillin targets are different in different bacteria would also argue against the feasibility of a universal β-lactam antibiotic.

Acknowledgments. We thank M. A. Ondetti and J. L. Strominger for their interest and encouragement during some of the studies described and J. Baumann and S. Krupa for typing the manuscript.

References

Abraham EP, Chain E (1940) An enzyme from bacteria able to destroy penicillin. Nature 146:837

Albers-Schönberg G, Arison BH, Hensens OD, Hirshfield J, Hoogsten K, Kaczka EA, Rhodes RE, Kahan JS, Kahan FM, Ratcliffe RW, Walton E, Ruswinkel LJ, Morin RB, Christensen BG (1978) Structure and absolute configuration of thienamycin. J Am Chem Soc 100:6491–6499

Ambler RP (1975) The amino acid sequence of *Staphylococcus aureus* penicillinase. Biochem J 151:197–218

Ambler RP, Meadway R (1969) Chemical nature of bacterial penicillinase. Nature 222:24–26

Ambler RP, Scott GK (1978) Partial amino acid sequence of penicillinase coded by *Escherichia coli* plasmid R6K. Proc Natl Acad Sci USA 75:3732–3736

Anderson ES, Datta N (1965) Resistance to penicillins and its transfer in *Enterobacteriaceae*. Lancet i:407–409

Anderson JS, Meadow PM, Haskin MA, Strominger JL (1966) Biosynthesis of the peptidoglycan of bacterial cell walls. I. Utilization of uridine diphosphate acetylmuramyl pentapeptide and uridine diphosphate acetylglucosamine for peptidoglycan synthesis by particulate enzymes from *Staphylococcus aureus* and *Micrococcus lysodeikticus*. Arch Biochem Biophys 116:487–515

Aoki H, Sakai H, Kohsaka M, Konomi T, Hosoda J, Kubochi Y, Iguchi R, Imanaka H (1976) Nocardicin A, a new monocyclic β-lactam antibiotic. I. Discovery, isolation and characterization. J Antibiot (Tokyo) 29:492–500

Appelbaum PC, Chatterton SA (1978) Susceptibility of anaerobic bacteria to ten antimicrobial agents. Antimicrob Agents Chemother 14:371–376

Beck BD, Park JT (1976) Activity of three murein hydrolases during the cell division cycle of *Escherichia coli* K-12 as measured in toluene-treated cells. J Bacteriol 126:1250–1260

Blobel G, Dobberstein B (1975) Transfer of proteins across membranes. I. Presence of proteolytically processed and unprocessed nascent immunologlobulin light chains on membrane-bound ribosomes of murine myeloma. J Cell Biol 67:835–851

Blumberg PM, Strominger JL (1972a) Five penicillin-binding components occur in *Bacillus subtilis* membranes. J Biol Chem 247:8107–8113

Blumberg PM, Strominger JL (1972b) Isolation by affinity chromatography of the penicillin-binding components from membranes of *Bacillus subtilis*. Proc Natl Acad Sci USA 69:3751–3755

Blumberg PM, Strominger JL (1974) Interaction of penicillin with the bacterial cell: penicillin binding proteins and penicillin-sensitive enzymes. Bacteriol Rev 38:291–335

Blumberg PM, Yocum RR, Willoughby E, Strominger JL (1974) Binding of [^{14}C] penicillin G to the membrane-bound and purified D-alanine carboxypeptidases from *Bacillus stearothermophilus* and *Bacillus subtilis* and its release. J Biol Chem 249:6828–6835

Bobrowski MM, Matthew M, Barth PT, Datta N, Glinter NJ, Jacob AE, Kontomichalou P, Dale JW, Smith JT (1976) A plasmid-determined β-lactamase indistinguishable from the chromosomal β-lactamase of *E. coli*. J Bacteriol 125:149–159

Bonner WM, Laskey RA (1974) A film detection method for tritium labelled proteins and nucleic acids in polyacrylamide gels. Eur J Biochem 46:83–88
Boyd DB (1977) Transition state structures of a dipeptide related to the mode of action of β-lactam antibiotics. Proc Natl Acad Sci USA 74:5239–5243
Braun V, Rehn K (1969) Chemical characterization, spatial distribution, and function of a lipoprotein (murein-lipoprotein) of the *Escherichia coli* cell wall. The specific effect of trypsin on membrane structure. Eur J Biochem 10:426–438
Braun V, Bosch V, Hantke K, Schaller K (1974) Structure and biosynthesis of functionally defined areas of the *Escherichia coli* outer membrane. Ann NY Acad Sci 235:66–82
Bristow AF, Virden R (1978) Preferential nitration with tetranitromethane of a specific tyrosine residue in penicillinase from *Staphylococcus aureus* PCl. Biochem J 169:381–388
Britz ML, Wilkinson RG (1978) Purification and properties of β-lactamase from *Bacteroides fragilis*. Antimicrob Agents Chemother 13:373–382
Broad DF, Smith JT (1979) Release of enzymes from bacteria. J Pharm Pharmacol [Suppl] 31:30P
Brown AG, Corbett DF, Englington AJ, Howarth TT (1977) Structures of olivanic acid derivatives MM4550 and MM12902; two new fused β-lactams isolated from *Streptomyces olivaceus*. J Chem Soc Chem Common 1977:523–525
Bryan LE, Shahrabadi MS, VanDenElzen HM (1974) Gentamicin resistance in *Pseudomonas aeruginosa:* R-factor-mediated resistance. Antimicrob Agents Chemother 6:191–199
Buchanan CE, Strominger JL (1976) Altered penicillin-binding components in penicillin-resistant mutants of *Bacillus subtilis*. Proc Natl Acad Sci USA 73:1816–1820
Burman LG, Nordström K, Boman HK (1968) Resistance of *Escherichia coli* to penicillins. V. Physiological comparison of two isogenic strains, one with chromosomally and one with episomally mediated ampicillin resistance. J Bacteriol 96:438–446
Bush K, Bonner DP, Sykes RB (1980) Izumenolide – a novel β-lactamase inhibitor produced by *Micromonospora* II Biological Studies. J Antibiot (Tokyo) 33:1262–1269
Butterworth D, Cole M, Hanscomb G, Rolinson GN (1979) Olivanic acids, a family of beta-lactam antibiotics with beta-lactamase inhibitory properties produced by *Streptomyces* species. 1. Detection, properties and fermentation studies. J Antibiot (Tokyo) 32:287–294
Carpenter CV, Goyer S, Neuhaus FC (1976) Steric effects on penicillin-sensitive peptidoglycan synthesis in membrane-wall system for *Gaffkya homari*. Biochemistry 15:3146–3152
Cartwright SJ, Coulson AFW (1979) Semisynthetic penicillinase inactivator. Nature 278:360–361
Catlin W (1975) Iodometric detection of *Haemophilus influenza* β-lactamase: rapid presumptive test for ampicillin resistance. Antimicrob Agents Chemother 7:265–270
Charnas RL, Fisher J, Knowles JR (1978) Chemical studies on the inactivation of *Escherichia coli* R-TEM β-lactamase by clavulanic acid. Biochemistry 17:2185–2189
Chase HA (1980) Purification of four penicillin-binding proteins from *Bacillus megaterium*. J Gen Microbiol 117:211–224
Chase HA, Shepherd ST, Reynolds PE (1977) Studies on the penicillin-binding components of *Bacillus megaterium*. FEBS Lett 76:199–203
Chase HA, Reynolds PE, Ward JB (1978) Purification and characterization of the penicillin-binding protein that is the lethal target of penicillin in *Bacillus megaterium* and *Bacillus licheniformis*. Eur J Biochem 88:275–285
Citri N, Pollock MR (1966) The biochemistry and function of beta-lactamase (penicillinase). Adv Enzymol 28:237–323
Citri N, Samuni A, Zyk N (1976) Acquisition of substrate-specific parameters during the catalytic reaction of pennicillinase. Proc Natl Acad Sci USA 73:1048–1052
Citri N, Zyk N (1965) The interaction of penicillinase with penicillins. IV: Structural aspects of catalytic and non-catalytic interactions. Biochim Biophys Acta 99:427–441
Cocks GT, Wilson AC (1972) Enzyme evolution in *Enterobacteriaceae*. J Bacteriol 110:793–802

Cole M (1969a) Hydrolysis of penicillins and related compounds by the cell-bound penicillin acylase of *Escherichia coli*. Biochem J 115:733–739
Cole M (1969b) Deacylation of acylamino compounds other than penicillins by the cell-bound penicillin acylase of *Escherichia coli*. Biochem J 115:741–745
Cole M, Savidge T, Vanderhaeghe H (1975) Penicillin acylase (assay). Methods Enzymol 25:698–705
Coley J, Tarelli E, Archibald AR, Baddiley J (1978) The linkage between teichoic acid and peptidoglycan in bacterial cells. FEBS Lett 88:1–9
Cornelis G, Abraham EP (1975) β-Lactamases from *Yersinia enterocolitica*. J Gen Microbiol 87:273–284
Costerton JW, Cheng KJ (1975) The role of the bacterial cell envelope in antibiotic resistance. J Antimicrob Chemother 1:363–377
Couillard M, Letarte R, Pechere JC, Morin C (1979) Need of a combination of methods for identifying beta-lactamases: the case of *Enterobacter*. 19th Intersci Conf Antimicrob Agents Chemother, Oct 1–5, 1979, Abstract 31. Am Soc Microbiol, Washington DC
Coyette J, Ghuysen JM, Binot F, Adriaens P, Meeschaert B, Vanderhaege H (1977) Interactions between β-lactam antibiotics and isolated membranes of *Streptococcus faecalis* ATCC 9790. Eur J Biochem 75:231–239
Coyette J, Ghuysen J-M, Fontana R (1978) Solubilization and isolation of the membrane-bound DD-carboxypeptidase of *Streptococcus faecalis* ATCC 9790. Eur J Biochem 88:297–305
Coyette J, Ghuysen J-M, Fontana R (1980) The penicillin-binding proteins in *Streptococcus faecalis* ATCC 9790. Eur J Biochem 110:445–456
Crane LJ, Bettinger GE, Lampen JO (1973) Affinity chromatography purification of penicillinase of *Bacillus licheniformis* 749/C and its use to measure turnover of the cell-bound enzyme. Biochem Biophys Res Commun 50:220–227
Curtis NAC, Orr D, Ross GW, Boulton MG (1979a) Competition of β-lactam antibiotics for the penicillin-binding proteins of *Pseudomonas aeruginosa*, *Enterobacter cloacae*, *Klebsiella aerogenes*, *Proteus rettgeri*, and *Escherichia coli*: comparison with antibacterial activity and effects upon bacterial morphology. Antimicrob Agents Chemother 16:325–328
Curtis NAC, Ross GW, Boulton MG (1979b) Effect of 7-α methoxy substitution of cephalosporins upon their affinity for the penicillin-binding proteins of *E. coli* K12: comparison with antibacterial activity and inhibition of membrane-bound model transpeptidase activity. J Antimicrob Chemother 5:391–398
Curtis NAC, Boulton MG, Orr D, Ross GW (1980) The competition of α-sulfocephalosporins for the penicillin-binding proteins of *Escherichia coli* K12 and *Pseudomonas aeruginosa* – comparison with effects upon morphology. J Antimicrob Chemother 6:189–196
Curtis SJ, Strominger JL (1978) Effects of sulfhydryl reagents on the binding and release of penicillin G by D-alanine carboxypeptidase 1A of *Escherichia coli*. J Biol Chem 253:2584–2588
Dale JW (1971) Characterization of the β-lactamase specified by the resistance factor R-1818 in *E. coli* K-12 and other gram-negative bacteria. Biochem J 123:501–508
Dale JW (1975) An inducible β-lactamase in a strain of *Escherichia coli*. Antonie van Leeuwenhoek 41:59–68
Dale JW, Smith JT (1971) The purification and properties of the β-lactamase specified by the resistance factor R-1818 in *Escherichia coli* and *Proteus mirabilis*. Biochem J 123:493–500
Dale JW, Smith JT (1974) R-factor-mediated β-lactamases that hydrolyze oxacillin: evidence for two distinct groups. J Bacteriol 119:351–356
Dale JW, Smith JT (1976) The dimeric nature of an R-factor mediated β-lactamase. Biochem Biophys Res Commun 68:1000–1005
Daneo-Moore L, Coyette J, Sayare M, Boothby D, Schockman GD (1975) Turnover of the cell wall peptidoglycan of *Lactobacillus acidophilus*. The presence of a fraction immune to turnover. J Biol Chem 250:1348–1353

Darland G, Birnbaum J (1977) Cefoxitin resistance to β-lactamase: a major factor for susceptibility to *Bacteroides fragilis* to the antibiotic. Anitmicrob Agents Chemother 11:725–734
Datta N, Kontomichalou P (1965) Penicillinase synthesis controlled by infectious R-factors in *Enterobacteriaceae*. Nature 208:239–241
Datta N, Richmond MH (1966) The purification and properties of a penicillinase whose synthesis is mediated by an R-factor in *Escherichia coli*. Biochem J 98:204–209
Davies RB, Abraham EP (1974) Metal cofactor requirements of β-lactamase II. Biochem J 143:129–135
Davies RB, Abraham EP, Melling J (1974a) Separation, purification and properties of β-lactamase I and β-lactamase II from *Bacillus cereus* 569/H/9. Biochem J 143:115–127
Davies RB, Abraham EP, Dalgleish DG (1974b) Conformational changes in the extracellular β-lactamase I from *Bacillus cereus* 569/H/9. Biochem J 143:137–141
Davies RB, Abraham EP, Fleming J, Pollock MR (1975) Comparison of β-lactamase II from *Bacillus cereus* 569/H/9 with a β-lactamase from *Bacillus cereus* 5/B/6. Biochem J 145:409–411
Davis RH, Linder R, Salton MRJ (1978) Solubilization and characterization of the partially purified penicillin sensitive D-alanine carboxypeptidase of *Neisseria gonorrhoeae*. Microbios 21:69–80
DeBell RM, Hickey TM, Uddin DE (1978) Partial characterization of a beta-lactamase from *Vibrio parahaemolyticus* by a new automated microiodometric technique. Antimicrob Agents Chemother 13:165–169
DelBene VE, Farra E, Weinrich EA, Brunson JW, Rubens CE (1979) β-lactamase, β-lactam resistance, and extrachromosomal DNA in anaerobic bacteria. In: S. Mitsuhashi (ed) Microbial drug resistance. University Park Press, Baltimore, p 301
Durkin J-P, Viswanantha T (1978) Clavulanic acid inhibition of beta-lactamase I from *Bacillus cereus* 569/HH. J Antibiot (Tokyo) 31:1162–1169
Durkin J-P, Dimitrenko GI, Viswanantha T (1977) Reversibility of ampicillin-induced and nitrite-induced inactivation of beta-lactamase 1. Can J Biochem 55:453–457
Dyke KGH (1979) β-Lactamases of *Staphylococcus aureus*. In: Hamilton-Miller JMT, Smith JT (eds) Beta-lactamases. Academic Press, London New York, pp 291–310
English AR, Retsema JA, Girard AE, Lynch JE, Barth WE (1978) CP-45,889, a beta-lactamase inhibitor that extends the antibacterial spectrum of beta lactams: initial bacteriological characterization. Antimicrob Agents Chemother 14:414–419
Farrar EW, Krause JM (1970) Relationship between β-lactamase activity and resistance of enterobacter to cephalothin. Infect Immunol 2:610–616
Farrar EW, Newsome JK (1973) Mechanism of synergistic effects of β-lactam antibiotic combinations on gram-negative bacilli. Antimicrob Agents Chemother 4:109–114
Fein JE, Rogers HJ (1976) Autolytic enzyme-deficient mutants of *Bacillus subtilis* 168. J Bacteriol 127:1427–1442
Finegold SM, Sutter VL (1972) Antimicrobial susceptibility of anaerobic gram-negative bacilli. In: MacPhee T (ed) Host resistance to commensal bacteria. Churchill Livingston, Edinburgh, p 275
Fisher JF, Knowles JR (1980) The inactivation of β-lactamase by mechanism-based reagents. In: Sandler M (ed) Enzyme inhibitors as drugs. MacMillan, London, pp 209–218
Fisher J, Charnas RL, Knowles JR (1978) Kinetic studies on the inactivation of *Escherichia coli* R-TEM β-lactamase by clavulanic acid. Biochemistry 17:2180–2184
Fisher J, Belasco JG, Khosla S, Knowles JR (1980) β-Lactamase proceeds via an acyl intermediate. Interaction of the *Escherichia coli* R-TEM enzyme with cefoxitin. Biochemistry 19:2895–2901
Fleming PC, Goldner M, Glass DG (1963) Observations on the nature, distribution and significance of cephalosporinase. Lancet i:1399–1401
Fox GE, Stackebrandt E, Hespell RB (1980) The phylogeny of prokaryotes. Science 209:457–463
Frere JM, Ghuysen J-M, Perkins HR, Nieto M (1973a) Molecular weight and amino acid composition of the exocellular DD-carboxypeptidase-transpeptidase of *Streptomyces* R61. Biochem J 135:463–468

Frere JM, Ghuysen J-M, Perkins HR, Nieto M (1973 b) Kinetics of concomitant transfer and hydrolysis reactions catalyzed by the exocellular DD-carboxypeptidase-transpeptidase of *Streptomyces* R61. Biochem J 135:483–492

Frere JM, Leyh-Bouille M, Ghuysen J-M, Perkins HR (1974 a) Interaction between β-lactam antibiotics and exocellular DD-carboxypeptidase-transpeptidase of *Streptomyces* R61. Eur J Biochem 50:203–214

Frere JM, Moreno R, Ghuysen J-M, Perkins RH, Dierickx L, Delcambe L (1974 b) Molecular weight, amino acid composition and physiochemical properties of the exocellular DD-carboxypeptidase of *Streptomyces* R39. Biochem J 143:233–240

Frere JM, Ghuysen J-M, Degelaen J, Loffet A, Perkins HR (1975 a) Fragmentation of benzylpenicillin after interaction with exocellular DD-carboxypeptidase-transpeptidase of *Streptomyces* R61 and R39. Nature 258:168–170

Frere JM, Ghuysen J-M, Iwatsubo M (1975 b) Kinetics of interaction between exocellular DD-carboxypeptidase-transpeptidase from *Streptomyces* R61 and β-lactam antibiotics. A choice of models. Eur J Biochem 57:343–351

Frere JM, Duez C, Ghuysen J-M, Vanderkerkhove J (1976) Occurrence of a serine residue in the penicillin-binding site of the exocellular DD-carboxypeptidase-transpeptidase from *Streptomyces* R61. FEBS Lett 70:257–260

Frere JM, Geurts F, Ghuysen J-M (1978) The exocellular DD-carboxypeptidase-endopeptidase of *Streptomyces albus* G. Interaction with β-lactam antibiotics. Biochem J 175:801–805

Fruton JS (1971) Pepsin. In: Boyer PD (ed) Hydrolysis: peptide bonds, the enzymes, 3rd edn, vol III. Academic Press, New York, p 157

Fuad N, Frere JM, Ghuysen JM, Duez C, Iwatsubo M (1976) Mode of interaction between β-lactam antibiotics and the exocellular DD-carboxypeptidase-transpeptidase from *Streptomyces* R39. Biochem J 155:623–629

Fujii-Kuriyama Y, Yamamoto M, Sugawara S (1977) Purification and properties of β-lactamase from *Proteus morganii.* J Bacteriol 131:726–734

Fukagawa Y, Kubo K, Ishikura T, Kouno K (1980 a) Deacylation of PS-5, a new β-lactam compound. 1. Microbial deacylation of PS-5. J Antibiot (Tokyo) 33:343–348

Fukagawa Y, Takei T, Ishikura T (1980 b) Inhibition of β-lactamase of *Bacillus licheniformis* 749/C by compound PS-5, a new β-lactam antibiotic. Biochem J 185:177–188

Fung J, MacAlister TJ, Rothfield LI (1978) Role of murein lipoprotein in morphogenesis of the bacterial division septum: phenotypic similarity of lky D and lpo mutants. J Bacteriol 133:1467–1471

Furth A (1975) Purification and properties of a constitutive β-lactamase from *Pseudomonas aeruginosa* strain Dalgleish. Biochim Biophys Acta 377:431–443

Garber N, Friedman J (1970) β-Lactamase and the resistance of *Pseudomonas aeruginosa* to various penicillins and cephalosporins. J Gen Microbiol 64:343–352

Georgopapadakou NH, Liu FY (1980 a) Penicillin-binding proteins in bacteria. Antimicrob Agents Chemother 18:148–157

Georgopapadakou NH, Liu FY (1980 b) Binding of β-lactam antibiotics to penicillin-binding proteins of *Staphylococcus aureus* and *Streptococcus faecalis* – relation to antibacterial activity. Antimicrob Agents Chemother 18:834–836

Georgopapadakou NH, Hammarstrom S, Strominger JL (1977) Isolation of the penicillin-binding peptide from D-alanine carboxypeptidase of *Bacillus subtilis*. Proc Natl Acad Sci USA 74:1009–1012

Georgopapadakou NH, Liu FY, Ondetti MA (1979) Comparison of D and L isomers in 7-substituted cephalosporins. 19th Intersci Conf Antimicrob Agents Chemother, Oct 1–5, 1979, Abstract 567. Am Soc Microbiol, Washington DC

Georgopapadakou NH, Liu FY, Ryono DE, Neubeck R, Ondetti MA (1981 a) Chemical modifications of *Streptomyces* R61 DD-carboxypeptidase active site. Eur J Biochem 115:53–57

Georgopapadakou NH, Liu FY, Ryono DE, Neubeck R, Gordon EM, Pluscec J, Szabo E, Ondetti MA (1981 b) A simple and sensitive assay for DD-carboxypeptidase. Manuscript in preparation

Georgopapadakou NH, Smith SA, Cimarusti CM (1982) Interaction between monobactams and *Streptomyces* R61 DD-carboxypeptidase. Eur J Biochem 124:507–512
Ghuysen J-M (1977) The bacterial DD-carboxypeptidase-transpeptidase enzyme system. A new insight into the mode of action of penicillin. In: Brown WE (ed) E R Squibb lectures on chemistry of microbial products. University of Tokyo Press, Tokyo
Ghuysen J-M, Shockman GD (1973) Biosynthesis of peptidoglycan. In: Leive L (ed) Bacterial membranes and walls. Dekker, New York, pp 37–117
Ghuysen J-M, Frere JM, Bouille M, Coyette J, Dusart J, Nguyen-Disteche M (1979) Use of model enzymes in the determination of the mode of action of penicillins and Δ^3-cephalosporins. Annu Rev Biochem 48:73–101
Ghuysen J-M, Frere JM, Leyh-Bouille M (1980) Mechanistic properties and functioning of DD-carboxypeptidases. In: Mitsuhashi S (ed) β-lactam antibiotics, vol 3. Japan Sci Soc, Tokyo
Giles AF, Reynolds PE (1979) *Bacillus megaterium* resistance accompanied by a compensatory change in penicillin-binding proteins. Nature 28:167–168
Glaser L, Lindsay B (1977) Relation between cell-wall turnover and cell growth in *Bacillus subtilis*. J Bacteriol 13:610–619
Goddell EW, Schwarz U (1977) Enzymes synthesizing and hydrolyzing murein in *Escherichia coli*. Eur J Biochem 81:205–210
Gorecki M, Bar-Eli A, Burstein Y, Patchornik A, Chain EB (1975) Purification of D-alanine carboxypeptidase from *Escherichia coli* B on a penicillin-Sepharose column. Biochem J 147:131–137
Grimont PA, Grimont F (1978) The genus *Serratia*. Annu Rev Microbiol 32:221–248
Hackenbeck R, Tarpay M, Tomasz A (1980) Multiple changes of penicillin-binding proteins in penicillin-resistant clinical isolates of *Streptococcus pneumoniae*. Antimicrob Agents Chemother 17:364–371
Hamilton-Miller JMT, Smith JT, Knox R (1965) Interaction of cephaloridine with penicillinase-producing gram-negative bacteria. Nature 208:235–237
Hammarstrom S, Strominger JL (1975) Degradation of penicillin G to phenylacetylglycine by D-alanine carboxypeptidase from *Bacillus stearothermophilus*. Proc Natl Acad Sci USA 72:3463–3467
Hammes WP, Kandler O (1976) Biosynthesis of peptidoglycan in *Gaffkya homari*. The incorporation of peptidoglycan into cell wall and the direction of transpeptidation. Eur J Biochem 70:97–106
Harmon SA, Baldwin JN (1964) Nature of the determinant controlling penicillinase production in *Staphylococcus aureus*. J Bacteriol 87:593–597
Hedges RW, Jacob AE (1974) Transposition of ampicillin resistance from RP4 to other replicons. Mol Gen Genet 132:31–40
Hedges RW, Matthew M (1979) Acquisition by *Escherichia coli* of plasmid-borne β-lactamases normally confined to *Pseudomonas* spp. Plasmid 2:169–178
Hedges RW, Datta N, Kontomichalou P, Smith JT (1974) Molecular specificities of R-factor determined beta-lactamases: correlation with plasmid compatibility. J Bacteriol 117:56–62
Hennessey TD (1967) Inducible β-lactamase in *Enterobacter*. J Gen Microbiol 49:277–285
Ho PPK, Towner RD, Indelicato JM, Spitzer WA, Koppel GA (1972) Biochemical and microbiological studies on 6-substituted penicillins. J Antibiot (Tokyo) 25:627–628
Ho PPK, Towner RD, Indelicato JM, Wilham WJ, Spitzer AW, Koppel GA (1973) Biochemical and microbiological studies on 7-methoxy-cephalosporins. J Antibiot (Tokyo) 26:313–314
Hood JD, Box SJ, Verrall MS (1979) Olivanic acids, a family of beta-lactam antibiotics with beta-lactamase inhibitory properties produced by *Streptomyces* species. 2. Isolation and characterization of the olivanic acids MM-4550, MM-13902 and MM-17880 from *Streptomyces olivaceus*. J Antibiot (Tokyo) 32:295–304
Horikawa S, Ogawara H (1980) Penicillin-binding proteins in *Bacillus subtilis*. The effects on penicillin-binding proteins and the antibacterial activities of β-lactams. J Antibiot (Tokyo) 33:614–619
Howarth TT, Brown AG, King TJ (1976) Clavulanic acid, a novel β-lactam isolated from *Streptomyces clavuligerus*. J Chem Soc Chem Commun 1976:266–267

Imsande JJ (1970) Regulation of penicillinase synthesis: evidence for a unified model. J Bacteriol 101:173–180

Izaki K, Matsuhashi M, Strominger JL (1968) Biosynthesis of the peptidoglycan of bacterial cell walls. XIII. Peptidoglycan transpeptidase and D-alanine carboxypeptidase: penicillin sensitive enzymatic reaction in strains of *Escherichia coli*. J Biol Chem 243:3180–3292

Izui K, Nielsen JBK, Caulfield MP, Lampen JO (1980) Large exopenicillinase, initial extracellular form detected in cultures of *Bacillus licheniformis*. Biochemistry 19:1882–1886

Jacoby GA, Matthew M (1979) The distribution of β-lactamases on *Pseudomonas* plasmids. Plasmid 2:41–47

Jannson JAT (1965) A direct spectrophotometric assay for penicillin β-lactamase (penicillinase). Biochim Biophys Acta 99:171–172

Johnson K, Dusart J, Campbell JN, Ghuysen J-M (1973) Exocellular β-lactamases of *Streptomyces albus* G and strains R39 and K11. Antimicrob Agents Chemother 3:289–298

Jones RM, Fuchs PC (1976) Identification and antimicrobial susceptibility of 250 *Bacteroides fragilis* subspecies tested by broth micro dilution method. Antimicrob Agents Chemother 9:719–721

Jorgensen JH, Lee JC, Alexander GA (1977) Rapid penicillinase paper strip test for detection of β-lactamase producing *Haemophilus influenzae* and *Neisseria gonorrhoeae*. Antimicrob Agents Chemother 11:1087–1088

Kahan FM, Kropp H (1980) An antibacterial composition of thienamycin-type compound and a diepeptidase inhibitor. European Patent Application 09587C

Kaminsky ZC (1963) Effect of related anionic detergents on staphylococcal penicillinase. J Bacteriol 85:1182–1183

Kasik JE (1979) Mycobacterial β-lactamases. In: Hamilton-Miller JMT, Smith JT (eds) Beta-lactamases. Academic Press, London New York, pp 339–350

Kasik JE, Peacham L (1968) Properties of β-lactamases produced by three species of *Mycobacteria*. Biochem J 197:675–682

Kiener PA, Waley SG (1977) Substrate induced deactivation of penicillinases. Studies of β-lactamase I by hydrogen exchange. Biochem J 165:279–285

Kiener PA, Waley SG (1978) Reversible inhibitors of penicillinases. Biochem J 169:197–204

Kleppe G, Strominger JL (1979) Studies of the high molecular weight penicillin-binding proteins of *Bacillus subtilis*. J Biol Chem 254:4856–4862

Knott-Hunziker V, Waley SG, Orlek BS, Sammes PG (1979) Penicillinase active sites. Labeling of serine-44 in beta-lactamase I by 6-beta-bromo-penicillanic acid. FEBS Lett 9:59–61

Knox JR, Kelly JA, Moews PG, Murthy NS (1976) 5.5 Å crystallographic structure of penicillin β-lactamase and radius of gyration in solution. J Mol Biol 104:865–875

Kogut M, Pollock MR, Tridgell EJ (1956) Purification of penicillin-induced penicillinase of *Bacillus cereus* NRRL 569: a comparison of its properties with those of a similarly purified penicillinase produced spontaneously by a constitutive mutant. Biochem J 62:391–401

Koyasu S, Fukuda A, Okada Y (1980) The penicillin-binding proteins of *Caulobacter crescentus*. J Biochem 87:363–366

Kozarich JW, Strominger JL (1978) A membrane enzyme from *Staphylococcus aureus* which catalyzes transpeptidase, carboxypeptidase, and penicillinase activities. J Biol Chem 253:1272–1278

Kuwabara S, Abraham EP (1967) Some properties of two extracellular β-lactamases from *Bacillus cereus* 569/H. Biochem J 103:27C–30C

Kuwabara S, Lloyd PH (1971) Protein and carbohydrate moieties of a preparation of β-lactamase II. Biochem J 124:215–220

Kusher DJ, Breuil C (1977) Pennicillinase (β-lactamase) formation by blue-green algae. Arch Microbiol 112:219–223

Labia R, Barthelémy M (1977) Problèmes de la determination des points isoélectriques des β-lactamases. CR Acad Sci [D] (Paris) 284:1729–1732

Labia R, Peduzzi J (1978) Cinétique de l'inhibition de beta-lactamases par l'acide clavulanique. Biochim Biophys Acta 596:572–579

Laemmli UK (1970) Cleavage of structural proteins during assembly of the head of bacteriophage T4. Nature 227:680–685
Lampen JO (1978) Phospholipoproteins in enzyme excretion by bacteria. In: Stanier RY, Rogers HJ, Ward T (eds) Relations between structure and function in the prokaryotic cell. Cambridge University Press, New York, pp 231–247
Lee B (1971) Conformation of penicillin as a transition-state analog of the substrate of peptidoglycan transpeptidase. J Mol Biol 61:463–469
Letarte R, Devaud-Felix M, Pechere JC, Allard-Leprohon D (1977) Enzymatic and immunological characterization of a new cephalosporinase from *Enterobacter Aerogenes*. Antimicrob Agents Chemother 12:301–305
Leung T, Williams JD (1978) Beta-lactamases of subspecies of *Bacteroides fragilis*. J Antimicrob Chemother 4:47–54
Leyh-Bouille M, Coyette J, Ghuysen J-M, Idczak J, Perkins HR, Nieto M (1971) Penicillin-sensitive DD-carboxypeptidases from *Streptomyces* strain R61. Biochemistry 10:2163–2170
Leyh-Bouille M, Nakel M, Frere JM, Johnson K, Ghuysen J-M, Nieto M, Perkins HR (1972) Penicillin sensitive DD-carboxypeptidases from *Streptomyces* strains R39 and K11. Biochemistry 11:1290–1298
Lugtenberg EJJ, deHaas-Menger L, Ruyters WHM (1972) Murein synthesis and identification of cell wall precursors of temperature-sensitive lysis mutants of *Escherichia coli*. J Bacteriol 109:326–335
Lund F, Tybring L (1972) 6β-Amidinopenicillanic acids – a new group of antibiotics. Nature N Biol 236:135–137
Makover SD, Wright RB, Telep E (1980) Penicillin binding proteins in *Haemophilus influenzae*. In: 80th American society for microbiology meeting. May 11–16, Abstract K189. Am Soc Microbiol, Washington DC
Marquet A, Nieto M, Diaz-Maurino T (1976) Membrane-bound DD-carboxypeptidase and transpeptidase activities from *Bacillus megaterium* KM at pH 7. Eur J Biochem 68:581–589
Marshall MJ, Ross GW, Chanter KW, Harris MA (1972) Comparison of the substrate specificities of the β-lactamases from *Klebsiella aerogenes* 1082E and *Enterobacter cloacae* P99. Appl Microbiol 23:765–769
Martin HH, Maskos C, Burger R (1975) D-alanyl-D-alanine carboxypeptidase in the bacterial form and L-form of *Proteus mirabilis*. Eur J Biochem 55:465–473
Martin WJ, Gardner M, Washington JA II (1972) In vitro antimicrobial susceptibility of anaerobic bacteria isolated from clinical specimens. Antimicrob Agents Chemother 1:148–158
Matsuhashi M, Maruyama IN, Takagaki Y, Tamaki S, Nishimura Y, Hirota Y (1978) Isolation of a mutant of *Escherichia coli* lacking penicillin-sensitive D-alanine carboxypeptidase IA. Proc Natl Acad Sci USA 75:2631–2635
Matsuhashi M, Tamaki S, Nakajima S, Nakagawa J, Tomioka S, Takagaki Y (1979) Properties and functions of penicillin-binding proteins and related enzymes in *Escherichia coli*. In: Matsuhashi S (ed) Microbial drug resistance, vol 2. Japan Sci Soc and Univ Park, Tokyo, pp 389–404
Matthew M (1975) Isoelectric focusing studies of β-lactamases. In: Arbuthnott JP, Beeley JA (eds) Isoelectric focusing. Butterworths, London, pp 248–253
Matthew M (1978) Properties of the β-lactamase specified by the pseudomonas plasmid R151. FEMS Microbiol Lett 4:241–244
Matthew M (1979) Plasmid-mediated β-lactamases of gram-negative bacteria: properties and distribution. J Antimicrob Chemother 5:349–358
Matthew M, Harris AM (1976) Identification of β-lactamases by analytical isoelectric focusing: correlation with bacterial taxonomy. J Gen Microbiol 94:55–67
Matthew M, Sykes RB (1977) Properties of the β-lactamase specified by the pseudomonas plasmid RPL11. J Bacteril 132:341–345
Matthew M, Harris AM, Marshall MJ, Ross GE (1975) The use of analytical isoelectric focusing for detection and identification of β-lactamases. J Gen Microbiol 88:169–178
Matthew M, Hedges RW, Smith JT (1979) Types of β-lactamase determined by plasmids in gram-negative bacteria. J Bacteriol 138:657–662

Mays DL, Sangest FK, Cautrell WC, Evans WG (1975) Hydroxylamine determination of cephalosporins. Anal Chem 47:2229–2234
Medeiros AA, Mandel MD (1979) In vivo acquired resistance to β-lactam antibiotics due to hyperproduction of β-lactamase. 79th annual ASM meeting, Oct 1–5, 1979, Abstract A32. Am Soc Microbiol, Washington DC
Medeiros AA, Ximenez J, Blickstein-Goldworm K, O'Brien TF, Acar J (1979) β-lactamases of ampicillin-resistant *Escherichia coli* from Brazil, France, and the United States. In: Nelson JD, Grassi C (eds) Current chemotherapy and infectious disease. American Society for Microbiology, Washington DC, p 761
Mehta RJ, Nash CH (1978) β-lactamase activity in yeast. J Antibiot (Tokyo) 31:239–240
Melchior NH, Blom J, Tybring L, Birch-Andersen A (1973) Light and electron microscopy of the early response of *Escherichia coli* to 6β-amidino-penicillanic acid (FL1060). Acta Pathol Microbiol Scand [B] 81:393–407
McArthur HAI, Reynolds PE (1979a) The solubilization of the membrane bound D-alanyl-D-alanine carboxypeptidase of *Bacillus coagulans* NCIB 9365. Biochim Biophys Acta 568:395–407
McArthur HAI, Reynolds PE (1979b) Peptidoglycan carboxypeptidase and endopeptidase activities of *Bacillus coagulans* NCIB 9365. J Gen Microbiol 111:327–335
McArthur HAI, Reynolds PE (1980) Purification and properties of the D-alanyl-D-alanine carboxypeptidase of *Bacillus coagulans* NCIB 9365. Biochim Biophys Acta 612:107–118
Mirelman D, Sharon N (1972) Biosynthesis of peptidoglycan by a cell wall preparation of *Staphylococcus aureus* and its inhibition by penicillin. Biochem Biophys Res Commun 46:1909–1017
Mirelman D, Nuchamowitz Y (1979a) Biosynthesis of peptidoglycan in *Pseudomonas aeruginosa*. 1. The incorporation of peptidoglycan into the cell wall. Eur J Biochem 94:541–548
Mirelman D, Nuchamowitz Y (1979b) Biosynthesis of peptidoglycan in *Pseudomonas aeruginosa*. 2. Mode of action of β-lactam antibiotics. Eur J Biochem 94:549–556
Mirelman D, Yashouv-Gan Y, Nuchamowitz Y, Rozenhak S, Ron EZ (1978) Murein biosynthesis during a synchronous cell cycle of *Escherichia coli* B. J Bacteriol 134:458–461
Moore BA, Jevons S, Brammer KW (1979) Peptidoglycan transpeptidase inhibition in *Pseudomonas aeruginosa* and *Escherichia coli* by penicillins and cephalosporins. Antimicrob Agents Chemother 15:513–517
Morohoshi T, Saito T (1977) β-Lactamase and β-lactam antibiotics resistance in *Acinetobacter anitratum* (syn: *A. calcoaceticus*). J Antibiot (Tokyo) 30.969–973
Murray PR, Rosenblatt JE (1977) Penicillin resistance and penicillinase production in clinical isolates of *Bacteroides melaninogenicus*. Antimicrob Agents Chemother 11:605–608
Nagarajan R (1972) β-Lactam antibiotics from *Streptomyces*. In: Flynn EH (ed) Cephalosporins and penicillins, chemistry and biology. Academic Press, New York London, pp 636–661
Nagarajan R, Boeck LD, Golman M et al. (1971) β-Lactam antibiotics from *Streptomyces*. J Am Chem Soc 93:2308–2310
Nakagawa J, Tamaki S, Matsuhashi M (1979) Purified penicillin binding proteins 1Bs from *Escherichia coli* membrane showing activities of both peptidoglycan polymerase and peptidoglycan crosslinking enzyme. Agric Biol Chem 43:1379–1380
Neu HC, Heppel LA (1965) The release of enzymes from *Escherichia coli* by osmotic shock during the formation of spheroplasts. J Biol Chem 240:3685–3692
Neuhaus FC, Goyer S, Neuhaus DW (1977) Growth inhibition of *Escherichia coli* W by D-norvalyl-D-alanine: an analogue of D-alanine in position 4 of the peptide subunit of peptidoglycan. Antimicrob Agents Chemother 11:638–644
Newsome SWB, Sykes RB, Richmond MH (1970) Detection of a β-lactamase markedly active against carbenicillin in a strain of *Pseudomonas aeruginosa*. J Bacteriol 101:1079–1080
Newton GGF, Abraham EP (1956) Isolation of cephalosporin C, a penicillin-like antibiotic containing D-α-aminoadipic acid. Biochem J 62:651–658
Newton GGF, Abraham EP, Kiwabara S (1967) Preliminary observations on the formation and breakdown of cephalosporoic acids. In: Hobby GL (ed) Antimicrob Agents Chemother. Amer Soc Microbiol, Washington DC, p 449

Nguyen-Disteche M, Ghuysen J-M, Pollock JJ, Reynolds P, Perkins HR, Coyette J, Salton MRJ (1974a) Enzymes involved in wall peptide cross-linking in *Escherichia coli* K12, strain 44. Eur J Biochem 41:447–455
Nguyen-Disteche M, Pollock JJ, Ghuysen J-M, Puig J, Reynolds P, Perkins HR, Coyette J, Salton MRJ (1974b) Sensitivity to ampicillin and cephalothin of enzymes involved in wall peptide crosslinking in *Escherichia coli* K12, strain 44. Eur J Biochem 41:457–463
Nieto M, Perkins HR, Frere JM, Ghuysen J-M (1973) Fluorescence and circular dichroism studies on the *Streptomyces* R61 DD-carboxypeptidase-transpeptidase. Biochem J 135:493–505
Nikaido H, Nakae T (1979) The outer membrane of gram-negative bacteria. In: Rose AH, Morris JG (eds) Advances in microbial physiology, vol 20. Academic Press, London New York, pp 163–250
Nishida M, Mine Y, Nonoyama S, Kojo H, Goto S, Kuwahara S (1977) Nocardicin A, a new monocyclic antibiotic III. In vitro evaluation. J Antibiot (Tokyo) 30:917–925
Nishino T, Kozarich JW, Strominger JL (1977) Kinetic evidence for an acyl-enzyme intermediate in D-alanine carboxypeptidases of *Bacillus subtilis* and *Bacillus stearothermophilus*. J Biol Chem 252:2934–2939
Nishiura T, Kawada Y, Shiomi Y, O'Hara K, Kono M (1978) Microbial degradation of cephalothin by cephalothin-susceptible *E. coli*. Antimicrob Agents Chemother 13:1036–1039
Noguchi H, Matsuhashi M, Mitsuhashi S (1979) Comparative studies of penicillin-binding proteins in *Pseudomonas aeruginosa* and *Escherichia coli*. Eur J Biochem 100:41–49
Nolan RD, Hildebrandt JF (1979) Comparison of the penicillin-binding proteins of different strains of *Neisseria gonorrhoeae*. Antimicrob Agents Chemother 16:336–340
Nordström K, Sykes RB (1974) Induction kinetics of beta-lactamase biosynthesis in *Pseudomonas aeruginosa*. Antimicrob Agents Chemother 6:734–740
Normark S, Edlund T, Grundström T, Bergström S, Wolf-Watz H (1977) *Escherichia coli* K-12 mutants hyperproducing chromosomal beta-lactamase by gene repetitions. J Bacteriol 132:912–922
Novick RP (1963) Analysis by transduction of mutations affecting penicillinase formation in *Staphylococcus aureus*. J Gen Microbiol 33:121–136
O'Callaghan CH, Morris A, Kirby S, Shingler AH (1972) Novel method for detection of *β*-lactamases by using a chromogenic cephalosporin substrate. Antimicrob Agents Chemother 1:283–288
Ochiai K, Yamanaka T, Kimura K, Sawada O (1959) Studies on inheritance of drug resistance between *Shigella* strains and *Escherichia coli* strains. Nihon Iji Shimpo 861:34–46
Odugbemi TO, Hafiz S, McEntegart MG (1977) Penicillinase-producing *Neisseria gonorrhoeae:* detection by starch paper technique. Br Med J ii:500
Ofek I, Beachey EH (1980) Bacterial adherence. Annu Rev Int Med 25:503–532
Ogawara H (1975) Production and property of beta-lactamases in *Streptomyces*. Antimicrob Agents Chemother 8:402–408
Ogawara H, Horikawa S (1979) Purification of *β*-lactamase from *Streptomyces cellulosae* by affinity chromatography on Blue Sepharose. J Antiobiot (Tokyo) 32:1328–1335
Ogawara H, Horikawa S (1980) Penicillin-binding proteins of *Streptomyces cocaoi*, *Streptomyces olivaceus* and *Streptomyces clavuligerus*. Antimicrob Agents Chemother 17:1–7
Ogawara H, Nozaki S (1977) Effect of acriflavine on the production of *β*-lactamase in *Streptomyces*. J Antibiot (Tokyo) 30:337–338
Ogawara H, Maeda K, Umezawa H (1972) A *β*-lactamase of *Escherichia coli*. Biochim Biophys Acta 289:203–211
Ogawara H, Horikawa S, Shimada-Miyoshi S, Yasuzawa K (1978) Production and property of beta-lactamases in *Streptomyces:* Comparison of the strains isolated newly and thirty years ago. Antimicrob Agents Chemother 13:865–870
Ogawara T, Umezawa H (1975) *Bacillus cereus* *β*-lactamase. Reaction with *N*-bromosuccinimide and the properties of the product. Biochim Biophys Acta 391:437–447
Ohmori H, Azuma A, Suzuki Y, Hashimoto (1977) Factors involved in beta-lactam resistance in *Pseudomonas aeruginosa*. Antimicrob Agents Chemother 12:537–539
Ohya S, Yamazaki M, Sugawara S, Matsuhashi M (1979) Penicillin-binding proteins in *Proteus* species. J Bacteriol 137:474–479

Okamura K, Hirata S, Okmura Y, Fukagawa Y, Shimauchi Y, Kouno K, Ishikura T, Lein J (1978). PS-5, a new β-lactam antibiotic from *Streptomyces*. J Antibiot (Tokyo) 31:480–482

Olsson B, Dornbusch K, Nord CE (1977) Susceptibility to beta-lactam antibiotics and production of beta-lactamase in *Bacteroides fragilis*. Med Microbiol Immunol (Berl) 163:183–194

Olsson-Liljequist B, Dornbusch K, Nord CE (1979) Immunological characterization of beta-lactamases from *Bacteroides fragilis*. 19th Intersci Conf Antimicrob Agents Chemother, Oct 1–5, 1979, Abstract 26. Am Soc Microbiol, Washington DC

Pain RH, Virden R (1979) The structural and conformational basis of β-lactamase activity. In: Hamilton-Miller JMT, Smith JT (eds) Beta-lactamases. Academic Press, London New York, pp 141–180

Park JT (1952) Uridine-5′-pyrophosphate derivatives. I. Isolation from *Staphylococcus aureus*. J Biol Chem 194:877–884

Patil GV, Day RA (1973) Involvement of a carboxyl group in the active site of *Bacillus cereus* 569/H penicillinase (β-lactamase II). Biochim Biophys Acta 293:490–493

Perkins HR, Nieto M, Frere JM, Leyh-Bouille M, Ghuysen J-M (1973) *Streptomyces* DD-carboxypeptidases as transpeptidases. The specificity for amino compounds acting as carboxyl acceptors. Biochem J 131:707–718

Petrocheilou V, Sykes RB, Richmond MH (1977) Novel R-plasmid-mediated beta-lactamase from *Klebsiella aerogenes*. Antimicrob Agents Chemother 12:126–128

Phillipon A, Paul G, Labia G, Neuot P (1976) Distinction entre des β-lactamases immunotypes 1 et 2 de Pitton grâce à une nouvelle β-lactamine. Ann Microbiol (Paris) 127A:487–491

Pitton JS (1972) Mechanisms of bacterial resistance to antibiotics. In: Adrian RH (ed) Review of physiology, vol 65. Springer, Berlin Heidelberg New York, pp 15–93

Pollock JJ, Nguyen-Disteche M, Ghuysen J-M, Coyette J, Linder R, Salton MRJ, Kim KS, Perkins HR, Reynolds P (1974) Fractionation of the DD-carboxypeptidase-transpeptidase activities solubilized from membranes of *Escherichia coli* K12, strain 44. Eur J Biochem 41:439–446

Pollock MR (1965) Purification and properties of penicillinase from two strains of *Bacillus licheniformis:* A chemical, physiochemical and physiological comparison. Biochem J 94:666–675

Pollock MR (1971) The function and evolution of penicillinase. Proc Soc Lond [Biol] 179:385–401

Pooley HM, Schlaeppi J-M, Karamata D (1978) Localized insertion of new cell wall in *Bacillus subtilis*. Nature 274:264–266

Pratt RF, Loosemore MJ (1978) 6-Beta-bromopenicillanic acid, a potent beta-lactamase inhibitor. Proc Natl. Acad Sci USA 75:4145–4149

Pratt RF, Anderson EG, Odeh I (1980) Certain monocyclic β-lactams are β-lactamase substrates: Nocardicin A and desthiobenzylpenicillin. Biochem Biophys Res Commun 93:1266–1273

Presslitz JE (1978) Mode of action of a structurally novel beta-lactam. Antimicrob Agents Chemother 14:144–150

Presslitz JE, Ray VA (1975) DD-carboxypeptidase and peptidoglycan transpeptidase from *Pseudomonas aeruginosa*. Antimicrob Agents Chemother 7:578–581

Rando RR (1975) On the mechanism of action of antibiotics which act as irreversible enzyme inhibitors. Biochem Pharmacol 24:1153–1160

Rasmussen JR, Strominger JL (1978) Utilization of a depsipeptide substrate for trapping acyl-enzyme intermediates of penicillin-sensitive D-alanine carboxypeptidases. Proc Natl Acad Sci USA 75:84–88

Reading C, Cole M (1977) Clavulanic acid: A beta-lactamase inhibiting beta-lactam from *Streptomyces clavuligerus*. Antimicrob Agents Chemother 11:852–857

Reading C, Hepburn P (1979) The inhibition of staphylococcal β-lactamase by clavulanic acid. Biochem J 179:67–76

Reynolds PE, Shepherd ST, Chase HA (1978) Identification of the binding protein which may be the target of penicillin action in *Bacillus megaterium*. Nature 271:568–570

Richmond MH (1963) Purification and properties of the exopenicillinase from *Staphylococcus aureus*. Biochem J 88:452–459
Richmond MH (1965) Wild type variants of exopenicillinase from *Staphylococcus aureus*. Biochem J 94:584–593
Richmond MH, Sykes RB (1973) The β-lactamases of gram-negative bacteria and their possible physiological role. In: Rose AH, Tempest DW (eds) Advances in microbial physiology, vol 9. Academic Press, London New York, pp 31–88
Rogers HJ (1970) Bacterial growth and the cell envelope. Bacteriol Rev 34:194–214
Rogers HJ, Forsberg CW (1971) Role of autolysins in the killing of bacteria by some bactericidal antibiotics. J Bacteriol 108:1235–1243
Roupas A, Pitton JS (1974) R-factor-mediated and chromosomal resistance to ampicillin in *Escherichia coli*. Antimicrob Agents Chemother 5:186–191
Sabath LD, Jago M, Abraham EP (1965) Cephalosporinase and penicillinase activities of a β-lactamase from *Pseudomonas pyocyanea*. Biochem J 96:739–752
Salyers AA, Wang J, Williams TD (1977) β-Lactamase activity in strains of *Bacteroides melaninogenicus* and *Bacteroides oralis*. Antimicrob Agents Chemother 11:142–146
Samuni A (1975) A direct spectrophotometric assay and determination of Michaelis constants for the beta-lactamase reaction. Anal Biochem 63:17–26
Samuni A, Meyer AY (1978) Conformation patterns in penicillins and the penicillin-penicillinase interaction. Mol Pharmacol 14:704–709
Sawada Y, Yaginuma S, Tai M, Iyobe S, Mitsuhashi S (1975) Resistance to β-lactam antibiotics in *Pseudomonas aeruginosa*. In: Mitsuhashi S, Hashimoto H (eds) Microbial drug resistance. Univ Tokyo Press, Tokyo, pp 391–397
Sawai T, Mitsuhashi S, Yamagishi S (1968) Drug resistance of enteric bacteria. XIV. Comparison of β-lactamases in gram-negative rod bacteria resistant to α-aminobenzylpenicillin. Jpn J Microbiol 12:423–434
Sawai T, Saito T, Mitsuhashi S (1970) A stereoisomer of benzylpenicillin as substrate and inducer for β-lactamases. J Antibiot (Tokyo) 23:488–492
Sawai T, Yamagishi S, Mitsuhashi S (1973) Penicillinases of *Klebsiella pneumoniae* and their phylogenetic relationship to penicillinases mediated by R-factors. J Bacteriol 115:1045–1054
Schenkein DP, Pratt RF (1980) Phenylpropynal, a specific, irreversible, non-beta-lactam inhibitor of beta-lactamases. J Biol Chem 255:45–48
Schilf W, Martin HH (1980) Purification of two DD-carboxypeptidases/transpeptidases with different penicillin sensitivities from *Proteus mirabilis*. Eur J Biochem 105:361–370
Schilf W, Frere P, Frere J-M, Martin HH, Ghuysen J-M, Adriaens P, Meesschaert B (1978) Interaction between penicillin and the DD-carboxypeptidase of the unstable L-form of *Proteus mirabilis* strain 19. Eur J Biochem 85:325–330
Schleifer KH, Kandler O (1972) Peptidoglycan types of bacterial cell walls and their taxonomic implications. Bacteriol Rev 36:407–477
Schwartz JL, Schwartz SP (1979) Production of β-lactamase by non-*Streptomyces* Actinomycetales. Antimicrob Agents Chemother 15:123–125
Scott GK (1973) Structure and mechanism of β-lactamase from *Escherichia coli*. Biochem Soc Trans 1:159–162
Shepherd ST, Chase HA, Reynolds PR (1977) The separation and properties of two penicillin-binding proteins from *Salmonella typhimurium*. Eur J Biochem 78:521–532
Sherratt DJ, Collins JF (1973) Analysis by transformation of the penicillinase system in *Bacillus licheniformis* 749/C. J Gen Microbiol 76:217–230
Sherrill JM, McCarthy LR (1979) Cephalosporinase activity within the *Bacteroides fragilis* group and in strains of *B. melaninogenicus* and *B. oralis*. 19th Intersci Conf Antimicrob Agents and Chemotherapy, 1–5 Oct, 1979, Abstract 28. Am Soc Microbiol, Washington DC
Shockman GD, Daneo-Moore L, Higgins ML (1974) Problems of cell wall and membrane growth, enlargement, and division. Ann NY Acad Sci 235:161–197
Simons K, Servas M, Garoff H, Helenius A (1978) Membrane-bound and secreted forms of penicillinase from *Bacillus licheniformis*. J Mol Biol 126:673–690

Smith JT (1963) Penicillinase and ampicillin resistance in a strain of *Escherichia coli.* J Gen Microbiol 30:299–306 (1963)
Smith JT, Wyatt JM (1974) Relation of R factor and chromosomal β-lactamase with the periplasmic space. J Bacteriol 117:931–939
Smith JT, Bremmer DA, Datta N (1974) Ampicillin resistance of *Shigella sonnei.* Antimicrob Agents Chemother 6:418–421
Smith JT, Hamilton-Miller MJT (1963) Penicillinases from gram-positive and gram-negative bacteria: a thermodynamic difference. Nature 197:769–770
Spratt BG (1975) Distinct penicillin-binding proteins involved in the division, elongation and shape of *Escherichia coli* K12. Proc Natl Acad Sci USA 72:2999–3003
Spratt BG (1977a) Properties of the penicillin-binding proteins of *Escherichia coli* k 12. Eur J Biochem 72:341–352
Spratt BG (1977b) Comparison of the binding properties of two 6β-amidinopenicillanic acid derivatives that differ in their physiological effects on *Escherichia coli.* Antimicrob Agents Chemother 11:161–166
Spratt BG (1978) Mechanism of action of penicillin. Sci Progr Oxford 65:101–128
Spratt BG (1979) Identification of the killing targets for β-lactam antibiotics in *Escherichia coli.* In: Matsuhashi (ed) Microbial drug resistance, vol 2. Japan Sci Soc, Univ Park, Tokyo, pp 349–361
Spratt BG, Pardee AB (1975) Penicillin-binding proteins and cell-shape in *E. coli.* Nature 254:516–517
Spratt BG, Strominger JL (1976) Indentification of the major penicillin-binding proteins of *Escherichia coli* as D-alanine carboxypeptidase IA. J Bacteriol 127:660–663
Spratt BG, Jobanputra U, Schwarz U (1977) Mutants of *Escherichia coli* which lack a component of penicillin-binding protein 1 are viable. FEBS Lett 79:374–378
Stapley EO, Cassidy P, Currie SA, Daoust D, Goegelman R, Hernandez S, Jackson M, Mata JM, Miller AK, Monaghan RL, Tunac JB, Zimmerman SB, Hendlin D (1977) Epithienamycins: biological studies of a new family of β-lactam antibiotics. In: 17th Intersci Conf Antimicrob Agents Chemother, 12–14 Oct, 1977, Abstract 80. Am Soc Microbiol, Washington DC
Suginaka H, Blumberg PM, Strominger JL (1972) Multiple penicillin binding components in *Bacillus subtilis, Bacillus cereus, Staphylococcus aureus* and *Escherichia coli.* J Biol Chem 247:5279–5288
Sutcliffe JG (1978) Nucleotide sequence of the ampicillin resistance gene of *Escherichia coli* plasmid pBR322. Proc Natl Acad Sci USA 75:3737–3741
Suzuki H, Nishimura Y, Hirota Y (1978) On the process of cellular division in *Escherichia coli:* A series of mutants of *E. coli* altered in the penicillin-binding properties. Proc Natl Acad Sci USA 75:664–668
Suzuki H, vanHeijenoort Y, Tamura T, Mizoguchi J, Hirota Y, vanHeijenoort J (1980) In vitro peptidoglycan polymerization catalyzed by penicillin binding protein 1b of *Escherichia coli* K12. FEBS Lett 110:245–249
Sykes RB, Bush K (1982) Physiology, biochemistry and inactivation of β-lactamases. In: Gorman M, Morin RB (eds) β-Lactam antibiotics, chemistry and biology. Academic Press, New York Vol. 3:155–207
Sykes RB, Matthew M (1976) The β-lactamases of gram-negative bacteria on their role in resistance to β-lactam antibiotics. J Antimicrob Chemother 2:115–157
Sykes RB, Matthew M (1979) Detection, assay and immunology of β-lactamases. In: Hamilton-Miller JMT, Smith JT (eds) Beta-lactamases. Academic Press, London New York, pp 17–49
Sykes RB, Percival A (1978) Studies on gonococcal β-lactamases. In: Brooks GF, Gotschlick EC, Holmes KK, Sawyer WD, Yound FE (eds) Immunobiology of *Neisseria gonorrhoeae.* Am Soc Microbiol, Washington DC, p 68
Sykes RB, Richmond MH (1970) Intergeneric transfer of a β-lactamase gene between *Ps. aeruginosa* and *E. coli.* Nature 226:952–954
Sykes RB, Richmond MH (1971) R-factors, beta-lactamase and carbenicillin-resistant *Pseudomonas aeruginosa.* Lancet ii:342–344

Sykes RB, Smith JT (1979) Biochemical aspects of β-lactamases from gram-negative organisms. In: Hamilton-Miller JMT, Smith JT (eds) Beta-lactamases. Academic Press, London New York, pp 369–401
Sykes RB, Matthew M, O'Callaghan CH (1975) R-factor mediated β-lactamase production by *Haemophilus influenzae*. J Med Microbiol 8:437–441
Sykes RB, Bonner DP, Bush K, Georgopapadakou NH (1982) Azthreonam (SQ 26,776), a synthetic monobactam specifically active against aerobic Gram-negative bacteria. Antimicrob Agents Chemother 21:85–92
Szewczuk A, Siewinski M, Slowinska R (1980) Colorimetric assay of penicillin amidase activity using phenylacetylaminobenzoic acid as substrate. Anal Biochem 103:166–169
Tally FP, O'Keefe JP, Sullivan NM, Gorbach SL (1977) Inactivation of cephalosporins by *Bacteroides fragilis*. Proc 10th int congr chemother vol 1, pp 487–489
Tamaki S, Nakajima S, Matsuhashi M (1977) Thermosensitive mutation in *Escherichia coli* simultaneously causing defects in penicillin-binding protein-1Bs and in enzyme activity for peptidoglycan synthesis in vitro. Proc Natl Acad Sci USA 74:5472–5476
Tamaki S, Nakagawa J, Maruyama IN, Matsuhashi M (1978) Supersensitivity to β-lactam antibiotics in *Escherichia coli* caused by D-alanine carboxypeptidase 1A mutation. Agric Biol Chem 42:2147–2150
Tamaki S, Matsuzawa H, Matsuhashi M (1980) Cluster of *mrd* A and *mrd* B genes responsible for the rod shape and mecillinam sensitivity of *Escherichia coli*. J Bacteriol 141:52–57
Tamura T, Imae Y, Strominger JL (1976) Purification to homogeneity and properties of two D-alanine carboxypeptidases I from *Escherichia coli*. J Biol Chem 251:414–423
Thatcher DR (1975) The partial amino acid sequence of the extracelllar β-lactamase I of *Bacillus cereus* 569/H. Biochem J 147:313–326
Thomas R (1979) The microbial metabolism of penicillin V sulfoxide and its its possible relevance to the mode of action of penicillin. JCS Chem Commun 1979:1176–1177
Tipper DJ, Strominger JL (1965) Mechanism of action of penicillins: a proposal based on their structural similarity to acyl-D-alanyl-D-alanine. Proc Natl Acad Sci USA 54:1133–1141
Tomasz A, Waks S (1975) Mechanism of action of penicillin: Triggering of the pneumococcal autolytic enzyme by inhibition of cell wall synthesis. Proc Nat Acad Sci USA 72:4162–4166
Umbreit JN, Strominger JL (1973) D-Alanine carboxypeptidase from *Bacillus subtilis* membranes. I. Purification and characterization. J Biol Chem 248:6759–6766
Vesterberg O (1973) Isoelectric focusing of proteins in thin layers of polyacrylamide gel. Sci Tools 20:22–28
Virden R, Bristow AF, Pain RH (1978) Reversible inhibition of penicillinase by quinacillin. Evaluation of mechanisms involving two conformational states of the enzyme. Biochem Biophys Res Commun 82:951–956
VonDaehne W (1980) 6β-Halopenicillanic acids, a group of β-lactamase inhibitors.J Antibiot (Tokyo) 33:451–452
Vosberg H-P, Hoffman-Berling H (1971) DNA synthesis in nucleotide-permeable *Escherichia coli* cells. I. Preparation and properties of ether-treated cells. J Mol Biol 58:739–759
Waley SG (1974) A spectrophotometric assay for β-lactamase action on penicillins. Biochem J 139:789–790
Waley SG (1975) The pH-dependence and group modification of β-lactamase I. Biochem J 149:547–551
Wallace RJ, Vance P, Weissfeld A, Martin R (1978) Beta-lactamase production and resistance of beta-lactam antibiotics in *Nocardia*. Antimicrob Agents Chemother 14:704–709
Waxman DJ, Strominger JL (1979) Cephalosporin-sensitive penicillin-binding proteins of *Staphylococcus aureus* and *Bacillus subtilis* active in the conversion of ^{14}C-penicillin to ^{14}C-phenylacetylglycine. J Biol Chem 254:2056–2061
Waxman DJ, Strominger JL (1980) Sequence of active-site peptides from the penicillin-sensitive D-alanine carboxypeptidase of *Bacillus subtilis*. Mechanism of penicillin action and sequence homology to beta-lactamases. J Biol Chem 255:3964–3976

Waxman DJ, Yocum RR, Strominger JL (1980) Penicillins and cephalosporins are active site-directed acylating agents. Evidence in support of the substrate-analog hypothesis. Philos Trans R Soc (Lond) B289–271

Weston A, Ward JB, Perkins HR (1977) Biosynthesis of peptidoglycan in wall plus membrane preparations from *Micrococcus luteus:* Direction of chain extension, lengths of chains and effect of penicillin on cross-linking. J Gen Microbiol 99:171–181

Williamson R, Hackenbeck R, Tomasz A (1980) The penicillin-binding proteins of *Streptococcus pneumoniae* grown under lysis permissive and lysis-protective (tolerant) conditions. FEMS Microbiol Lett 7:127–131

Wust J, Wilkins TD (1978) Effect of clavulanic acid on anaerobic bacteria resistant to beta-lactam antibiotics. Antimicrob Agents Chemother 13:130–133

Yaginuma S, Sawai T, Ono H, Yamagishi S, Mitsuhashi S (1973) Biochemical properties of a cephalosporin β-lactamase from *Pseudomonas aeruginosa.* Jpn J Microbiol 17:141–149

Yamagishi S, O'Hara K, Sawai T, Mitsuhashi S (1979) The purification and properties of penicillin β-lactamases mediated by transmissible R-factors in *Escherichia coli.* J Biochem 66:11–20

Yamamoto S, Lampen JO (1976) Purification of plasma membrane penicillinase from *Bacillus licheniformis* 749/C and comparison with exoenzyme. J Biol Chem 251:4095–4101

Yamasaki M, Aono R, Tamura G (1976) FL1060 binding protein of *Escherichia coli* is probably under the control of adenosine 3′,5′-cyclic monophosphate. Agric Biol Chem 40:1665–1667

Yano K, Suzaki K, Saito M, Toda M, Saito T, Mitsuhashi S (1979) In vitro and in vivo antibacterial activities of YM-09330, a new cephamycin derivative. 19th intersci conf antimicrob agents chemother, 1–5 Oct 1979, Abstract 564. Am Soc Microbiol, Washington DC

Yocum RR, Blumberg PM, Strominger JL (1974) Purification and characterization of the thermophilic D-alanine carboxypeptidase from membranes of *Bacillus stearothermophilus.* J Biol Chem 249:4863–4871

Yocum RR, Waxman DJ, Rasmussen JR, Strominger JL (1979) Mechanism of penicillin action: penicillin and substrate bind covalently to the same active site serine in two bacterial D-alanine carboxypeptidases. Proc Natl Acad Sci USA 76:2730–2734

Yoshida T, Norisada M, Matsuura S, Nagata W, Kuwabara S (1978) 6059-S, a new parenterally active 1-oxacephalosporin: (1) Microbiological studies. In: 18th intersci conf antimicrob agents chemother, 4–6 Oct 1978, Abstract 151. Am Soc Microbiol, Washington DC

Young FR, Mayer L (1979) Genetic determinants of microbial resistance to antibiotics Rev Infect Dis 1:55–62

Zyk N, Citri N (1968) The interaction of penicillinase with penicillins. VII. Effect of specific antibodies on conformative response. Biochim Biophys Acta 159:327–339

CHAPTER 13

In Vitro and In Vivo Laboratory Evaluation of β-Lactam Antibiotics

A. K. MILLER

A. Historical

I. Penicillins

The use of molds to treat cuts and injuries (FLOREY 1949) can be traced back in records of folk medicine to ancient Egypt where "crumbs of a moldy wheaten loaf" were used to treat scalp infections (BÖTTCHER 1964). The agent being used was indoubtedly a penicillin.

The first laboratory evaluation of "penicillin" occurred long before this name had been used for a specific agent. In 1871 Joseph Lister, in his laboratory diary, described studies directed toward finding a nonpoisonous antiseptic substance. In one experiment, he added bacteria to jars containing either sparse or dense growths of *Penicillium*. Later he noted the abundance of actively moving organisms in jars with little *Penicillium*, and motionless organisms in jars with dense growths of the mold (BÖTTCHER 1964; SELWYN 1979). GRATIA and DATH (1924, 1925) reported their observations of the bacteriolytic properties of "certain molds", including a *Penicillium*. In 1876 John Tyndall, intent on discrediting spontaneous generation, described the "struggle for existence between Bacteria and the *Penicillium*" (quoted in WELCH and MARTÍ-IBÁÑEZ 1960). Apparently none of these workers pursued these observations of the effects of mold growth on bacteria.

In 1928, the now often described "accidental contamination" by a mold on a plate of staphylococci was observed by Alexander Fleming. Perhaps because he was studying lysozyme, an enzyme he had isolated from white blood cells and had shown to be capable of destroying bacteria, he was particularly interested in the ability of the mold to lyse the staphylococcal colonies. In any event, he made further studies of the inhibitory activities of this fungus that now had been identified as a *Penicillium*. To demonstrate the inhibitory activity that was present in the culture medium on which the fungus grew, Fleming used the "ditch" or "trench" plate. On one side of a hardened, uninoculated agar plate a strip of agar was removed aseptically leaving a trench, into which was poured agar mixed with the *Penicillium* broth filtrate that Fleming now called "penicillin." When this had hardened, cultures of various organisms were streaked at right angles from the filled trench to the edge of the plate. The inhibitory substance, diffusing from the trench through the agar, prevented the growth of the organisms sensitive to it. After incubation, examination of the plate showed which organisms were insensitive to the agent because they grew all the way to the trench, and which were sensitive because their growth was inhibited by penicillin. The degree of sensitivity of a culture was indicated by the extent of the area of no-growth. Fleming titrated this inhibition by making serial dilutions of penicillin in broth, seeding each tube of dilution with the test culture, incubating, and then examining the tubes for growth.

By these two procedures, the agar plate and the broth dilution, the first spectrum-of-activity tests of penicillin were performed. FLEMING (1929) reported that penicillin activity was very marked on the pyogenic cocci and the diphtheria group of bacilli, but that many bacteria, such as the coli-typhoid group, the influenza-bacillus group, and the enterococcus were quite insensitive. Fleming further evaluated his "antiseptic agent," examining the influence of the culture medium and other factors on its production, studying its solubility and stability, determining the influence of temperature, filtration, and pH on its activity, measuring its effect on leukocytes and determining its rate of killing of staphylococci.

Fleming used penicillin as a tool in in vitro tests to aid in the isolation of specific bacteria from the mixtures normally found in human saliva, sputum, nasal mucus, and throat swabs. He paid tribute to this use of the agent by entitling his 1929 paper "On the antibacterial action of cultures of a Penicillium, with special reference to their use in the isolation of *B. Influenzae.*" Included in the paper are details of work on cultures made from the throats of 25 nurses hospitalized for "influenza." Also included is reference to some in vivo work that determined that penicillin was not toxic when given intravenously to a rabbit or intraperitoneally to a mouse, and further showed that it had no ill effect when used to irrigate "large infected surfaces in man" or to irrigate the human conjunctiva every hour for a day. He suggested that penicillin might be an efficient agent "for application to, or injection into, areas infected with penicillin-sensitive microbes."

Although Fleming himself was unable to proceed with the isolation of pure material, he did maintain his culture. Several years later, the biochemists Raistrick and colleagues, working with this culture, were able to isolate penicillin and to determine under what conditions the agent was "moderately stable" (CLUTTERBUCK et al. 1932). These workers used a Seitz filtered culture in a tube dilution test to confirm the activity of penicillin against *Bacterium coli* and *Haemophilus influenza.* As a check on the titration in the fluid medium, each bacterial culture was streaked on a plate of solid medium containing a single concentration of the sterile filtrate.

REID (1935), also working with Fleming's culture (because a large number of molds he tested had not produced the inhibitory agent), added his confirmation of the "selective activity" of penicillin. His test procedure was to pour into one-half of a divided petri dish nutrient agar containing the filtrate, and into the other half the same agar without the filtrate. After the agars had hardened, bacterial cultures were streaked across the two halves on the plate. Growth on the half of the plate containing only nutrient agar was evidence of no error in streaking. Absence of growth on the other half indicated the presence of an inhibitory substance. Reid studied some of the properties of the inhibitory substance, but was unable to isolate it by dialysis, absorption, or distillation of the culture filtrate.

Penicillin finally was isolated and concentrated into a reasonably stable, if not pure, form by a group working with Florey. In their first publication (CHAIN et al. 1940), they reported briefly on the chemotherapeutic activity of their concentrate, mentioning an in vitro spectrum that included the anaerobes *Clostridium welchii, Clostridium septique*, and *Clostridium oedematiens*, in vivo therapy tests in mice infected with streptococci, staphylococci or *Clostridium septique*, and pharmacological studies (effect on leukocytes, on blood pressure, heart beat, and respiration, as well as absorption and excretion and tolerance to subcutaneous and intravenous injections) on mice, rats, or cats. These observations were expanded in their subsequent paper (ABRAHAM et al. 1941). Details of growing *Penicillium*, of producing, isolating, concentrating and storing the antibiotic are given. To follow penicillin production and determine activity, a cylinder-plate assay procedure using *Staphylococcus aureus* was developed to replace the serial dilution method used by FLEMING (1929). The plate assay was faster and required only a small amount of test material that did not have to be sterile. A tube dilution test was used to study the spectrum of activity, and other tests were devised to study the effects, if any, of serum, whole blood, pus, tissue autolysates and peptones on penicillin activity in vitro. A culture of *Staphylococcus aureus*, passaged through penicillin-containing broth, adapted to penicillin, but this resistance was not associated with the destruction of the antibiotic. ABRAHAM and CHAIN had reported earlier (1940) on a penicillin-destroying enzyme, which they named penicillinase. They had isolated the enzyme from "*Bacterium coli*," from an unidentified gram-negative rod, and also from *Micrococcus lysodeikticus*, and stated that "the presence or absence of the enzyme in a bacterium may not be the sole factor determining its insensitivity or sensitivity to penicillin."

The effect of penicillin on the morphology of many bacterial cells – an extreme elongation of cells in the presence of subinhibitory concentration of the antibiotic – also had been reported earlier by GARDNER (1940). Both he and ABRAHAM et al. (1941) commented on the therapeutic implications of this effect. These latter authors not only included laboratory studies of absorption and excretion of penicillin by mice, rats, cats, and rabbits but also reported such studies in man. Their monumental paper concludes by giving the case histories of the first ten patients to receive this remarkable antibiotic. Five of the patients received the drug intravenously for the treatment of staphylococcal or streptococcal infections; an infant was treated by mouth for a persistent staphylococcal infection, and the remaining four patients were treated locally for eye infections. "In all these cases," the final sentence states, "a favorable therapeutic response was obtained."

So, in the early 1940s penicillin was evaluated and established as a clinically useful agent. Its properties were almost unbelievable; it was extremely active against some important disease-producing bacteria and it was essentially nontoxic to the patient. But there were deficiencies. Its spectrum of activity included few gram-negative organisms; its acid instability resulted in poor absorption when given orally; its destruction by penicillinase reduced its activity against organisms producing this enzyme, and it was excreted rapidly. As new and improved penicillins were sought, testing investigated these points in particular. In addition, although penicillin is remarkably nontoxic, clinical evidence was beginning to show that it possessed definite allergenic properties (KOLODNY and DENHOFF 1946; CALVERT and SMITH 1955; ROSENTHAL 1958). It was hoped that newly isolated or derived agents would not elicit such responses.

As work on the production, isolation, and purification of Fleming's penicillin continued, there proved to be not one, but a family of at least four penicillins produced naturally. Although all were quite similar, penicillin G (benzylpenicillin) was considered to have the most desirable properties, and was the one developed for therapeutic use. Other so-called "natural penicillins" were produced by the *Penicillium* depending on the constituents in the broth on which the mold was growing. The production of a number of such biosynthetic penicillins was described by BEHRENS et al. (1948). Many of these were evaluated to compare their activities with those of penicillin G. One of them, phenoxymethylpenicillin, later called penicillin V, was studied by BRANDL et al. (1953), who reported that, after oral administration, concentrations of penicillin V in the blood exceeded those of penicillin G. Although the antibacterial spectra of penicillin G and V vary somewhat (GARROD 1960a, b), as do some aspects of their pharmacology and toxicity (ANDERSON et al. 1955), the outstanding difference is the considerably greater absorption of V over G after oral administration (WRIGHT et al. 1955; WHITE et al. 1955; DIDING and FRISK 1955; HEATLEY 1956). Clinical trials showed the antibiotic to be effective therapeutically (MARTIN et al. 1955) and to be of value for oral therapy against moderately severe infections caused by sensitive organisms (GARROD 1960b).

By the time this first orally effective penicillin was being used widely, the isolation of the penicillin nucleus (BATCHELOR et al. 1959) provided the means of preparing semisynthetic penicillins by the addition of sidechains to the nucleus. Of the thousands of such compounds that were prepared in the 1960s and 1970s, only a few have been introduced into clinical practice. These have been developed because, in relation to penicillin G, laboratory evaluations showed them to be more acid resistant, more resistant to destruction by penicillinase, or to have a broader spectrum of activity.

One of the first of the penicillinase-resistant compounds was methicillin, which must be injected. Then came the acid-resistant, penicillinase-resistant oxacillin, cloxacillin, and flucloxacillin, which can be used orally. Other orally effective penicillins are pivampicillin, amoxycillin, and ampicillin, these having a spectrum of activity that includes some gram-negative organisms. Carbenicillin was the first penicillin that showed activity against *Pseudomonas;* others are ticarcillin, subenicillin, and others under development.

II. Cephalosporins

The discovery and development of penicillin stimulated the search for new and different antibiotic agents. Among those seeking was Brotzu, in Sardinia. ABRAHAM and LODER (1972) describe Brotzu's demonstration of activity against the growth of both gram-positive and gram-negative organisms by material produced on an agar plate by a *Cephalosporium*. Both crude filtrates and crude concentrates of the antibiotic were used clinically with some success in the treatment of boils and abscesses, brucellosis, and typhoid fever. Unable himself to do the work of developing the antibiotic, Brotzu arranged eventually to have his antibiotic-producing culture sent to Florey in 1948 (FLOREY 1955). Three "cephalosporins" were described by workers in his laboratory; cephalosporin P, later shown to be a steroid, cephalosporin N, later shown to be a penicillin identical to synnematin B, and cephalosporin C. Cephalosporin C, recognized only during the purification studies of penicillin N (NEWTON and ABRAHAM 1955, 1956), was of particular interest because it was resistant to destruction by penicillinase (but not by a new enzyme they called C-cephalosporinase). The antibiotic was not highly active against bacteria, but its spectrum of activity was wide. Moreover, it was remarkably nontoxic when given intravenously to mice, and therapeutically effective by the subcutaneous route for mice infected with a *Streptococcus* (FLOREY 1955) and even with a penicillin-resistant *Staphylococcus* (FLOREY 1956). These early in vivo experiments were carried out on a very small scale, as were those with penicillin, undoubtedly because of the scarcity of test material. Often three mice constituted a test group. For the *Staphylococcus* test just mentioned, however, there were 14 control mice and five mice in each of three treatment groups.

One further early observation concerning cephalosporin C was that, under certain conditions in vitro it competed with penicillin for penicillinase (ABRAHAM and NEWTON 1956). An effort to demonstrate this effect in vivo was not successful when a combination of penicillin with a small amount of cephalosporin C was used to treat an infection with a penicillinase-producing *Staphylococcus* (FLOREY 1956); however, the amount of cephalosporin C needed for protection was reduced 50%–75% when given with an equal, but ineffective, amount of penicillin G (ABRAHAM 1962). ABRAHAM and LODER (1972) summarize the work involved in developing cephalosporin C and isolating its nucleus to allow the chemical manipulations resulting in the production of the injectables cephalothin (CHAUVETTE et al. 1962a, b), cephaloridine (MUGGLETON et al. 1964), cefazolin (NISHIDA et al. 1969), and cefamandole (WICK and PRESTON 1972), and the orally active cephaloglycin (WICK and BONIECE 1965) and cephalexin (WICK 1967). Many other cephalosporins are in the process of evaluation or development; some have a greater intrinsic activity, some a greater spectrum of activity which includes *Pseudomonas;* some differ in their susceptibility to enzymatic degradation; and some differ in the extent of their binding to serum in comparison with products now available for therapy. The test procedures used for these evaluations, while based on those used in the development of the penicillins, have been refined, modified, and adapted to the particular attribute and compound being studied.

O'CALLAGHAN (1979) has described the newer cephalosporins and discusses their relationships with the earlier compounds in a comprehensive review. Of the newer agents, cefuroxime is available commercially in Great Britain, and others such as cefotaxime (HR 756), cefsulodin (SCE 129, CGP 7174E), cefotiam (SCE 963, CPG 14221 E), and cefmetazole (CS 1170) are under intensive study.

III. Cephamycins (7-α-Methoxy Cephalosporins)

The cephamycins are β-lactam antibiotics produced by actinomycetes and structurally similar to cephalosporins. They were discovered in the course of programs looking for new antibiotics. STAPLEY et al. (1972) first described a family of cephamycins, designated A, B, and C. NAGARAJAN et al. (1971) listed the compound Stapley et al. designated C as one of the β-lactam antibiotics produced by a *Streptomyces*. The cephamycins showed some interesting activities. All were resistant to destruction by β-lactamases (DAOUST et al. 1973); cephamycin A had a broad spectrum of activity, while B and C were narrow in spectrum, being active mostly against gram-negative organisms. An agar dilution test for obtaining minimal inhibitory concentration data and the mouse protection tests for therapeutic efficacies showed cephamycin C to be more active than cephalosporin C against gram-negative organisms both in vitro and in vivo. In addition, it was active against cephalosporin-resistant organisms (MILLER et al. 1972a, b). Other in vitro tests demonstrated cephamycin C to be bactericidal in its activity, and to show little change in endpoint with increased inoculum size. It was remarkably nontoxic when given to mice. Since the use of probenecid did not enhance the therapeutic effectiveness nor result in increased concentrations of cephamycin C in the sera of treated mice, this agent was judged to be excreted mainly by glomerular filtration as is cephalosporin C and cephaloridine (see Sect. B.III.1.c).

The lack of broad-spectrum activity shown by cephamycin C led to efforts to modify its structure. The chemistry used to prepare semisynthetic cephalosporins was not applicable to the cephamycins. It was necessary, therefore, to develop new procedures (KARADY et al. 1972) to produce semisynthetic cephamycin compounds. One of these, now used clinically, is cefoxitin. It was shown to be resistant to destruction by β-lactamases, to be essentially nontoxic and to have a broad spectrum of activity in vitro and in vivo against pathogenic bacteria, including anaerobes (STAPLEY et al. 1979; BIRNBAUM et al. 1978, 1979).

Other cephamycins are under study and development such as cefmetazole (CS 1170) (NAKAO et al. 1976) and the oxacepham called moxalactam (6059S, LY 127935) (YOSHIDA et al. 1980; WISE et al. 1979; NEU et al. 1979a). In laboratory tests these have greater intrinsic activity than has cefoxitin with moxalactam including *Pseudomonas aeruginosa* in its spectrum.

IV. β-Lactams of Novel Structure

Thienamycin, a β-lactam antibiotic with an unusual structure, has been shown in the laboratory to be highly active both in vitro and in vivo against a broad spectrum of gram-positive and gram-negative organisms including *Pseudomonas* (KROPP et al. 1976). TALLEY et al. (1978) and WEAVER et al. (1979), using microserial broth dilutions, confirmed the in vitro activity, including that against anaerobes and organisms resistant to other drugs. The sensitivity of the β-lactam of thienamycin to certain chemical reactions required precautions in the use of the antibiotic for in vitro studies (KAHAN et al. 1979). Recently WILDONGER et al. (1979) described a more stable derivative of thienamycin that retained the parent antibiotics's broad spectrum of activity and its resistance to destruction by β-lactamase (KROPP et al. 1980).

Clavulanic acid, an avid β-lactamase inhibitor (BROWN et al. 1976) is being developed not for use as an antibiotic agent, but to be used synergistically with β-lactamase-labile agents to control organisms producing this enzyme. Laboratory evaluations, using agar, broth, or microtiter broth dilution technique have shown such synergistic activity in vitro against a number of gram-positive and gram-negative organisms, including some anaerobes (READING and COLE 1977; JACKSON et al. 1978; WÜST and WILKINS 1978; WISE et al. 1978; DUMON et al. 1979), and in vivo in mouse protection (HUNTER et al. 1978) and renal infection tests (HEEREMA et al. 1979). Preliminary clinical tests have been reported, indicating effective therapy with amoxycillin-clavulanic acid preparations (GOLDSTEIN et al. 1979; NINANE et al. 1978).

Laboratory studies have been reported recently on another β-lactamase inhibitor, CP-45899. ENGLISH et al. (1978) and RETSEMA et al. (1980) used agar and broth dilution tests, broth checkerboard square procedures, and mouse protection tests to demonstrate the ability of CP-45899 to extend the spectrum of β-lactam antibiotics in vitro and in vivo. The inhibitor used alone is only weakly antibacterial except against *Neisseria gonorrhoeae*. This observation was confirmed by WISE et al. (1980) in their studies comparing the in vitro activities of CP-45899 and clavulanic acid. In general, the activities of the two compounds are quite similar.

Other β-lactams of unusual structure are the epithienamycins, nocardicin A, and the olivanic acid derivatives. The epithienamycins (CASSIDY et al. 1977; STAPLEY et al. 1977) are a family of antibiotics structurally related to thienamycin. Broad spectrum in activity, they are somewhat less active than thienamycin against *Staphylococcus aureus* and show a wide variation in their β-lactamase susceptibility. Nocardicin A has a good gram-negative spectrum including *Pseudomonas* both in vitro, and in vivo in mouse protection tests (NISHIDA et al. 1977; MINE et al. 1977). Several olivanic acid derivatives are reported to have broad-spectrum antibacterial activity and to be potent β-lactamase inhibitors (BROWN et al. 1977, 1979).

B. β-Lactam Laboratory Evaluation Procedures

I. Introduction

The first laboratory evaluation of the compound later called penicillin was, as described in Sect. A.I, FLEMING's observation in 1929 of the inhibition of growth around a colony of a mold contaminant on a plate of *Staphylococcus*. A test for inhibition of growth of various bacteria on an agar plate is still one of the first procedures used in screening potential activity during the development of a new antibacterial chemotherapeutic antibiotic. Indeed, spectrum of activity may distinguish β-lactam antibiotics from each other as much as do the differences in their chemical structures.

The degree and extent of activity of an antibiotic have important implications for its possible therapeutic use. So do many other attributes and activities that will be examined first in the laboratory. These include, for example, determining the effect on in vitro activity of pH, temperature, serum, minerals, or other ingredients of the test media; the stability of the β-lactam agent to β-lactamases; the influence of the inoculum size of the test organisms on inhibitory endpoints; whether at "useful" concentrations the agent acts mainly by inhibiting growth, or by destroying the microorganism; how fast it acts; what its mode of action is; whether microorganisms readily become resistant to it; whether it acts synergistically with other agents; how such laboratory observations should be interpreted in terms of therapeutic significance.

No matter how active or interesting the agent is in vitro, it will be of little practical value as a therapeutic agent if it is not active in vivo. Therefore, while these in vitro studies are in progress, preliminary in vivo tests are begun, usually using the mouse as the test animal. These investigations will examine such points as whether the spectrum and relative degree of activity seen in vitro are also seen in vivo; whether the compound is effective by the oral route; whether it can be detected in serum, urine, and other tissues; whether it is toxic, is long acting, and is therapeutic as well as protective.

Some of the tests used in the laboratory evaluation of β-lactam and other antibiotics are discussed below. As a matter of convenience, they are divided into in vitro and in vivo catagories.

II. In Vitro Test Procedures

1. Spectrum of Activity and Sensitivity Tests

As mentioned above, the degree and extent of its activity are of major importance in the initial assessment of an antibiotic. Methods used in studying β-lactam agents include those listed below.

a) Trench and Streak Tests

The trench or ditch test used by FLEMING in 1929 and the streak plate procedure used by REID in 1935 with penicillin (see Sect. A.I) are rarely used now. For a more commonly used agar streak test, the antibiotic is mixed with melted, cooled agar, which is then poured immediately into petri dishes. When set, the surface is inoculated with the test organisms. As described and used for penicillin testing by CLUTTERBUCK et al. (1932), this method measures the activity of a single concentration of the antibiotic.

b) Paper Strip Method

The principle of the ditch test is applied in the paper strip method. Here the organisms are streaked on the surface of an agar plate. A filter-paper strip saturated with the test antibiotic is placed at right angles across the streaks and the plate is incubated. In this case, the antibiotic diffuses away from the paper into the agar. Interpretation of sensitivity depends on the degree of inhibition of growth near the strip.

c) Agar Cup-Plate Method

For many years, reservoirs for solutions in the testing of antiseptics and disinfectants consisted of circular wells cut into the surface of seeded agar (ROSE and MILLER 1939). Rather than using such wells, ABRAHAM et al. (1941) placed specially prepared short cylinders of glass tubing on the surface of the seeded agar. The cylinders were filled with solutions of the antibiotic that then diffused into the agar, inhibiting the growth of the test organism. This procedure can be used both to assay the potency of known agents, or to measure activity of unknown materials. Cylinders, of stainless steel rather than glass, are still in use today, but in highly controlled and standardized procedures to determine the antibiotic potencies of market products as well as those of physiologic fluids and laboratory stock solutions.

d) Disc Test

The cup method described in Sect. c) was replaced in some laboratories by a filter paper disc modification (VINCENT and VINCENT 1944) for determining antibiotic potency. BONDI et al. (1947) used discs to determine the susceptibility of clinical cultures to antibiotics. For this purpose the filter paper disc is dipped into a solution of the antibiotic, excess solution is removed by touching the disc against the wall of the antibiotic-containing tube, and the saturated disc is placed on the surface of the inoculated plates. Similar procedures are used today in antibiotic screening and development programs.

e) Minimal Inhibitory Concentration (MIC)

α) Broth Dilution Test. To determine the degree of penicillin activity FLEMING (1929) used a broth tube-dilution test. Such a test is commonly used to determine the minimal inhibitory concentration (MIC) of a test compound. Serial dilutions (usually but not necessarily twofold) of the antibiotic are made in, or added to, broth that is distributed to series of tubes. Each tube in a series then is inoculated with a test organism. After suitable incubation, the tubes are examined and the endpoint recorded as the lowest concentration of antibiotic that prevents visible growth. Such broth dilution tube tests can be used to determine both the spectrum and the MIC of an antibiotic as was done, for example, for cephaloridine by MUGGLETON et al. (1964). Recently, the broth MIC test has been miniaturized and automated to save both time and material. The microtiter systems make use of plastic trays of small wells into which test materials are placed by hand-held or machine-operated dispenser and diluting equipment. The total content of each well is 0.2 ml or less, depending on the system used. The endpoints are read manually or electronically. Other automated systems use small vials or tubes with a series of dilutions to obtain MIC values; some use one or two concentrations of the test materials, measure and plot the growth of the organisms, and calculate and record the MIC from the growth curve. The automated microtiter was used, for example, by BODEY and WEAVER (1976) in their studies of cefamandole. Such microdilution techniques have been developed for use in testing anaerobic bacteria (ROTILIE et al. 1975; MURRAY and CHRISTMAN 1978).

The culture media, conditions of incubation, and other factors of any of the MIC methods may be modified to accommodate the test to the special growth requirements of specific organisms. Other variations permit studying the effect of inoculum size, pH, or medium ingredients (see Sect. B.II.7).

β) Agar Dilution Test. Agar plates containing, usually, twofold dilutions of test antibiotics are inoculated by streaking (BRUMFITT et al. 1974; NISHIDA et al. 1969) or by depositing on the surface a drop of culture by means of a loop (KATO et al. 1978) or some mechanical inoculum replicator such as that described by STEERS et al. (1959). Such a replicator device allows depositing 20 or more organisms on a single plate at one time. These multiple inoculators are commonly used as, for example, by THADEPALLI et al. (1979), who compared the activities of some penicillins and cephalosporins against 900 clinical isolates, and by O'CALLAGHAN et al. (1976a, b) in their work with cefuroxime. As in the broth tests, conditions of the agar-dilution test may be modified to provide special information.

Standard methods for both agar and broth dilution tests have been proposed by ERRICSON and SHERRIS (1971).

γ) Gradient Plate Test. In serial dilution series, the antibiotic concentration decreases stepwise according to the dilution increment used. Szybalski (in BRYSON and SZYBALSKI 1952) devised a method to prepare agar plates having a very gradual proportional increase of the antibiotic concentration along one axis – the gradient axis. A bottom layer of plain agar is poured and allowed to harden while the plate is so slanted that the entire bottom is just covered with agar. The second, antibiotic-containing, layer is poured over the hardened layer while the plate is in a normal horizontal position. The antibiotic diffuses downward and becomes diluted in proportion to the thickness of the two layers, forming a gradient of concentration that remains stable for several days. Standardized bacterial cultures are streaked parallel to the concentration gradient axis. After incubation, the endpoints are calculated from the proportion of the length of growth of the streak and the concentration of the antibiotic added to the agar (WICK 1972). In the initial studies with cephalothin GODZESKI et al. (1961, 1963) used this procedure particularly because of the ease of detecting small differences between different antibiotics, and because it gave some indication of the nature of inhibition, as demonstrated by sharpness of the endpoint at the termination of the streak. Other gradient plate procedures and modifications are discussed by HARTMAN (1968), who feels the potential of the gradient plate in diagnostic bacteriology has not been realized.

f) Minimal Bactericidal (or Lethal) Concentrations (MBC, MLC)

All of the tests in Sect. e measure the ability of the antibiotic to inhibit growth. The question arises as to whether the agent is only, or mainly, inhibitory, i.e., bacteriostatic, in its action, or whether it actually kills the microorganism and is therefore a bactericidal agent. If it is bacteriostatic at therapeutically used concentrations, the defense mechanisms of the infected host may eliminate the organism whose growth is being inhibited by the antibiotic. Should, however, the antibiotic agent be eliminated or inactivated before the infective organisms are destroyed, there is the possibility that the surviving bacteria may grow and cause reinfection or relapse.

Almost every antibacterial agent is bactericidal at some concentration, and bacteriostatic at other, lesser concentrations. A comparison or ratio between such -cidal and -static concentrations permits designation of the predominant in vitro activity. If the MBC/MIC ratio is small, say 2 or 4, the agent is said to be mainly bactericidal in action; if the difference is large (16-fold or more) the designation bacteriostatic is assigned.

β-Lactam antibiotics may cause the lysis of bacteria. A clear distinction between three types of antimicrobial effects of penicillins (inhibition of growth, killing of bacteria, and lysis) has been demonstrated. Such studies are reviewed by TOMASZ (1979) and in Chapt. 2 of this volume. A consideration of the antibiotic concentrations achieved during therapy at the site of infection in a host may indicate the probable type of action of the agent during treatment.

To determine in vitro the lowest concentration of antibiotic that kills rather than merely inhibits the growth of an organism, subcultures are made on agar plates from tubes of broth MIC tests. The interpretation of bactericidal activity is specified variously by different workers as the lowest concentration of antibiotic from which no colonies are detected after incubation (WALLICK and HENDLIN 1974; GOERING et al. 1978) or the lowest concentration from which only a few, say fewer than three viable colonies, are recovered (ADAMS et al. 1976). If actual plate counts of the original inoculum and the surviving organisms are made, the percentage kill can be calculated. The bactericidal concentration is that amount that killed 99.9% of the original inoculum (BARRY and SABATH 1974). Endpoints may also be determined by subculturing from broth MIC tubes to other broth tubes. Absence of growth in the subculture tube indicates the bactericidal action of the antibiotic in the MIC tube (NAUMANN 1966). In all of these tests, consideration must be given to the concentration of antibiotic as well as to the amount of the original inoculum that could be carried over to the subculture tube or plate.

2. Speed of Action Test

Viable counts are determined at intervals during the incubation of antibiotic-containing broth cultures of the test organism (MILLER et al. 1972a). NISHIDA et al. (1977) performed such tests on both growing and stationary phase populations of *Pseudomonas*. Against growing cells, both carbenicillin and nocardicin A were active; against cells from the stationary phase, only nocardicin showed some, though relatively weak, activity. Such observations recall the report by HOBBY et al. (1942) that penicillin appears to be an effective agent only when active bacterial multiplication is taking place.

3. Susceptibility Disc Test

Antibiotic-containing diffusion discs have been used for many years to determine the probable susceptibility of a clinically isolated organism to therapy. Filter paper discs containing the test antibiotic are available commercially. Government regulations and controls have helped standardize the content and potencies of the antibiotics in discs produced by different manufacturers. The producing companies provide clear instructions for the proper storage of the discs. Test procedures and interpretations have also been standardized and controlled. In 1966 BAUER et al. published the procedure, now commonly called the Bauer-Kirby or the Kirby-Bauer test, to determine the antibiotic susceptibility of aerobic, rapidly growing organisms. A modification of this procedure and its interpretation is described in the package circular of all antimicrobial discs sold in the United States. The National Committee for Clinical Laboratory Standards (NCCLS 1975 and supplement, to be published) has published this method in a handbook that includes detailed instructions for performing and interpreting the test. Briefly, dried plates of Mueller-Hinton agar are inoculated with a standardized suspension of the test organisms. Antibiotic-containing discs are placed on the inoculated surface. After incubation the diameters of the zones of inhibition are read and recorded. It is important to realize that zones around discs containing different drugs are not to be compared to determine the relative activity of these drugs. A zone size interpretive chart is used to determine whether the organism being tested is resistant, susceptible, or intermediate in its sensitivity to the antibiotic. Specified control cultures, included in each test, must produce prescribed endpoints to assure the validity of the test. A thorough discussion of the preparation, control, and use of such antibiotic discs has been written by RIPPERE (1980). He comments not only on the commercially available discs but also on those being prepared in a research laboratory.

The primary purpose of this disc susceptibility test is to enable the selection of those antibiotic agents that could be used therapeutically for inhibition of the microorganism. For this purpose an infection caused by a "susceptible" organism should be amenable to treatment by that agent used at the recommended dosage, infections by strains of "intermediate sensitivity" may respond to high dosages of the agent, while infections caused by "resistant" strains would not be expected to respond to therapy by this agent (NCCLS 1975).

To simplify routine susceptibility testing, the disc of a single representative of each group of antimicrobial agents often is used as a "class disc" (NCCLS 1975, p. 2). Cephalothin was used as the class disc for the earlier cephalosporin agents. With the introduction of cefamandole, cefoxitin, and cefuroxime however, it became obvious that differences in spectrum required the inclusion of discs of these antibiotics in addition to that of cephalothin for accurate assessment of susceptibility (BARRY et al. 1979; O'CALLAGHAN et al. 1976b; STAPLEY et al. 1979; NCCLS 1975, supplement, to be published). This will of course be true for the newer agents (SUTHERLAND and ROLINSON 1978) such as those active against *Pseudomonas*.

The clinical importance of this concern over class discs lies in the fact, mentioned above, that the zone diameters are reported in terms of "susceptible" to "resistant" by referring to an interpretive chart. Such charts are based on the assumption that there is a relationship between the zone size and the MIC of susceptible organisms, and that the "susceptible" designation takes into consideration the amount of antibiotic achieved in the body by recommended therapeutic doses. A class cephalothin disc, for example, might designate as resistant an organism such as *Legionella pneumophila* that is "susceptible" to a cefoxitin or cefuroxime disc.

The amount of antibiotic that should be used in sensitivity discs is determined by plotting zone sizes from discs containing various amounts of the antibiotic against MIC values. A linear relationship is plotted mathematically to obtain a "regression line." From such lines the decision is made that determines which disc concentration and which zone diameters shall be used on the charts for the susceptibility determinations. Discussions on the regression curve are found in BROWN and BLOWERS (1978) and ACAR (1980).

4. Interaction and Synergy Tests

The clinical significance of laboratory demonstrations of interactions between two drugs is often questioned. Tests for synergy, potentiation, or antagonism, however, are performed and the data produced are taken into consideration when the probable therapeutic usefulness of an antibiotic is being discussed.

The classic test for interaction applies antibiotic-containing discs or filter paper strips placed in proximity to each other on seeded agar plates. Observation of the enhancement or suppression of growth inhibition in the area of overlapping diffusion is interpreted as synergy or antagonism respectively (DYE 1956). Perhaps more sophisticated is the "checkerboard square" test, in which each of a series of broth or agar dilution concentrations of one agent is combined with each of the series of dilutions of the second agent. This method has been used for many years (PATTE et al. 1958; SABATH et al. 1966) and has now been adapted to automated equipment, using multipoint inoculators on agar plates, or microtiter techniques for broth tests. The growth responses of such tests are plotted in the form of isobolograms to determine the type of interaction. Such an agar-incorporation technique was used by SLACK et al. (1979) to study the interaction of cefsulodin and gentamicin and of cefsulodin and cefuroxime against *Pseudomonas aeruginosa*. Synergistic, additive, indifferent or antagonistic interactions were observed, depending on the strain of organism tested.

The interaction of fixed combinations of two agents can be tested using appropriate controls in speed of action tests (Sect. B.II.2) or the MIC tests (Sect. B.II.e) described above. An MIC method was used by TYBRING and MELCHIOR (1975) to show synergy between mecillinam and ampicillin, while NEU (1976) studied the synergistic activity of mecillinam and a number of β-lactam antibiotics by four different methods – the checkerboard square test in broth, the checkerboard square test in agar, fixed ratios in broth, and titrating in agar one antibiotic in the presence of a constant concentration of the other.

The use of one agent directed against β-lactamases to synergize the antibacterial action of a more potent but enzyme-sensitive second agent has long been studied. Combinations of enzyme-resistant methicillin, cloxacillin, or nafcillin with ampicillin or cephalosporins were moderately successful in laboratory tests (GREENWOOD and O'GRADY 1975) and in clinical trials (SABATH et al. 1967). More potent enzyme inhibitors are the novel β-lactam agents clavulanic acid and CP-45899. As discussed in Sect. A.IV, clavulanic acid has been shown to be synergistic with enzyme-labile agents both in the laboratory and clinically. At the time of writing, only laboratory studies have been reported for CP-45899. KROGSTAD and MOELLERING (1980) have reviewed those and other methods of testing antibiotic interactions, and also have discussed the mechanisms of such interactions. They list the following presently known interactions resulting in synergism: sequential inhibition of a common biochemical pathway, as with mecillinam or vancomycin plus β-lactams; inhibition of or decreased production of β-lactamase, as with clavulanic acid or chloramphenicol plus penicillin; sequential inhibition of cell wall synthesis, again as mecillinam or vancomycin plus β-lactams; and the use of a β-lactam to permit the increased entry of aminoglycosides, as with penicillin plus streptomycin or carbenicillin plus gentamicin. Other possible interactions are mentioned.

5. Effect on Morphology

FLEMING (1929) first described the bacteriolytic action of penicillin. GARDNER (1940) reported the extreme elongation of bacterial cells in subinhibitory concentrations of penicillin (see Sect. A.I) and commented on its possible chemotherapeutic significance. Such elongation, or filament formation, is caused by subinhibitory concentrations of many β-lactam antibiotics. LORIAN (1980) includes a section on in vitro techniques in his review of the effects of subminimum inhibitory concentrations of antibiotics on bacteria. These include a relatively simple screening method using a cover glass print of the edge of a zone of inhibition on a disc diffusion plate. The cover glass, pressed gently along the edge of the zone, is removed, stained, and examined microscopically to observe the organisms transferred from the plate to the cover glass. In the membrane technique, organisms are grown on a filter membrane placed on the surface of an agar plate. The membrane can then be transferred to antibiotic-containing agar plates for various time periods of growth before being returned to drug-free agar for examination. This membrane procedure has been used by LORIAN (1975) in his studies on the effect of such sub-MIC of penicillin on staphylococci. GRASSI et al. (1980) used this same method to show that short exposures to sub-MIC of penicillin and some non-β-lactam agents did not substantially modify the MIC for his test bacteria, nor was there a modification of the emergence of "one-step" mutants resistant to the antibiotics. ZIMMERMAN and STAPLEY (1976) examined the morphology of bacterial cells grown in antibiotic-containing broth. Using a non-β-lactamase-producing *Enterobacter cloacae* and a number of β-lactam antibiotics, they noted a possible relationship between filament induction and the molecular nature of the constituents in the 7- or 6-position of the β-lactams. LORIAN (1980) suggests that determining the MAC (the lowest concentration of an antibacterial agent that can affect bacterial structure) may have significance because of the known good clinical response of patients whose sera contained considerably less than the MIC of a therapeutic agent.

6. Procedures Using Anaerobes

For many years the difficulties and lack of standardization of anaerobic test methods resulted in such procedures not being included in routine evaluations. With the introduction of more manageable equipment and the publication of standardized methodology (SUTTER et al. 1975; HOLDEMAN et al. 1977) such tests became more common and led to an increased awareness of the importance of anaerobic organisms as human pathogens. Many of the penicillins and cephalosporins inhibit the growth of most of the anaerobic cocci, *Clostridium* sp. and the gram-negative anaerobic bacilli except for *Bacteroides fragilis*. This latter organism, the anaerobe most frequently isolated from human infections, is only moderately sensitive to the currently available cephalosporins probably because it produces a potent β-lactamase. Cefoxitin, a cephamycin, resistant to the *Bacteroides fragilis* lactamase (DARLAND and BIRNBAUM 1977), is highly active against this organism (WATT 1979), as are the newer 7-methoxycephalosporins (DORNBUSCH et al. 1980).

In vitro anaerobic test procedures used in studying the β-lactam antibiotics include agar and broth dilution as well as agar diffusion tests using anaerobic jars (WERNER et al. 1979) or glove boxes for incubation (ROY et al. 1977). WILKINS and THIEL (1973) introduced a broth-disc method. Commercial discs are used as the source of the antibiotic. The antibiotic is allowed to elute from the disc into broth which is then inoculated and incubated to determine the growth of the test organism. All procedures are carried out anaerobically, and only a single concentration of antibiotic is tested. KURZYNSKI et al. (1976) modified this method to allow the aerobic incubation of the disc-containing tubes, JORGENSEN et al. (1980) modified it by changing the culture medium but incubating anaerobically, and WEST and

WILKINS (1980) modified the original method to use aerobically prepared medium that after inoculation was overlaid with vaspar. In each case, only a single concentration of the antibiotic agent was tested.

In an effort to standardize test procedures so that reproducible results could be obtained routinely, a working group for the National Committee for Clinical Laboratory Standards, after studying currently used methods, suggested an agar dilution test. A collaborative study was conducted in 10 laboratories where the MIC values of six antibiotics were determined against 10 bacterial strains on Wilkins-Chalgren agar prepared by three manufacturers (SUTTER et al. 1979). The method proved to be sufficiently reproducible to allow recommendation of the procedure as a reference method (NCCLS 1979).

ROSENBLATT et al. (1979) compared several anaerobic susceptibility test procedures and found good agreement between a microdilution broth test and the NCCLS proposed procedure. The Wilkins-Thiel broth-disc test showed a number of discrepancies with the NCCLS test, particularly with tetracycline. JORGENSEN et al. (1980) also reported that their modified broth-disc test results compared favorably with those from the NCCLS method except for tetracycline.

7. Factors Influencing In Vitro Tests

It is extremely important to standardize and control test procedures because of the many factors that can influence the end results. WICK (1972) describes how differences in the test procedures resulted in conflicting results in the early in vitro studies of cephalothin. The influence of culture medium ingredients, pH, inoculation, incubation, and the reading of zones on the reproducibility of disc methods of sensitivity testing are some of the factors discussed by BROWN and BLOWERS (1978) in their review of such test methods. THRUPP (1980) describes the effect of some of these and other factors influencing susceptibility tests run in liquid media.

The size of the inoculum is of extreme importance when the test strains may produce antibiotic-destroying enzymes such as β-lactamases. GARROD (1960a) credits Pamela M. Waterworth with devising the heavy inoculum method used to study resistant staphylococci. CLEELAND and GRUNBERG (1980) also comment on inoculum size as well as on incubation time, the effect of serum binding, the need to adjust test conditions as much as possible to approximate in vivo conditions, and the proper maintenance of test cultures.

The influence of test techniques on results obtained for some β-lactam compounds is the subject of several recent papers (RYLANDER et al. 1979; MASUDA et al. 1979).

8. Enzymes and Resistance to β-Lactam Antibiotics

Many bacteria produce enzymes capable of degrading β-lactam antibiotics. Such organisms may or may not be resistant to the antibacterial action of these agents. The distinction between "penicillinase" and "cephalosporinase" was noted by NEWTON and ABRAHAM (1955) (Sect. A.II) and ABRAHAM and CHAIN (1940) stated, as quoted in Sect. A.I above, that the production of a β-lactamase was not the sole factor determining bacterial sensitivity to the β-lactam antibiotics. SABATH and

FINLAND (1967) showed that β-lactamase and bacterial resistance do not always correlate, and said that information about "other factors" determining resistance was, at that time, only fragmentary. ONISHI et al. (1974) discussed the complexity of the relationship between β-lactamase and basic tolerance. O'CALLAGHAN (1979) points out that unless a β-lactamase-resistant antibiotic can penetrate the bacterial cell wall, it cannot inhibit the growth of the lactamase-producing organism, and DORNBUSCH et al. (1980) speculate that the resistance of some few strains of *Bacteroides* to lactamase-resistant cephamycins may be of intrinsic nature because of changes in the cell wall.

There are many β-lactam-degrading enzymes produced by bacteria (SYKES and MATTHEW 1976, 1979). These and their significance to β-lactam antibiotics are discussed in Chap. 12 of this volume.

9. Automation and Miniaturization

Reference has been made in Sects. B.II.1.e and B.II.4 to the use of automated or miniaturized in vitro laboratory procedures. A number of the systems used for such tests are available commercially ("Autobac I" and "Autobac MIC," Pfizer Inc; "MS 2," Abbott; "Autotiter," Canalco Inc; "MIC-2000," Dynatech Laboratories; "Micro Media," Micro Media Laboratories; " Sensititer," Gibco). Some of these make use of special antibiotic-containing discs, called elution discs. The agent is eluted from the disc into a fluid medium, rather than diffusing from the disc into agar as in the disc-diffusion susceptibility test. Inoculated broth and the test discs are dispensed, resulting growth is monitored, and endpoints calculated, all automatically in ways varying with the test system. In other procedures, culture medium is dispensed and antibiotic dilutions made automatically in, for example, microdilution trays. The serial dilutions may then be seeded automatically. After incubation and the reading and recording of the MIC, subcultures for MBC readings can be made automatically. Serially diluted antibiotics may be dispensed into microdilution trays that are stored frozen until needed. Such frozen trays are available commercially, as are trays in which the antibiotic dilutions have been dried by lyophilization. A discussion of these systems and procedures for their use are given in THORNSBERRY's recent review (1980).

10. In Vitro Models to Simulate In Vivo Conditions

Although determining bacterial sensitivities or minimal inhibitory concentrations is the conventional way to assess the potential therapeutic efficacy of antibiotics, it is generally agreed that the procedures used do not reproduce the in vivo situation in which the agent will be used. In the body, for example, after intermittent doses the antibiotic concentration changes with time. Depending on the rapidity of elimination from the host, the antibiotic is in contact with the infecting organism for a much shorter time than is the case in an MIC test.

To simulate the variation of antibiotic concentration in the blood stream following therapy, NISHIDA et al. (1976) devised an assay procedure to determine bactericidal activity in periodically modified antibiotic concentrations. This in vitro pharmacokinetic model was used by LEITNER et al. (1979) to compare the bactericidal activity of three orally active cephalosporins. The authors of this latter study suggested that, in the blood stream, isoactive antibiotics with divergent pharmacokinetic properties may differ in efficacy if the susceptibility of the infecting organism is concentration dependent within the range of drug concentrations occurring in serum.

GRASSO et al. (1978) also described an in vitro model to study the effect of the antibiotic concentration and the rate of elimination of cephalosporins on antibacterial activity. In their system, the antibiotic concentration is modified by the addition of diluent at a constant rate by means of a peristaltic pump. It is of interest that they observed bacterial regrowth when antibiotic concentrations fell below MIC levels. The interval required for regrowth depended, essentially, on the elimination rate of the antibiotic. Studies carried out in a medium containing 4% albumin suggested that, for the cephalosporins and organisms tested, a longer half-life might be more useful than higher peak levels.

It should be noted that in both these procedures, the cultures are diluted along with the antibiotics. Both LEITNER et al. (1979) and GRASSO et al. (1978) comment on this fact and its influence on the test results.

ANDERSON et al. (1980) used the human urinary bladder model described in 1979 (ANDERSON et al.) to compare the activities of amoxycillin and ampicillin against clinical isolates of *Escherichia coli*. Human urine is used as the culture medium, and a pump transfers materials into the culture chamber which is automatically "emptied" every 4 h. Samples are withdrawn during the test period to determine viable cell counts. The test data, showing amoxycillin to be more rapidly bactericidal than ampicillin although their MIC values were similar, were judged to reflect clinical responses. The authors discuss the advantages of their model over previously described systems, but point out that they have not simulated cyclical changes in urinary antibiotic concentrations found in patients taking repeated doses of antibiotic.

III. In Vivo Test Procedures

The initial animal tests for therapeutic activity of β-lactam and other antibiotics almost always are done with mice. The mouse protection test has been used for many years in the study of chemotherapeutic materials and a large background of information on procedures and the therapeutic activity of known agents has been compiled. General principles of in vivo testing, matters concerned with the infection, the test cultures and test methods and their interpretation are discussed by MILLER (1971) and by CLEELAND and GRUNBERG (1980).

During the course of evaluating an antibiotic agent, animal tests are begun as soon as possible since it is well known that compounds active in vitro are not always active in vivo. When therapeutic activity has been shown, principles demonstrated in vitro are studied in vivo if at all possible. Some of the procedures used to evaluate β-lactam antibiotics are mentioned below.

1. Mouse Protection Test

As the name implies this test is a prophylactic, not a therapeutic one. Groups of mice are infected intraperitoneally with an acutely fatal dose of the test bacterium.

Treatment begins immediately, or at least within an hour, and may be repeated one or more times with the next 6–24 h. The infecting, or challenge, dose is such that all the unprotected control animals die within 24–48 h. The treated mice, several groups given logarithmically spaced dilutions of the antibiotic, will be observed for a longer time, usually 7 days after the infection, before the test is considered complete. Survival records of the final day of the test are used to calculate the amount of drug that would protect 50% of the infected, treated animals, a dose designated the PD_{50} (protective dose for 50% survival) or ED_{50} (the effective dose for 50% survival). Since the injecting dose also was titrated, and a plate count made to determine the number of organisms injected, the LD_{50} (lethal dose of bacteria for death of 50% of the infected untreated mice) also can be calculated, and from that figure the number of LD_{50}s used to challenge the test animals. Uninfected mice given the antibiotic provide data to calculate the TD_{50} (toxic dose for 50% of the uninfected, treated mice) if the test agent is indeed toxic at the concentrations used. A positive control, that is, the inclusion in the test of an agent known to protect against the test organism, checks the validity of the test, as does the inclusion of a group of "stress control" animals. These latter may be animals given appropriate doses of sterile mucin to determine that the batch of mice used in the test are capable of surviving the stress of the test's handling and injecting procedures.

The route of therapy used for parenterally effective drugs may be intramuscular or, more convenient in routine testing, subcutaneous. Experience has shown that PD_{50} values for these two routes generally are similar. Orally effective drugs are given to the mouse by gavage, using a syringe fitted with a blunt-tipped needle. Other routes of treatment (or infection) can be used, i.e., intranasal, intracranial, intravenous, or topical, to investigate special properties of the drug.

As for the in vitro tests, it is important to standardize and control in vivo test procedures as much as possible, to aid in the reproducibility of test results. As shown by MILLER (1971) the ED_{50} and the LD_{50} values for mouse protection tests can be remarkably constant when the cultures and test conditions are controlled properly. The influence of the size of the challenge dose and the route of therapy are also illustrated and discussed.

As an aid in judging the significance of mouse test data it is wise to examine the reported procedures to determine, for example, the number of LD_{50}s in the challenge, the number of mice in a group, the dosage increment used, the length of the observation time, the number and type of controls, the number of replicate tests included in any average figure and the range of variation among replicates.

a) Spectrum of Activity

One of the first questions asked about a new agent is whether in vivo activity can be demonstrated, and, if so, by what route. These questions can be answered easily by using as the infecting organism one known to be sensitive in vitro to the new antibiotic. If activity at a nontoxic concentration of the agent can be demonstrated, the spectrum of in vitro activity is checked as much as possible in vivo. Unfortunately, not all bacteria can be used in mouse protection tests. Some strains have a very low degree of infectivity for the mouse, even when a stressing agent is used to lower the animal's resistance. For some bacteria, acute infections can be established only by using such a large challenge dose that the amount of "foreign protein" being injected is a matter of concern. In such cases the injection of a similar dose of killed bacteria into control animals is used to determine the toxicity of the "infecting" dose. Although it is not possible to test in vivo all the organisms tested in vitro, the reverse usually is not true. Strains used in vivo should be checked for susceptibility in vitro, with proper precaution for their pathogenicity.

b) Interaction and Synergy Tests

The mouse protection test can be used to study the interaction of two antibiotic agents. It will be recalled that FLOREY (1956) attempted to demonstrate in vivo the cephalosporin C competition with penicillin for penicillinase. Although the test was not clear cut, ABRAHAM (1962) reported the potentiation of cephalosporin C therapy by penicillin (Sect. A.II). HUNTER et al. (1978) used conventional mouse protection tests to show the ability of clavulanic acid to protect amoxycillin from destruction by β-lactamase. MILLER and VERWEY (1954), by titrating penicillin in the presence of fixed amounts of sulfonamides, demonstrated synergy for these agents in streptococcal-infected mice. MILLER et al. (1958) reported the broadened spectrum of in vivo activity of combinations of novobiocin and penicillin. For this, mice were given a mixed infection containing both streptococci and penicillin-resistant staphylococci. An amount of penicillin G that was ineffective against the *Staphylococcus* but could protect against the *Streptococcus* was combined with an amount of novobiocin ineffective against the *Streptococcus* but effective against the *Staphylococcus*. All the mice given the mixed infection were protected by this combination of individually ineffective drugs.

A partial, rather than a complete, checkerboard square test for synergy is used in in vivo studies. One of two agents is titrated in the presence of constant amounts (estimated to be 40%, 20%, 10%, and 0%) of the effective dose of the other agent. The second agent then is titrated in the presence of constant amounts of the first, or each of two agents may be administered alone and combined in fixed ratios. This latter procedure was used by GRUNBERG et al. (1976) to show synergy in vivo between mecillinam and other antibiotics.

c) Pharmacological Information

Mouse protection tests automatically provide preliminary pharmacological data in terms of toxicity and absorption. When therapy is given orally, protection indicates absorption from the gastrointestinal tract. The degree of absorption is indicated by a ratio of the parenteral and oral ED_{50} values. Cephalexin, for example, is about as effective orally as it is parenterally in mouse protection tests, indicative of its excellent absorption. For cephradine, also well absorped, GADEBUSCH et al. (1972) showed subcutaneous-oral ED_{50} ratios in mice of 1:1 to 1:3.

Blood, urine and other tissue samples, taken from treated mice, may be assayed to determine the distribution of the antibiotic in the body.

Information on the manner of urinary excretion of β-lactam antibiotics can be obtained by determining the effect of probenecid on the antibiotic concentration in the serum of treated mice or on the therapeutic effectiveness of the agent. Probenecid blocks renal tubular but not glomerular excretion. Its use with cephalothin and other antibiotics that are excreted mainly by renal tubular secretion results in an increase in the peak concentration and persistence of these agents in the serum. There is no similar enhancement of cephaloridine or other antibiotics that are excreted mainly by glomerular filtration. The use of probenecid in mouse tests to indicate the manner of excretion has been reported by MILLER et al. (1972b, 1974) and by RYAN et al. (1976), and the demonstration that the probenecid-produced increases in antibiotic concentrations in mice are therapeutically useful has been demonstrated by MILLER et al. (1972b, 1974) and by MATTIE and KUNST (1978).

The biliary excretion of some cephalosporins and their derivatives was examined in cannulated rats by WRIGHT and LINE (1980). They point out the effect of the molecular weight of the compound on the degree of biliary excretion; above a threshold molecular weight of about 450, biliary excretion increased in a "generally progressive way, becoming the principal route of excretion of the higher-molecular-weight derivatives." This effect should be taken into consideration when agents for human use are evaluated in this test procedure.

A method using rats to assess the degree of pain associated with the injection of β-lactam antibiotics has been developed (CELOZZI et al. 1980). Each antibiotic is injected into the subplantar tissue of a hind paw of each of eight rats. At intervals between 3 and 15 min after the injection, each animal is observed for 1 min, and the number of paw-licking responses noted and recorded. The observations are compiled and the data treated statistically to compare the response of the treated with that of control animals. Test results of the known agents studied correlated with clinical observations.

Measurements for the pharmacokinetics and for the toxicity of β-lactam antibiotics are subjects of Chaps. 15 and 16 of this volume.

d) Effect on Morphology

The in vivo bacteriolytic activity of two related β-lactam antibiotics was studied by COMBER et al. (1977a). Samples of blood or peritoneal washings of infected, treated animals were obtained, assayed for antibiotic content, and examined microscopically to observe bacterial morphology. At comparable concentrations, amoxycillin had greater bacteriolytic activity in vivo than did ampicillin. This observation suggested a probable explanation for the superior in vivo activity of amoxycillin compared with that of ampicillin (see Sects. B.II.10 and B.IV).

2. Specialized Test Procedures

In addition to the mouse protection and pharmacological tests mentioned above, other procedures are performed to obtain specific information. For example, withholding therapy after infection or withholding infection after therapy can be used to measure curative or long-acting properties respectively (MILLER 1971). Some other tests using special techniques to evaluate β-lactam antibiotics are discussed below.

a) Pyelonephritis or Urinary Tract Infection Tests

MILLER (1971) mentions a number of rat and mouse models used to investigate urinary tract infections and discusses some of the factors affecting these tests and their interpretation. COMBER et al. (1977 b) describe the use of their mouse model and COMMINCHAU et al. (1976) explain their procedure for establishing a chronic pyelonephritis in rats. In both tests, a "stressing agent" is used to aid in establishing the infection. In the mouse test, infection by the intravenous route was followed by several daily intramuscular injections of iron sorbitol citrate to promote the growth of the organism in the kidney. Therapy starts after the first iron sorbitol citrate injection and continues for 4 days. Treated and control mice are killed, starting 7 days after infection, and the kidneys examined both macroscopically and by bacterial counts of homogenates for evidence of the infection. The chronic infection in rats is established after lowering host resistance by weekly intramuscular injections of estradiolundecylate. After the first week, the infecting organism is instilled directly into the bladder. A second infecting dose is given a week later and 10 days after that, treatment is begun. At the completion of the test, the animals are killed and infection assessed by bacterial counts of kidney homogenates.

ZAK et al. (1980) did not use a stressing agent in the pyelonephritis test in their studies of β-lactam agents. The infecting organisms were injected directly into the parenchyma of the rat kidney. After therapy and the completion of the experiment, bacterial recoveries were made from kidney homogenates. Interestingly, they injected a non-β-lactamase producing organism into one kidney and its enzyme-producing mutant into the other. Cefotiam and cefuroxime treatment reduced the count in both kidneys, while ampicillin treatment was effective only in the kidney infected with the β-lactamase-negative strain. MATTIE et al. (1973) and MATTIE and KUNST (1978) produced an infection in the renal parenchyma of mice by injecting *Staphylococcus aureus* intravenously. Therapy, in these cases with β-lactam agents, was given shortly after infection. The animals were killed 24 or 30 h after infection and bacterial counts were made of kidney homogenates. These studies investigated the effect of serum binding and demonstrated the potentiation of antibiotic activity by probenecid. ZAK et al. (1978) injected *Pseudomonas aeruginosa* intravenously into mice conditioned by an intravenous injection of carrageenan. The resulting renal infection was lethal to untreated mice. When therapy was used, it was started 1 h after infection and continued for 5 days. Two days later, surviving animals were killed and the number of viable organisms in the kidneys was determined. Thus both percent survival and "sterilization" of the kidney could be reported.

b) Experimental Meningitis

β-Lactam antibiotics have been tested for efficacy in experimental meningitis caused by a number of organisms. In the majority of tests, the experimental animal has been the rabbit, and the infection has been given intravenously or intracisternally, usually following a cisternal tap. For example, an intravenous infection with *Streptococcus pneumoniae* type III, following a cisternal tap, was used by BEATY and WALTERS (1979). SCHELD et al. (1979) injected *Escherichia coli* or *Klebsiella pneumoniae* intracisternally, BEAM and ALLEN (1980) used *Escherichia coli* and PERFECT et al. (1980), *Haemophilus influenzae* B as the infecting organism intracisternally. The method of restraining and handling the animals differed, but in all cases meningitis of varying severities developed.

The infant rat was used by MOXON et al. (1977) in their work with ampicillin treatment of *Haemophilus influenzae* B. Animals infected intranasally first develop a bacteremia and those with 10^4 or more organisms/ml blood (determined by culture) develop meningitis that produces about a 10% mortality. A mouse model described by TSAI et al. (1975) induces a fatal pneumococcal meningitis by injecting the organism intracranially through the right orbital surface of the zygomatic bone.

c) Enterococcal Endocarditis

Combinations of penicillins or cephalosporins with aminoglycosides have been tested for synergy against enterococcal endocarditis in rabbits. A reproducible endocarditis with vegatations on the aortic valve can be established by the intravenous injection of the test organisms into rabbits that have had a cannula inserted through the right carotid artery into the left ventricle. Such a procedure was used, for example, by CARRIZOSA and KAYE (1976) and by LINCOLN et al. (1977). The infection can be followed by culturing blood samples and, at the completion of the test, by removing, weighing and culturing the aortic vegetations.

d) Penetration into Extravascular Tissues

For an antibiotic agent to be effective therapeutically it must reach the site of infection. Often this site is an avascular abscess. BARZA and WEINSTEIN (1974) and BARZA et al. (1974a, b) studied the penetration of antibiotics into fibrin clots implanted subcutaneously in rabbits. They felt the level of ampicillin in the clot after an intravenous injection of the antibiotic resembled that found in abscesses established in the same animal. Working with some penicillins, they demonstrated in the clots higher concentration of weakly serum-bound antibiotics than of strongly bound agents. The influence of the dosage schedule, intermittent bolus or continuous infusion, and the effect of probenecid on antibiotic concentrations also could be shown.

Devices other than clots may be implanted in rabbits, for example, Visking chambers (PETERSON and GERDING 1978) or diffusion chambers (GEORGOPOULOS and SCHULTZE 1980) from which accumulated fluids can be withdrawn for study. Rather than using chambers, TARYLE et al. (1980) collected normal pleural fluid from the treated rabbits and created a sterile inflammatory exudative pleural effusion that could then be infected to cause an empyema.

These and other methods have been devised to create situations somewhat resembling those in which agents will be used clinically, and to provide information not always obtainable from mouse protection tests.

Recently RYAN (1979) suggested a simple and novel method for measuring concentrations of antibiotics in tissue fluids. In mice, lengths of sterilized cotton threads were inserted under depilated skin, one thread per mouse. Twentyfour hours later the test antibiotic, in this case cefuroxime, was injected intraperitoneally. At given times after the dose, the thread was removed and assayed by a specially devised procedure. A blood sample taken from the mouse at the time the thread was withdrawn, also was assayed. Comparison then could be made of serum and tissue concentrations. Ryan adapted this method for use in human volunteers, and concluded from his study that the "thread technique provides a convenient and well tolerated method which will be useful for determining extravascular concentrations of antibiotics in experimental animals and human volunteers."

e) Others

Other in vivo test procedures used for examining β-lactam antibiotics include intradermal infections to study local lesions, keratitis for eye infections, and osteomyelitis for bone infections. As examples, FROST and VALIANT (1964) used a penicillin-resistant *Staphylococcus* to produce a local lesion for treatment with cephalosporin derivatives. Their paper includes a statistical procedure for evaluating the test data. ZAK et al. (1980) used cefotiam as the test agent in an experimental keratitis in guinea pigs (using the procedure of DAVIS and CHANDLER 1975) and NORDEN and KENNEDY (1970, 1971) included cephalothin in the treatment agents for a *Staphylococcus aureus* induced osteomyelitis in rabbits. In this latter model, although lincomycin-treated rabbits had less severe bone disease than did cephalothin-treated animals, both agents were effective. Their data were interpreted to indicate that there was not a simple relationship between the level of antibiotic in bone and the likelihood of its sterilizing that tissue.

3. Tests Using Anaerobes

WILKINS and SMITH (1974) described a mouse test using for infection a strain of *Fusobacterium necrophorum* that had been isolated from a case of sheepfoot rot. This strain not only caused the formation of abscesses in the mouse but also was sufficiently virulent to permit the use of death or survival of the mouse as the measure of effectiveness of the therapeutic agent tested. KUCK (1975) used a strain of *F. necrophorum* isolated from a human clinical case and capable of producing lesions in mice. The effectiveness of therapy of the subcutaneously induced infection was based on the number of mice in the test group that showed no macroscopic lesions at the completion of the observation period.

Deep-seated abscesses were produced in mice infected with a mixture of *F. necrophorum* and *F. nucleatum*, but β-lactam antibiotics were not tested in this model (HILL 1977). Nor were they tested in the mixed aerobic and anaerobic organism intraabdominal infection established in rats by the inplantation of capsules containing rat stool flora. In this test, to establish an animal model that simulated the septic complications occurring after colonic perforation, WEINSTEIN et al. (1974) implanted gelatin capsules containing pooled rat colonic contents and barium sulfate into the pelvic region of rats. Animals surviving an initial peritonitis developed discrete intraabdominal abscesses. The initial lethality is the result primarily of coliform bacteremia, while the abscess formation probably results from synergy between anaerobes and facultative bacteria (ONDERDONK et al. 1976). Such an infection has been used by LOUIE et al. (1977) to test cephalosporins.

A procedure using *Bacteroides fragilis* as the sole infecting agent in mice has not yet been published.

IV. In Vitro–In Vivo Relationships

Although in many instances in vivo activity can be predicted from in vitro test results, this is not always true. Such predictions are particularly difficult when the relative in vitro activities of several agents are compared with their relative activities in vivo. A recent demonstration of this is the work reported by GOERING et al. (1978). Regardless of the comparative in vitro activity of BL-S786, cephalothin, cefamandole, and cefoxitin, BL-S 786 was the most effective drug in the treatment of mice lethally infected with Enterobacteriaceae. COMBER et al. (1975) showed that amoxycillin was more active in mouse protection tests than was ampicillin, despite the equivalency of their MIC values against the infecting organism (see Sect. B.III.1.d). KUNST and MATTIE (1978) developed a thigh lesion model in which inhibition of the growth of the injected bacteria by an antibiotic could be measured quantitatively and so was felt to be comparable with growth inhibition in vitro. After establishing the infection, the test antibiotics were injected, concentrations in the blood were followed and later plotted to determine the "area under the curve," and the antibacterial activity was estimated from bacterial counts made of homogenized thighs. Protein binding of the test agents also was taken into consideration. Their data from a study of cefazolin and cephradine suggested that the prediction of antibacterial activity in vivo solely on the basis of in vitro data and pharmacokinetic parameters is not reliable.

MILLER et al. (1979) used agar MIC, mouse protection tests, and β-lactamase activities to study the activities of four β-lactam antibiotics against each of 12 gram-negative and three gram-positive bacterial cultures. The relative in vitro activities quite accurately predicted the relative in vivo efficacies for cefoxitin versus cefazolin, but not for cefoxitin versus cefamandole or cefoxitin versus cephalothin.

Despite these descrepancies, the accumulation of in vitro data is indeed an important function of the laboratory evaluation of an antibiotic. Valuable information pointing the way to improvements and the development of ever-better agents can be obtained from such data. Just as the interpretation of the information must be tempered with the knowledge that it comes from in vitro tests, so the interpretation of laboratory animal data must be influenced by the knowledge that they come, after all, from animal tests. Most of the infections studied bear no relation to infections in man, nor are the treatment schedules and doses those that would be used in clinical practice. It is particularly difficult, in preliminary laboratory evaluations, to know what allowances, if any, to make for possible pharmacokinetic differences between human and animal processing of the drug. Nevertheless, animal models are of value in the development of, and in predicting the probable clinical usefulness of, antibiotic agents, as has been shown by years of experience.

C. Representative β-Lactam Agents

β-Lactam agents commercially available at the time of writing, as well as some in development, are listed in Tables 1–6. Practically all are bactericidal in action at therapeutic concentrations, are, unless otherwise designated, remarkably nontoxic, and are excreted mainly by urinary tubular secretion. Although the percent protein binding is listed, it must be pointed out that the significance of this figure in terms of therapeutic efficacy is not clear (ROLINSON and SUTHERLAND 1965; WARREN 1965/1966). The percent figures listed in the tables are those for binding to human serum since the degree of binding may vary depending on the kind of serum (as well as on the test procedure) used.

Results of tests to determine stability to enzymatic hydrolysis are also influenced by the test procedure used. The "stability" or "lability" of a compound

Table 1. Natural and semisynthetic penicillins

Name	In vitro spectrum	Susceptibility to penicillinase	% Protein binding	Comment
Penicillin G	Standard [a]	Labile [b]	60 [c]	Not orally active
Penicillin V	Poor G− [d]	Labile [d]	79 [c]	Orally active [e]
Phenethicillin	Mostly G+ [d]	Modestly stable [h]	62 [c]	Oral: better than penicillin V [e]
Propicillin	Mostly G+ [f]	Modestly stable [h]	89 [g]	Oral: better than penicillin V [h]
Methicillin	Mostly pen-resistant staph [i]	Stable [i]	40 [f]	Not oral [j]
Nafcillin	Less than pen G; greater than methicillin [j]	Stable [f]	90 [c]	Oral absorption erratic? [f] Biliary recycling [k]

[a] See text
[b] Abraham and Chain (1940)
[c] Kunin (1967)
[d] Garrod (1960a, b)
[e] Knudsen and Rolinson (1959)
[f] Garrod and O'Grady (1971)
[g] Bond et al. (1963)
[h] Williamson et al. (1961)
[i] Rolinson et al. (1960)
[j] Marcy and Klein (1970)
[k] Warren (1965/1966)
G−, gram-negative; G+, gram-positive; pen, penicillin

Table 2. Isoxazoyl penicillins

Name	In vitro spectrum	Susceptibility to penicillinase	% Protein binding	Comments
Oxacillin	Poor G− [a, b]	Stable [b]	93 [c]	Orally active [b]
Cloxacillin	Poor G− [a, b]	Stable [b]	94 [c]	Better absorbed than oxacillin [b]
Dicloxacillin	Poor G− [a, b]	Stable [b]	97 [c]	Better absorbed than cloxacillin [c]
Flucloxacillin	Poor G− [a, c]	Stable [c]	95 [c]	Equal to or better than dicloxacillin [c]

[a] See text
[b] Marcy and Klein (1970)
[c] Sutherland et al. (1970b)
G−, gram-negative

is sometimes listed as a matter of degree. An inoculum effect (sharp increases in MIC with increasing inocula) is often interpreted to indicate the production, by cells, of enzymes capable of destroying the agent. Both cefotiam and cefsulodin (see Table 4) show such inoculum effects, although both are listed as stable to destruction by cephalosporinase.

The "standard in vitro spectrum" reflects the generalization that penicillins are active against aerobic non-penicillinase-producing staphylococci, pneumococci, streptococci (except *Streptococcus fecalis*), *Neisseria* and *Haemophilus* and many of the anaerobes except for *Bacteroides fragilis*. Most of the Enterobacteriaceae are refractory to penicillins. The penicillinase-resistant methicillin and nafcillin listed in Table 1 are less active than penicillin G except against penicillin-resistant staphylococci. This also is generally true for the orally active penicillinase-stable isoxazoyl penicillins listed in Table 2.

Table 3. Broad spectrum penicillins

Name	In vitro spectrum	Susceptibility to penicillinase	% Protein binding	Comment
Ampicillin	Nonpenase G+ & G−[a, b]	Labile[c]	25[d]	Orally active, good vs. nonpenase *Haemophilus*[c]
Hetacillin	Nonpenase[e] G+ & G−	Labile[e]		Orally active, hydrolyzes in vitro[e] to ampicillin
Amoxycillin	Nonpenase[f] G+ &G−	Labile[f]	17[f]	Activity and oral[g] absorption better than ampicillin
Pivampicillin	Nonpenase[a, b] G+ & G−	Labile		Completely hydrolyzes to and better absorbed than ampicillin[h]
Not orally active				
Carbenicillin	Low G+, nonpenase G−[e]	Labile[e]	47[f]	Good *Pseudomonas* and indol-positive *Proteus*[e] in high dosage
Ticarcillin	As carbenicillin[i]	Mostly labile[i]	45[i]	Better than carbenicillin against *Pseudomonas*[j]
Sulbenicillin	As carbenicillin[k]	Labile[k]	28[k]	Active against *Pseudomonas*[k]
Mezlocillin	Good G−[l]	Mostly labile[l]		Better than carbenicillin against *Pseudomonas*[l]
Piperacillin	Broad, high activity[m]	Labile[n]		Better than carbenicillin against *Pseudomonas*[n]

[a] See text
[b] MARCY and KLEIN (1970)
[c] GARROD and O'GRADY (1971)
[d] KUNIN (1967)
[e] THRUPP (1974)
[f] SUTHERLAND and ROLINSON (1970)
[g] ROLINSON (1973)
[h] VON DAEHNE et al. (1970)
[i] SUTHERLAND et al. (1970a)
[j] ACRED et al. (1970)
[k] TSUCHIYA et al. (1971)
[l] BODEY and PAN (1977)
[m] VERBIST (1978)
[n] UEO et al. (1977)
penase, penicillinase; G+, gram-positive; G−, gram-negative

The "broad spectrum" penicillins in Table 3 are active against some non-penicillinase-producing gram-negative organisms, but are not always so active as penicillin G against the "standard" gram-positive bacteria. Recently, penicillins active against *Pseudomonas* (Table 3) have been announced. These agents are not necessarily resistant to staphylococcal penicillinase, but are able in some way to control *Pseudomonas*.

Table 4. Injectable cephalosporins

Name	In vitro spectrum	Susceptibility to cephalosporinase	% Protein binding	Comment
Cephalothin	Standard[a]	Labile[b]	65[c]	Deacetylated in vivo[b]
Cephapirin	Standard[d]	Labile[d]	50[e]	Deacetylated in vivo[e]
Cephacetrile	Standard[e]	Labile[e]	40[e]	Deacetylated in vivo[e]
Cephaloridine	Standard[e]	Labile[e]	20[e]	Little tubular excretion[f], potentially nephrotoxic[d]
Cefazolin	Improved G– [g]	Labile[d]	74[g]	Little tubular excretion[d], biliary excretion[d]
Cefamandole	Improved G– [h]	Stable[h]	74[d]	In vitro/in vivo discrepancies[i]
Cefuroxime	Improved G– [j]	Stable[j]	33[j]	Excretion glomerular[n], some tubular[d]
Cefotaxime (HR756)	Improved G– [k]	Stable[d]	38[k]	Some *Pseudomonas* and *B. fragilis* activity[k]
Cefotiam (SCE963), CGP 14221E)	Broad-spectrum[l] high activity	Stable[l] but inoculum effect	40[d]	Includes *Haemophilus*[b]
Cefsulodin (SCE129, CGP 7174E)	Narrow[m, o]	Stable[d] but inoculum effect	30[d]	Better than carbenicillin against *Pseudomonas*

[a] See text
[b] WICK (1972)
[c] KIND et al. (1968)
[d] O'CALLAGHAN (1979)
[e] CABANA et al. (1976)
[f] MOELLERING and SWARTZ (1976)
[g] NISHIDA et al. (1969)
[h] WICK and PRESTON (1972)
[i] GOERING et al. (1978)
[j] O'CALLAGHAN et al. (1976a, b)
[k] NEU et al. (1979b)
[l] TSUCHIYA et al. (1978b)
[m] TSUCHIYA et al. (1978a)
[n] RYAN et al. (1976)
[o] SLACK et al. (1979)
G–, gram-negative

The "standard in vitro spectrum" of the cephalosporins includes penicillinase-producing, but not necessarily cephalosporinase-producing organisms. In general, their spectrum of activity includes the aerobic gram-positive organisms, except for *Streptococcus fecalis*, and many gram-negative organisms, except for the cephalosporinase-producing *Enterobacter*, indole-positive *Proteus*, *Providencia*, *Serratia*, and *Pseudomonas* and the anaerobe *Bacteroides fragilis*. Table 4 lists the conventional injectable cephalosporins and some more recently introduced agents that show cephalosporinase-resistance and improved activity against gram-negative organisms. In the first group, cephapirin and cephacetrile are essentially equivalent to cephalothin, and all three are metabolized in the body to some extent to a deacetylated form having less antibacterial activity than the parent compound. Ce-

Table 5. Oral cephalosporins

Name	In vitro spectrum	Susceptibility to cephalosporinase	% Protein binding	Comment
Cephaloglycin	Standard[a, b]	Modestly stable[c]	35[c]	Deacetylated in vivo[c]
Cephalexin	Standard[c]	Stable[c]	15[d]	
Cephradine	Standard[e]	Stable[e]	10[e]	Equivalent to cephalexin[c]
Cefadroxil	Standard[f]	Stable[f]	20[f]	Longer half-life than cephalexin[f]

[a] See text.
[b] WICK and BONIECE (1965)
[c] O'CALLAGHAN (1979)
[d] KIND et al. (1968)
[e] GADEBUSCH et al. (1972)
[f] BUCK and PRICE (1977)

Table 6. 7-α-Methoxycephalosporins, and oxacephem

Name	In vitro spectrum	Susceptibility to cephalosporinase	% Protein binding	Comments
Cefoxitin	Improved G–[a, b]	Stable[c]	65[d]	Active against *B. fragilis*[e]
Cefmetazole (CS 1170)	Improved activity[f]	Stable[g]	85[h]	Active against *B. fragilis*[f]
SQ 14,359	Improved activity[i]	Stable[i]		*B. fragilis ?*[f]
SKF 73678	Improved activity[j]	Stable[j]		*B. fragilis*[j]
Moxalactam (6059S, LY127935)	Improved G–[k, n]	Stable[l]	38[m]	*Pseudomonas*[l] and *B. fragilis*

[a] See text.
[b] WALLICK and HENDLIN (1974)
[c] ONISHI et al. (1974)
[d] MOELLERING and SWARTZ (1976)
[e] WATT (1979)
[f] O'CALLAGHAN (1979)
[g] SUGAWARA et al. (1976)
[h] TACHIBANA et al. (1980)
[i] GADEBUSCH et al. (1978)
[j] URI et al. (1978)
[k] NEU et al. (1979a)
[l] YOSHIDA et al. (1980)
[m] MATSUURA et al. (1978)
[n] WEAVER et al. (1980)
G–, gram-negative

phaloridine, more active than cephalothin against gram-positives, can cause some nephrotoxicity. Cefazolin, with high intrinsic in vitro activity and producing high and prolonged activity in the serum, is said to have substantial biliary (SHIBATA and FUJII 1970) in addition to urinary excretion, and may have the potential for nephrotoxicity (O'CALLAGHAN 1979). Cefuroxime, not yet available in the United States, is, along with cefoxitin (Table 6), resistant to the rather unusual β-lactamase of the Legionnaires' disease organism *Legionella pneumophila* (O'CALLAGHAN 1979; THORNSBERRY et al. 1978; FU and NEW 1979). Several of the newer injectable cephalosporins are active against *Pseudomonas*.

Of the orally active cephalosporins listed in Table 5, cephalexin is more active and metabolically stable than cephaloglycin. Cephradine and cefadroxil are essentially equivalent to cephalexin, although cefadroxil has a longer serum half-life and slower excretion rate than the other two agents (BUCK and PRICE 1977). As was the case for the penicillins, the orally active cephalosporins generally have less intrinsic activity than do the injectable agents.

Of the 7-α-methoxycephalosporins (Table 6), only cefoxitin is available commercially. It has shown good activity clinically against gram-positive and gram-negative aerobic and anaerobic organisms including β-lactamase producers. In the laboratory it also has shown resistance to destruction by β-lactamases including those of *Legionella pneumophila* (FU and NEU 1979) and *Bacteroides fragilis* (DARLAND and BIRNBAUM 1977, TALLY et al. 1979). The newer 7-α-methoxy compounds, including the 1-oxacephalosporin, moxalactam, have greater intrinsic activity in vitro than does cefoxitin. All these compounds are β-lactamase stable and have activity against *Bacteroides fragilis*. The oxacephem also inhibits the growth of *Pseudomonas* (YOSHIDA et al. 1980; REIMER et al. 1980; LANG et al. 1980).

Many other β-lactam antibiotics are currently under study. Undoubtedly, some not mentioned here will be available commercially by the time this volume is published, and other agents with even more potentially exciting attributes will be under development. Certainly many of the procedures enumerated here will be used in testing these compounds, and just as certainly new technology and improved methodology will permit more accurate estimates of the probable value of the compounds.

The final decision regarding the therapeutic effectiveness of an antibiotic depends, of course, on its performance in the clinic. Such a clinical examination, however, is made only of an agent whose potential efficacy was first demonstrated in the laboratory. Many of the procedures used in these laboratory studies have been mentioned and referenced here. Hopefully this review will not only be helpful to those already working in this important field, but will stimulate others to become involved in the interesting and challenging study of the in vitro and in vivo evaluation of antibiotic agents.

References

Abraham EP (1962) The cephalosporins. Pharmacol Rev 14:473–500

Abraham EP, Chain E (1940) An enzyme from bacteria able to destroy penicillin. Nature 146:837

Abraham EP, Loder PB (1972) Cephalosporin C. In: Flynn EH (ed) Cephalosporins and penicillins: chemistry and biology. Academic Press, New York London, pp 3–11

Abraham EP, Newton GGF (1956) A comparison of the action of penicillinase on benzylpenicillin and cephalosporin N and the competitive inhibition of penicillinase by cephalosporin C. Biochem J 63:628–634

Abraham EP, Chain E, Fletcher CM, Gardner AD, Heatley NG, Jennings MA, Florey HW (1941) Further observations on penicillin. Lancet II:177–189

Acar JF (1980) The disc susceptibility test. In: Lorian V (ed) Antibiotics in laboratory medicine. Williams and Wilkins, Baltimore London, pp 24–54

Acred P, Hunter PA, Mizen L, Rolinson GN (1970) α-Carboxy-3-thienylmethylpenicillin (BL 2288), a new semisynthetic penicillin: in vivo evaluation. In: Hobby GL (ed) Antimicrobial agents and chemotherapy. American Society for Microbiology, Bethesda, MD, p 396

Adams HG, Stillwell GA, Turck M (1976) In vitro evaluation of cefoxitin and cefamandole. Antimicrob Agents Chemother 9:1019–1024

Anderson JD, Eftekhar F, Aird MY, Hammond J (1979) Role of bacterial growth rates in the epidemiology and pathogenesis of urinary infections in women. J Clin Microbiol 10:766–771
Anderson JD, Johnson KR, Aird MY (1980) Comparison of amoxicillin and ampicillin activities in a continuous culture model of the human urinary bladder. Antimicrob Agents Chemother 17:554–557
Anderson RC, Lee CC, Worth HM, Chen KK (1955) Pharmacologic and toxicologic studies with penicillin V. In: Welch H, Marti-Ibáñez F (eds) Antibiotic annual. Medical Encyclopedia, New York, pp 540–548
Barry AL, Sabath LD (1974) Special tests: Bactericidal activity and activity of antimicrobics in combination. In: Lennette EH, Spaulding EH, Truant JP (eds) Manual of clinical microbiology, 2nd edn. American Society for Microbiology, Washington DC, pp 431–435
Barry AL, Schoenknecht FD, Shadomy S, Sherris JC, Thornsberry C, Washington JA, Kammer RB (1979) Interpretive criteria for cefamandole and cephalothin disk diffusion susceptibility tests. Antimicrob Agents Chemother 15:140–141
Barza M, Weinstein L (1974) Penetration of antibiotics into fibrin loci in vivo. I. Comparison of penetration of ampicillin into fibrin clots, abscesses and "interstitial fluid." J Infect Dis 129:59–65
Barza M, Samuelson T, Weinstein L (1974a) Penetration of antibiotics into fibrin loci in vivo. II. Comparison of nine antibiotics: Effect of dose and degree of protein binding. J Infect Dis 129:66–72
Barza M, Brusch J, Bergeron MG, Weinstein L (1974b) Penetration of antibiotics into fibrin loci in vivo. III. Intermittent vs continuous infusion and the effect of probenecid. J Infect Dis 129:73–78
Batchelor FR, Doyle FP, Nayler JHC, Rolinson GN (1959) Synthesis of penicillin: 6-aminopenicillanic acid in penicillin fermentations. Nature 183:257–258
Bauer AW, Kirby WMM, Sherris JC, Turck M (1966) Antibiotic susceptibility by a standardized single disc method. Am J Clin Pathol 45:493–496
Beam Jr TR, Allen JC (1980) Comparison of cefamandole, cephalothin, ampicillin, and chloramphenicol in experimental *Escherichia coli* meningitis. Antimicrob Agents Chemother 17:37–42
Beaty HN, Walters E (1979) Pharmacokinetics of cefamandole and ampicillin in experimental meningitis. Antimicrob Agents Chemother 16:584–588
Behrens OK, Corse J, Edwards JP, Garrison L, Jones RG, Soper QF, van Abeele FR, Whitehead CW (1948) Biosynthesis of penicillins. IV. New crystalline biosynthetic penicillins. J Biol Chem 175:793–809
Birnbaum J, Stapley EO, Miller AK, Wallick H, Hendlin D, Woodruff HB (1978) Cefoxitin, a semi-synthetic cephamycin: a microbiological overview. J Antimicrob Chemother [Suppl B] 4:15–32
Birnbaum J, Stapley EO, Miller AK, Celozzi E, Wallick H, Pelak BA, Zimmerman SB, Hendlin D, Woodruff HB (1979) Development of the semi-synthetic cephamycin, cefoxitin as a clinical candidate. Infection [Suppl 1] 7:S13–S20
Bodey GP, Pan T (1977) Mezlocillin: in vitro studies of a new broad spectrum penicillin. Antimicrob Agents Chemother 11:74–79
Bodey GP, Weaver S (1976) In vitro studies of cefamandole. Antimicrob Agents Chemother 9:452–457
Bond JM, Lightbrown JW, Barber M, Waterworth PM (1963) A comparison of four phenoxypenicillins. Br Med J 2:956–961
Bondi A, Spaulding EH, Smith DE, Dietz CC (1947) A routine method for the rapid determination of susceptibility to penicillin and other antibiotics. Am J Med Sci 213:221–225
Böttcher HM (1964) Wonder drugs. A history of antibiotics. JB Lippincott, Philadelphia New York, p 36; pp 130–131
Brandl E, Giovannini M, Margreiter H (1953) Untersuchungen über das saurestabile, oral wirksame phenoxymethyl penicillin (penicillin V). Wien Med Wochenschr 103:602–607
Brown AG, Butterworth D, Cole M, Hanscomb G, Hood JD, Reading C, Rolinson GN (1976) Naturally occurring β-lactamase inhibitors with antibacterial activity. J Antibiot 29:668–669

Brown AG, Corbett DF, Eglington AJ, Howarth TT (1977) Structures of olivanic acid derivatives MM 4550 and MM 13902; two new, fused β-lactams isolated from *Streptomyces olivaceus*. J Chem Soc Chem Comm 1977:523–525
Brown AG, Corbett DF, Eglington AJ, Howarth TT (1979) Structures of olivanic acid derivatives MM 22380, MM 22381, MM 22382, and MM 22383; four new antibiotics isolated from *Streptomyces olivaceus*. J Antibiot 32:961–963
Brown D, Blowers R (1978) Disc methods of sensitivity testing and other semiquantitative methods. In: Reeve DS, Phillips I, Williams JD, Wise R (eds) Laboratory methods in antimicrobial chemotherapy. Churchill Livingstone, Edinburgh London New York, pp 8–30
Brumfitt W, Kosmidis J, Hamilton-Miller JMT, Gilchrist JNG (1974) Cefoxitin and Cephalothin: Antimicrobial activity, human pharmacokinetics and toxicology. Antimicrob Agents Chemother 6:290–299
Buck RE, Price KE (1977) Cefadroxil, a new broad-spectrum cephalosporin. Antimicrob Agents Chemother 11:324–330
Bryson V, Syzbalski W (1952) Microbial selection. Science 116:45–51
Cabana BE, VanHarken DR, Hottendorf GH (1976) Comparative pharmacokinetics and metabolism of cephapirin in laboratory animals and humans. Antimicrob Agents Chemother 10:307–317
Calvert RJ, Smith E (1955) Penicillin anaphylactoid shock. Br Med J 2:302–305
Carrizosa J, Kaye D (1976) Antibiotic synergism in enterococcal endocarditis. J Lab Clin Med 88:132–141
Cassidy PJ, Stapley EO, Goegelman R, Miller TW, Arison B, Albers-Schonberg G, Zimmerman SB, Birnbaum J (1977) Isolation and identification of epithienamycins. 17th intersc conf antimicrob agents chemother, Abstract 81. Am Soc Microbiol, Washington DC
Celozzi E, Lotti VJ, Stapley EO, Miller AK (1980) An animal model for assessing pain-on-injection of antibiotics. J Pharmacol Methods 4:285–289
Chain E, Florey HW, Gardner AD, Heatley NG, Jennings MA, Orr-Ewing J, Sanders AG (1940) Penicillin as a chemotherapeutic agent. Lancet II:226–228
Chauvette RR, Flynn EH, Jackson BG, Lavagnino ER, Morin RB, Mueller RA, Pioch RP, Roeske RW, Ryan CW, Spencer JL, van Heyningen E (1962a) Chemistry of cephalosporin antibiotics. II. Preparation of a new class of antibiotics and the relation of structure to activity. J Am Chem Soc 84:3401–3402
Chauvette RR, Flynn EH, Jackson BG, Lavagnino ER, Morin RB, Mueller RA, Pioch RP, Roeske RW, Ryan CW, Spencer JL, van Heyningen E (1962b) Structure-activity relationships among 7-acylamidocephalosporanic acids. In: Sylvester JC (ed) Antimicrobial agents chemother. American Society for Microbiology, Ann Arbor, MI, pp 687–694
Cleeland R, Grunberg E (1980) Laboratory evaluation of new antibiotics in vitro and in experimental animal infections. In: Lorian V (ed) Antibiotics in laboratory medicine. Williams and Wilkins, Baltimore London, pp 506–548
Clutterbuck PW, Lovell R, Raistrick H (1932) CCXXVII Studies in the biochemistry of microorganisms. XXVI. The formation from glucose by members of the *Penicillium chrysogenum* series of a pigment, an alkaline-soluble protein and penicillin – the antibacterial substance of Fleming. Biochem J 26:1907–1918
Comber KR, Osborne CD, Sutherland R (1975) Comparative effects of amoxycillin and ampicillin in the treatment of experimental mouse infections. Antimicrob Agents Chemother 7:179–185
Comber KR, Boon RJ, Sutherland R (1977a) Comparative effects of amoxycillin and ampicillin on the morphology of *Escherichia coli* in vivo and correlation with activity. Antimicrob Agents Chemother 12:736–744
Comber KR, Basker MJ, Osborne CD, Sutherland R (1977b) Synergy between ticarcillin and tobramycin against *Pseudomonas aeruginosa* and *Enterobacteriaceae* in vitro and in vivo. Antimicrob Agents Chemother 11:956–964
Commichau R, Freiesleben H, Sack K, Krüger CH, Henkel W (1976) Chronic *E. coli* nephritis in rats. Model for assessment of activity of antimicrobial agents. In: Williams JD, Geddes AM (eds) Chemotherapy, vol 2. Plenum, New York London, pp 311–316

Daoust DR, Onishi HR, Wallick H, Hendlin D, Stapley EO (1973) Cephamycins, a new family of β-lactam antibiotics: antibacterial activity and resistance to β-lactam degradation. Antimicrob Agents Chemother 3:254–261

Darland G, Birnbaum J (1977) Cefoxitin resistance to β-lactamase: a major factor for susceptibility of *Bacteroides fragilis* to the antibiotic. Antimicrob Agents Chemother 11:725–734

Davis SD, Chandler JW (1975) Experimental keratitis due to *Pseudomonas aeruginosa:* model for evaluation of antimicrobial drugs. Antimicrob Agents Chemother 8:350–355

Diding N-Å, Frisk AR (1955) Some properties of phenoxymethyl penicillin (penicillin V). In: Hobby (ed) Antibiotics annual. American Society for Microbiology, Bethesda, MD, pp 529–533

Dornbusch K, Olsson-Liljequist, Nord CE (1980) Antibacterial activity of new β-lactam antibiotics on cefoxitin-resistant strains of *Bacteroides fragilis*. J Antimicrob Chemother 6:207–216

Dumon L, Adriaens P, Arné J, Eyssen H (1979) Effect of clavulanic acid on the minimum inhibitory concentration of benzylpenicillin, ampicillin, carbenicillin, or cephalothin against clinical isolates resistant to beta-lactam antibiotics. Antimicrob Agents Chemother 15:315–317

Dye WE (1956) An agar diffusion method for studying the bacteriostatic action of combinations of antimicrobial agents. In: Welch H, Martí-Ibáñez F (eds) Antibiotics annual 1955–1956. Medical Encyclopedia, New York, pp 374–382

English AE, Retsema JA, Girard AE, Lynch JE, Barth WE (1978) CP-45,899, a beta-lactamase inhibitor that extends the antibacterial spectrum of beta-lactams: initial bacteriological characterization. Antimicrob Agents Chemother 14:414–419

Ericsson HM, Sherris JC (1971) Antimicrobial sensitivity testing. Report of an international collaborative study. Acta Pathol Microbiol Scand [B] [Suppl] 217:1–90

Fleming A (1929) On the antibacterial action of cultures of a penicillium, with special reference to their use in the isolation of *B. influenzae*. Br J Exp Pathol 10:226–236

Florey HW (1949) Historical introduction. In: Florey HW, Chain E, Heatley NG, Jennings MA, Sanders AG, Abraham EP, Florey ME (eds) Antibiotics, a survey of penicillin, streptomycin, and other antimicrobial substances from fungi, actinomycetes, bacteria, and plants, vol I. Oxford University Press, London New York, pp 1–3

Florey HW (1955) Antibiotic products of a versatile fungus. Arch Intern Med 43:480–490

Florey HW (1956) The medical aspects of the development of resistance to antibiotics. G Microbiol 2:361–370

Frost BM, Valiant ME (1964) An evaluation of cephalosporin derivatives in vitro and in experimental infections. J Pathol Bacteriol 88:125–136

Fu KP, Neu HC (1979) Inactivation of β-lactam antibiotics by *Legionella pneumophila*. Antimicrob Agents Chemother 16:561–564

Gadebusch HH, Miraglia GJ, Busch HI, Goodwin G, Pan S, Renz K (1972) Cephradine – A new orally absorbed cephalosporin antibiotic. Antimicrob Antineoplast Chemother 1/2:1059–1062

Gadebusch HH, Schwind R, Lukaszow P, Whitney R, McRipley RJ (1978) Cephamycin derivatives: comparison of the in vitro and in vivo antibacterial activities of SQ 14,359, CS-1170 and cefoxitin. J Antibiot 1046–1058

Gardner AD (1940) Morphological effects of penicillin on bacteria. Nature 146:837–838

Garrod LP (1960a) Relative antibacterial activity of three penicillins. Br Med J 1:527–529

Garrod LP (1960b) The relative antibacterial activity of four penicillins. Br Med J 2:1695–1696

Garrod LP, O'Grady F (1971) Antibiotics and chemotherapy, 3rd edn. Livingstone, Edinburgh London, p 90

Georgopoulos A, Schütze E (1980) Concentrations of various antibiotics in serum and fluids accumulated in diffusion chambers implanted in various sites in rabbits. Antimicrob Agents Chemother 17:779–783

Godzeski CW, Brown C, Pavey D, McGowen J (1961) In vitro examination of levopenicillin. In: Finland M, Savage GM (eds) Antimicrobial agents and chemotherapy. American Society for Microbiology, Bethesda, MD, pp 547–554

Godzeski CW, Brier G, Pavey DE (1963) Cephalothin, a new cephalosporin with a broad antibacterial spectrum. I. In vitro studies employing the gradient plate technique. Appl Microbiol 11:122–127
Goering RV, Sanders CC, Sanders Jr WE (1978) Comparison of BL-S 786 with cephalothin, cefamandole, and cefoxitin in vitro and in treatment of experimental infections in mice. J Antibiot 31:363–372
Goldstein FW, Kitzis MD, Acar JF (1979) Effect of clavulanic acid and amoxycillin formulation against β-lactamase producing gram-negative bacteria in urinary tract infections. J Antimicrob Chemother 5:705–709
Grassi GG, Ferrara A, Navone A, Sala P (1980) Effect of subinhibitory concentration of antibiotics on the emergence of drug resistant bacteria in vitro. J Antimicrob Chemother 6:217–223
Grasso S, Meinardi G, Carneri I de, Tamassia V (1978) New in vitro model to study the effect of antibiotic concentration and rate of elimination on antibacterial activity. Antimicrob Agents Chemother 13:570–576
Gratia A, Dath S (1924) Propriétés bactériolytiques de certaines Moisissures. C R Soc Biol (Paris) 91:1442–1443
Gratia A, Dath S (1925) Moisissures et microbes bactériophages. C R Soc Biol (Paris) 92:461–462
Greenwood D, O'Grady F (1975) Potent combinations of β-lactam antibiotics using the β-lactamase inhibition principle. Chemotherapy 21:330–341
Grunberg E, Cleeland R, Beskid G, DeLorenzo WF (1976). In vivo synergy between 6β-amidinopenicillanic acid derivatives and other antibiotics. Antimicrob Agents Chemother 9:589–594
Hartman PA (1968) Gradient methods. In: Miniaturized microbiological methods. Academic Press, New York London, pp 155–158
Heatley NG (1956) Comparative serum concentration and excretion experiments with benzyl penicillin (G) and phenoxymethyl penicillin (V) on a single subject. Antibiot Med 2:33–41
Heerema MS, Musher DM, Williams Jr TW (1979) Clavulanic acid and penicillin in treatment of *Staphylococcal aureus* renal infection in mice. Antimicrob Agents Chemother 16:798–800
Hill GB (1977) Therapeutic evaluation of minocycline and tetracycline for mixed anaerobic infection in mice. Antimicrob Agents Chemother 11:625–630
Hobby GL, Meyer K, Chaffee E (1942) Observations on the mechanism of action of penicillin. Proc Soc Exp Biol Med 50:281–285
Holdeman LV, Cato EP, Moore WEC (1977) Anaerobe lab manual, 4th edn. Virginia Polytechnic Institute and State University, Blacksburg VA
Hunter PA, Reading C, Witting DA (1978) In vitro and in vivo properties of BRL 14151, a novel beta-lactam with beta-lactamase-inhibiting properties. In: Siegenthaler W, Lüthy R (eds) Current chemotherapy, vol 1. Proceedings 10th international congress of chemotherapy. American Society for Microbiology, Bethesda MD, pp 478–480
Jackson RT, Harris LF, Alford RH (1978) Sodium clavulanate potentiation of cephalosporin activity versus cephalothin-resistant *Klebsiella pneumoniae*. In: Siegenthaler W, Lüthy R (eds) Current chemotherapy, vol 1. Proceedings 10th international congress chemotherapy. American Society for Microbiology, Bethesda MD, pp 480–482
Jorgensen JH, Alexander GA, Johnson JE (1980) Practical anaerobic broth-disc elution susceptibility test. Antimicrob Agent Chemother 17:740–742
Kahan JS, Kahan FM, Goegelman R, Currie SA, Jackson M, Stapley EO, Miller TW, Miller AK, Hendlin D, Mochales S, Hernandez S, Woodruff HB, Birnbaum J (1979) Thienamycin, a new β-lactam antibiotic. I. Discovery, taxonomy, isolation and physical properties. J Antibiot 32:1–12
Karady S, Pines SH, Weinstock LM, Roberts FE, Brenner GS, Hoinowski AM, Cheng TY, Sletzinger M (1972) Semisynthetic cephalosporins via a novel acyl exchange reaction. J Am Chem Soc 94:1410–1411
Kato T, Kurashige S, Chabbert YA, Mitsuhashi S (1978) Determination of the ID_{50} values of antibacterial agents in agar. J Antibiot 31:1299–1303

Kind AC, Kestle KG, Standiford HC, Kirby WMM (1968) Laboratory and clinical experience with cephalexin. In: Hobby GL (ed) Antimicrobial agents and chemotherapy. American Society for Microbiology, Bethesda MD, pp 361–365
Knudsen ET, Rolinson GN (1959) Absorption and excretion studies of the potassium salt of 6 (α-phenoxypropionamido) penicillanic acid. Lancet II:1105-1109
Kolodny MH, Denhoff E (1946) Reactions in penicillin therapy. JAMA 130:1058–1061
Krogstad DJ, Moellering RC Jr (1980) Combinations of antibiotics, mechanisms of interaction against bacteria. In: Lorian V (ed) Antibiotics in laboratory medicine. Williams and Wilkins, Baltimore London, pp 298–341
Kropp H, Kahan JS, Kahan FM, Sundelof J, Darland G, Birnbaum J (1976) Thienamycin. A new β-lactam antibiotic. II. In vitro and in vivo evaluation. In: 16th intersc conf antimicrob agents chemother, abstract 228. Am Soc Microbiol, Washington DC
Kropp H, Sundelof J, Kahan JS, Kahan FM, Birnbaum J (1980) MK 0787 (N-formimidoyl-thienamycin): evaluation of in vitro and in vivo activity. Antimicrob Agents Chemother 17:993–1000
Kuck NA (1975) Effects of minocycline and other antibiotics on *Fusobacterium necrophorum* infections in mice. Antimicrob Agents Chemother 7:421–425
Kunin CM (1967) Clinical significance of protein binding of penicillins. Ann NY Acad Sci 145:282–289
Kunst MW, Mattie H (1978) Cefazolin and cephradine: relationship between antibacterial activity in vitro and in mice experimentally infected with *Escherichia coli*. J Infect Dis 137:391–402
Kurzynski TA, Yrios JW, Helstad AG, Field CR (1976) Aerobically incubated thioglycollate broth disc method for antibiotic susceptibility testing of anaerobes. Antimicrob Agents Chemother 10:727–732
Lang SDR, Edwards DJ, Durack DT (1980) Comparison of cefoperazone, cefotaxime and moxalactam (LY 127935) against aerobic gram-negative bacilli. Antimicrob Agents Chemother 17:488–493
Leitner F, Goodhines RA, Buck RE, Price KE (1979) Bactericidal activity of cefadroxil, cephalexin, and cephradine in an in vitro pharmacokinetic model. J Antibiot 32:718–732
Lincoln LJ, Weinstein AJ, Gallagher M, Abrutyn E (1977) Penicillinase-resistant penicillins plus gentamicin in experimental enterococcal endocarditis. Antimicrob Agents Chemother 12:484–489
Lorian V (1975) Some effects of subinhibitory concentrations of penicillin on the structure and division of staphylococci. Antimicrob Agents Chemother 7:864–870
Lorian V (1980) Effects of subminimum inhibitory concentrations of antibiotics on bacteria. In: Lorian V (ed) Antibiotics in laboratory medicine. Williams and Wilkins, Baltimore London, pp 342–408
Louie TJ, Onderdonk AB, Gorbach SL, Bartlett JG (1977). Therapy for experimental intraabdominal sepsis: Comparison of four cephalosporins with clindamycin plus gentamicin. J Infect Dis [Suppl] 135:S18–S22
Marcy SM, Klein JO (1970) The isoxazolyl penicillins: oxacillin, cloxacillin, and dicloxacillin. Med Clin North Am 54:1127–1143
Martin WJ, Nichols DR, Heilman FR (1955) Penicillin V, a new type of penicillin: preliminary clinical and laboratory observations. Proc Staff Meet Mayo Clin 30:467–476
Masuda G, Yajima T, Nakamura K, Yanagishita T, Hayashi H (1979) Comparative bactericidal activities of beta-lactam antibiotics determined in agar and broth media. J Antibiot 32:1168–1173
Matsuura S, Yoshida T, Sugeno K, Harada Y, Harada M, Kuwahara S (1978) 6059-S, a new parenterally active 1-oxacephalosporin: (2) pharmacological studies. In: 18th intersc conf antimicrob agents chemother, abstract 152. Am Soc Microbiol, Washington DC
Mattie H, Kunst MW (1978) Animal models for the assessment of potentiation of antibiotics by probenecid and by host resistance. Infection [Suppl 1] 6:S36–S37
Mattie H, Goslings WRO, Noach EL (1973) Cloxacillin and nafcillin: serum binding and its relationship to antibacterial effect in mice. J Infect Dis 128:170–177

Miller AK (1971) In vivo evaluation of antibacterial chemotherapeutic substances. In: Perlman D (ed) Advances in applied microbiology, vol 14. Academic Press, New York London, pp 151–183
Miller AK, Verwey WF (1954) Effect of probenecid on combined penicillin and triple sulfonamides therapy of experimental streptococcal infections. Antibiot Chemother 4:169–172
Miller AK, Baron BJ, Verwey WF, Keller DG (1958) Novobiocin-penicillin combinations. II. Broadened spectrum of activity of combinations of novobiocin and penicillin. In: Welch H, Martı-Ibáñez F (eds) Antibiotics annual. Medical Encyclopedia, New York, pp 38–42
Miller AK, Celozzi E, Pelak BA, Stapley EO, Hendlin D (1972a) Cephamycins, a new family of β-lactam antibiotics. III. In vitro studies. Antimicrob Agents Chemother 2:281–286
Miller AK, Celozzi E, Kong Y, Pelak BA, Kropp H, Stapley EO, Hendlin D (1972b) Cephamycins, a new family of β-lactam antibiotics. IV. In vivo studies. Antimicrob Agents Chemother 2:287–290
Miller AK, Celozzi E, Kong Y, Pelak BA, Hendlin D, Stapley EO (1974) Cefoxitin, a semisynthetic cephamycin antibiotic: in vivo evaluation. Antimicrob Agents Chemother 5:33–37
Miller AK, Celozzi E, Pelak BA, Birnbaum J, Stapley EO (1979) Correlation of in vitro susceptibility with in vivo efficacy in mice for cefoxitin in comparison with cephalosporins. J Antimicrob Chemother 5:569–579
Mine Y, Nonoyama S, Kojo H, Fukada S, Nishida M (1977) Nocardicin A, a new monocyclic β-lactam antibiotic. V. In vivo evaluation. J Antibiot 30:932–937
Moellering RC, Swartz MN (1976) The newer cephalosporins. N Engl J Med 294:24–28
Moxon ER, Medeiros AA, O'Brien TF (1977) Beta-lactamase effect on ampicillin treatment of *Haemophilus influenzae* B bacteremia and meningitis in infant rats. Antimicrob Agents Chemother 12:461–464
Muggleton PW, O'Callaghan CH, Sevens WK (1964) Laboratory evaluation of a new antibiotic-cephaloridine (ceporin). Br Med J II:1234–1237
Murray PR, Christman JL (1978) Anaerobic susceptibility tests. Evaluation of the stability of antimicrobials in Wilkins-Chalgren broth and the effect of media prereduction. J Antibiot 31:1296–1298
Nagarajan R, Boeck LD, Gorman M, Hamill RL, Higgins CE, Hoehn MM, Stark WM, Whitney JG (1971) β-Lactam antibiotics from *Streptomyces*. J Am Chem Soc 93:2308–2310
Nakao H, Yanagisawa H, Shimizu B, Kaneko M, Nagano M, Sugawara S (1976) A new semisynthetic 7-α-methoxycephalosporin, CS 1170: 7β[[(cyanomethyl)thio]acetamido]-7α-methoxy-3-[[(1-methyl-1H-tetrazol-5-yl)thio]methyl]-3-cephem-4-carboxylic acid. J Antibiot 29:554–558
Naumann P (1966) Bakteriologische und pharmakologische Eigenschaften der neuen Cephalosporic-Antibiotica I Cephalothin 1 Mitteilung. Arzneim Forsch (Drug Res) 16:818–825
NCCLS (1975, suppl to be published) Approved Standard ASM-2. Performance standards for antimicrobial disc susceptibility tests. National Committee for Clinical Laboratory Standards, Villanova, PA
NCCLS (1979) Proposed Standard: PSM 11. Proposed reference dilution procedure for antimicrobic susceptibility testing of anaerobic bacteria. National Committee for Clinical Laboratory Standards, Villanova, PA
Neu HC (1976) Synergism of mecillinam, a beta-amidinopenicillanic acid derivative, combined with beta-lactam antibiotics. Antimicrob Agents Chemother 10:535–542
Neu HC, Aswapokee N, Fu KP, Aswapokee P (1979a) Antibacterial activity of a new 1-oxacephalosporin compared with that of other β-lactam compounds. Antimicrob Agents Chemother 16:141–149
Neu HC, Aswapokee N, Aswapokee P, Fu KP (1979b) HR 756, a new cephalosporin active against gram-positive and gram-negative aerobic and anaerobic bacteria. Antimicrob Agents Chemother 15:273–281

Newton GGF, Abraham EP (1955) Cephalosporin C, a new antibiotic containing sulfur and D-α-aminoadipic acid. Nature 175:548
Newton GGF, Abraham EP (1956) Isolation of cephalosporin C, a penicillin-like antibiotic containing D-α-aminoadipic acid. Biochem J 62:651–658
Ninane G, Joly J, Kraytman M, Piot P (1978) Bronchopulmonary infection due to β-lactamase-producing *Branhamella catarrhalis* treated with amoxycillin/clavulanic acid. Lancet 2:257
Nishida M, Matsubara T, Murakawa T, Mine Y, Yokota Y, Kuwahara S, Goto S (1969) In vitro and in vivo evaluation of cefazolin, a new cephalosporin C derivative. In: Hobby GL (ed) Antimicrobial agents and chemotherapy. American Society Microbiology, Bethesda MD, pp 236–243
Nishida M, Murakawa T, Kamimura T, Okada N, Sakamoto H, Kukada S, Nakamoto S, Yokota Y, Miki K (1976) Laboratory evaluation of FR 10612, a new oral cephalosporin derivative. J Antibiot 29:444–459
Nishida M, Mine Y, Nonoyawa S, Kojo H, Goto S, Kuwahara S (1977) Nocardin A, a new monocyclic β-lactam antibiotic. III. In vitro evaluation. J Antibiot 30:917–925
Norden CW, Kennedy E (1970) Experimental osteomyelitis. I. A description of the model. J Infect Dis 122:410–418
Norden CW, Kennedy E (1971) Experimental osteomyelitis. II. Therapeutic trials and measurement of antibiotic levels in bone. J Infect Dis 124:565–571
O'Callaghan CH (1979) Description and classification of the newer cephalosporins and their relationship with the established compounds. J Antimicrob Chemother 5:635–671
O'Callaghan CH, Sykes RB, Ryan DM, Foord RD, Muggleton PW (1976a) Cefuroxime – a new cephalosporin antibiotic. J Antibiot 29:29–37
O'Callaghan CH, Sykes RB, Griffiths A, Thornton JE (1976b) Cefuroxime, a new cephalosporin antibiotic: activity in vitro. Antimicrob Agents Chemother 9:511–519
Onderdonk AB, Bartlett JG, Louie T, Sullivan-Seigler N, Gorbach SL (1976) Microbial synergy in experimental intra-abdominal abscesses. Infect Immun 13:22–26
Onishi HR, Daoust DR, Zimmerman SB, Hendlin D, Stapley EO (1974) Cefoxitin, a semisynthetic cephamycin antibiotic: resistance to β-lactamase inactivation. Antimicrob Agents Chemother 5:38–48
Patte JC, Hirsch H, Chabbert Y (1958) Etude des courbes d'effet bacteriostatique des associations d'antibiotiques. Ann Inst Pasteur (Paris) 94:621–625
Peterson LR, Gerding DN (1978) Prediction of cefazolin penetration into high and low-protein-containing extravascular fluid: new method for performing simultaneous studies. Antimicrob Agents Chemother 14:533–538
Perfect JR, Land SDR, Durack DT (1980) Comparison of cotrimoxazole, ampicillin, and chloramphenicol in the treatment of experimental *Haemophilus influenzae* Type B meningitis. Antimicrob Agents Chemother 17:43–48
Reading C, Cole M (1977) Clavulanic acid: a beta-lactamase-inhibiting beta-lactam from *Streptomyces clavuligerus*. Antimicrob Agents Chemother 11:852–857
Reid RD (1935) Some properties of a bacterial-inhibitory substance produced by a mold. J Bacteriol 29:215–220
Reimer LG, Mirrett S, Reller LB (1980) Comparison of in vitro activity of moxalactam (LY 127935) with cefazolin, amikacin, tobramycin, carbenicillin, piperacillin, and ticarcillin against 420 blood culture isolates. Antimicrob Agents Chemother 17:412–416
Retsema JA, English AR, Girard AE (1980) CP 45,899 in combination with penicillin or ampicillin against penicillin-resistant *Staphylococcus*, *Haemophilus influenzae* and *Bacteroides*. Antimicrob Agents Chemother 17:615–622
Rippere RA (1980) Preparation and control of antibiotic susceptibility discs and other devices containing antibiotics. In: Lorian V (ed) Antibiotics in laboratory medicine. Williams and Wilkins, Baltimore London, pp 549–572
Rolinson GN (1973) Laboratory evaluation of amoxycillin. Chemotherapy [Suppl] 18:1–10
Rolinson GN, Sutherland R (1965) The binding of antibiotics to serum protein. Br J Pharmacol 25:638–650
Rolinson GN, Stevens S, Batchelor FR, Wood JC, Chain EB (1960) Bacteriological studies on a new penicillin-BRL 1241. Lancet II:564–567

Rose SB, Miller RE (1939) Studies with the agar cup-plate method. I. A standardized agar cup-plate technique. J Bacteriol 38:525–537

Rosenblatt JE, Muray PR, Sonnenwirth AC, Joyce JL (1979) Comparison of anaerobic results obtained by different methods. Antimicrob Agents Chemother 15:351–355

Rosenthal A (1958) Follow-up study of fatal penicillin reactions. JAMA 167:1118–1121

Rotilie CA, Fass RJ, Prior RB, Perkins RL (1975) Microdilution technique for antimicrobial susceptibility testing of anaerobic bacteria. Antimicrob Agents Chemother 7:311–315

Roy I, Bach V, Thadepalli H (1977) In vitro activity of ticarcillin against anaerobic bacteria compared with that of carbenicillin and penicillin. Antimicrob Agents Chemother 11:258–261

Ryan DM (1979) Implanted cotton threads; a novel method measuring concentrations of antibiotics in tissue fluid. J Antimicrob Chemother 5:735–739

Ryan DM, O'Callaghan CH, Muggleton PW (1976) Cefuroxime, a new cephalosporin antibiotic: activity in vivo. Antimicrob Agents Chemother 9:520–525

Rylander M, Brorson J-E, Johnsson J, Norrby R (1979) Comparison between agar and broth minimum inhibitory concentrations of cefamandole, cefoxitin and cefuroxime. Antimicrob Agents Chemother 15:572–579

Sabath LD, Finland M (1967) Resistance of penicillins and cephalosporins to beta-lactamases from gram-negative bacilli: some correlations with antibacterial activity. Ann NY Acad Sci 145:237–247

Sabath LD, McCall CE, Steigbigel NH, Finland M (1966) Synergistic penicillin combinations for treatment of human urinary-tract infections. In: Hobby GL (ed) Antimicrobial agents and chemotherapy. American Society for Microbiology, Bethesda MD, pp 149–155

Sabath LD, Elder HA, McCall CE, Finland M (1967) Synergistic combinations of penicillins in the treatment of bacteriuria. N Engl J Med 277:232–238

Scheld WM, Fink FN, Fletcher DD, Sande MA (1979) Mecillinam-ampicillin synergism in experimental *Enterobacteriaceae* meningitis. Antimicrob Agents Chemother 16:271–276

Selwyn S (1979) Pioneer work on the "penicillin phenomenon," 1870–1876. J Antimicrob Chemother 5:249–255

Shibata K, Fujii M (1970) Clinical studies of cefazolin in the surgical field. In: Hobby GL (ed) Antimicrobial agents and chemotherapy. American Society for Microbiology, Bethesda MD, pp 467–472

Slack MPE, Wheldon DB, Swann RA, Perks E (1979) Cefsulodin, a cephalosporin with specific antipseudomonal activity; in vitro studies of the drug alone and in combination. J Antimicrob Chemother 5:687–691

Stapley EO, Jackson M, Hernandez S, Zimmerman SB, Currie SA, Mochales S, Mata JM, Woodruff HB, Hendlin D (1972) Cephamycins, a new family of β-lactam antibiotics. I. Production by actinomycetes, including *Streptomyces lactamdurams* sp. n. Antimicrob Agents Chemother 2:122–131

Stapley EO, Cassidy PJ, Currie SA, Daoust D, Goegelman R, Hernandez S, Jackson M, Mata JM, Miller AK, Monaghan RL, Tunac JB, Zimmerman SB, Hendlin D (1977) Epithienamycins: Biological studies of a new family of β-lactam antibiotics. In: 17th intersc conf antimicrob agents chemother, abstract 80. Am Soc Microbiol, Washington DC

Stapley EO, Birnbaum J, Miller AK, Wallick H, Hendlin D, Woodruff HB (1979) Cefoxitin and cephamycins: Microbiological studies. Rev Infect Dis 1:73–87

Steers E, Foltz EL, Graves BS (1959) An inocula replicating apparatus for routine testing of bacterial susceptibility to antibiotics. Antibiot Chemother 9:307–311

Sugawara S, Tajima M, Igarashi I, Ohya S, Utsui Y (1976) CS 1170, a new cephalosporin derivative. II. In vitro and in vivo antibacterial activities. In: 16th intersc conf antimicrob agents chemother, abstract 231. Am Soc Microbiol, Washington DC

Sutherland R, Rolinson GN (1970) α-Amino-p-hydroxybenzyl-penicillin (BRL 2333), a new semisynthetic penicillin: in vitro evaluation. In: Hobby GL (ed) Antimicrobial agents and chemotherapy. American Society for Microbiology, Bethesda MD, pp 411–415

Sutherland R, Rolinson GN (1978) Penicillins and cephalosporins. In: Reeves DS, Phillips I, Williams JD, Wise R (eds) Laboratory methods in antimicrobial chemotherapy. Churchill Livingstone, Edinburgh New York London, pp 76–78
Sutherland R, Burnett J, Rolinson GN (1970a) α-Carboxy-3-thienylmethylpenicillin (BRL 2288) a new semisynthetic penicillin: In vitro evaluation. In: Hobby GL (ed) Antimicrobial agents and chemotherapy. American Society for Microbiology, Bethesda MD, pp 390–395
Sutherland R, Croyden EAP, Rolinson GN (1970b) Flucloxacillin, a new isoxazolyl penicillin, compared with oxacillin, cloxacillin, and dicloxicillin. Br Med J 4:455–460
Sutter VL, Vargo VL, Finegold SM (1975) Wadsworth. Anaerobic bacteriology manual, 2nd edn. University of California Los Angeles Extention division, Los Angeles
Sutter VL, Barry AL, Wilkins TD, Zabransky RJ (1979) Collaborative evaluation of a proposed reference dilution method of susceptibility testing of anaerobic bacteria. Antimicrob Agents Chemother 16:495–502
Sykes RB, Matthew M (1976) The β-lactamases of gram-negative bacteria and their role in resistance to β-lactam antibiotics. J Antimicrob Chemother 2:115–157
Sykes RB, Matthews M (1979) Detection, assay and immunology of β-lactamases. In: Hamilton-Miller JMT, Smith JT (eds) Beta-Lactamases. Academic Press, London New York, pp 17–49
Tachibana A, Komiya M, Kikuchi Y, Yano K, Mashimo K (1980) Pharmacological studies on YM 09330, a new parenteral cephamycin derivative. In: Nelson JD, Grassi C (eds) Current chemotherapy and infectious disease, vol 1. American Society for Microbiology, Washington DC, pp 273–275
Tally FP, Jacobus NV, Gorbach SL (1978) In vitro activity of thienamycin. Antimicrob Agents Chemotherapy 14:436–438
Tally FP, O'Keefe JP, Sullivan NM, Gorbach SL (1979) Inactivation of cephalosporins by *Bacteroides*. Antimicrob Agents Chemother 16:565–571
Taryle DA, Good Jr JT, Reller LB, Sahn SA (1980) Penetration of cephradine into normal, inflammatory, and infected pleural fluids in rabbits. J Antimicrob Chemother 6:143–149
Thadepalli H, Roy I, Bach VT, Webb D (1979) In vitro activity of mezlocillin and its related compounds against aerobic and anaerobic bacteria. Antimicrob Agents Chemother 15:487–490
Thornsberry C (1980) Automation in antibiotic susceptibility testing. In: Lorian V (ed) Antibiotics in laboratory medicine. Williams and Wilkins, Baltimore London, pp 193–205
Thornsberry C, Baker CN, Kirren LA (1978) In vitro activity of antimicrobial agents on Legionnaires' disease bacterium. Antimicrob Agents Chemother 13:78–80
Thrupp L (1974) Newer cephalosporins and "expanded-spectrum" penicillins. In: Elliott HW, Okun R, George R (eds) Annual review of pharmacology. Annual Reviews, Palo Alto, pp 435–467
Thrupp LD (1980) Susceptibility testing of antibiotics in liquid media. In: Lorian V (ed) Antibiotics in laboratory medicine. Williams and Wilkins, Baltimore London, pp 73–113
Tomasz A (1979) The mechanism of the irreversible antimicrobial effects of penicillins. How the beta-lactam antibiotics kill and lyse bacteria. In: Starr MP, Ingraham JL, Raffel S (eds) Annual review microbiology, vol 33. Annual Reviews, Palo Alto, pp 113–137
Tsai YH, Williams EB, Hirth RS, Price KE (1975) Pneumococcal meningitis – therapeutic studies in mice. Chemotherapy 21:342–357
Tsuchiya K, Oishi T, Iwagishi C, Iwahi T (1971) In vitro antibacterial activity of disodium α-sulfobenzylpenicillin. J Antibiot 24:607–619
Tsuchiya K, Kondo M, Nagatowo H (1978a) SCE-129, antipseudomonal cephalosporin: in vitro and in vivo antibacterial activities. Antimicrob Agents Chemother 13:137–145
Tsuchiya K, Kida M, Kondo M, Ono H, Takeuchi M, Nishi T (1978b) SCE-963, a new broad-spectrum cephalosporin: in vitro and in vivo antibacterial activities. Antimicrob Agents Chemother 14:551–568
Tybring L, Melchior NH (1975) Mecillinam (FL 1060), a 6-β-amidinopenicillanic acid derivative: bactericidal action and synergy in vitro. Antimicrob Agents Chemother 8:271–276

Ueo K, Fukuoka Y, Hayashi T, Yasuda T, Taki H, Tai M, Watanabe Y, Saikawa I, Mitsuhashi S (1977) In vitro and in vivo antibacterial activity of T 1220, a new semisynthetic penicillin. Antimicrob Agents Chemother 12:455–460

Uri JV, Actor P, Guarini JR, Phillips L, Pitkin D, Demarinis RM, Weisbach JA (1978) Biological and chemotherapeutic studies on three semisynthetic cephamycins. J Antibiot 31:82–91

Verbist L (1978) In vitro activity of piperacillin, a new semisynthetic penicillin with an unusually broad spectrum of activity. Antimicrob Agents Chemother 13:349–357

Vincent JG, Vincent HW (1944) Filter paper modification of the Oxford cup penicillin determination. Proc Soc Exp Biol Med 55:162–164

von Daehne W, Godfredsen WO, Roholt K, Tybring L (1970) Pivampicillin, a new orally active ampicillin ester. In: Hobby GL (ed) Antimicrobial agents and chemotherapy. American Society for Microbiology, Bethesda MD, pp 431–437

Wallick H, Hendlin D (1974) Cefoxitin, a semisynthetic cephamycin antibiotic: susceptibility studies. Antimicrob Agents Chemother 5:25–32

Warren G (1965/66) The prognostic significance of penicillin serum levels and protein binding in clinical medicine. A review of current studies. Chemotherapy 10:339–358

Watt B (1979) Antibiotic susceptibility of anaerobic bacteria. J Inf [Suppl 1] 1:39–48

Weaver SS, Bodey GP, LeBlanc BM (1979) Thienamycin: New beta-lactam antibiotic with potent broad-spectrum activity. Antimicrob Agents Chemother 15:518–521

Weaver SS, LeBlanc BM, Bodey GP (1980) In vitro studies of 1-oxacephalosporin (LY 127935), a new beta-lactam antibiotic. Antimicrob Agents Chemother 17:92–95

Weinstein WM, Onderdonk AB, Bartlett JG, Gorwood SL (1974) Experimental intra-abdominal abscesses in rats: development of an experimental model. Infect Immun 10:1250–1255

Welch H, Martí-Ibáñez F (1960) The story of antibiotics. In: The antibiotic saga. Medical Encyclopedia, New York, p 19

Werner H, Krasemann C, Ungerechts J (1979) Cefoxitin-Empfindlichkeit von Cephalosporinase-positiven und -negativen Bacteroidaceae. Infection [Suppl 1] 7:S43–S46

West SEH, Wilkins TD (1980) Vaspar broth-disk procedure for antibiotic susceptibility testing of anaerobic bacteria. Antimicrob Agents Chemother 17:288–291

White AC, Couch RA, Foster F, Calloway J, Hunter W, Knight V (1955) Absorption and antimicrobial activity of penicillin V (phenoxymethyl penicillin). In: Welch H, Martí-Ibáñez F (eds) Antibiotics annual. Medical Encyclopedia, New York, pp 490–500

Wick WE (1967) Cephalexin, a new orally absorbed cephalosporin antibiotic. Appl Microbiol 15:765–769

Wick WE (1972) Biological evaluation. In: Flynn EH (ed) Cephalosporins and penicillins. Chemistry and biology. Academic Press, New York London, p 499

Wick WE, Boniece WS (1965) In vitro and in vivo laboratory evaluation of cephaloglycin and cephaloridine. Appl Microbiol 13:248–253

Wick WE, Preston DA (1972) Biological properties of three 3-heterocyclic-thiomethyl cephalosporin antibiotics. Antimicrob Agents Chemother. 1:221–234

Wildonger KJ, Leanza WJ, Miller TW, Christensen BG (1979) N-acetimidoyl and N-formimidoyl thienamycin – chemically stable, broad spectrum derivatives. In: 19th intersc conf antimicrob agents chemother, abstract 232. Am Soc Microbiol, Washington DC

Wilkins TD, Smith LDS (1974) Chemotherapy of an experimental *Fusobacterium (sphaerophorus) necrophorum* infection in mice. Antimicrob Agents Chemother 5:658–662

Wilkins TD, Thiel T (1973) Modified broth-disc method for testing the antibiotic susceptibility of anaerobic bacteria. Antimicrob Agents Chemother 3:350–356

Williamson GM, Morrison JK, Stevens KJ (1961) A new synthetic penicillin. Lancet 1:847–850

Wise R, Andrews JM, Bedford KA (1978) In vitro study of clavulanic acid in combination with penicillin, amoxycillin, and carbenicillin. Antimicrob Agents Chemother 13:389–393

Wise R, Andrews JM, Bedford KA (1979) LY 127935, a novel oxa-β-lactam: an in vitro comparison with other β-lactam antibiotics. Antimicrob Agents Chemother 16:341–345

Wise R, Andrews JM, Bedford KA (1980) Clavulanic acid and CP-45,899: a comparison of their in vitro activity in combination with penicillins. J Antimicrob Chemother 6:197–206

Wright WE, Line VD (1980) Biliary excretion in rats: influence of molecular weight. Antimicrob Agents Chemother 17:842–846
Wright WW, Kirshbaum A, Arret A, Putnam LE, Welch W (1955) Serum concentrations and urinary excretion following oral administration of penicillin V and comparison with penicillin G. Antibiot Med 1:490–495
Wüst J, Wilkins TD (1978) Effect of clavulanic acid on anaerobic bacteria resistant to beta-lactam antibiotics. Antimicrob Agents Chemother 13:130–133
Yoshida T, Matsuura S, Mayama M, Kameda Y, Kuwahara S (1980) Moxalactam (6059-S) a novel 1-oxa-β-lactam with an expanded antibacterial spectrum: laboratory evaluation. Antimicrob Agents Chemother 17:302–312
Zak O, Kradolfer F, Konopka EA, Kunz S, Batt E (1978) CGP 7174/E (Takeda SCE 129): activity against systemic and urinary tract infections in mice and rats. In: Siegenthaler W, Lüthy R (eds) Current chemotherapy and infectious disease. Proceedings 10th international congress chemotherapy, vol 1. American Society for Microbiology, Bethesda MD, pp 846–848
Zak O, Konopka EA, Tosch W, Zimmerman W, Kunz S, Fehlmann H, Kradolfer F (1980) Experimental studies of cefotiam (CGP 14221/E). In: Nelson JD, Grassi C (eds) Current chemotherapy and infectious disease, vol 1. American Society for Microbiology, Washington, DC, pp 223–225
Zimmerman SB, Stapley EO (1976) Relative morphological effects induced by cefoxitin and other beta-lactam antibiotics in vitro. Antimicrob Agents Chemother 9:318–326

CHAPTER 14

β-Lactam Antibiotics: Structure-Activity Relationships

J. R. E. Hoover

A. Introduction: Scope

The enormous clinical and commercial importance of the β-lactam antibiotics has sustained a worldwide research effort directed at examining the effects of structural modifications on their biological properties for well over three decades (Moyer and Coghill 1946). This effort has been bolstered by the propensity of these chemical systems to exhibit improved biological activities with appropriate structural changes. As a consequence the β-lactams now rank with the most extensively varied and most thoroughly studied substances in the field of medicinal chemistry. Each position of the penicillin and cephalosporin rings has undergone alterations, with the exception of the 4(5)-bridgehead nitrogen atom, and although the clavulanic acids, penems, carbapenems, and monobactams have been known for 5 years or less, a large proportion of the conceivable modifications of these structures have been disclosed in publications and patents.

Fortunately, surveys of the field appeared quite early (Florey et al. 1949; Clarke et al. 1949), and they have been followed by a continuous and growing stream of reviews which now deal with all aspects of β-lactam chemistry and biology. Especially thorough analyses of earlier penicillin and cephalosporin structure–activity relationships are included in the following references: Stewart 1965; Doyle and Nayler 1964; Van Heyningen 1967; Sassiver and Lewis 1970; Price 1970; Gorman and Ryan 1972; Nayler 1973. More recent developments, including the newer β-lactam classes, are reviewed in references such as: Price 1977; Webber and Ott 1977; Hoover and Dunn 1979; O'Callaghan 1979; Neu 1979; Mandell 1979; Cooper 1980; Jung et al. 1980; Gregory 1981; Morin and Gorman 1982. The organization of this chapter and the selection of the data to be included herein takes into account the broad scope of this field and its earlier reviews. It also recognizes the therapeutic basis for much of the work that has been carried out. Results leading to clinical applications are emphasized and structure–activity relationships are examined with emphasis on recent developments. Access to details of earlier studies which provided the groundwork for structure–activity relationships of current interest is available through the cited reviews.

I. Structure

Figure 1 illustrates the essential structural features of the majority of the β-lactams included in this chapter. It should serve as a guide to structure, identification and position numbering in the text which follows. Although the diversity of structure

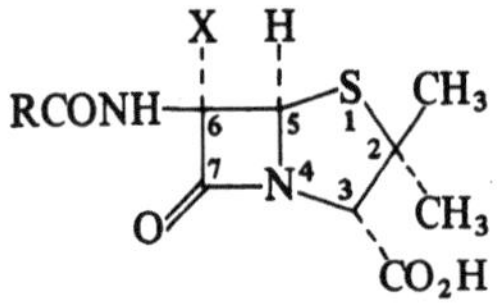

Penicillins (X = H)
Temocillin (X = OCH_3)

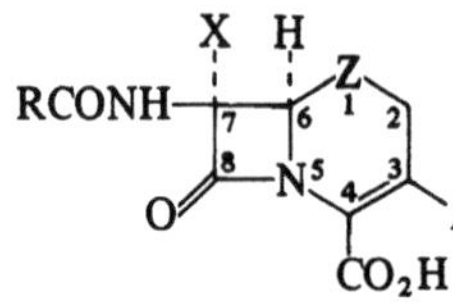

Cephalosporins (X=H, Z=S)
Cephamycins (X=OCH_3, Z=S)
1–Oxacephalosporins (X=H, OCH_3, Z=O)

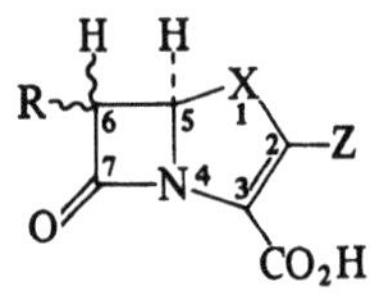

1–(Carba)penems:
Thienamycins (X=CH_2)
Olivanic acids (X=CH_2)
Penems (X=S)

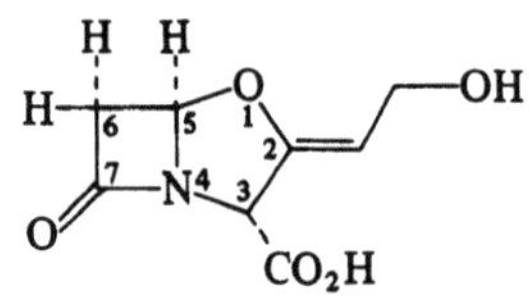

Clavulanic acids

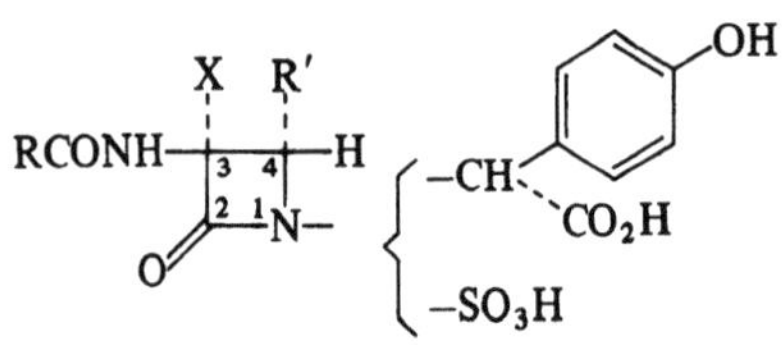

Nocardicins
Sulfazecins
Monobactams
(X=H, OCH_3; R′=H, CH_3)

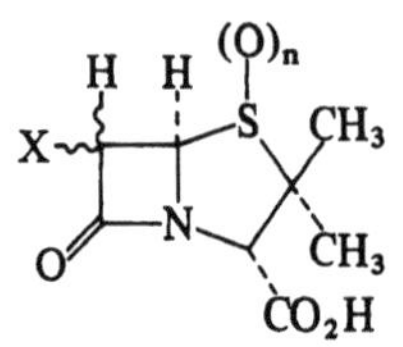

Penams:
Sulfones (n=2)
6–Halo (n=0, 2)

Fig. 1. β-Lactam antibiotics of (potential) clinical interest

requires use of the more cumbersome systematic nomenclature for archival and retrieval purposes (HOOVER and DUNN 1979, p. 86) the trivial names indicated are used here when they are unambiguous. As might be expected, SAR studies have not only varied the type of substituent attached to the β-lactam ring system, but also the size and atom content of the rings, the position and configuration of the ring junctures and the configuration of substituent attachment. In light of such broad variation it would be useful to look for some commonality of structure as a starting point for the comparisons that follow.

The β-lactams produced in nature and many of the more active synthetic products do share a number of structural similarities. All have the four-membered lactam ring. With the exception of the nocardicins and monobactams, the β-lactam ring is fused through the nitrogen and the adjacent tetrahedral carbon atoms to a second ring. The stereochemistry around the β-lactam ring of the penicillins and the cephalosporins is the same in both series; the asymmetric centers at C-5 and C-6 in the penicillins correspond to those at C-6 and C-7 in the cephalosporins. Thus the absolute configuration of the amide-bearing carbon atoms (C-6, C-7) and the carbon atoms at the ring junctions (C-5, C-6) is *R* in both cases. This makes the hydrogen atoms attached to these two carbons *cis* and placed on the α-side of the fused ring systems, which are folded along the C-5(6) to N-4(5) axis. The ring-juncture stereochemistry of clavulanic acid and the natural carbapenems (thienamycin and its analogs) is the same as that of the penicillins and cephalosporins; the absolute configuration of the ring-junction carbon atom is *R*. This position is without substituent on natural β-lactams and synthetic analogs with biological activity.

A feature common to nearly all is the carboxyl group on a carbon atom attached to the lactam nitrogen. In those systems (penicillins, clavulanic acid, 2-cephems) where the carbon atom carrying the carboxyl group is tetrahedral the absolute configuration is *S*, placing the carboxyl on the α-side of the ring system. Although the nocardicins do not have the fused-ring arrangement the acylamino- and carboxyl-carrying carbon atoms both have configurations congruent with the corresponding stereochemical centers of the other known structures in this group. The monobactams constitute a notable exception to the requirement for a properly positioned carboxyl group.

The substitution pattern on the β-lactam ring carbon opposite the nitrogen atom (the 6-position of penicillins, carbapenems, and clavulanic acid; the 7-position of oxacephalosporins and cephamycins) is heterotypic. For the penicillins and cephalosporins a 6(7)β-acylamino group or its equivalent (see mecillinam) appears necessary for significant antibiotic activity, and manipulation of this side-chain has provided a route to most of the useful therapeutic agents. In the light of this, the relatively low antibacterial activity of clavulanic acid (no 6-position substituent) is not too surprising but the high level of antibiotic activity exhibited by thienamycin and its congeners (6-hydroxyethyl substituent, either α or β) is unexpected. This apparent anomaly illustrates the interrelationship of chemical reactivity of the β-lactam ring with biological activity. The level of reactivity achieved with the carbapenem ring system appears to obviate the need for additional activation through the 6(7)-acylamino group required by the penam and cephem ring systems (Woodward 1949, 1980). This concept of an optimal level of chemical reactivity for good antibiotic activity is illustrated at several points in the following discussion.

II. Activity

The essential activity of the β-lactams is the inhibition (usually bactericidal) of bacteria, presumably by influencing in some way the complex and dynamic processes involved in bacterial cell-wall construction and maintenance. The nearly universal unit of in vitro antibacterial activity for the initial comparison of β-lactam analogs is the minimum inhibitory concentration (MIC) determined using appropriate microorganisms under a variety of conditions (see Chap. 13). This is a very practical unit of measure since it provides a relatively accurate first estimate of the ability of the compound to kill the target microorganism, provided it is handled appropriately by the host. However, it has long been obvious that the MIC is the end expression of many specific interactions between the compound and the organism. These vary in their degree of contribution to the final outcome so that direct comparisons of MIC values over a broad range of structural variations do not always provide trends which permit a high level of predictability for proposed new analogs.

Other chapters in this volume examine in some detail the extensive and growing body of knowledge that deals with the way the target organism takes up, processes and interacts with the antibiotic, and the consequences thereof. Three major factors have emerged that can profoundly influence the MIC that a given β-lactam exhibits against a specific organism: (1) production of β-lactamase(s) (quantity, type, location) by the organism and susceptibility of the antibiotic to inactivation by these enzymes (Chap. 12); (2) affinity of the β-lactam for the target enzyme(s) essential to cell-wall maintenance, reflected in the degree and distribution of binding of the antibiotic to the penicillin-binding proteins (PBP) of the bacterial cytoplasmic membrane (Chap. 2); and (3) relative ability of the antibiotic to penetrate the outer cell membrane of the gram-negative bacteria (Chap. 13). Studies based on each of these factors now provide more specific quantitation of structure–activity relationships amongst the β-lactams, but such data are still limited in comparison with those from MIC value comparisons.

The β-lactams are, for the most part, broad-spectrum antibiotics. Thus, SAR comparisons frequently include MIC data for a relatively large number of species and strains. Total in vitro data published for a clinical product can encompass MIC values numbering into the thousands, including clinical isolates and laboratory strains of bacteria. For the sake of manageability, the data included here have been restricted largely to laboratory strains and an effort has been made to maintain as consistently as the reported data permit similar groups of bacteria from table to table. It should be kept in mind that a broad review of structure–activity relationships combines results from many laboratories. While the species names may be the same in some comparisons, the strains and conditions used may not be. In consideration of this, values for standards from each laboratory are included, where available, in order to provide a better basis for comparing the reported MIC values.

The foundation for the interest in β-lactam antibiotics is clinical utility. Thus an examination of structure–activity relationships requires the inclusion of some pharmacokinetic characteristics as well. From a clinical standpoint significant improvement in the β-lactam antibiotics has been achieved through control of the behaviour of these substances in terms of serum levels (peak and duration, by parenteral and oral routes), tissue distribution, urinary excretion, metabolism, serum and tissue binding, serum and tissue inactivation and biliary excretion. Comparisons using this type of data are included where this seems appropriate. Of course, measurements of protective effectiveness in laboratory animals (PD_{50}, ED_{50}, mg/kg) are widely used to reflect ultimate expression of in vitro activity and pharmacokinetic handling, thus predicting (sometimes imperfectly) potential clinical usefulness in man.

B. Clinically Useful Penicillins

Penicillins that are now available for clinical use in the various world markets, or are under clinical evaluation are listed in Table 1 and Fig. 2. Except for the 6-disubstituted amidino analog mecillinam, and several penicillin pro-drugs (e.g., acy-

Table 1. Penicillins for clinical use

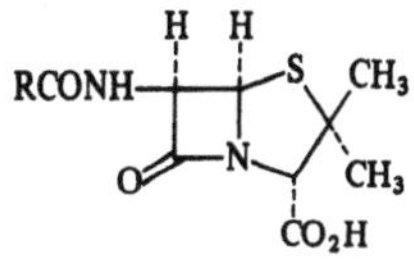

1. *Natural, biosynthetic and related penicillins*

Benzylpenicillin	$C_6H_5CH_2-$
Phenoxymethylpenicillin	$C_6H_5OCH_2-$
Phenethicillin	$C_6H_5OCH(CH_3)-$
Propicillin	$C_6H_5OCH(C_2H_5)-$
Clometocillin	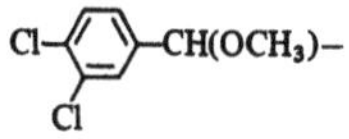
Azidocillin	$C_6H_5CH(N_3)-$

2. *Penicillinase–resistant penicillins*

Methicillin	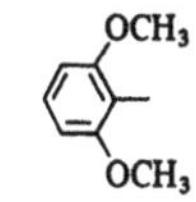
Nafcillin	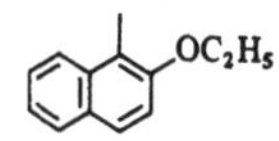
Oxacillins	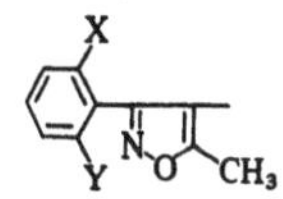

	X	Y
Oxacillin	H	H
Cloxacillin	Cl	H
Dicloxacillin	Cl	Cl
Flucloxacillin	Cl	F

3. *α–Aminopenicillins*

Ampicillin	D–$C_6H_5CH(NH_2)-$
Bacampicillin	$(-CH(CH_3)OCO_2C_2H_5$ ester)
Pivampicillin	$(-CH_2OCOC(CH_3)_3$ ester)
Hetacillin	(acetonide)
Metampicillin	$C_6H_5CH(N{=}CH_2)-$
Amoxicillin	D–$HOC_6H_4CH(NH_2)-$
Epicillin	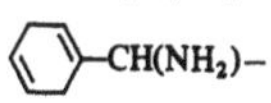
Cyclacillin	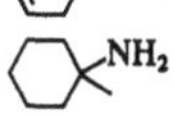

4. *α–Carboxy and α–sulfopenicillins*

Carbenicillin	$C_6H_5CH(CO_2H)-$
Carfecillin	(α–phenyl ester)
Carindacillin	(α–indanyl ester)
Ticarcillin	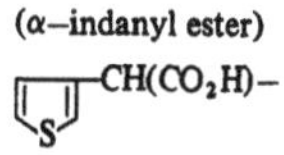
Sulbenicillin	$C_6H_5CH(SO_3H)-$
Suncillin	$C_6H_5CH(NHSO_3H)-$

5. *N–Acylampicillins*

See Fig. 2 — $C_6H_5CH(NHCOZ)-$
(Z=Guanidino, Cycloureido and Heterocyclic groups)

6. *Amidinopenicillanic acids*

Mecillinam	$RCONH = (CH_2)_6NCH{=}N-$
Promecillinam	$(-CH_2OCOC(CH_3)_3$ ester)

loxymethyl esters of ampicillin with improved oral absorption), all have been obtained by varying the 6-acyl group. Other modifications of the structure have not yet produced agents that have found use in the clinic. (However, see Sect. B.III.5.) Indeed, the side-chains that provide high levels of antibacterial activity fall within the narrow structural constraints of carboxamides; the sulfonamide, phosphoramide, imide, urea, thiourea, and urethane side-chains do not confer advantageous biological properties (SHEEHAN and HOFF 1957; PERRON et al. 1961, 1962; KOE et al. 1963; NAITO et al. 1965). Most, though not all, of the side-chains of interest are derived from *mono-* or *di*-substituted acetic acids. These relatively narrow structural changes have resulted in several major improvements over the early natural and biosynthetic derivatives including: (a) greater acid stability accompanied by

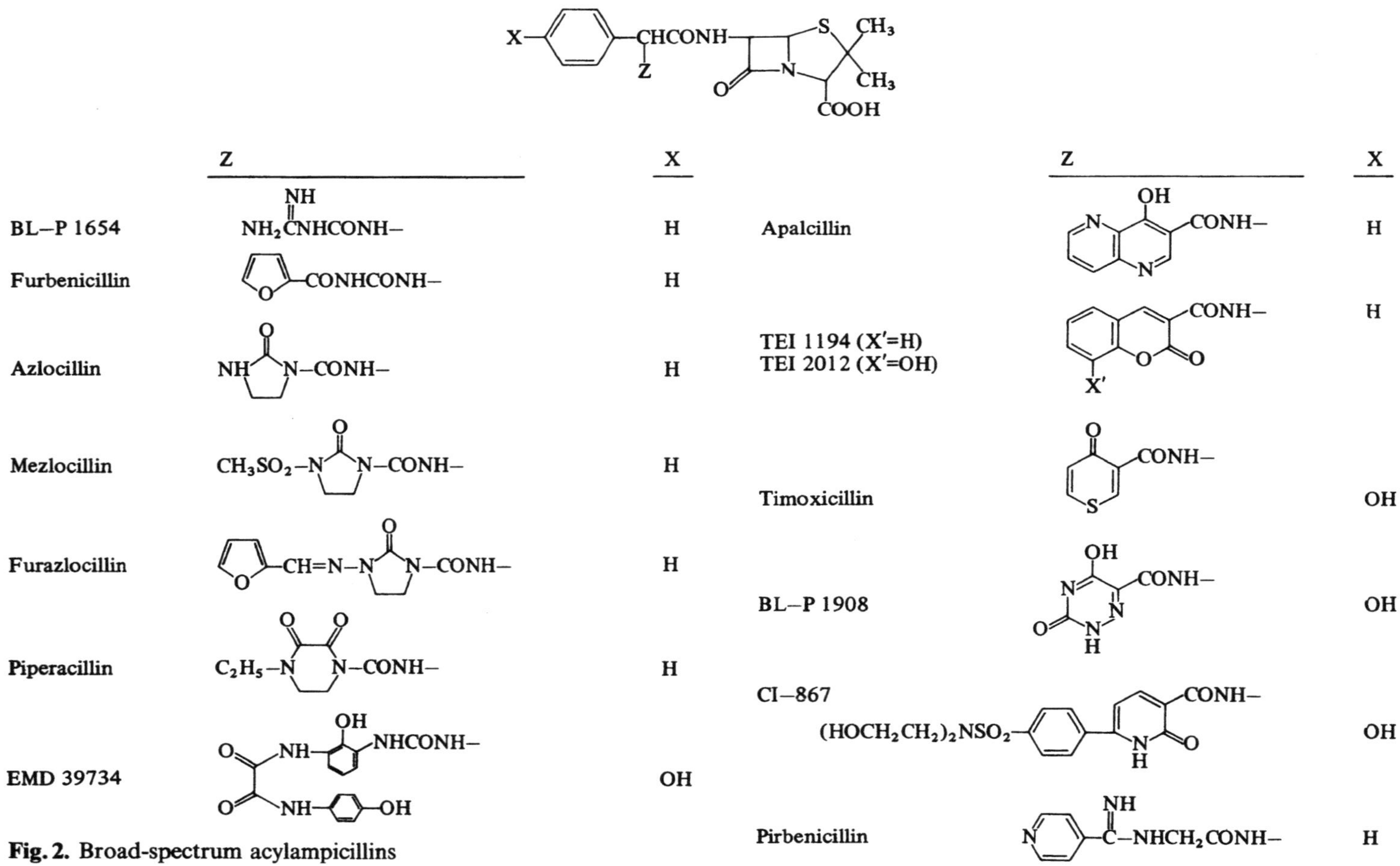

Fig. 2. Broad-spectrum acylampicillins

better oral absorption, (b) resistance to staphylococcal penicillinase, and (c) a broader spectrum of in vitro activity against gram-negative bacteria. The discussion of the penicillins which follows is organized according to the categories listed in Table 1.

I. Natural, Biosynthetic, and Related Penicillins

Benzylpenicillin was one of the first of the fifty or so biosynthetic penicillins that were obtained through unaided fermentations, or by the addition of appropriate precursors to the fermentation mixtures. It was selected for commercial development on the basis of fermentation yield and in vitro/in vivo performance. Its dominance in therapy throughout the antibiotic era makes it the appropriate standard on which to base SAR relationships among the penicillins. Table 2 lists typical MIC values obtained with benzylpenicillin against a representative group of gram-positive and gram-negative bacteria. This penicillin exhibits high intrinsic activity

Table 2. Typical minimum inhibitory concentrations (MIC) of benzylpenicillin, cephalothin, cefoxitin and cefotaxime against bacteria

	MIC (μg/ml)			
Organism	*Benzylpenicillin*	*Cephalothin*	*Cefoxitin*	*Cefotaxime*
Staphylococcus aureus (S)	0.02–0.06	0.05–2	3	1.6
Staphylococcus aureus (R)	7.5–>100	0.1–0.8	6	1.6
Streptococcus pyogenes	0.008–0.016	0.03–0.05	–	–
Streptococcus pneumoniae	0.006–0.015	0.02–0.15	–	–
Streptococcus faecalis	1.25–4	25–>100	>100	>100
Corynebacterium diphtheriae	0.03–3	0.16–0.63	–	–
Neisseria gonorrhoeae	0.03–0.1	0.25–0.5	0.4	–
Neisseria meningitidis	0.03	0.12–0.5	–	–
Hemophilis influenzae	0.5–3	2–8	3	–
Escherichia coli (S)	16–>125	2–8	3	0.1
Escherichia coli (R)	>100	>100	6	0.1
Klebsiella pneumoniae (S)	25	2	2	0.1
Klebsiella pneumoniae (R)	>100	>100	3	0.4
Proteus mirabilis	6–32	3	6	0.1
Proteus morganii	>100	>100	50	0.1
Shigella sonnei	16	4–8	–	0.1
Salmonella typhi	2.5–16	0.5–2	–	0.3
Enterobacter cloacae	50	50	50	0.2
Serratia marcescens	>100	>100	12	0.1
Pseudomonas aeruginosa	>200	>200	>200	25
Clostridium perfringens	0.5	–	–	0.2
Bacteroides fragilis	32	90	7	25

Sources: Kucers and Bennett, 1975; Barker and Prescott, 1973; SK&F, unpublished data; S=non–β–lactamase producers; R=β–lactamase producers.

against aerobic gram-positive bacilli and many, but not all, gram-positive and gram-negative cocci, including *Neisseria*, *Hemophilus*, *Brucella* sp., and *Pasturella multocida*, and *Trepenoma pallidum*. Its activity extends to most gram-positive and gram-negative anaerobes except *Bacteroides fragilis*, which is susceptible to only high levels of the antibiotic. Most aerobic gram-negative bacilli are considered resistant to useful levels, although strains of several species among the Enterobacteriaceae, notably *Escherichia coli*, *Proteus mirabilis*, *Salmonella*, and *Shigella* species, are sometimes susceptible at higher concentrations of the antibiotic (Table 2). In addition to its relatively narrow spectrum of activity, benzylpenicillin appears to be inactivated by all β-lactamases. This accounts, in part, for its poor performance against many of the gram-negative bacteria. Furthermore, the chemical reactivity of its β-lactam ring gives rise to extensive degradation (penicillic acid, penicillenic acid, pH 2 and 4, respectively) in the acidic milieu of the stomach, resulting in erratic oral absorption, thus requiring oral doses five times the recommended parenteral dose for assured therapeutic effectiveness (MARTIN 1967). Much of the research on the penicillins has been directed toward obviating these specific shortcomings. The degree of success of this work is reflected in the classification of clinically used penicillins listed in Table 1.

The biosynthetic penicillins were obtained by procedures which permit only incorporation of acetic acids with a single substituent on the α-carbon, although the group attached to the acetyl carbon can be fairly complicated (SOPER et al. 1948). As a consequence the biological differences between these analogs are relatively minor, the most significant being increased acid stability for phenoxymethylpenicillin (MCCARTHY and FINLAND 1960). This penicillin and others with a hetero atom on the α-carbon of the side-chain have better stability towards acids than has, for example, benzylpenicillin. The hetero atom reduces the interaction of the side-chain amide carbonyl with the β-lactam group that results in the rearrangement to penicillic and penicillenic acids. This stabilizing effect is readily seen in a comparison of the rate of inactivation (pH 1.3 and 35 °C in 50% aqueous ethanol) of phenoxymethylpenicillin with that of benzylpenicillin and three analogs with hetero atoms on the α-carbon of benzylpenicillin (DOYLE et al. 1961 a). Half-life values ($t_{1/2}$) were as follows: benzylpenicillin, 3.5 min; α-OMe, 77 min; phenoxymethylpenicillin, 160 min; α-Cl, 300 min; $\alpha-NH_3^+$, 660 min.

The improved acid stability of phenoxymethylpenicillin is reflected in increased absorption compared to benzylpenicillin when administered per os (typically 60% versus 20%; peak serum levels for 500-mg dose, orally, in man: 4 versus 2 µg/ml). This effect of the α-hetero atom extends to other important analogs such as ampicillin ($\alpha-NH_3^+$), as already seen, and the oxacillins. However, acid stability per se is not a guarantee of good oral absorption. The cephalosporins, which generally have a greater degree of stability toward acids than the penicillins, are virtually unabsorbed by the oral route. Exceptions to this are certain cephalosporins with phenylglycine-like side chains. These analogs, along with the amphoteric penicillins such as amoxicillin and cyclacillin appear to be absorbed by passive diffusion at high concentrations and by carrier-mediated transport at lower concentrations (rat intestine; QUAY 1972; KIMURA et al. 1978; TSUJI et al. 1979). This role of the side chain in oral absorption is examined further in a later section on oral cephalosporins.

Although the availability of 6-aminopenicillanic acid provided unlimited latitude in varying the acylamino side chain, the first semisynthetic penicillins to be introduced in commerce (phenethicillin, propicillin, phenbenicillin, clometocillin; see for example PERRON et al. 1960; VANDERHAEGHE et al. 1962) were α-aryloxyalkyl penicillins. Clometocillin is the analogous 3,4-dichloro-α-methoxybenzylpenicillin. Claims for therapeutic superiority were based on in vitro activities very similar to those of phenoxymethylpenicillin, coupled with more efficient oral absorption. For example, the 1-h serum concentrations (μg/ml) in a human crossover study for phenoxymethylpenicillin, phenethicillin, and propicillin (250-mg dose) were 1.63, 5.26, and 6.22, respectively (WILLIAMSON et al. 1961). Unfortunately, the more effective oral absorption is accompanied by greater serum binding (LYNN 1965). Because of the greater steric bulk of the di-substituted acetic acid side chains, these analogs were also found to be slightly more resistant than phenoxymethylpenicillin to staphylococcal penicillinase. This advantage is insignificant in the light of more recent work.

II. Penicillinase-Resistant Penicillins

Recognition of the important function of β-lactamases in bacterial resistance has shaped much of the structure modification and testing of the penicillins and cephalosporins. The *r*-plasmid mediated staphylococcal penicillinases (Chap. 12) were the first of the β-lactamases recognized to be clinically important. In comparison with the myriad penicillinases and cephalosporinases produced by gram-negative bacteria, the staphylococcal penicillinases exhibit comparatively narrow substrate and inhibition profiles. Consequently, the susceptibility of benzylpenicillin and its congeners to inactivation by this penicillinase can now be reversed in several ways. They include lowering the sensitivity of the β-lactam to the enzyme by increasing steric hindrance around the carbon atom attached to the amide carbonyl group (e.g., methicillin, oxacillins), and expanding the annelated sulfur-containing ring to the 6-membered dihydrothiazine ring of the cephalosporins. Alternatively, it is possible to protect the susceptible penicillin (benzylpenicillin, ampicillin) by co-introduction of an inhibitor of the β-lactamase (methicillin, nafcillin, oxacillin, clavulanic acid, carbapenems; Sect. D.III).

Resistance to inactivation by penicillinase is of little value unless the molecule retains a useful level of in vitro antibiotic activity and appropriate pharmacokinetic properties. Unfortunately, many of the structural changes which confer resistance to inactivation are accompanied by a corresponding reduction of the desired biological activities. Essentially all of the penicillins reported to have significant levels of staphylococcal penicillinase resistance carry acyl side-chains in which the α-carbon atom is quaternary, either through multiple substitution or by incorporation into an aromatic or heterocyclic ring. The effect of simply increasing the level of substitution on methylpenicillin is illustrated at the top of Tables 3 and 4. Resistance to staphylococcal penicillinase becomes effective only when the α-carbon is completely substituted by groupings of sufficient bulk (BRAIN et al. 1962; DOYLE and NAYLER 1966). Bulk at the β-carbon is ineffective. The introduction of the large hydrophobic group to achieve β-lactamase stability is accompanied by a

Table 3. Effect of side chain on susceptibility to penicillinase

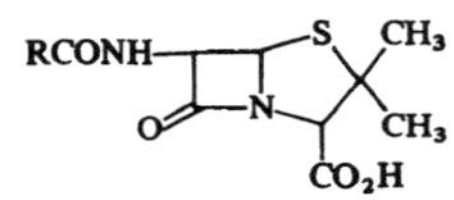

Resistant			Susceptible		
Ph_3C–	Ph_2HetC	Ph_2RC–	$(CH_3)_3C$–	Ph_3CCH_2–	Ph_2CH–
PhR_2C–	$Ph_2(RO)_2C$	$Ph_2(RS)_2C$	Cl_3C–	$PhCH_2$–	$PhOCH_2$–

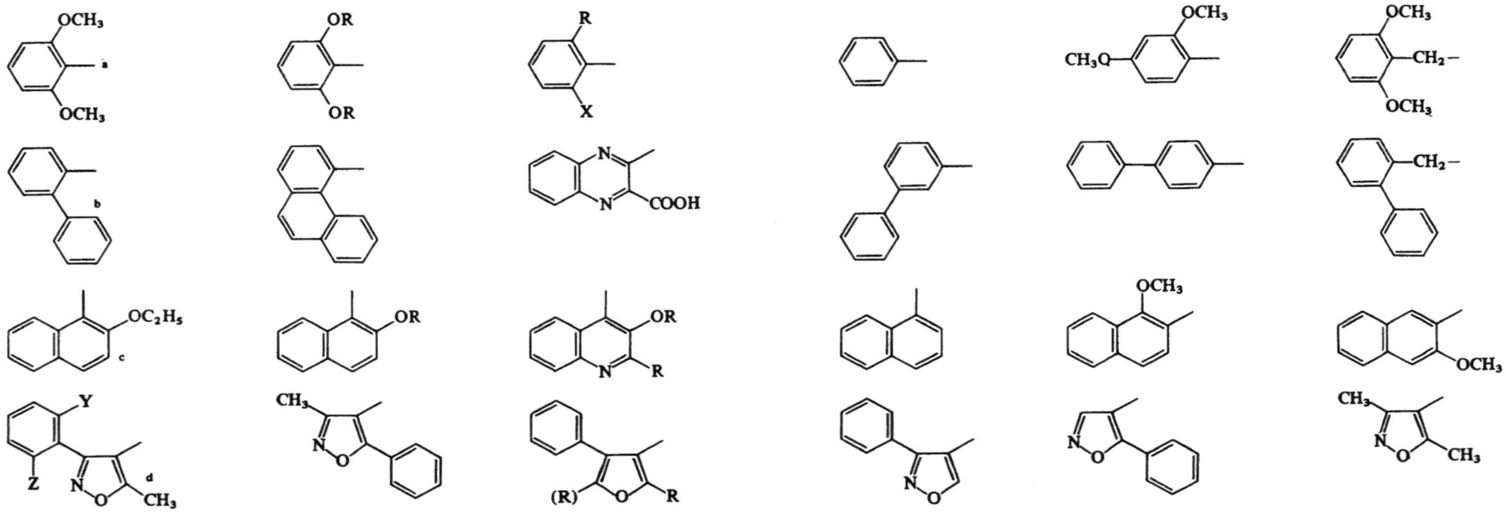

[a]Methicillin. [b]Diphenicillin. [c]Nafcillin. [d]Oxacillins. [e]Quinacillin. Ph = C_6H_5; Het = 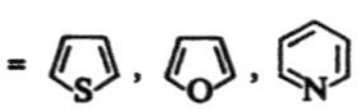
X = Br, Cl, NO_2, etc.; Y, Z = Cl, F; R = CH_3, C_2H_5, $C_6H_5CH_2$, etc.

Table 4. In vitro activities of selected penicillins against sensitive and penicillinase–producing *Staphylococcus aureus*

	MIC (μg/ml)	
Penicillin	*Sensitive*	*Resistant*
Benzylpenicillin	0.005–0.05	5–>250
Diphenylmethylpenicillin	0.05	250
Triphenylmethylpenicillin	0.3	0.3–0.6
Phenylpenicillin	0.1–0.25	>250
Methicillin	0.5–2.5	1.25–3.7
3,5–Dimethyl–4–isoxazolyl penicillin	0.25	>250
3–Phenyl–4–isoxazolyl penicillin	0.1	5–250
Oxacillins[a]	0.1–0.5	0.25–1.5
1–Naphthylpenicillin	0.1	12.5–25
Nafcillin	0.2	0.6
Diphenicillin	0.2	0.5
Quinacillin	0.5	0.5

Sources: Hoover and Dunn 1979; Nayler 1973.
[a])Oxacillin, cloxacillin, dicloxacillin, flucloxacillin.

lower level and a narrower spectrum of antibiotic activity. Still triphenylmethyl penicillin retains sufficient activity to qualify as a candidate for therapeutic use (Table 4). However, its in vitro activity is greatly diminished in the presence of serum, and it fails to protect laboratory animals against bacterial infection. Consequently, analogs of this type have not found commercial utility.

Penicillins in which the α-carbon atom of the side chain is incorporated into an aromatic or heterocyclic ring have provided the successful approaches to the clinically effective agents that are penicillinase resistant. Per se, this structural change does not improve penicillinase resistance and the in vitro activity is significantly reduced (Table 4). Phenylpenicillin and 3,5-dimethyl-4-isoxazolylpenicillins have only 5%–10% of the in vitro activity of benzylpenicillin against staphylococci (Price 1970) and their activities are confined to gram-positive bacteria that do not produce penicillinase. Substitution at the meta and para positions of phenylpenicillin does not greatly affect antibacterial activity or penicillinase susceptibility. However, by placing substituents on the ortho positions, there is little further loss in intrinsic activity, but penicillinase resistance improves profoundly (methicillin, Tables 3 and 4). Similar effects are observed when the phenyl ring is changed to a heterocyclic one such as isoxazole (oxacillins), 3-furyl (Hanson et al. 1965), 4-isothiazolyl (Micetich and Raap 1968; Grant et al. 1965), 5-pyrazolyl (Koczka et al. 1970) and sydnon-5-yl (Pala et al. 1969).

The size of the ring plays an important role in determining the ability of the ortho substituents to confer penicillinase resistance on the structure. Phenyl penicillins and equivalent heterocyclic analogs have marked stability to penicillinase when both ortho positions are occupied by any of a large variety of substituents (Doyle et al. 1962a; Brain et al. 1963). In fact with a six-membered ring (or a fused ring system of equivalent or greater bulk, e.g., quinacillin) a single ortho substituent of proper type can be sufficient for good penicillinase resistance. Thus o-biphenylylpenicillin (diphenicillin) is stable toward penicillinase but the analogous meta and para analogs, as well as o-biphenylylmethylpenicillin, are susceptible (Tables 3 and 4) (Dolan et al. 1962; Hoover et al. 1964). Other aromatic or heterocyclic ring systems, and even a cyclohexyl ring, can substitute for either benzene ring in o-biphenylylpenicillin, provided they meet specific structural requirements (Stedman et al. 1964; Chow et al. 1966).

When a five-membered heterocyclic ring is attached to the amide carbonyl group bulkier substituents are required for significant resistance to penicillinase inactivation. Thus, neither a single ortho phenyl group nor two ortho methyl groups confer penicillinase resistance on the isoxazolylpenicillin molecule. Predictably, total substituent size influences the opposed balance of in vitro activity and penicillinase resistance. Optimal activity and resistance are obtained with a phenyl and methyl substituent (oxacillin; Doyle et al. 1961b, 1963a). The phenyl group can be replaced by other aromatic rings (furyl, thienyl) but larger (naphthyl) or more polar (4-pyridyl) rings lower the in vitro activity. Replacement of the methyl (or ethyl) group by larger alkyl groups (isopropyl, *t*-butyl) or phenyl results in retention of penicillinase resistance, but lowered in vitro activity (Doyle et al. 1963b). The phenyl and methyl groups can be interchanged on the isoxazole ring with retention of resistance and activity. The rather definite substituent requirements also apply to the other five-membered heterocyclic analogs mentioned. The 2-alkoxy-1-naphthylpenicillins (nafcillin) can be viewed as analogs of methicillin in which a fused ring contributes the steric effect supplied by one of the o-methoxy groups of methicillin. These penicillins and their corresponding quinoline analogs are stable to penicillinase, whereas the less hindered 1-naphthyl, 3-methoxy-2-naphthyl- and 4-quinolinylpenicillins are sensitive to the enzyme (Rosenman and Warren 1962; Brain et al. 1963).

Methicillin (2,6-dimethoxyphenylpenicillin) was the first penicillinase-resistant penicillin to be used clinically. Its in vitro activity against *S. aureus* is poor relative to penicillin G (Table 4); it is unstable to acids, and must be given by injection. However, it is markedly nontoxic, it is bactericidal at concentrations very near to its bacteriostatic level and it exhibits a low level of serum binding. Nafcillin (2-ethoxy-1-naphthylpenicillin) is more active in vitro than methicillin and it is more stable to acid but its oral absorption is erratic and low serum levels obtained by intramuscular injection make intravenous administration preferable. Four 3-phenyl-5-methyl-4-isoxazolylpenicillins are available for clinical use: oxacillin, cloxacillin, dicloxacillin and flucloxacillin (Table 1). Their in vitro activities against susceptible and resistant staphylococci are roughly the same, and superior to that of methicillin: they are stable to acid (see above) and are readily absorbed from the gastrointestinal tract. The halogenation of the ortho positions of the phenyl group progressively doubles the efficiency of oral absorption. However, all of these penicillins are extensively bound to serum proteins (93%, 94%, 97%, and 95%, respectively, as opposed to 49% for methicillin) (Nayler 1973).

Table 5. Typical MIC values for four broad–spectrum penicillins and benzylpenicillin against laboratory strains of gram–positive and gram–negative bacteria

	MIC (μg/ml)				
	Benzylpenicillin	*Ampicillin*	*Carbenicillin*	*Piperacillin*	*Mecillinam*
S. aureus (S)	0.02	0.05	1.5	0.8	(5)
S. aureus (R)	>250	>250	25	>100	(>100)
S. pyogenes	0.01	0.02	0.5	–	(0.5)
S. faecalis	3.0	1.5	50	3	(>100)
N. gonorrhoeae	0.01	0.03	0.3	–	(0.16)
H. influenzae	0.5	0.5	0.5	–	(16)
E. coli	100	3	6	2	0.4
K. pneumoniae	250	250	250	12	2
S. typhi	10	1.5	5	–	0.8
Sh. sonnei	50	2.5	3	–	0.8
P. mirabilis	5	1.5	2.5	0.2	25
Proteus (indole +)	>250	250	5	–	–
P. vulgaris	>500	>500	12	6	100
E. cloacae	50	–	125	3	–
Enterobacter sp.	>500	>500	50	3	2
S. marcescens	>500	>500	100	12	100
Providencia sp.	>500	>500	12	6	100
Ps. aeruginosa	>500	>500	50	3	100

Sources: ROLINSON and SUTHERLAND 1973; SK&F Unpublished data; NEU 1979; LUND and TYBRING 1971 (note values in parentheses are IC_{50} values).

III. Broad-Spectrum Penicillins

Except for a few genera like *Neisseria, Hemophilus, Brucella, Pasteurella,* and anaerobes other than *Bacteroides,* the older penicillins are intrinsically less active against gram-negative than against gram-positive bacteria. These differences in sensitivity, already apparent in benzylpenicillin, are accentuated in the modifications which provide staphylococcal penicillinase stability. Such agents (methicillin, oxacillins) are essentially devoid of gram-negative activity. However, by appropriate manipulation of the 6β-substituents, penicillins have been developed which extend the spectrum of antibiotic activity to include many genera of Enterobacteriaceae insensitive to benzylpenicillin; and a growing number of analogs now exhibit significant activity against *Pseudomonas aeruginosa* and other genera that in the past have been especially insensitive to β-lactam antibiotics. Improvement of gram-negative activity has been accomplished for the most part by appropriate substitution of the α-carbon of the 6 β-side chain of benzylpenicillin or closely related analogs, the exceptions being mecillinam and some (4-pyridinio)amino penicillanic acids (*vide infra*). These analogs can be classified into four structural groups which are exemplified by ampicillin, carbenicillin, piperacillin and mecillinam in Table 5.

1. α-Aminopenicillins

Relatively early studies on the penicillins suggested that introduction of hydrophilic groups on the side-chain can result in improved gram-negative activity. Thus, while penicillin N (6-D-aminoadipoyl side-chain) is 100 times less active than benzylpenicillin against gram-positive bacteria, it is several times more active than penicillin G against coliform bacilli and certain other gram-negative organisms (Heatley and Florey 1953). Acylation of the amino group improves gram-positive activity and lowers gram-negative activity (Newton and Abraham 1954).

Table 6 lists analogs selected to illustrate than many α-substituents on benzylpenicillin reduce activity against gram-negative bacteria (exemplified here by MIC values against *E. coli*), but certain polar substituents, notably amino, hydroxyl, carboxyl and sulfonyl, increase gram-negative activity. This trend is reversed by alkylation (methoxy, methylamino, carbenicillin esters) or simple acylation (*N*-formyl, *N*-acetyl, etc.). These relationships imply that the interplay of lipophilicity versus hydrophilicity influences the balance of gram-positive to gram-negative activity (Hansch and Steward 1964). Obviously, this is not the sole explanation. The stereochemistry of attachment of the α-substituent plays a role in the activity observed for both the α-hydroxy and α-amino analogs. In both cases the L-isomers are only about as active as benzylpenicillin against gram-negative bacteria (Table 6). The D-isomer is required for increased activity (Nayler 1973; Long and Nayler 1972; e.g., MICs for D- versus L-epimers of ampicillin: *E. coli* 2.5 versus 12.5 μg/ml; *Klebsiella pneumoniae*, 1.6 versus 12.5 μg/ml; *S. typhosa*, 1.6 versus 12.5 μg/ml). This stereochemical specificity implies side-chain participation in receptor site binding (PBP binding comparisons are not yet available) or outer membrane transport.

Ampicillin is D-α-aminobenzylpenicillin (Tables 1, 5 and 6). It is the second most widely used penicillin in medical practice (Doyle et al. 1962b; Neu 1975). Its activity and β-lactamase sensitivity closely parallels that of benzylpenicillin against gram-positive bacteria and the gram-negative cocci. However, its activity against gram-negative bacilli extends to include some strains of *E. coli* and most *Salmonella, Shigella sp.*, and *Proteus mirabilis*. Most species of *Klebsiella*, indole-positive *Proteus*, *Serratia*, *Pseudomonas* and *B. fragilis* are insensitive. As indicated earlier, the α-amino group not only broadens the antibacterial spectrum, but it also increases the stability of the penicillin toward acids. Thus, ampicillin is well absorbed orally (peak serum level at 2 h approximately 2–6 μg/ml with 500-mg dose in humans) and serum levels are measurable after 4–6 h. It can be injected intramuscularly and intravenously as well. These pharmacokinetic properties contribute to its wide clinical use.

The success of ampicillin has led to many structural variations designed to improve its biological properties, and this has resulted in the development of several analogs and a number of pro-drug derivatives. Analogs include epicillin (the 1,4-cyclohexadienyl analog of ampicillin; Table 1; Dolfini et al. 1971) and cyclacillin (1-aminocyclohexylpenicillin, Table 1, Rosenman et al. 1968). Both penicillins have antibacterial spectra similar to that of ampicillin, but they appear to be absorbed more rapidly from the gastrointestinal tract (Schaedler and Warren 1980). The possible advantages of this in terms of lowered liability for disturbance of the commensal microflora of the lower bowel has recently been reviewed (Sel-

Table 6. Selected examples of the effect of lipophilic and hydrophilic α-substituents on the gram-positive and gram-negative activities of benzylpenicillin

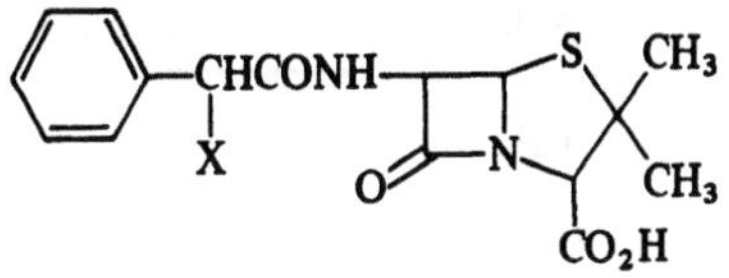

	MIC (μg/ml)		
X	*S. aureus*	*E. coli*	*Ps. aeruginosa*
H–	0.02	25	>500
Cl (D,L)	0.02	125	>500
CH_3 (D,L)	0.05	25	>500
OCH_3 (D,L)	0.02	125	>500
N_3 (D)	0.02	125	>500
$N(CH_3)_2$ (D,L)	0.25	125	>500
$NHCH_3$ (D,L)	0.01	25	>500
OH (D)	0.05	5	>500
OH (L)	0.1	25	>500
NH_2 (D)	0.05	2.5	>500
NH_2 (L)	0.1	12.5	>500
CH_2NH_2 (D)	0.25	2.5	>500
NHCHO (D)	0.1	12.5	>500
$NHCOCH_3$ (D)	0.5	62.5	>500
$NHCOCH_2NH_2$ (D)	1.25	5	>500
$NHCONH_2$ (D)	0.25	5	500
$NHCONHCOCH_3$ (D)	0.5	50	25
$NHSO_3H$ (D)	1.25	125	125
$CONH_2$ (D,L)	0.1	25	>500
COOH (D L)	2.5	5	50
SO_2NH_2 (D,L)	0.25	25	>500
SO_3H (D,L)	2.5	2.5	50

Source: NAYLER 1973

WYN 1979). Amoxicillin (Table 1) is the p-hydroxy derivative of ampicillin (LONG and NAYLER 1972). For broad-spectrum penicillins such as ampicillin, a second substituent, whether on the benzene ring or the α-carbon atom, tends to reduce gram-negative activity (EKSTROM et al. 1965). An important exception is the introduction of a hydroxyl group at the meta or para position (o-hydroxyl also reduces activity). Thus amoxicillin has essentially the same in vitro activity as ampicillin, and it produces similar serum levels on injection. However, orally it gives higher serum levels and better urinary recovery than ampicillin (Table 7; NEU and WINDSHELL 1971 a). Many additional analogs of ampicillin have been studied. The benzene ring has been replaced by heterocyclic rings such as thiophene (PRICE et al.

Table 7. Oral absorption of ampicillin, amoxicillin and ampicillin esters

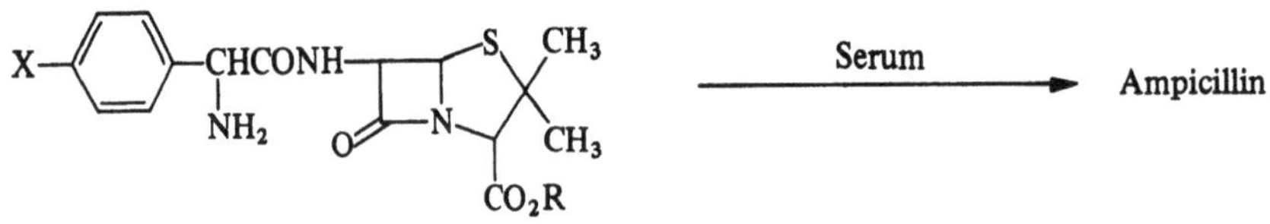

	R	*Oral dose* *mg*	*moles*	*Serum peak* (*μg/ml*)	*Peak ratio*	*Urinary recovery* (*%*)
Ampicillin (X=H)	H	278	0.8	3.7	1	45
		(250)	(0.7)	(2.2)	(1)	(35)
Pivampicillin	$-CH_2OCOC(CH_3)_3$	398	0.8	7.1	1.9	65
Bacampicillin	$-CH(CH_3)OCOOC_2H_5$	400	0.8	8.2	2.2	71
Talampicillin	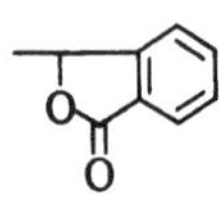	(371)	(0.7)	(5.7)	(2.6)	(54)
Amoxicillin (X=OH)	H	291	0.8	7.7	2.1	74

Sources: Shiobara et al. 1974; Sjovall et al. 1978.

1969 a), isothiazole (Raap 1971) and thiazole (Hatanaka and Ishimaru 1973) with little change in biological properties. Homologation to 6-(D- or L-phenylalanyl-amino) penicillanic acid lowers the gram-positive activity and results in gram-negative activity intermediate between ampicillin and benzylpenicillin. Insertion of a methylene between the amino group and the α-carbon atom gives betacin (Table 6; $X=CH_2NH_2$) with retention of gram-negative activity but lowered oral absorption (Acocella et al. 1965).

Two types of pro-drug forms of ampicillin have been developed to improve serum levels of free ampicillin on oral administration: carbonyl adducts involving the α-amino group and esters of the carboxyl group. Both types are inactive in vitro and release ampicillin after ingestion. The adducts include hetacillin (acetone) and metampicillin (formaldehyde). The pharmacokinetic behavior of the esters (pivampicillin, bacampicillin and talampicillin) is compared with that of ampicillin and amoxicillin in Table 7. Primary references to these agents can be obtained from prior reviews (e.g., Hoover and Dunn 1979; Price 1977). Sarmoxicillin is the most recent entry to this group. It is the combined acetone adduct and methoxymethyl ester of amoxicillin (Anon 1979).

2. α-Carboxy and α-Sulfopenicillins

The broadened antibacterial activity exhibited by the aminopenicillins just described does not extend to *Ps. aeruginosa* or a number of newly emerging, highly resistant, pathogenic enteric bacteria such as *Serratia*, *Providencia* and *Citrobacter* sp. Table 6 contains examples which suggest two methods to achieve this. While most of the penicillins in the table – including those active against *E. coli* – are inactive against *Ps. aeruginosa*, measurable MIC values (50–500 μg/ml) are observed, with some complex acylampicillins (see next section), and, with the three benzylpenicillins that have a strongly acidic function (carboxylic, sulfamic, sulfonic acid) on the α-carbon atom of the side chain. The effect on in vitro activity of placing an acidic group on the α-carbon can be seen in the MIC values reported for carbenicillin (ACRED et al. 1967; KIRBY et al. 1970) in Table 5. Typical of penicillins and cephalosporins, the presence of a highly ionic group of this type on the molecule reduces gram-positive activity, but in this case gram-negative activity is extended to include not only species susceptible to ampicillin [*E. coli* (partial), *Salmonella*, *Shigella*, *P. mirabilis*], but also several that are not usually susceptible to the latter, for example, indole-positive *Proteus*, *Pseudomonas*, some *Enterobacter*, *Providencia*, and *Serratia* species, and many *Bacteroides fragilis* strains. Most *Klebsiella* species remain insensitive. For many of the susceptible species, high concentrations of the antibiotic are required; often the MIC values range from 50 to 100 μg/ml. However, carbenicillin is regarded as a life-saving antibiotic, especially for the treatment of infections caused by *Ps. aeuroginosa*. The low in vitro activity requires intravenous infusion of impressively high amounts of the drug. Fortunately it has a very low level of toxicity since serum levels in excess of 150 μg/ml are frequently attained by infusing dosages up to 100 mg/kg over short periods of time (1–2 h).

The side chain of carbenicillin is racemic; the D- and L-isomers, when separated, have essentially the same level of activity and they undergo rapid interconversion. This derivative of phenylmalonic acid has poor acid stability and must be given by injection. Some decarboxylation to benzylpenicillin occurs. Many attempts have been made to improve stability and activity. The chemical stability can be improved by esterification of the side-chain α-carboxyl group. The indanyl (carindacillin) and phenyl (carfecillin) esters are available for clinical use (ENGLISH et al. 1972; CLAYTON et al. 1975). These esters are absorbed orally and hydrolyze rapidly in serum to carbenicillin. They are useful primarily for urinary tract infections since they do not provide adequate serum levels for treatment of systemic infections (WALLACE et al. 1971).

Structure–activity studies directed toward replacement of the phenyl group of cabenicillin with a heterocyclic ring have been more successful clinically than with ampicillin. Ticarcillin is the 3-thienyl analog of carbenicillin. Its in vitro spectrum closely resembles that of carbenicillin, but it is about twice as active against most strains of *Ps. aeruginosa*. This better therapeutic effectiveness is also observed in vivo (BODEY and DEERAKE 1971; NEU and WINSHELL 1971b; ACRED et al. 1971). Replacement of the side chain carboxyl of carbenicillin with a sulfonic acid group (sulbenicillin) results in better chemical stability, but the two penicillins have almost the same in vitro antibacterial activity and very similar pharmacokinetic properties (TSUCHIYA et al. 1971; MORIMOTO et al. 1972; YAMAZAKI and TSUCHIYA 1971). As expected, benzylpenicillins with other acidic α-substituents have been found to have similar properties. Suncillin (α-sulfoaminobenzylpenicillin) has an α-sulfamic acid substituent with in vitro activity against *Ps. aeruginosa* strains similar to that of carbenicillin, but it is less active against some other gram-negative genera (PRICE et al. 1969b; BARZA et al. 1971). The benzylpenicillin analog with an α-(5-tetrazolyl) group has been found to resemble carbenicillin in vitro, but is less active in vivo (ESSERY 1969). As with ampicillin the carbenicillin side chain has been homologated and hetero atoms have been inserted between the α-carbon and the ring with reduction in activity versus *Ps. aeruginosa.*

3. Acylampicillins

The most recent structure–activity research on the penicillins has been largely directed toward the other method for increasing the level of in vitro activity against species now moderately susceptible to carbenicillin and ampicillin. This research has concentrated on the synthesis of ampicillin or amoxicillin derivatives in which the α-amino group carries a relatively complex acyl moiety. The deleterious effect of simple acylation of the amino group of ampicillin on gram-negative activity was noted earlier. However, the analogs listed in Table 6 supply a hint that acylation involving more complex groupings can, in fact, increase activity against gram-negative bacteria (e.g., the D-α-ureido and acetylureido analogs). Extension of this observation has produced a large number of agents which exhibit a sufficiently impressive spectrum of activity against gram-positive and gram-negative bacteria to qualify them for evaluation as candidates for clinical use. The structural features and generic designations of some of the more thoroughly studied of these analogs are summarized in Fig. 2. Approximately half of these penicillins have an α-ureido grouping; of these all but one have an additional carbonyl group or its equivalent (guanidyl) on the N-3 atom. Appopriate substitution of this nitrogen atom, improves activity and toxicity (KOENIG et al. 1977). The structural relationships of the remaining analogs to the acylurea types, or to each other, are not obvious. In spite of their apparent diversity of structure, these penicillins exhibit relatively similar antimicrobial spectra. Their broad-spectrum activities, illustrated by the MIC values listed for piperacillin in Table 5, extends to *Ps. aeruginosa* as well as Enterobacteriaceae such as *K. pneumoniae* strains resistant to carbenicillin and ampicillin, *Enterobacter*, *Serratra* and *Providencia* sp. Activity against gram-positive bacteria is retained, but resistance to staphylococcal penicillinase is absent. The collective similarities of these penicillins can be seen in the compilation of MIC 50% values for nine analogs against the representative gram-negative bacteria listed in Table 8. These data are single-point comparisons extracted from a number of different evaluations of the in vitro activities of the penicillins against clinical isolates. To provide some basis for the comparisons the MIC values of carbenicillin used as a control in each experiment are included in parenthesis. This table should provide a means for comparing the activities of the analogs in a general sense, but a suitably accurate assessment of the in vitro effectiveness of these penicillins requires consultation of the original articles. As a group these agents exhibit activities against *Ps. aeruginosa* 2–20 times better than that of carbenicillin. MIC values against the usually insensitive *Klebsiella* species are reduced to clinically achievable serum levels in most cases. Individual variations within the group serve as potential attributes for clinical promotion. The acylampicillins have generally acceptable pharmacokinetic properties although individual variations in handling and toxicity in laboratory animals might be expected to prevent several from achieving clinical acceptability (for example, GOTTSCHLICH et al. 1980; BERGAN 1978). High and prolonged serum levels are attainable [e.g., piperacillin, 2 g i.v.: 126 μg/ml at 15 min,

Table 8. Comparative in vitro activities of nine acylampicillins against clinical isolates of gram–negative bacteria

			MIC_{50} (μg/ml)						
	Ref.	*n*	*Ps. aeruginosa*	*E. coli*	*Klebsiella sp.*	*P. mirabilis*	*Proteus sp.*	*Enterobacter sp.*	*S. marcescens*
Azlocillin	a	50	12.5(50)	6.2(3.1)	50(>200)	3.1(0.8)	25(1.6)	25(6.2)	25(12.5)
Mezlocillin	a	50	25(50)	3.1(3.1)	12.5(>200)	0.8(0.8)	3.1(1.6)	3.1(6.2)	6.2(12.5)
Piperacillin	a	50	6.2(50)	1.6(3.1)	25(>200)	0.4(0.8)	1.6(1.6)	3.1(6.2)	3.1(12.5)
Furazlocillin	g	25–74	2(32)	0.5(8)	2(256)	0.5(0.5)	0.5(0.5)	–	–
Apalcillin	b,c	50	0.8(50)	0.2(3.1)	3.1(>200)	0.2(0.2)	–	50(>200)	3.1(12.5)
Pirbenicillin	d	20–30	7.8(62)	3.1(6.2)	50(>200)	3.1(0.8)	3.1(0.8)	6.2(6.2)	12.5(3.1)
CI–867	a	50	3.1(50)	3.1(3.1)	25(>200)	3.1(0.8)	6.2(1.6)	3.1(6.2)	12.5(12.5)
BL–P 1654	e	50	6.2(50)	3.1(6.2)	25(>200)	0.2(0.2)	50(1.6)	100(50)	12.5(25)
BL–P 1908	f	20–101	1 (64)	16(4)	>64(>256)	1(0.5)	>64(4)	4(>64)	–

Sources: [a]WEAVER and BODEY 1980. [b]BODEY and LE BLANC 1978. [c]BODEY et al. 1978. [d]RETSEMA et al. 1976. [e]STEWART and BODEY 1977. [f]FUCHS et al. 1977. [g]WISE et al. 1978. MIC_{50}: minimum concentration of antibiotic inhibiting 50% of strains tested. Values in parentheses: MIC_{50} for carbenicillin in same tests. Values from b and c estimated from graphs. See sources for methods and conditions used.

Table 9. Penicillin binding protein affinities for wild–type and permeability mutants of *E. coli* K12 and *Ps. aeruginosa* K799

	MIC (μg/ml)		I_{50}(μg/ml)[a]						
Antibiotic	*Wild type*	*Permeab. mutant*	*1A*	*1B*	*2*	*3*	*4*	*5*	*6*
Ps. aeruginosa									
Carbenicillin	8	0.02	0.08	0.26	–	0.04	0.54	>10	1.6
Azlocillin	2	0.01	0.10	0.47	–	0.02	0.04	4.2	0.08
E. coli									
Benzylpenicillin	16	1.6	0.5	3.0	0.8	0.9	1.0	24	19
Ampicillin	3.2	0.5	1.4	3.9	0.7	0.9	2.0	140	9
Amoxicillin	3.2	1.6	0.7	2.2	0.9	4.1	2.5	110	9
Carbenicillin	2	1	2.1	5.0	4.0	2.1	3.5	130	120
Mezlocillin	6.4	0.025	1.5	8.0	0.9	0.02	>25	>25	>25
Mecillinam	0.05	–	>500	>500	0.04	>500	>500	>500	>500

Sources: CURTIS et al. 1979; ZIMMERMAN 1980; SPRATT 1977,1980. [a])Concentration of penicillin required to reduce ^{14}C–benzyl penicillin binding to PBPs by 50%. Values (I_{50}) given are for wild type, those for permeability mutant were essentially the same (within experimental error.)

20 μg/ml at 2 h (BERGAN 1978); azlocillin, 2 g i.v.: 60 μg/ml at 1 h, 6 μg/ml at 4 h (NEU 1979)].

Unfortunately, members of this class of penicillins exhibit several properties which cast some doubt on their long-range utility. Some analogs exhibit a marked spread between the minimum inhibitory concentration and the minimum bactericidal concentration, especially for *Pseudomonas* [e.g., BL-P 1654 (KURTZ et al. 1975); BL-P 1908 (FUCHS et al. 1977)]. This appears to be less of a problem for others; piperacillin and pirbenicillin have MBC values only 2- to 4-fold greater than the MIC values (KUCK and REDIN 1978; RETSEMA et al. 1976). While improved in vitro activity is observed against *Ps. aeruginosa* strains susceptible to carbenicillin, those which have acquired resistance to the latter are usually likewise resistant to the acylampicillins (VERBIST 1978, 1979). A more ubiquitous problem is the effect of innoculum size on the in vitro activities of these penicillins. Almost uniformly, the acylampicillins undergo significant reduction in in vitro activity when the innoculum size is increased from 10^5 to 10^7 CFU (STEWART and BODEY 1977; BODEY et al. 1978; BODEY and LEBLANC 1978; WEAVER and BODEY 1980; KUCK and REDIN 1978).

The mechanism for the extended activity against *Pseudomonas* and the Enterobacteriaceae indicated is not yet clearly defined. These penicillins obviously lack resistance to staphylococcal penicillinase. Observations on resistance to gram-negative *β*-lactamases are conflicting but suggest that this is not a major factor in determining their high level of activity against the carbenicillin-sensitive *Pseudomonas* strains, and the like (O'CALLAGHAN 1980; FU and NEU 1978b).

The level and distribution of binding of azlocillin to the PBPs of *Ps. aeruginosa* and the binding of mezlocillin to the PBPs of *E. coli* have been compared with that of several penicillins including carbenicillin (CURTIS et al. 1979; ZIMMERMAN 1980). Some of these data are listed in Table 9. The differences between the binding of mezlocillin and carbenicillin to the PBP 3 of the *E. coli* strain may relate, in part, to their differences in intrinsic activity against Enterobacteriaceae such as *Klebsiella* since CURTIS et al. (1980a) found good correlation in the binding profiles of *E. coli*, *E. cloacae*, *K. pneumoniae* and *P. rettgeri*. But this difference, reflected in the nearly equal MIC and I_{50} values for each compound against the permeability mutant, is small compared to the differences between the MICs of these penicillins against the wild strain. Thus, it is probably safe to assume that permeability of the outer membrane is a major factor for the differences in intrinsic activity in this case; and more so in the case with *Klebsiella* species where greater differences in MIC, in the reverse sense, are observed. The same considerations seem to apply to *Ps. aeruginosa*. In this case, there appears to be little difference between carbenicillin and azlocillin in the binding to the essential PBPs, which correlates with the MIC values for the permeable mutant, and the MIC values against the wild type are significantly higher. Thus, these data strongly suggest that the permeability of the outer membrane of *Ps. aeruginosa* is a major factor in the level of susceptibility of this species to these antibiotics.

4. 6-Acylamino Alternatives: Quaternary Heterocyclic Aminopenicillanic Acids and 6-Amidinopenicillanic Acids

The 6β-amidinopenicillanic acids constitute the one known exception to the rule that clinically useful activity among the penicillins requires an appropriate 6β-acylamino substituent. A new group of quaternary (4-pyridino)amino penicillanic and cephalosporanic acids may soon provide a second example (HANNAH et al. 1982). Like many other significant developments in the β-lactam antibiotic field, the discovery of biological utility for this type of penicillin resulted from a serendipitous observation. The synthetic intermediate 6β-dimethylformamidinopenicillanic acid (Table 10, $Z=(CH_3)_2N-$, $X=H$) was prepared in an attempt to modify the penicillin structure by opening of the thiazolidine ring. This chemical approach was unsuccessful, but the intermediate was found to have antibacterial activity (LUND 1977). The synthesis and testing of many analogs of this amidino penicillin led to the selection of mecillinam (6β-[(hexahydro-1*H*-azepin-1-yl)-methyleneamino]penicillanic acid; FL 1060; Table 1) for clinical use. Typical in vitro activities of mecillinam are listed in Table 5 for comparison with those of the penicillins already discussed. Mecillinam is considerably different from conventional penicillins in antibacterial spectrum. It has poor activity against gram-positive bacteria, and *H. influenza*, and *Neisseria* sp. do not exhibit the extreme sensitivity observed with benzylpenicillin and ampicillin. However, it is very active against *E. coli*, inhibiting many strains that produce plasmid-mediated β-lactamases even though it is hydrolyzed by these enzymes. This activity may be explained, in part, by its low affinity for the β-lactamase. It is also active against many *Klebsiella*, *Enterobacter* and *Citrobacter* species, as well as ampicillin-resistant species of *Shigella* and *Salmonella*. Activity against *Proteus* sp. (both *P. mirabilis* and indole-positive *Proteus*) is variable, and it is inactive against *Ps. aeruginosa* and *B. fragilis*. Par-

Table 10. Structure–activity relationships of 6–β–amidinopenicillin analogs

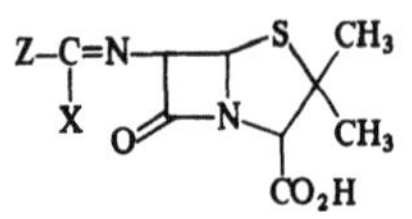

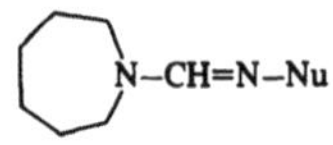

Z	*X*	*S. aureus*	*E. coli*
$(CH_3)_2N$–	H	1.6	0.5
$(CH_3)_2N$–	C_6H_5	10	>100
$(CH_3)_2N$–	C_3H_7	2	>100
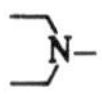	H	5	0.1
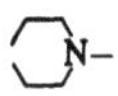	H	7.9	0.16
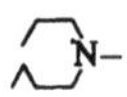	H	10	0.16
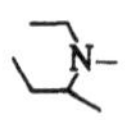	H	40	0.16
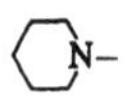	H	2	0.05
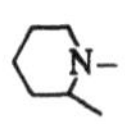	H	7.9	0.05
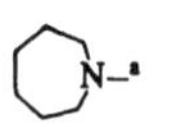 [a]	H	6.3	0.016
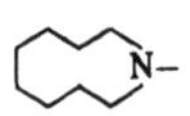	H	16	0.063
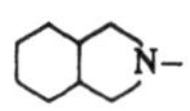	H	32	0.025
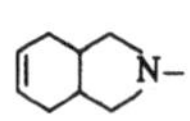	H	5	0.16
$CH_3(NH_2COCH_2)N$–	H	4	6.3
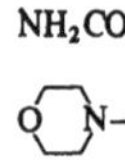	H	0.63	5.0
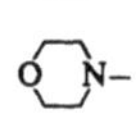	C_5H_{11}	0.16	100
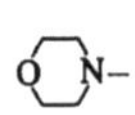	C_7H_{15}	0.5	>100
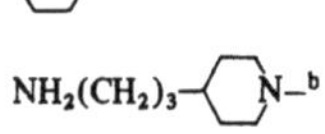 [b]	H	–	0.016

Nu	*S. aureus*	*E. coli*
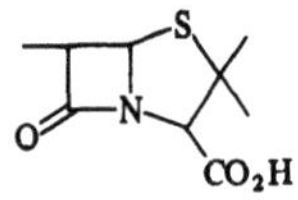	6.3	0.016
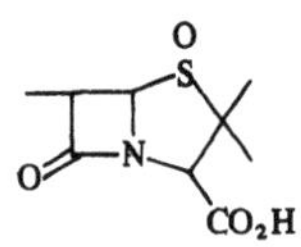	>100	1
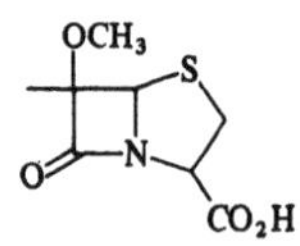	16	100
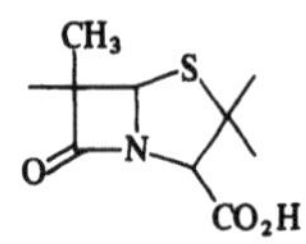	>100	79
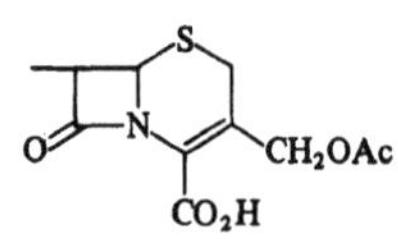	20	5.0
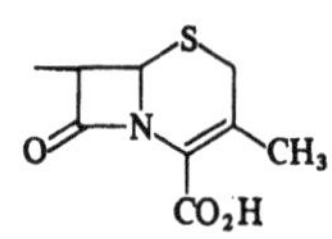	>100	>100
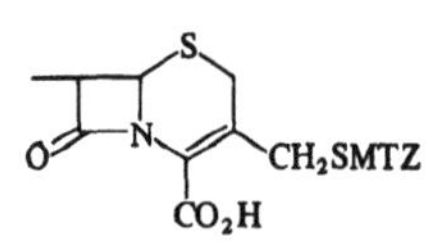	6.3	1.6

Z	*X*	*S. aureus*	*E. coli*
$(CH_2{=}CHCH_2)_2N$–	H	1.6	0.5
$CH_3(C_6H_5)N$–	H	1.3	10
$CH_3(C_6H_5CH_2)N$–	H	1	0.5

Source: LUND 1977. Note in vitro activities reported are IC_{50} values, not MIC values; SMTZ=4–thio–2–methyl–1, 2, 4–thiadiazole. [a]Mecillinam. [b]BINDERUP 1980.

enterally, mecillinam exhibits pharmacokinetic properties similar to those of ampicillin. While it is stable toward acids (BALTZER et al. 1979), it is not appreciably absorbed by the oral route (ROHOLT et al. 1975). The pivaloyloxymethyl ester (Table 1) is well absorbed orally and is hydrolyzed in the process to give clinically effective levels of the parent antibiotic (GAMBERTOGLIO et al. 1980). The properties of mecillinam have been extensively reviewed (GEDDES and WISE 1977).

Table 11. Synergy of mecillinam with ampicillin in vitro and in mouse protection tests

	MIC (μg/ml total conc.); PD_{50} (mg/kg, in parentheses)		
	Mecillinam	*50/50 Mixture*	*Ampicillin*
E. coli	0.01 (8.8)	0.03 (<1.0)	3 (6.2)
K. pneumoniae	30 (33)	3 (4.4)	>100 (6.2)
P. vulgaris	30	10	>100

Source: TYBRING and MELCHIOR 1975

In the extensive study of structure–activity relationships that led to the selection of mecillinam, *S. aureus* and *E. coli* were used as indicators of the level of gram-positive and gram-negative activity of the analogs. This study (LUND 1977) produced the following general conclusions for formamidino analogs illustrated by the selected examples included in Table 10. With *n*-alkyl groups on the amidino nitrogen atom optimal gram-negative activity is seen with a total of four to eight carbon atoms regardless of their distribution. Alkyl group variation has a smaller and less predictable effect on gram-positive activity, except that branching next to the nitrogen atom lowers it. Conversely, introduction of unsaturation improves gram-positive activity, but lowers gram-negative activity, as does introduction of aromatic or heterocyclic rings. Incorporation of the *n*-alkyl groups into a ring has little effect on gram-positive activity but gram-negative activity generally is improved three- to ten-fold. The total ring size is important since analogs with smaller, alkyl-substituted rings having the same total number of carbons are less active. Polar groups tend to lower activity, hetero atoms in the cyclic analogs have a variable effect, but properly placed, they can reverse the gram-positive–gram-negative activity ratio. An alkyl group on the amidine carbon atom abruptly reduces gram-negative activity, but increases gram-positive activity up to chain lengths of about five carbons. Modification of the nucleus (sulfoxide, 7α-substitution, 7β-amidino cephalosporins) reduces biological activity. In a recent patent a piperidine analog with a 4′-aminopropyl substituent was reported to have significantly better activity than mecillinam against gram-negative bacteria, including *Ps. aeruginosa* (BINDERUP 1980; compound (b), Table 10).

The profile of mecillinam binding to PBPs has been found to be unusual compared with almost all other β-lactam antibiotics in that it binds almost exclusively to PBP 2 of *E. coli* (PARK and BURMAN 1973; SPRATT 1977, 1980; CURTIS et al. 1979; see Table 9). This is reflected in the morphological changes of bacteria treated with mecillinam which form spherical cells (LUND and TYBRING 1971; GREENWOOD and O'GRADY 1973); and it very probably plays a role in the antibacterial spectral differences between mecillinam and other β-lactam antibiotics, both penicillins and cephalosporins. This property has been a useful tool in delineating the effects of binding to PBPs, changes in cell morphology, and killing by β-lactam antibiotics (SPRATT 1980). This phenomenon also relates to the fact that mecillinam has been found to act synergistically with other penicillins and with cephalosporins which bind more avidly to PBPs other than PBP 2 (TYBRING and MELCHIOR 1975; GRUNBERG et al. 1976). This synergism is illustrated with ampicillin in Table 11.

A second non-acyl type of substituent capable of conferring a high level of antibacterial activity on the penicillin and, in this case, the cephalosporin structures has recently been described. They are primarily 6(7)-[1-substituted-(4-pyridino)amino] substituents in which the pyridine ring nitrogen atom is quaternized, as exemplified in the following structure. Extensive SAR studies have produced penicillins (HANNAH et al. 1982) and cephalosporins (e.g., L-640867; KOUPAL et al. 1983) with in vitro activities equal to or better than that of mecillinam and in vivo effectiveness (L-640867) similar to that of cefotaxime (see below).

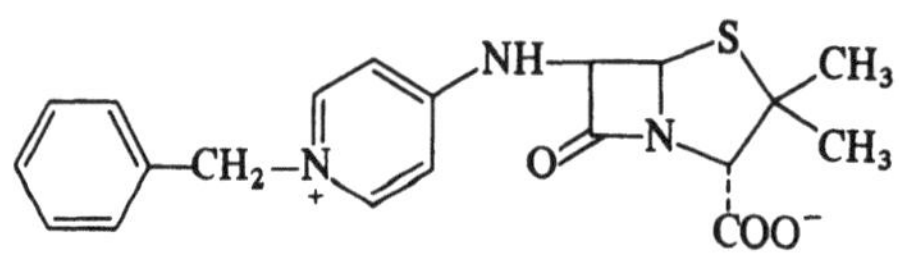

5. A 6α-Methoxy Penicillin (Temocillin)

Until recently, substitution of the 6α-position of the penicillin nucleus has been reported to result in virtual loss of in vitro antibacterial activity (see HOOVER and DUNN 1979 for a compilation of 6α-substituents reported and access references). One exception (BRL 17421, 6β-(2-carboxy-2-thien-3-ylacetamido)6α-methoxypenicillianic acid; SLOCOMBE et al. 1981; see Table 12) has now been described which is active against a wide range of Enterobacteriaceae including strains highly resistant to many penicillins and cephalosporins. This 6α-methoxy penicillin exhibits a very low level of activity against gram-positive bacteria, *Ps. aeruginosa* and anaerobes; activity against *H. influenzae* (0.2 μg/ml) and *N. gonorrhea* (0.5 μg/ml) is good. The poor gram-positive activity is not surprising since the molecule contains both a carboxyl group on the 6β-acyl side-chain and a 6α-methoxy group. The level of activity against *Ps. aeruginosa* is unexpectedly low.

Probably for the reasons advanced in the discussion of the cephamycins which follows later, this analog is highly resistant to inactivation by β-lactamases. Indeed, it has a wider spectrum of stability to these enzymes than the β-lactamase-resistant cephalosporins cefuroxime and cefoxitin. The compound shows no detectable hydrolysis by staphylococcal penicillinase or the class I–V (Richmond and Sykes classification, see below) β-lactamases from gram-negative bacteria. In contrast, cefuroxime exhibits variable susceptibility to all of these enzymes and cefoxitin is hydrolyzed by the chromosomally mediated class I cephalosporinases. This β-lactamase resistance is reflected in the favorable MIC values of temocillin compared to those of cefazolin generally and to the MIC values of cefoxitin against class I cephalosporinase-producers such as the *Enterobacter* sp. The comparative in vitro activity of temocillin is illustrated by the selected MIC values listed in Table 12.

Temocillin is well tolerated on injection intramuscularly or intravenously in man, and it produces high and prolonged serum levels (500 mg dose i.m.; serum peak, 48 μg/ml; $t_{1/2}$, 5.0–5.4 h). Urinary recovery (unmetabolized) ranges from 72% to 92%. The compound is strongly bound by serum (85%). In mice the protective effectiveness of temocillin is slightly poorer than that of cefazolin, cefuroxime, or cefoxitin in infections with non-β-lactamase-producing Enterobacteriaceae (e.g., comparative ED_{50} values vs. *E. coli* in mice dosed 1, 3, and 5 h postinfection: 15, 7, 4, and 8 mg/kg, respectively). This agent exhibits superior protectiveness

Table 12. Comparative in vitro activity of temocillin

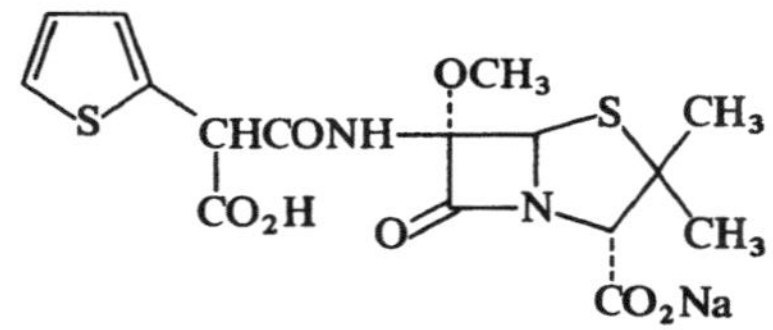

	Laboratory strains		Clinical isolates						
	Temocillin		Temocillin			Cefazolin		Cefoxitin	
Organism	Strain	MIC	N	MIC_{50}	Range	MIC_{50}	Range	MIC_{50}	Range
S.pyogenes	CN10	250	–	–	–	–	–	–	–
S. aureus	Oxford	250	–	–	–	–	–	–	–
S.faecalis	I	>500	–	–	–	–	–	–	–
N.gonorrhoeae	WHOvii	0.05	19	0.05	0.02–2.5	–	–	0.2	0.2–1.0
E.coli	J14	5.0	140	5.0	1.2–25	125	1.2–500	5.0	1.2–50
K. pneumoniae	A	2.5	112	2.5	1.2–25	5.0	1.2–>500	1.2	0.5–12.5
Proteus (indole +)	R276	1.2	19	2.5	0.5–5.0	500	0.5–>500	5.0	2.5–12.5
P. mirabilis	C977	1.2	19	2.5	2.5	5.0	5.0–>500	2.5	2.5–10
Enterobacter Sp.	N1	5.0	20	2.5	2.5–50	>500	50–>500	125	2.5–500
S. marcescens	–	–	48	12.5	2.5–500	>500	>500	25	5.0–125
Ps. aeruginosa	Dalgleish	250	–	–	–	–	–	–	–
B. fragilis	WSI	250	–	–	–	–	–	–	–

Source: SLOCOMBE et al. 1981. All MIC values are μg/ml, in agar using 10^5–10^6 CFU.

when β-lactamase-producers are used as the infectious agent (ED_{50} vs. *E. cloacae:* 22, >1,200, 60, and 840 mg/kg, respectively).

C. Clinically Useful Cephalosporins

Like the penicillins these agents usually have a low level of toxicity, and cross-allergenicity is sufficiently low to allow their use in penicillin-sensitive patients (DASH 1975). They are bactericidal at concentrations close to their MICs and resistant to staphylococcal β-lactamase, as illustrated in Table 13 by the higher MIC values for penicillins than for cephalosporins against the penicillin-resistant *S. aureus* strain. Natural cephalosporins such as cephalosporin C exhibit a better ratio of gram-negative to gram-positive activity, but the intrinsic antibacterial activities of cephalosporins tend to be lower than those of the corresponding penicillins (compare susceptible *S. aureus* MIC values of the penicillins with the resistant *S. aureus* MIC values of the cephalosporins. The activity of the cephalosporins against penicillin-susceptible *S. aureus* is not significantly different from that listed for the resistant strain). Differences in intrinsic activity (independent of permeability and β-lactamase inactivation factors) between penicillins and cephalosporins can be correlated with affinity of binding to the membrane enzymes vital to cell wall construction and maintenance by comparing Tables 9 and 14. These tables include the I_{50} values for the binding of penicillins (Table 9) and cephalosporins (Table 14) to PBPs of *E. coli* K 12 (DCO) as determined by CURTIS et al. (1979). It can be seen that the I_{50} values for the binding of benzylpenicillin, ampicillin, and amoxicillin to the PBPs (1 B, 2, 3) considered essential for cell-wall maintenance are significantly lower (0.8–4.1 μg/ml) than those for cephalothin, cephapirin, cefazolin (1–37 μg/ml) and, especially, cephalexin (8–>250 μg/ml). While the relationship between PBP binding and intrinsic activity is relatively good (SPRATT 1978), correlations at the next level, namely, in terms of the contribution of chemical reactivity to in vitro activity, are less clear. This will be examined further when the effect of the 3-substituents on bioactivity is considered.

Although the cephalosporins are resistant to β-lactamases produced by gram-positive bacteria such as *S. aureus*, gram-negative β-lactamases which can hydrolyze the cephalosporins abound (RICHMOND and SYKES 1973; O'CALLAGHAN 1979, 1980). Thus cephalosporin research has been directed primarily along two lines: (1) Because of the inherently lower intrinsic activity of the ring system, and the emergence of β-lactamases as a significant factor in resistance to the cephalosporins, major objectives have been to increase intrinsic antibacterial activity and to broaden the spectrum of activity, partly by improving β-lactamase resistance. (2) These efforts have been accompanied by successful attempts to improve the pharmacokinetic properties of the early cephalosporins, especially with respect to better oral absorption and higher and more prolonged serum levels.

I. Basic Structure–Activity Relationships

The cephalosporins exhibit greater latitude for structural modifications that improve biological performance than the penicillins. With the exception of mecil-

Table 13. Representative in vitro activities of selected 7–acylamino–cephalosporanic acids and their corresponding penicillins

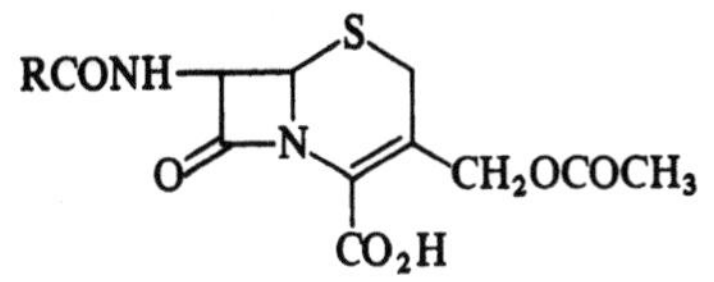

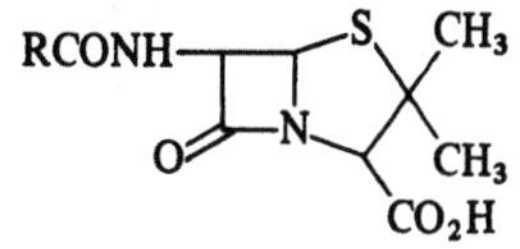

R	MIC (μg/ml)		MIC (μg/ml)		
	S. aureus (R)[a]	*E. coli*[a]	*S. aureus* (S)[b]	*S. aureus* (R)[a]	*E. coli*[b]
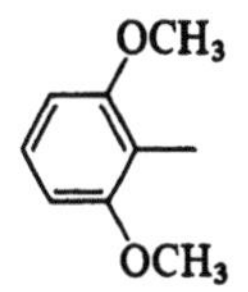	18	>200	0.5	3–14	in
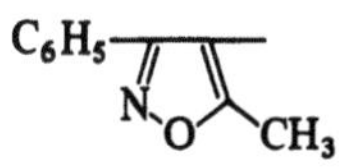	5.5	110	0.1	0.5–16	in
$C_6H_5CH_2$–	0.5[f]	27	0.02	160	25
$C_6H_5OCH_2$–	0.2[f]	140	0.02	150	62
$C_6H_5SCH_2$–	0.4	63	0.02	–	62
p–$CH_3OC_6H_4CH_2$–	0.4	110	–	–	–
p–$ClC_6H_4CH_2$–	<0.1	>200	–	–	–
$C_6H_5CH(CH_3)$–	3.0	100	0.05	–	25
$C_6H_5CH(Cl)$–	2.5	25	0.02	–	125
$C_6H_5CH(CO_2H)$–	6.3	88	0.25	170	5
$C_6H_5CH(NH_2)$–	3.1	3.5	0.05	180	2.5
$C_6H_5CH(OH)$–	1.5	5.6	0.05	–	5
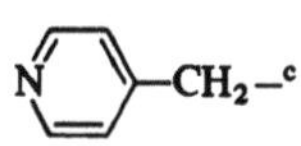 [c]	1.2	7.8	0.15	>10	32
NC–CH_2–	0.6	12	–	–	–
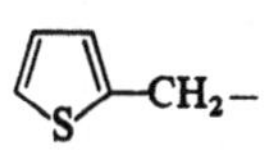	0.5	6.4	0.02	>20	12
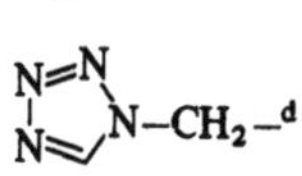 [d]	0.8	6	–	–	–
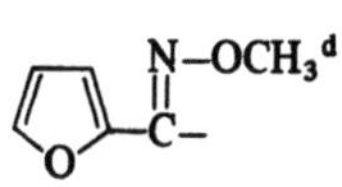 [d]	1.0	4	–	–	–
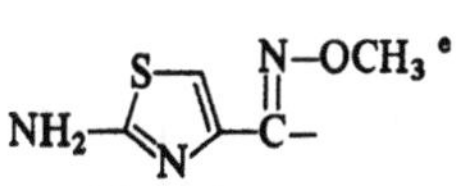 [e]	3.1	0.8	–	–	–

Sources: [a]) Gorman and Ryan 1972. [b]) Nayler 1973. [c]) Stedman et al. 1964. [d]) Weber and Ott 1977. [e]) Ochiai et al. 1981. [f]) SK&F unpublished data.

Table 14. Penicillin binding protein affinities for wild–type and permeability mutants of *E. coli* K12

	MIC (μg/ml)		I_{50} (μg/ml)[e]				
	Wild type	Permeab. mutant	1A	1B	2	3	4
Cephalexin	8	4	4	240	>250	8	30
Cefaclor	3.2	1.6	1	4.4	130	2	22
Cephalothin	1.6	0.8	<0.25	16	37	1	60
Cephapirin	6.4	3.2	<0.25	10	17	3.3	120
Cephaloridine	2	2	0.25	2.5	50	8	17
Cefazolin	4	4	<0.25	4.7	4.6	5.8	38
Cefamandole	1.6	0.1	<0.25	2.9	61	<0.25	38
Cefuroxime	2	0.1	0.12	1.6	13.7	0.09	200
Cefoxitin	4	2	0.1	3.9	>250	58	7
Cefotaxime	0.08	0.01	0.05	0.7	5	<0.05	30
Ceftriaxon[a]	—	—	<0.1	1.8	3.6	<0.1	>78
Cefsulodin	25	6.4	0.47	3.7	>250	>250	>250
Cefoperazone	0.4	0.05	0.5	1.5	0.9	0.05	>50
Cefotiam[b]	0.2	–	0.075	0.7	2.2	0.11	21
Carpetimycin A[c]	–	–	0.86	>20	5.1	>20	8.5
Carpetimycin B[c]	–	–	0.22	3.6	0.007	1.3	0.017
Thienamycin[d]	0.6	–	1.1		0.06	31	0.15
Clavulanic acid[d]	16	–	52		4.1	310	11

Sources: CURTIS et al. 1979, except: [a]WRIGHT et al. 1981; [b]NOZAKI et al. 1979; [c]NOZAKI et al. 1981; [d]SPRATT et al. 1977. [e]Concentration of antibiotic required to reduce ^{14}C–benzylpenicillin binding to PBP by 50%; compare Table 9. I_{50} values for PBPs 5 and 6 were >50 or >250 μg/ml except: cephalothin (60, 125), cefuroxime (>250, 18), thienamycin (1.0, 3.8) and clavulanic acid (21, 15), carpetimycins, PBP 5/6, not done.

linam, changes in the penicillin structure that have provided new clinically useful analogs are confined to variation of the 6β-acylamino side chain (but see Sects. B.III.4 and 5). With the cephalosporins, biological properties can be improved by varying the 3-substituent, as well as the 7β-acylamino group, and substitution of the 7α-position can increase β-lactamase stability with retention of useful biological activity over a broad range of 6β-acyl group variation. The new oxacephalosporin moxalactam demonstrates that replacement of the sulfur atom of the ring system by oxygen leads to significantly improved antimicrobial activity whereas this hetero atom exchange on the penicillin structure results in unimpressive activity against gram-negative bacteria and reduced activity against the gram-positive organisms (see Sect. C.V; cf. CAMA and CHRISTENSEN 1978b, and reference 44 therein). While the latitude for modification is broader, there are some constraints. Reactions involving the Δ^3-double bond, including its isomerization to the Δ^2-isomer, lowers activity, and the use of esters as pro-drugs has not been as successful with the cephalosporins as with the penicillins.

Table 15A. β–Lactamase–sensitive cephalosporins

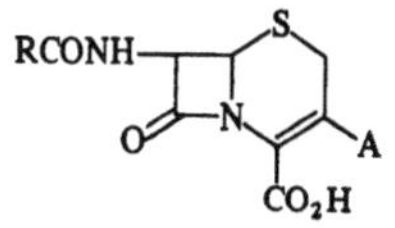

Parenteral

R	Generic name	A
Metabolically unstable		
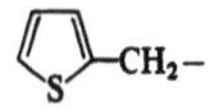	Cephalothin	$-CH_2OCOCH_3$
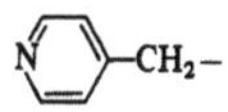	Cephapirin	$-CH_2OCOCH_3$
$N{\equiv}C{-}CH_2-$	Cephacetrile	$-CH_2OCOCH_3$
Metabolically stable		
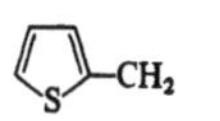	Cephaloridine	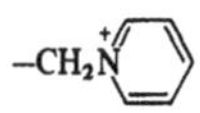
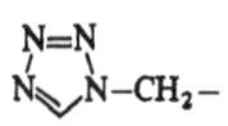	Cefazolin	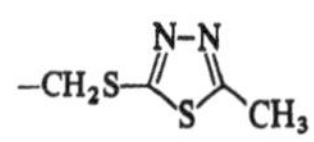
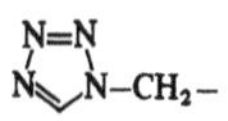	Ceftezole	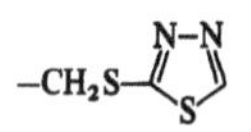
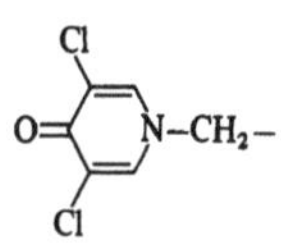	Cefazedone	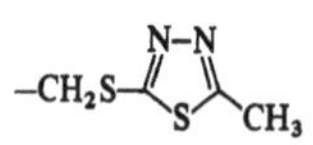
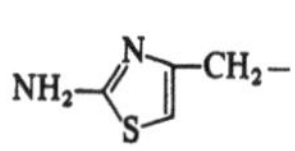	Cefotiam	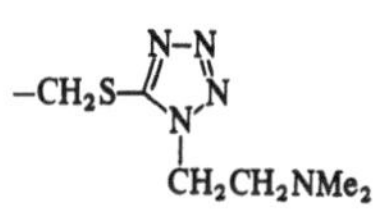
CF_3SCH_2-	Cefazaflur	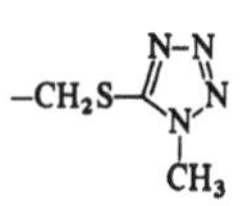
Improved pharmacokinetics		
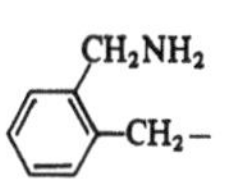	Ceforanide	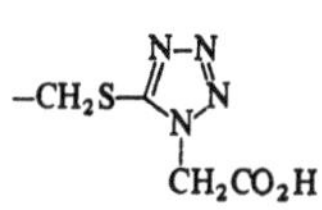

Oral

R	Generic name	A
Metabolically unstable		
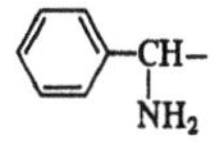	Cephaloglycin	$-CH_2OCOCH_3$
Metabolically stable		
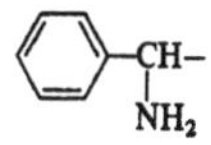	Cephalexin	$-CH_3$
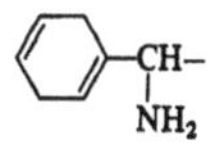	Cephradine	$-CH_3$
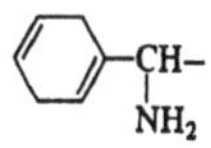	Cefroxadine	$-OCH_3$
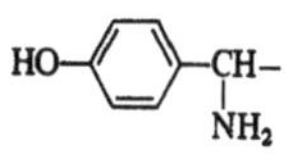	Cefadroxil	$-CH_3$
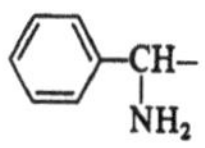	Cefaclor	–Cl
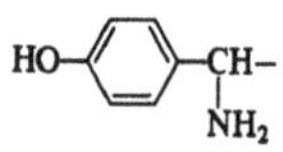	Cefatrizine	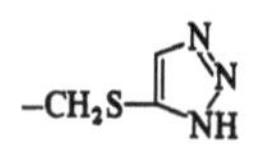
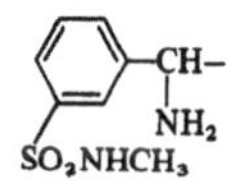	FR10612	$-CH_3$
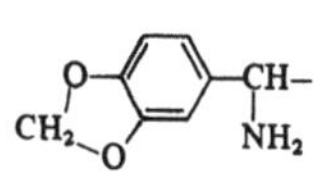	RMI19592	$-CH_3$
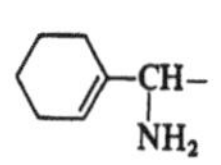	SCE100	$-CH_3$

The nature of the changes in biological properties that result from structural modifications depend to a large extent on which structural unit is involved. The nature of the 7β-acyl group largely determines the level and breadth of antibacterial activity; the effect on pharmacokinetic properties is less substantial with the narrow but very important exception of oral absorption of the 7-arylglycyl cephalosporins. Occasionally, changes at the 3-position have resulted in limited extension of the spectrum of activity (for example, susceptibility of some *Enterobacter* sp. to 3-(*N*-methyltetrazole)thiomethyl analogs, antipseudomonal activity of some 3-vinyl analogs, and extended spectrum of cefotiam, Table 21), but variations at this

Table 15B. β–Lactamase–resistant cephalosporins

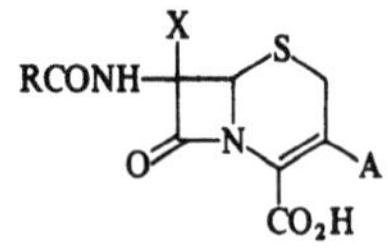

R	Generic name	A
Moderately resistant		
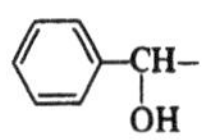	Cefamandole	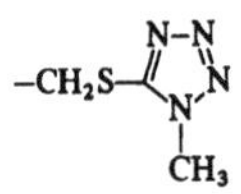
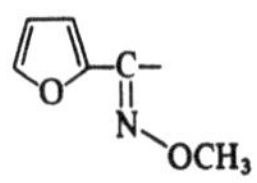	Cefuroxime	$-CH_2OCONH_2$
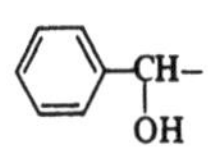	Cefonicid	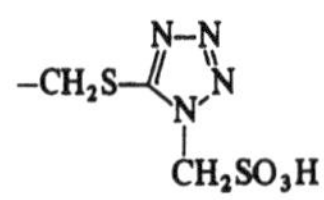
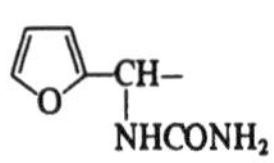	SQ69613	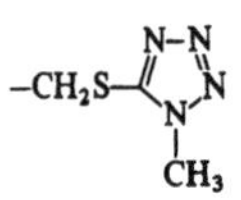
Cephamycins (7α–OCH$_3$)		
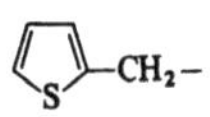	Cefoxitin	$-CH_2OCONH_2$
$NCCH_2SCH_2-$	Cefmetazole	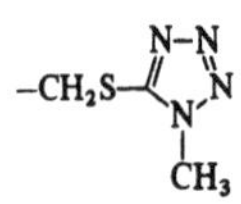
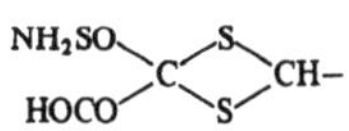	Cefotetan	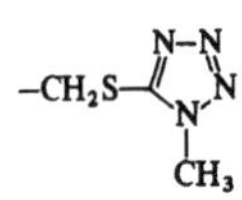
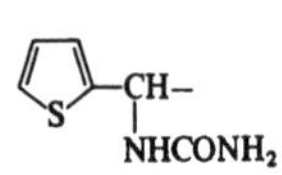	SQ14359	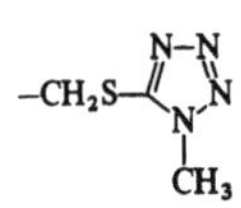
Oxacephalosporin: moxalactam		
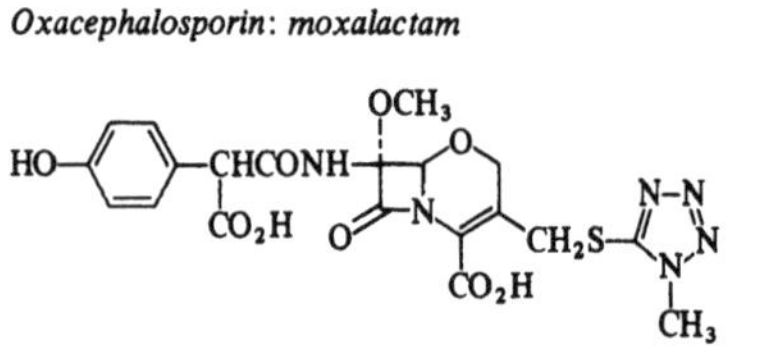		

R	Generic name	A
Highly resistant		
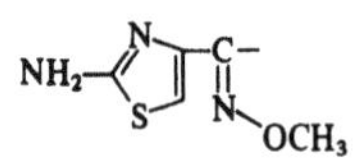	Cefotaxime	$-CH_2OCOCH_3$
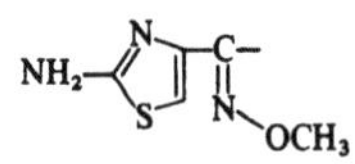	Ceftizoxime	–H
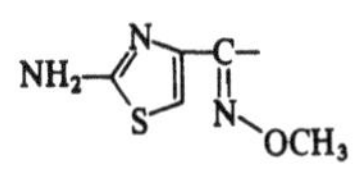	Cefmenoxime	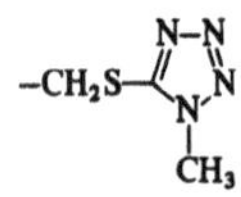
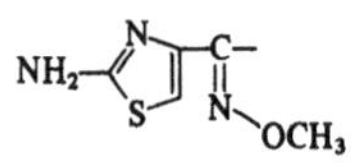	Ceftriaxon	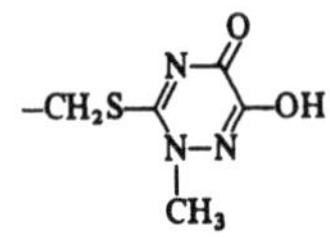
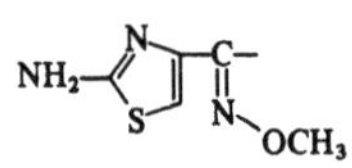	Cefodizime	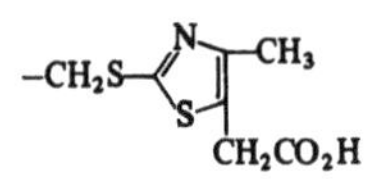
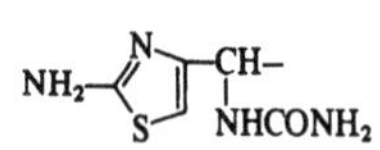	SQ81015	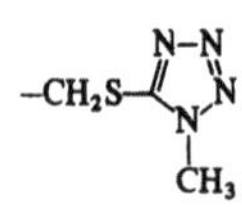
Resistant–activity includes Ps. aeruginosa		
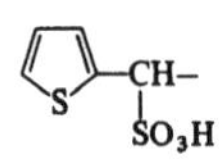	Cefsulodin	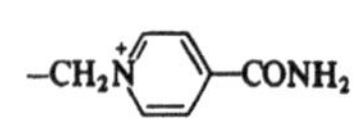
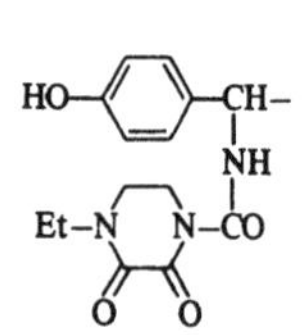	Cefoperazone	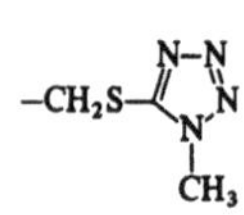
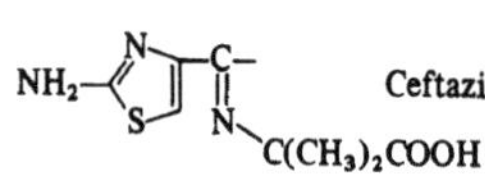	Ceftazidime	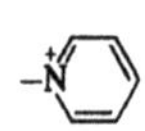
Orally absorbed		
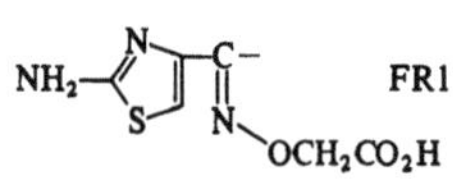	FR17027	$-CH{=}CH_2$

position have more influence on the level of activity and on metabolic and pharmacokinetic properties. Permissible variation of the third important locus of substituent modification, the 7α-position, is extremely narrow, consisting essentially of hydrogen (cephalosporins) and methoxy (cephamycins); the latter group plays a role only in increasing resistance to β-lactamase. As will be seen later, replacement of the ring sulfur atom by oxygen has little effect on the spectrum of activity, β-lactamase resistance or pharmacokinetic properties, but it increases significantly the level of activity over that of the sulfur-containing analog.

The degree of success for the extensive investment in structural modification of cephalosporins is reflected in Tables 15 A and 15 B, which list derivatives that are now clinically available, or have properties that make them candidates for such use. These tables should serve as a guide to structure and identity in the discussion which follows. The grouping of the cephalosporins in Tables 15 A and 15 B follows, to a large extent, the classification advanced by O'CALLAGHAN (1979). Thus, the analogs are divided according to relative resistance to inactivation by gram-negative β-lactamases, route of administration, and resistance to metabolic conversion. The differentiation of these analogs on the basis of β-lactamase resistance is not as sharp as the tables imply. Obviously, the overall gradation of resistance to these enzymes from bacteria which as a group produce different β-lactamases in variable amounts does not provide a rigorous basis for such classification. In addition, secondary characteristics which are important to cephalosporin use do not parallel β-lactamase resistance. Most notable are the cephalosporins which provide high and prolonged serum levels, and which range from susceptibility to β-lactamase to a high level of resistance to these enzymes (Sect. C.III.1).

II. β-Lactamase-Sensitive Cephalosporins

The parenteral cephalosporins listed in Table 15 A are similar in their antibacterial activities. These agents are active against most clinically important gram-positive organisms (except *S. faecalis*), *Neisseria* sp., and most strains of *E. coli*, *Klebsiella* sp., and *P. mirabilis*. Many of the other gram-negative rods including indole-positive *Proteus*, *Enterobacter*, *Providencia*, *Serratia*, and *Pseudomonas* species are resistant. *H. influenzae* is less susceptible to these cephalosporins than to the penicillins. Anaerobes such as *Clostridium* sp. are susceptible but most strains of *B. fragilis* are not inhibited. The in vitro activity of cephalothin was compared with that of benzylpenicillin in Table 2. With some minor variations this spectrum of activity is typical for the other members of this group except cefotiam (see below). These agents lack significant stability toward the β-lactamases of gram-negative bacteria and those with a 3′-acetoxy group are susceptible to metabolic hydrolysis. The studies on structure–activity relationships that have led to the development of the cephalosporins in this group have been thoroughly analyzed in the reviews cited earlier (see especially SASSIVER and LEWIS 1970; WEBBER and OTT 1977). Only a brief summary of the relationships which apply will be discussed here.

1. 7β-Acylamino Group Modifications

There is a fair correlation between the penicillins and cephalosporins with respect to activity against gram-positive and gram-negative bacteria. A few examples are given in Table 13 to illustrate the point. It can be seen that the general rules governing activity for the penicillins, discussed earlier, apply to some extent to the cephalosporins, notably reduction of activity when the α-carbon is multiply substituted or incorporated into a ring, the reduction of gram-negative activity when the lipophilicity of the side-chain is increased, and the enhancing effect of certain α-substituents (OH, NH_2) on gram-negative activity. Even with the small number of analogs presented in the table, however, it can be seen that good gram-negative activity is not a consistent characteristic of the cephalosporins in spite of early expectations based on the properties of the natural congeners. In fact, most cephalosporin analogs have relatively poor activity against gram-negative bacteria (see, for example, SASSIVER and LEWIS 1970), and only a few combine high intrinsic activity with a susceptibility spectrum broad enough to make then candidates for clinical use. Many of the cephalosporin acyl groups commonly associated with significant broad spectrum activity are listed in Table 16. Most of these side chains are still mono- or disubstituted acetyl groups, but the phenyl-linked acetic acid moiety found on a large proportion of the penicillins generally has additional α-carbon substitution (e.g., mandeloyl, phenylglycyl – side chains also found on the broad spectrum penicillins). The predominance of the (substituted) phenylacetyl group has been replaced by a larger incidence of acetyl groups linked, directly or through a sulfur atom, to heterocyclic rings (thiophene, tetrazole, sydnone, aminothiazole, etc.) or to small, frequently polar, groupings containing various hetero atoms (cyano, trifluoromethylthio, etc.). Notable departures from these general structures are the formyl group (of academic interest) and the α-oximino-containing side chains (cefuroxime, cefotaxime, etc.). The *syn* oximes are exceptional in providing β-lactamase resistance by multiple substitution of the α-carbon of the side chain without the usual reduction of in vitro activity that accompanies this manipulation. The quest for greater β-lactamase resistance has led to the construction of more complex 7-substituents based on acylation of the phenylglycine side chain similar to the acylaminopenicillins discussed in Sect. B.III.3.

It is not obvious why the side chains in Table 16 confer broad-spectrum activity on the cephalosporin structure while other similar acyl groups do not. Certainly the most popular analogy of β-lactams to the D-alanyl-D-alanine moiety involved in murein cross-linking (STROMINGER and TIPPER 1965; PARK 1966) does not provide much of a basis for explaining the frequently decisive influence of the 6(7)-acyl group on ultimate antimicrobial activity. Most of the knowledge concerning the contribution of the 7-acylamino group to activity has been obtained empirically by constructing and testing large groups of related analogs. The studies which attempt to correlate physical and chemical properties with biological activity have been directed primarily at differences in activity levels of penicillins and cephalosporins or the role of the 3-substituent (see Sect. C.II.3). Data which quantitate the actual contribution of the 7-acylamino side chains in chemical terms are few, since tools to differentiate the relative contribution to effectiveness of penetration, resistance to inactivation, active site coordination, and chemical reactivity have been lacking. Newer methods, which now measure binding to the PBPs of permeability mutants and their wild-type parents, others which quantitate susceptibility to β-lactamases, and better definition of the active sites of the enzymes involved, should provide the tools for delineating the roles of the 7-acylamino groups in more quantitative

Table 16. 7-Acyl groups that confer broad spectrum activity on the cephalosporin (cephamycin) structure

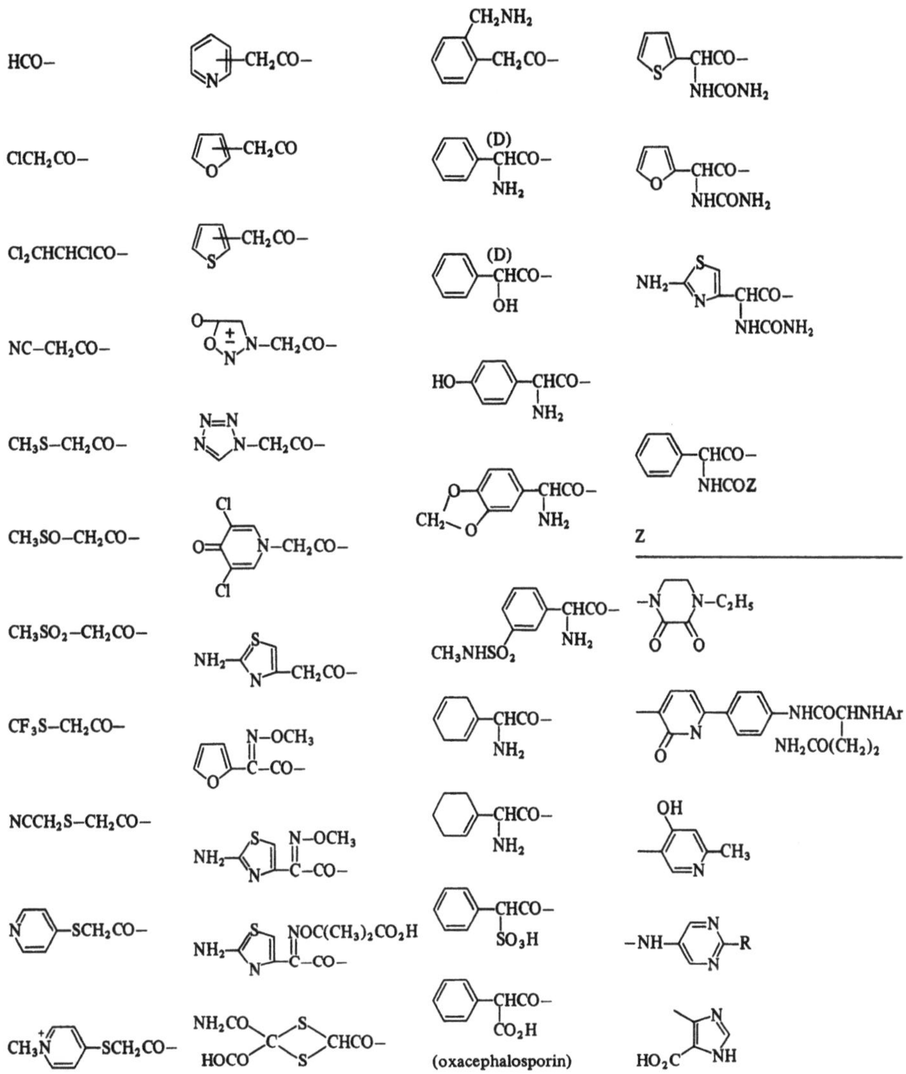

terms. The limited predictive power of the empirically derived data is underscored, for example, by the inability to predict the uniquely high efficacy of the 4-(2-aminothiazolyl) acetyl side chain in conferring antibacterial activity, which was discovered serendipitously (MORITA et al. 1980) after decades of research on 7-hetero-acetylaminocephalosporanic acids, many of which closely resembled the aminothiazole analogs. Table 17 illustrates this point. The generally superior gram-negative activity of the 7β-[4-(2-aminothiazolyl)acetylamino]cephalosporanic acid would not be anticipated from the activities of the other heterocyclic acetylamino analogs that accompany it in the table. Indeed, it was fortunate that the amino analog was synthesized and tested since the activity of the hydroxy derivative, which was apparently discovered first, is not particularly impressive. It

Table 17. In vitro activities of some heterocyclic acetylamino cephalosporanic acid analogs

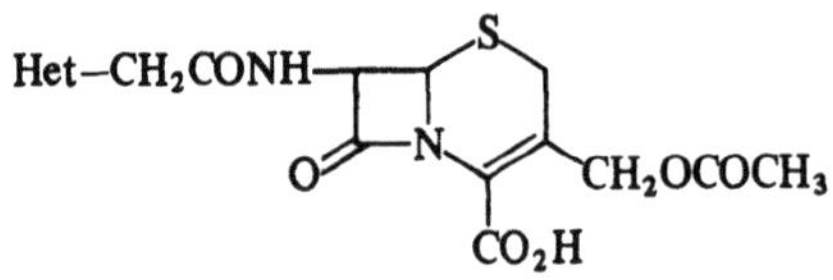

Het	Reference	MIC (μg/ml) *S. aureus* (R)	*E. coli*	*K. pneumoniae*	*E. cloacae*
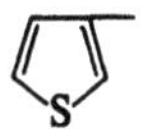	a	0.8	12	3.1	133
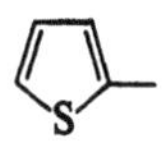	b	0.4	17	2	5
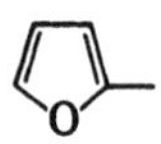	c	1	160	3.4	–
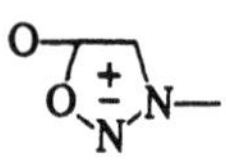	d	0.5	3.8	4.1	–
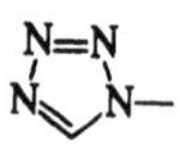	b	0.8	6	6	6
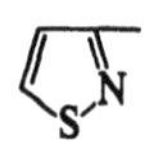	e	0.8	50	12.5	–
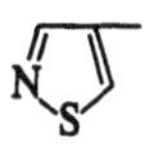	e	0.8	50	6.2	–
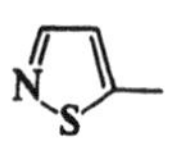	e	0.8	25	6.2	–
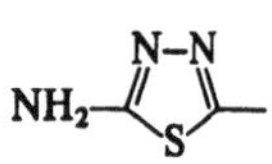	a	1.6	12.5	12.5	>200
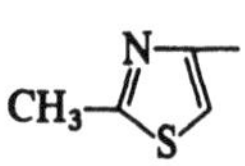	a	0.8	50	12.5	25
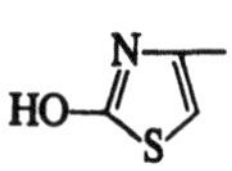	f	1.6	6.2	6.2	25
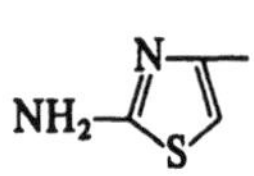	f	1.6	1.6	0.4	0.4

Sources: [a]SK&F unpublished data. [b]WEBER and OTT 1977. [c]GORMAN and RYAN 1972. [d]NATTO et al. 1968. [e]RAAP and MICETICH 1968. [f]NUMATA et al. 1978.

Table 18. Comparative in vitro activities of 3′–acetoxy cephalosporin analogs (cephalothin, cefotaxime) and their deacetyl metabolites

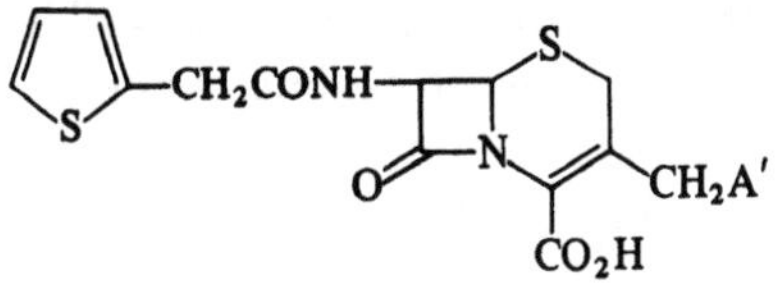

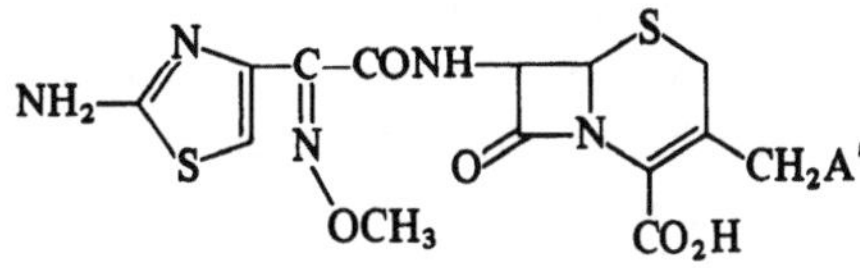

	MIC (μg/ml)[a]			Geometric mean MIC (μg/ml)[b]			
	Strain	A′=OCOCH₃	A′=OH	*n*	A′=OCOCH₃	A′=OH	Cefuroxime
S. aureus	3074	0.4	1.56	10	1.6	24.3	1.1
E. coli	EC–14	6.25	100	10	0.06	0.5	1.6
Klebsiella sp.	KA3	1.56	25	10	0.053	0.15	1.74
P. mirabilis	–	–	–	5	0.019	0.09	1.0
Proteus sp.	PR6	6.25	25	5	0.04	1.5	16
B. fragilis	–	–	–	10	4	12.9	8

Sources: [a]Wick 1966. [b]Wise et al. 1980a. Cephalothin comparisons are based on laboratory strains, cefotaxime comparisons use clinical isolates. Consult original article for MIC ranges, which are broad for *S. aureus* and *B. fragilis.*

should be observed that the improvement of gram-negative activity is not accompanied by improved activity against gram-positive bacteria. This is a characteristic of the analogs that have been derived from this structural lead.

The aminothiazolyl substituent has furnished a basis for a significant amount of recent research on cephalosporins, providing at least seven analogs with properties that are promising enough to make them candidates for clinical development (cefotiam, cefotaxime, ceftizoxime, cefmenoxime, ceftriaxon, ceftazidime, and SQ 81 015). Their structure–activity relationships are considered further at appropriate points in the following discussion.

2. Metabolic Stability

The 3-acetoxymethyl grouping, which is retained on four of the β-lactamase-sensitive cephalosporins (Table 15 A: cephalothin, cefapirin, cephacetrile, cephaloglycin) and the third-generation cephalosporin cefotaxime (Table 15 B; see below) is subject to metabolic hydrolysis to give the corresponding 3′-alcohol with antibacterial activity one-third to less than one-tenth that of the parent (Table 18). This can occur to a significant extent with all of the 3-acetoxymethyl analogs, including cefotaxime (Chauvette et al. 1963; Wick 1966; Wise et al. 1980 a). However, the result is different for cefotaxime than for the earlier cephalosporins. For the earlier analogs, the in vitro activity is lowered, and the serum half-life of the deacetyl analog is shorter, with the overall result that the half-life of the parent is relatively low (cephalothin, cephapirin: $t_{1/2}$, 30–40 min; cephacetrile: $t_{1/2}$, 80 min). While cefotaxime undergoes appreciable metabolic deacetylation the in vitro activity of the deacetyl derivative of cefotaxime against the Enterobacteriaceae, while lower, still compares favorably with that of other cephalosporins (Table 18 includes MIC values for cefuroxime); but activity against *S. aureus* and *B. fragilis* is poor. In contrast to the metabolite of cephalothin and its relatives, the serum half-life of the deacetyl metabolite of cefotaxime is longer than that of its parent so that at 4–7 h its serum levels can equal or surpass those of the remaining cefotaxime. Approximately half of the administered dose of cefotaxime is excreted into the urine as the parent and 20%–40% as the deacetyl metabolite (BAX et al. 1981; WISE et al. 1980a). This metabolic problem is obviated by replacing the 3-acetoxymethyl group in the various ways discussed next.

3. 3-Substituent Modifications

In addition to avoiding metabolic hydrolysis, modification of the 3-substituent can increase the intrinsic antibacterial activity and improve the pharmacokinetic properties of the cephalosporin analog. Thus, like the 7β-acylamino group, this substituent has been modified in many ways. The vast majority of such analogs have been obtained by displacement of the acetoxy group or its equivalent from acylaminocephalosporanic acid structures derived from natural sources, and thus they retain the methylene bridge between the new substituent and the 3-position of the dihydrothiazine ring. More recent chemical manipulations have provided a smaller number of derivatives lacking this 3-methylene carbon where the substituent is attached directly to the ring. These analogs have at the 3-position, for example, hydrogen (ceftizoxime), alkoxy (cefroxadine), halogen (cefaclor), vinyl, carboxyl, carbalkoxy, carboxamide, keto, sulfonate, and thioether groups (HOOVER and DUNN 1979; WEBBER and OTT 1977). A highly selected but representative group of 3-substituents that will serve as a guide in the following discussions are assembled in Table 19. MIC values for *S. aureus* and *E. coli* are listed to illustrate relative effects on gram-positive and gram-negative activity. The 7-acyl group is held constant even though some of these substituents are more effective with acyl side chains other than 2-thienylacetyl.

a) Esters

The natural 3-acetoxymethyl grouping can be hydrolyzed and other esters derived from 3′-deacetylcephalosporins can be obtained with some difficulty (BERGES 1975). The close homologous esters exhibit activities similar to those of the acetoxy analogs, but activity decreases with chain length while serum binding increases. The benzoyl ester displays good gram-positive but lowered gram-negative activity (Table 19). In general, these ester exchanges have been unprofitable with one exception. The carbamoyloxy moiety, which occurs naturally on some cephamycins, is retained on cefoxitin and has been incorporated into the cefuroxime molecule (Table 15B). In contrast to the 3′-acetoxy group the urethane is highly resistant to hydrolysis. This is illustrated by the recovery of unchanged cefoxitin versus that of the 3-acetoxy analog of cefoxitin in mouse and monkey (72% versus 11% and 93% versus 36%, respectively; STAPLEY et al. 1979a) and reflected, for example, by PD_{50} values in mice against *S. aureus*. The high urinary recovery of cefuroxime in man (97% in 24 h; FOORD 1976) and cefoxitin (86% in 2 h; FILLASTRE et al. 1978) with only slight metabolic conversion, also illustrates the resistance of the carba-

Table 19. Effects of selected 3–substituent modifications of 7–(2–thiopheneacetamido)–3–cephem–4–carboxylic acids on in vitro activity

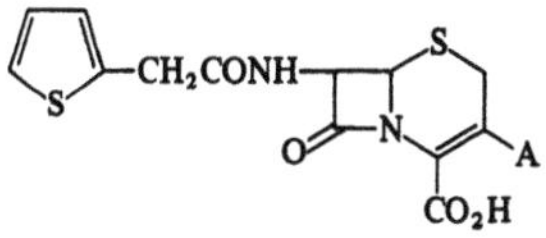

Average G–[c] MIC (μg/ml)	–TSE[c] (Kcal/mol)	A	MIC (μg/ml)[a,b] S. aureus	MIC (μg/ml)[a,b] E. coli	A	MIC (μg/ml)[a,b] S. aureus	MIC (μg/ml)[a,b] E. coli
57	129.5	$-CH_3$	3.8	>50	$-CH_2N_3$	0.4	43
49	131.0	$-CH_2OH$	4.0	130	$-CH_2NH_2$	4	>200
34	131.8	$-CH_2OCH_3$	0.5	39	$-CH_2SCSOC_2H_5$	1.0	106
31	132.1	$-CH_2SCH_3$	4	73	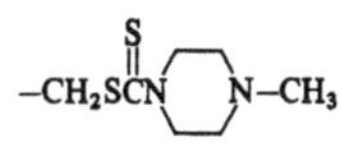	1.0	6
15	132.9	$-CH_2CN$	3	22	$-CH_2OCONHC_6H_5$	0.5	1.6
12	132.6	$-CH_2OCONH_2$	0.5	15	$-CH_2OCONHCH_3$	0.5	15
6	133.1	$-CH_2OCOCH_3$	0.5	6.4	$-CH_2OCOC_6H_5$	0.1	41
4	133.8	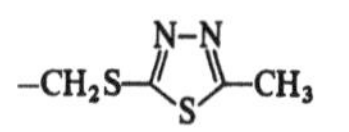	0.3	5.7	$-CH_2-SCOCH_3$	2.8	52
					$-CH_2-S(CNH)NH_2$	0.7	34
2	135.1	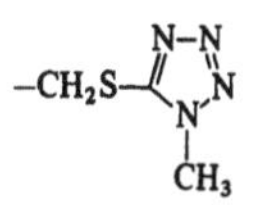	0.3	1.0	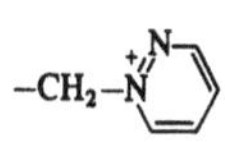	0.4	5
3	136.6	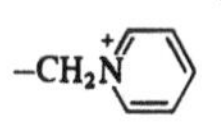	0.4	3.3	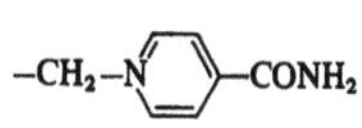	0.4	2.4
2	137.8	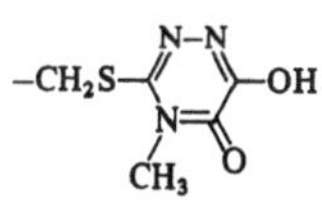	–	–	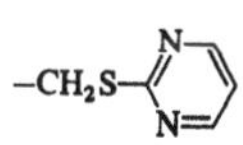	0.4	109
27	129.9	$-OCH_3$	>20	62	$-COCH_3$	>20	38
9	130.5	–H	8	20			
6	136.1	$-COOCH_3$	>20	16	–COOH	15	20
8	138.4	–Cl	13	24	–Br	14	31
15	139.4	$-CH=CHCO_2H$	12	26	$-CH=CH_2$	0.5	62
12	140.3	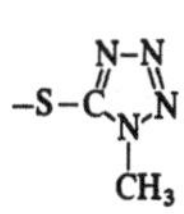	–	–		–	–

Sources: [a]GORMAN and RYAN 1972; [b]WEBBER and OTT 1977; [c]BOYD et al. 1980.

moyloxy methyl group to metabolic hydrolysis. *N*-Alkyl and aryl derivatives of 3-carbamoyloxymethyl cephalosporins exhibit in vitro activities similar to the unsubstituted parent (Table 19; GORMAN and RYAN 1972).

b) Nitrogen Nucleophiles

The early discovery that pyridine easily displaces the 3′-acetoxy group led to the marketing of cephaloridine (Table 15 A), the investigation of a large number of substituted 3-pyridiniummethyl cephalosporin analogs (SPENCER et al., 1967; SASSIVER and LEWIS 1970), and the introduction of other heterocyclic structures on the 3′-position. Cephaloridine has a spectrum of activity against gram-negative bacteria resembling that of cephalothin and excellent activity against gram-positive bacteria (Table 19). The pyridiniummethyl group provides the pharmacokinetic advantages of metabolic stability, water solubility, low serum binding, low pain on injection and good serum levels. Substitution of the pyridine ring and the introduction of other heterocyclic systems (e.g., pyrimidine) provides no advantage in terms of biological activity except for the 3-bromo and several 4-substituted analogs of cephaloridine. The 4-carbamoylpyridiniummethyl analog was found to be consistently the most active of this group, and it was assigned the generic name cephalonium (SPENCER et al. 1967). Unfortunately, emergence of nephrotoxicity for cephaloridine under certain dosage regimes has discouraged the use of this modification in cephalosporin structure design. Pyridiniummethyl groupings have now reappeared on the new cephalosporins cefsulodin and ceftazidime (Table 15 B). Introduction of other nitrogenous analogs [3′-azido, 3′-(acyl)amino, etc.] have not resulted in cephalosporin analogs with superior biological properties.

c) Sulfur Nucleophiles

Many displacements of the 3′-acetoxy groups by sulfur nucleophiles produce derivatives with undistinguished activities. Such analogs include those obtained by displacements with dithiocarbamates, xanthates, thiocarboxylic acids, thioureas, and thiosulfate (see HOOVER and DUNN 1979, for access references). While many of these analogs exhibit good activity against gram-positive bacteria, in most cases activity against gram-negative bacteria is poor (Table 19).

By far the most important displacements by sulfur nucleophiles have been those using heterocyclic thiols. Many of these reactions also generate thioethers with mediocre biological properties but, as with the 7-acylamino variations, a few result in enhancement of activity against gram-negative bacteria, and occasionally simultaneous improvement of such pharmacokinetic properties as height and duration of serum levels, are also observed. At least three cephalosporins of this type (cefazolin, cefamandole, and ceforanide) are now in clinical use and many of the analogs undergoing clinical evaluation carry the 3-heterocyclic thiomethyl grouping (Tables 15 A and 15 B). The relative effectiveness of various heterocyclic thiomethyl groups in improving biological properties is illustrated by the group of analogs listed in Table 20, which includes cefamandole. In this series most of the 3-heterocyclic thiomethylcephalosporins with a five-membered heterocyclic ring are less active than the analog with the 3-acetoxymethyl group. Indeed, many are less active than the deacetoxy (A = H) derivative. The methyltetrazole, thiadiazole,

Table 20. 3–Heterocyclicthiomethyl cephalosporins

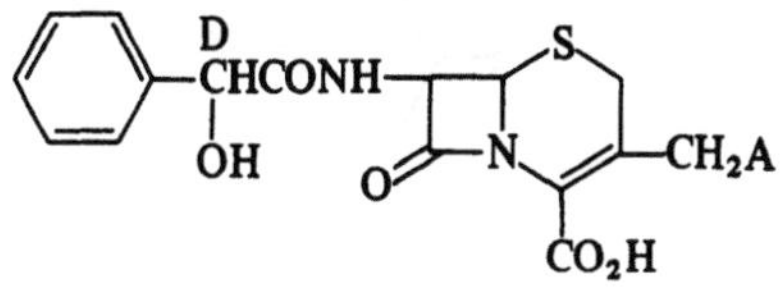

A	MIC (μg/ml) *S. aureus*	MIC (μg/ml) *E. coli*	PD_{50} s.c. (*E. coli* in mouse), mg/kg
–H	6.3	12.5	25
$-OCOCH_3$	1.6	1.6	6.2
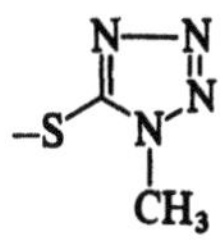	0.8	0.8	1.8
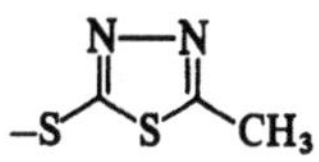	0.4	1.6	3.6
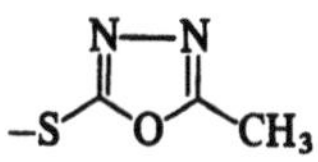	0.8	3.1	5.5
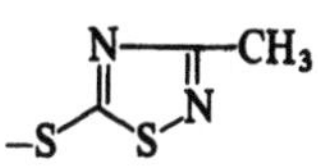	6.3	6.3	50
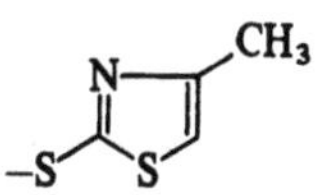	3.1	6.3	152
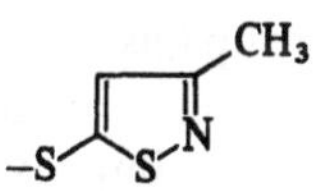	3.1	50	50
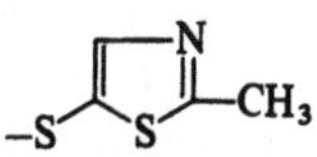	6.3	100	–
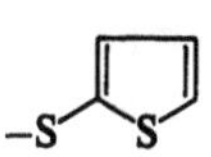	6.3	200	–
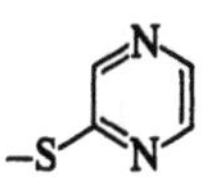	1.6	12.5	–

Source: Hoover and Dunn 1979.

and oxadiazole derivatives have the best antibacterial activities in vitro, and they exhibit the best PD_{50} values in infected mice. Similar trends are observed with 3-heterocyclic thiomethylcephalosporin analogs with many other side chains at the 7-position including additional mandeloyl (Berges et al. 1976), phenylglycyl (Dunn et al. 1976; Webber and Ott 1977), sydnone (Kurita et al. 1972), α-sulfo-

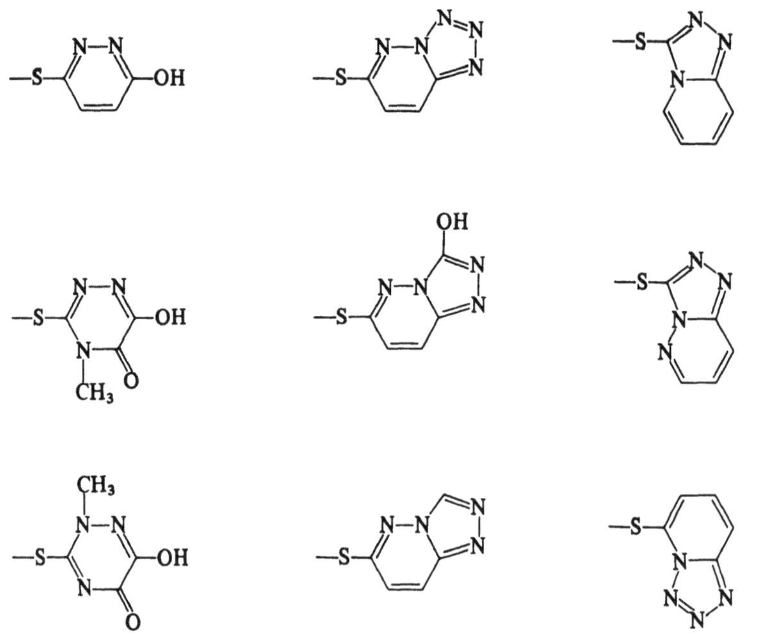

Fig. 3. Six-membered heterocyclic *thio* substitutes at the 3′ position

phenylacetyl (Nomura et al. 1974, 1975), vinylenethioacetyl (Nannino et al. 1981), and 4-(2-aminothiazole)acetyl (Ochiai et al. 1980c) analogs. The list in Table 20 is not exhaustive and other heterocyclic groups have been found to be as good as, or better than, those listed for enhancing biological characteristics (see, for example, Nomura et al. 1975). The 1,2,3-triazolethiomethyl group (cefatrizine) is nearly unique in providing a high level of in vitro activity with good oral absorption characteristics (Sect. C.III.2), and the tetrazolethiomethyl group has furnished many interesting analogs upon further modification, as described below. In general, the use of five-membered heterocyclic thiomethyl substituents to improve the biological properties of the cephalosporins has been more successful than the use of six-membered or larger rings (see Table 20), although several recent studies report derivatives of the latter type (Fig. 3) with good broad-spectrum activity. However, the results are less impressive than those described for the most active five-membered analogs (Naito et al. 1977a, b, c). The exception in this case is the 3-[2,5-dihydro-6-hydroxy-2-methyl-5-oxo-*as*-triazine-3-yl]thiomethyl group of the third generation cephalosporin ceftriaxon (Table 15 B). The activating effect of the isomeric 4-metyl-5-oxo-*as*-triazine substituent was indicated in Table 19 (see below).

Cefazolin was the first cephalosporin marketed with a 3-heterocyclic-thiomethyl substituent. It has a tetrazoleacetamide group at the 7-position (Table 15 A). Its spectrum of antibacterial activity is similar to cephalothin's, but it is more active against *E. coli* and *Klebsiella* species (Sabath et al. 1973). Its most important advantage is the production of serum levels on intramuscular or intravenous injection that are higher and longer than those for cephalothin or cephaloridine (see Sect. C.III.1).

Table 21. 2-Aminothiazole cephalosporins: effect of 3-substituents on antibiotic activity (cefotiam)

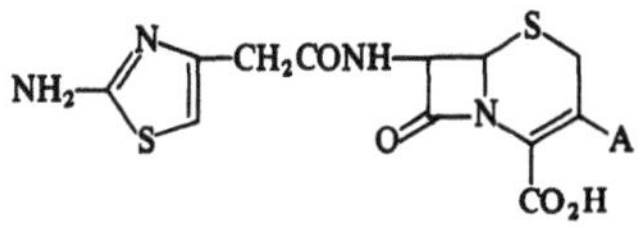

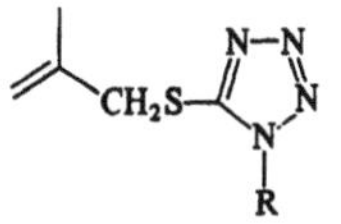

A	MIC (μg/ml) S. aureus (R) 1840	E. coli (S) JC-2	E. coli (R) T7	K. pneumoniae DT	P. morganii 3168	P. vulgaris 3988	ED_{50} E. coli mg/kg
Cefazolin	0.78	1.56	100	1.56	100	6.25	1.55
$-CH_2OCOCH_3$	1.56	1.56	50	0.39	50	0.39	–
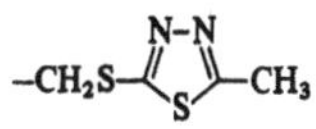	0.78	1.56	25	0.39	3.13	0.78	–
R							
$-CH_2CONMe_2$	1.56	1.56	25	≤0.2	25	≤0.2	–
$-CH_2CH_2NEt_2$	1.56	0.39	12.5	0.2	12.5	1.56	0.15
$-CH_2CH_2OH$	1.56	0.78	12.5	≤0.2	3.13	≤0.2	–
$-(CH_2)_3NMe_2$	0.78	0.39	6.25	0.39	3.13	0.39	–
$-CH_2CH_2NHMe$	0.78	0.39	3.13	≤0.2	6.25	0.39	–
$-CH_3$	0.78	0.39	6.25	≤0.1	3.13	0.39	0.11
$-CH_2CONH_2$	1.56	0.39	3.13	≤0.2	≤0.2	≤0.2	–
$CH_2CH_2NMe_2$ (cefotiam)	1.56	0.2	1.56	≤0.2	≤0.2	0.78	0.09

Source: NUMATA et al. 1978. See original article for description of test organisms and test conditions.

The superior performance of the methyltetrazolethiomethyl group has led to additional structural variations based on this heterocyclic ring, with the production of at least three new candidates for clinical use. Replacement of the methyl with an alkyl group carrying an acidic function (CH_2COOH, CH_2SO_3H, $CH_2CH_2NHSO_3H$) results in analogs which produce high and prolonged serum levels on injection (ceforanide, cefonicid, SK&F 88070 Sect. C.III.1). The effects of replacing the methyl by alkyl groups carrying nonacidic polar groups are illustrated in Table 21 which summarizes work by NUMATA et al. (1978) leading to the selection of cefotiam (Tables 21 and 15A) for clinical development. The activity trends observed with the structural variation in this series continue to argue for the high level of empiricism that has characterized cephalosporin research. It is not obvious why the diethylaminoethyl or dimethylaminopropyl analogs are less active than the methyl derivative while the dimethylaminoethyl analog (cefotiam) is more active. At any rate cefotiam is, overall, the most active against the enteric gram-negative bacteria of the group of analogs from which it evolved (Table 21) and it retains good gram-positive activity. In studies using both laboratory strains of bacteria and groups of clinical isolates, cefotiam was found to have in vitro activity equal to cefazolin or cephalothin against gram-positive organisms, but against *H. influenzae* and the usual Enterobacteriaceae it was about 10 times more potent (MIC values in the range of 0.2–0.78 μg/ml; compare Table 21). This spectrum includes some β-lactamase-producing strains, but against these organisms there is a pronounced inoculum effect (TSUCHIYA et al. 1978b). Cefotiam is inactive against *Serratia* and *Pseudomonas* species, as are the other cephalosporins in this group.

d) Effects of 3′-Substituents on In Vitro Activity

Differences in the intrinsic activities of the penicillin and cephalosporin structures have been attributed to the relative strain on the β-lactam ring resulting in different levels of chemical reactivity. The rôle of the 6(7)-acylamino group in increasing β-lactam ring reactivity has been examined (WOODWARD 1949, 1980) but, for the reasons mentioned above, little work has gone into quantitating this contribution. There have been a number of studies which attempt to relate bioactivity to the effect of the 3-substituent on β-lactam ring reactivity.

In the cephalosporins, the possibility for enamine resonance between the nitrogen atom's unshared electron pair and the olefinic π-orbital electrons provides an additional factor that contributes to the lability of the β-lactam amide group. The presence of enamine resonance is supported by the measurement of bond lengths using x-ray crystallography (SWEET and DAHL 1970). Further support is provided by correlation of the infrared absorption frequencies of the β-lactam with various 3′-substituents ($OCOCH_3$ vs. H, MORIN et al. 1969). This resonance form is one of those advanced to account for the facile S_N1 displacement of the 3′-acetoxy group. Whether the effects derive from the loss of the 3′-substituent, or only from its inductive effect on the β-lactam ring, the reactivity (rate of hydrolysis) of the β-lactam ring has been shown to correlate with the σ_I values of 3-methylene substituents (INDELICATO et al. 1974); and the rate of ring opening has been shown to be directly proportional to the intrinsic activity of cephalosporins against gram-negative bacteria (INDELICATO et al. 1977).

A more recent study has compared the correlation of averaged activity for several gram-negative bacteria with various parameters including: net atomic charge on C 8, the overlap population of the C 8–N 5 bond and the theoretical (CNDO/2) transition state energy of formation of the initial complex of the nucleophile, OH^-. Using cephems with various substituents at the 3-position, the latter was found to provide the best correlation. In essence, it is an approximation of the contribution of the 3-substituent to stabilization of the complex formed with the impinging hydroxyl ion (presumably representative of complex formation with the active sites of appropriate enzymes). Plots of these two values (average gram-negative MIC in μg/ml versus transition state energy in Kcal/mol) fall fairly accurately on a hyperbolic curve (BOYD and LUNN 1979; BOYD et al. 1980). The values obtained in this way, calculated from the published curves, are listed for the appropriate 3-substituents on the left side of Table 19. The leveling of the average MIC values beyond a point of increasing energy of formation (i.e., approximately 133 Kcal/mole) suggests that there is a limit to the activating influence of the 3-substituents.

III. Cephalosporins with Special Pharmacokinetic Properties

Improvement of the pharmacokinetic properties of the cephalosporins has been a major research concern. This has resulted in several parenteral cephalosporins which produce serum concentrations that are significantly higher and of longer duration than their close analogs, and another group of cephalosporins that are efficiently absorbed on oral administration.

Table 22. Pharmacokinetic properties of the cephalosporins

	Dose (g)	Serum peak (µg/ml)	$t_{1/2}$ (min)	Serum binding (%)	Urinary recovery (%)	Metabol-ism (%)	Volume of distribution (L)
Cephalothin	1	15–21	28–51	65–79	55–60	43	
Cefapirin	1	15–24	37–47	44–50	50–70	+	
Cefacetrile	1	22–23	33–90	33–36	80–90	+	
Cephaloridine	1	38–40	48–90	8–31	90	–	16
Cefazolin	1	38–76	90–153	74–86	86	–	10
Ceftezole	0.5	25	56	86	87	–	9
Cefazedone	0.5	17.5	150	92	79		9.3
Cefazaflur[a]	1	25–42	26–54	–	79–91	–	
Ceforanide	1	75	176	81	85	–	12
Cefamandole	1	20–35	55–90	67–80	80	–	12.8
Cefuroxime	1	34–40	65–82	28–38	97	–	13.5
Cefonicid[b]	1	98	277	91–98	98	–	
Cefotiam[c]	0.5	14	120	40–60	65		
Cefoxitin	1	20–28	41–48	50–73	87	5	8–12
Cefmetazole	0.5	29	60	85	66	–	
Cefotetan[d]	0.5	41	221	91	>80		
Cefotaxime	0.5	21.8	75	40	60–70	24	
Ceftizoxime[e]	0.5	13.7	104	31	60–80		23
Cefmenoxime[f]	0.5	10	54–72		~80		
Ceftriaxon[g,j]	0.5	50–85	480–600	83–96	60	–	10–12
Cefsulodin	0.5	21	90	30	70	–	13.5
Cefoperazone[h]	1	47	146	97	15–30		6.5
Ceftazidime[i]	0.5	23	96	17	48–88	–	
Moxalactam	0.5	21	120	38	84	–	12

Sources: For data not referenced see O'Callaghan 1979, Murray and Moellering 1979 and primary references cited therein. Other sources: [a]Actor et al. 1976a; Harvengt et al. 1977. [b]Pitkin et al. 1980. [c]Nakayama et al. 1977. [d]Nakagawa et al. 1980; Tachibana et al. 1980. [e]Srinivason and Neu 1980; Murakawa et al 1980. [f]Matsumoto et al. 1980. [g]Seddon et al. 1980; Wise et al. 1980d. [h]Reeves et al. 1980. [i]Acred et al. 1980. [j]Scully and Neu 1981. All data based on intramuscular dosing.

1. Cephalosporins with High and Prolonged Serum Levels

Most of the injectable cephalosporins can be given intravenously or intramuscularly, although some (e.g., cephalothin, cephapirin) are painful on intramuscular injection and are usually administered intravenously. Human i.m. pharmacokinetic properties of most of the cephalosporins listed in Tables 15 A and 15 B are summarized in Table 22. These data were obtained from intramuscular injections of 0.5- or 1-g doses in volunteers and come from many different laboratories. Cephalothin and its close analogs produce peak serum concentrations of 15–24 µg/ml in approximately 30 min to 1 h. The serum half-life is 0.5–1.5 h so that the levels tend to fall below clinically effective concentrations within 8 h. Thus 0.5- to 2-g doses are given at 4- to 6-h intervals. Cephaloridine produces a peak level (40 µg/ml) about double those of the 3′-acetoxy analogs, but the half-life is in the same range; it is given in 0.5- to 1.0-g doses every 6–8 h. It can be seen that many of the more recent cephalosporins have absorption characteristics which resemble those of cephaloridine.

Cefazolin has an in vitro antibacterial spectrum similar to that of cephalothin, but it exhibits peak serum levels and serum half-life values approximately 2–3 times those of the cephalosporins marketed before it. Replacement of the acetoxy group with a nonmetabolized substituent, as with cephaloridine, would account for part of the increase in height and duration of serum concentrations. The relatively high level of binding to serum proteins probably also contributes to the pharmacokinetic properties of cefazolin and later analogs. However, serum binding levels in laboratory animals do not always correlate closely with the height and duration of blood levels and it can be seen from Table 22 that many analogs with high human serum binding levels exhibit mediocre levels of the drug in the serum (metabolism, excretion, and biliary recycling are discussed in Chap. 15).

Three new cephalosporins produce unexpectedly high and prolonged serum levels (ceforanide, cefonicid, ceftriaxon). All three have an acidic heterocyclic thiomethyl grouping at the 3-position. However, this is not a characteristic of acidic 3-substituents generally. The structural requirements for producing the elevated serum concentrations observed are quite narrow with respect to the heterocyclic ring and the position of the acidic group. Table 23 summarizes a few of the structure–activity relationships in laboratory animals that led to the selection of cefonicid for clinical development (BERGES et al. 1976). In this case the usual tetrazole methyl group is replaced with an alkyl group carrying an acidic substituent (CO_2H, SO_3H). While there is broad latitude in the permissible variation of the 7-acyl groups, this improvement in serum levels is not observed with many other heterocyclic rings when they are substituted for the tetrazole. The position of the substituent on the tetrazole ring, the size of the alkyl bridge, and the pKa of the acidic function strongly influence the serum levels attained in mice. It can be seen that there is good correlation between the serum peak and half life values observed in mice and in humans where such data exist (cefazolin, cefamandole, cefonicid, ceforanide). All of these analogs have lower activity against gram-positive bacteria than corresponding derivatives with nonacidic 3-substituents. Ceforanide (GOTTSTEIN et al. 1976; LEITNER et al. 1976) is generally more active than cefazolin against Enterobacteriaceae susceptible to the latter, especially *E. coli*, *K. pneumoniae*, *Salmonella*, and *P. mirabilis*, but it is less active than cefamandole against resistant species like *Enterobacter* and indole-positive *Proteus* (ASAWAPOKEE et al. 1978). Cefonicid (BERGES et al. 1976; ACTOR et al. 1978) is very similar to cefamandole in its antibacterial activity and β-lactamase resistance pattern. Replacement of the carboxyl by a sulfonic acid group results in higher and longer serum levels. The 3-substituent of ceftriaxon (REINER et al. 1980) is acidic through the enolic 6-hydroxy-*as*-triazone moiety (Table 15B). The exquisite broad-spectrum activity of ceftriaxon resembles that of cefotaxime, with which it shares the same 7-acyl group (REINER et al. 1980; HINKLE and BODEY 1980a; WISE et al. 1980b).

The high and prolonged blood levels which these agents produce make them good candidates for prophylactic use, dosage regimens requiring less frequent injections (every 12–24 h), and single-dose treatment in some cases. Table 24 illustrates the prolonged effectiveness of cefonicid where good protection was observed in mice even when the drug was administered 6 h before infection. Cefonicid and ceftriaxon are highly active against *N. gonorrhoea*, including β-lactamase producers, making them good candidates for the use of single-dose regimens for treating gonorrhoea (ZAJAC et al. 1980; PITKIN et al. 1980). Single-dose treatment for some urinary tract infections has also been studied (YOSHIKAWA et al. 1980).

Table 23. Effect of acidic 3-substituents on serum levels of antibiotic

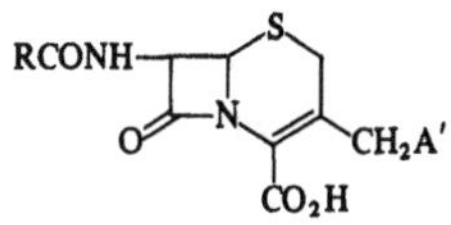

R	A'	MIC (μg/ml)		Mouse serum		Human serum	
		S. aureus	*E. coli*	Peak (μg/ml)	$t_{1/2}$ (min)	Peak (μg/ml)	$t_{1/2}$ (min)
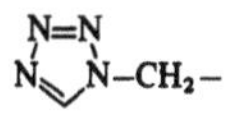	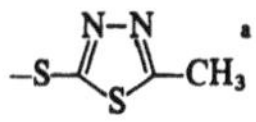 [a]	0.4	0.8	54	23	38–76	90
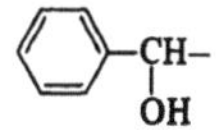	$-OCOCH_3$	1.6	3.1	26	24	–	–
	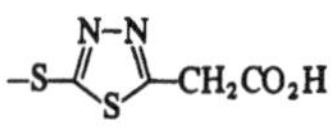	3.1	0.4	36	23	–	–
	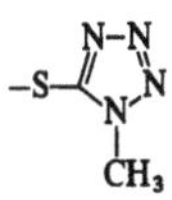 [b]	1.6	1.6	34	13	21	34
	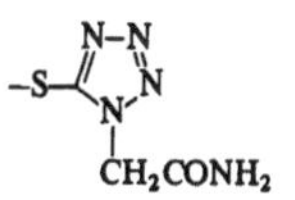	1.6	0.8	34	18	–	–
	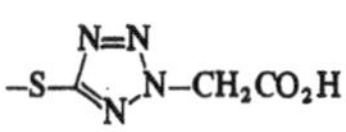	1.6	1.6	31	24	–	–
	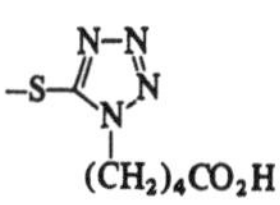	1.6	1.6	29	29	–	–
	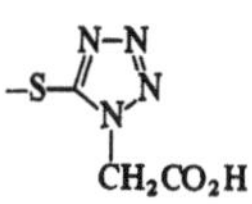	3.1	1.6	81	33	–	–
	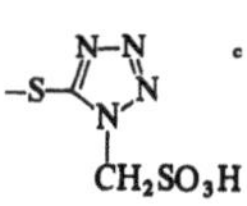 [c]	3.1	0.8	110	124	98	277
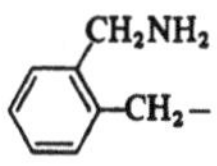	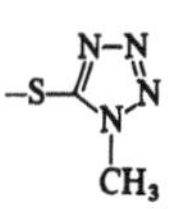	0.4	0.8	20	31	–	–
	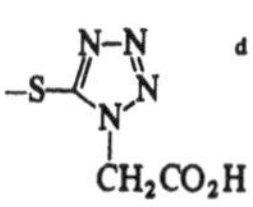 [d]	1.6	0.8	54	44	75	176
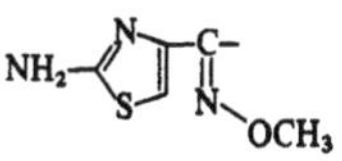	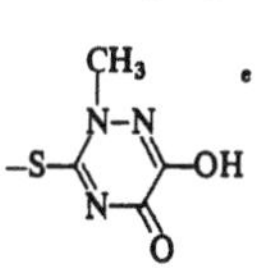 [e]	(4)	(0.12)	–	–	(50–85)	(480–600)

Sources: Berger et al. 1976; Shannon et al. 1980. For human serum values sources, see Table 22. [a]Cefazolin. [b]Cefamandole. [c]Cefonicid. [d]Ceforanide. [e]Cefatriaxon.

Table 24. Prophylactic effectiveness of a cephalosporin with prolonged serum levels

	ED_{50}(mg/kg) in mice							
	S. aureus 674		*E. coli* 12140		*K. pneumoniae* 4200		*P. mirabilis* 442	
	6h. Pre	1h. Post	6h. Pre	1h. Post	6h. Pre	1h. Post	6h. Pre	1h. Post
Cefonicid	65	8.1	3.1	0.7	3.1	0.6	2.1	0.3
Cefamandole	>100	15.5	>100	0.6	>100	1.3	>100	8.4
Cefoxitin	>100	40	>100	2.8	>100	4.1	>100	6.8

Source: GRAPPEL et al. 1980

2. Cephalosporins Absorbed Orally

Lack of oral activity, an almost universal characteristic of the cephalosporins, is unexpected since these compounds have distinctly better acid stability than the penicillins, and the latter are absorbed orally except when limited by acid instability. Because of the generality of this characteristic among the cephalosporins it is, likewise, unexpected that a few cephalosporins like cephalexin and cephradine (Table 15A) are absorbed with efficiencies greater (>88%) than for the penicillins. Essentially all of the cephalosporins that are known to combine broad-spectrum activity and good oral absorption have 7β-arylglycine side-chains. More specifically, the clinically useful cephalosporins (Table 15A) all involve the phenylglycine structure, with or without ring substituents or progressive levels of benzene ring hydrogenation. Good oral absorption of cephalosporins in humans has been ascribed to the presence of both the α-amino group on the 7β-acyl substituent and a small uncharged group at the 3-position (O'CALLAGHAN 1975). The one notable exception is cefatrizine (Table 15A) with a *lin*-triazolethiomethyl substituent at the 3-position.

Most of the cephalosporins in this group lack the 3′-leaving group found on the parenteral cephalosporins. The 3′-acetoxy group is retained on cephaloglycin. This combination with phenylglycine at the 7β-position renders cephaloglycin chemically unstable and relatively unsuitable as a clinical antibiotic (PITT et al. 1968). However, in line with the preceding discussion on the role of the 3′-substituent, deletion of the 3′-acetoxy group from the molecule profoundly lowers the antibacterial activity with most 7β-acyl side chains. This is reflected in the significant differences in MIC values between the 3-acetoxymethyl and 3-methyl analogs with a 7β-thienylacetylamino group as recorded in Table 25. There is a partial restoration of activity when groupings such as methoxy or methylthio are reintroduced on the 3-substituent (with lowered oral absorption; WEBBER et al. 1971). Alternatively, most of the broad-spectrum activity is restored when a D-mandeloylamino or D-phenylglycylamino group is placed at the 7β-position. As with the penicillins and most other β-lactams, side chains with the L-configuration confer significantly less activity on the molecule. The D-phenylglycine side chain combines broad-spectrum activity and oral absorption while the analogous α-hydroxy derivative is not absorbed significantly per os.

The enhancement of broad-spectrum activity for cephalosporins with 3-substituents of the type involved here appears to invoke a modified pattern of interaction with the enzymes involved in cell-wall maintenance. Thus, cephalexin and its

Table 25. Cephalosporins with oral activity *vs.* analogs with a 7β–thienylacetyl side chain

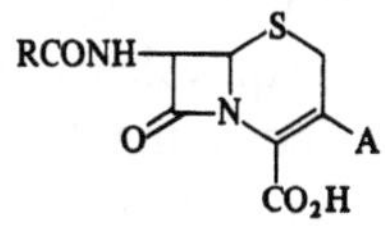

R	A	Source	MIC (μg/ml) *S. aureus*	*E. coli*	*K. pneumoniae*	*E. Aerogenes*
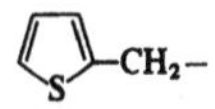	$-CH_2OCOCH_3$[g]	a	0.5	6.4	0.8	2.4
	$-CH_3$		3.8	>50	16	>50
	$-CH_2OCH_3$		0.5	39	43	12
	$-CH_2SCH_3$		3.1	>50	17	18
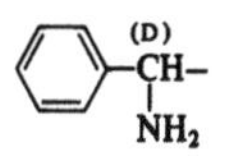	$-CH_2OCOCH_3$		3.1	3.5	1.0	3.5
	$-CH_3$[h]		4.8	9.7	6.6	6.4
	$-CH_2OCH_3$		0.6	4.1	1.9	1.4
	$-CH_2SCH_3$		1.4	3.6	1.8	1.4
	–H	b	10	14	6	8
	$-OCH_3$		9	6	6	6
	–Cl		6	1	0.6	0.6
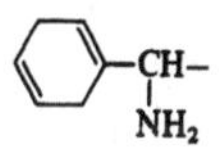	$-CH_3$[i]	c	3.1	9.4	9.4	9.4
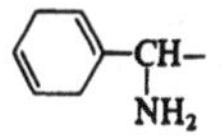	$-OCH_3$[j]	d	3.1	3.1	3.1	–
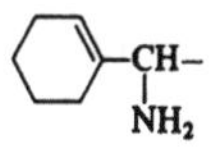	$-CH_3$[k]	e	3.1	50	12.5	–
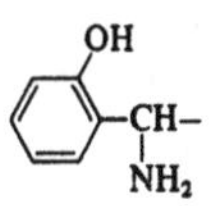	$-CH_3$	b	25	200	100	>200
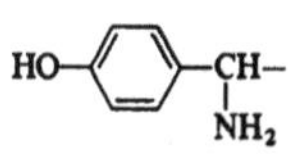	$-CH_3$[l]	f	3.1	13	25	25
	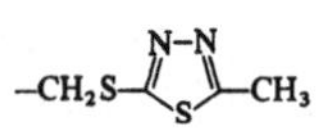		3.1	6.3	6.3	25
	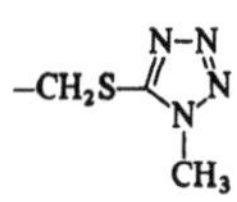		3.1	1.6	1.6	3.1
	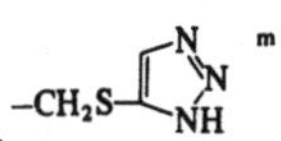 [m]		1.6	1.6	1.6	1.6

Sources: [a]GORMAN and RYAN 1972. [b]WEBBER and OTT 1977. [c]GADEBUSCH et al. 1972. [d]YASUDA et al. 1980. [e]YAMAZAKI et al. 1976. [f]DUNN et al. 1976. [g]Cephalothin. [h]Cephalexin. [i]Cephradine. [j]Cefroxadine. [k]SCE100. [l]Cefadroxil. [m]Cefatrizine.

analogs are still bactericidal but they have a slower killing rate than many 3′-substituted derivatives (MUGGLETON et al. 1969). This property is shared by cefaclor and other analogs of this series (SANDERS 1977). The slowness of killing for cephalexin may be attributed in part to poor kinetics of PBP binding and a binding pattern (I_{50} values PBP 1B, 2, 3: 240, >250, and 8 μg/ml, respectively; see Table 14) that results only in filamentation. Cefaclor binds PBP 1B nearly as efficiently as PBP3 (4.4 and 2 μg/ml, respectively) and its action results in relatively less filamentation. In a recent comparison of cephalosporins with different abilities to induce filamentation, all exhibited equivalent effectiveness in protecting mice infected intraperitoneally with *E. coli*, indicating that filamentation is not a determining factor in therapeutic efficacy (RYAN and MONSEY 1981).

Table 25 reflects attempts that have been made to increase intrinsic activity while retaining oral absorption in this series by replacing the 3-methyl group with other small substituents that are usually more polar (H, OCH_3, Cl). The analogs with hydrogen and methoxy at the 3-position have essentially the same activity as cephalexin. Introduction of chlorine increases activity against gram-negative bacteria that are susceptible to cephalexin 4- to 16-fold (clinical isolates; SANDERS 1977), with an accompanying increase in chemical instability as already indicated. None of the structural changes broadens the spectrum of activity, which parallels that of the β-lactamase-susceptible parenteral cephalosporins. This is surprising since cephalexin and cephradine have a relatively low, though measurable, rate of hydrolysis by *R*-plasmid mediated β-lactamases (SIMPSON et al. 1980; see Table 27).

Structural changes on the 7-acyl side chain produce analogs with activities equal to or less than that of cephalexin (Table 25). Thus, cephradine (dihydro-cephalexin) is slightly less active, but virtually indistinguishable, from cephalexin, while SCE 100 (the tetrahydro analog) has about the same activity against gram-positive bacteria but is only about one-fourth as active against the susceptible gram-negative organisms (YAMAZAKI and TSUCHIYA 1976). Introduction of an ortho-hydroxyl group drastically lowers activity, but a para-hydroxyl group lowers activity only slightly on cefadroxil and not at all on cefatrizine as compared to their unsubstituted analogs. The consequences of these structural manipulations on pharmacokinetic properties are reflected by the data in Table 26. The data contained in this table were again obtained in many different laboratories and, since oral absorption behaviour is less reproducible than that from intramuscular injection (O'CALLAGHAN et al. 1979), the information in this table should be used with some caution. Substitution of the phenyl group (4'-OH, cefadroxil; 3',4'-methylene dioxy, RMI 19592; 3'-methylaminosulfonate, FR 10612) tends to lower peak serum level concentrations but lengthens the serum half-life, so that higher serum levels are maintained with time, for example at 4 h after injection (Table 26).

Cefatrizine would seem to violate several of the generalities presented in the preceding discussion. This analog, with in vitro activity against gram-negative bacteria significantly better than that of cephalexin (e.g., MICs using an *E. coli* strain: 1.5 vs. 6–12 μg/ml), affords serum levels in mice, both subcutaneously and orally, that are approximately double those obtained with cephalexin (20 mg/kg dose: i.m. peak serum levels, 54 vs. 28 μg/ml; p.o. peak serum levels, 44 vs. 18 μg/ml). These exceptionally high serum levels are dependent on the presence of both a 3-(1,2,3-triazole-4-thiomethyl) substituent and a p-hydroxyl group on the phenylglycine side-chain at the 7-position. Peak serum concentrations in orally dosed mice for analogs without the p-hydroxyl group, or with a 2-methyl-1,2,3-thiadiazole or a 1-methyltetrazole ring in place of the 1,2,3-triazole moiety were 13, 24, and 7.6 μg/ml, respectively. The structure–activity studies that led to cefatrizine have been described (DUNN et al. 1976) and the role of the heterocyclic thiomethyl group in determining activity of 7-phenylglycine cephalosporins has been thoroughly reviewed

Table 26. Pharmacokinetic properties of orally absorbed cephalosporins

	Serum peak (μg/ml)	$t_{1/2}$ (min)	Serum binding (%)	Urinary recovery (%)	4–h Serum level (μg/ml)
Cephaloglycin	0–2.6	–	–	35	0.98
Cephalexin	13–20.7	36–54	10–17	88	1.05
Cephradine	11–22	31–58	6–20	100	0.96
Cefadroxine	12–14	45–75	9	88	~1
Cefadroxil	16.2	78	20	88	4.6
Cefaclor	10–23	30–60	–	51–72	<0.4
Cefatrizine	4.7–5.6[b]	86	58	35	2.7[b]
FR10612	8.8	120	13	89	7.3
RMI 19592[a]	11.8	70	–	86	–

Sources: See O'CALLAGHAN 1979; MURRAY and MOELLERING 1979, for references to primary data except; [a])BUSTRACK et al. 1980. All data were obtained using 0.5 g oral dose. [b])Values may be artifically low; see text.

(WEBBER and OTT 1977). Cefatrizine was found to produce serum levels in humans that are lower than predicted by the results in mice and other laboratory animals (ACTOR et al. 1976b). However, while this analog does not exhibit the chemical instability of cephaloglycin and cefaclor, it has been found, like cefaclor, to be unstable in serum (compare: O'CALLAGHAN 1978; NEU and FU 1978a; LAMB and FOGLESONG 1976). Thus, it appears likely that the human serum levels reported earlier for cefatrizine are artificially low. BROUGHALL et al. (1979) have reported that using techniques designed to prevent the decomposition of cephalosporins such as cefaclor and cefatrizine in serum samples, significantly higher blood concentrations and urinary recoveries in volunteers were obtained with this antibiotic.

A new entry which combines very broad-spectrum activity with good oral absorption characteristics, at least in laboratory animals, is FR 17027 (Table 15B). Administered orally, this 7-aminothiazole analog, with a vinyl group at the 3-position, produces peak serum levels in dogs equivalent to those obtained with amoxicillin, with a significantly longer half-life. This antibiotic is highly active against strains of gram-negative species resistant to cefaclor and cephalexin, but it is less active than cefaclor against staphylococci (TAKAYA et al. 1982).

Cephalexin and its several close analogs exhibit pharmacokinetic properties that do not require consideration of pro-drugs in their use. However, 3′-substituted derivatives, other than cefatrizine, frequently exhibit improved in vitro activity but disappointing absorption characteristics when administered per os. A few attempts to construct pro-drugs from such derivatives have been reported. The acetoxymethyl and pivaloyloxymethyl esters of cephaloglycin are inactive in vitro and produce higher serum levels and better urinary recovery of the parent antibiotic than unesterified cephaloglycin following oral administration to rats and humans (BINDERUP et al. 1971). Similarly, oral administration of the pivaloyloxymethyl, phthalidyl and acetoxymethyl esters of the 3-(5-methyl-(1,3,4-thiadiazol-2-yl)-thiomethyl analog of cephalexin to mice results in peak blood levels of the unesterified parent that are significantly higher than those obtained from the unesterified analog. These 3′-substituted analogs are more active than cephalexin in vitro against both *S. aureus* and Enterobacteriaceae. Unfortunately these esters tend to undergo double bond migration (Δ^3 to Δ^2) during synthesis requiring additional processing, and esters of phenylglycine cephalosporins are chemically unstable at physiological pH (WHEELER et al. 1977). The clinical utility of these agents is uncertain.

IV. β-Lactamase-Resistant Cephalosporins

The cephalosporins listed in Table 15B emphasize the importance of β-lactamase resistance in the continuing design of these molecules. Like the penicillins, significant improvement in resistance to β-lactamase hydrolysis has relied on manipulations which involve steric effects in the vicinity of the 6(7)β-amide grouping. (See O'CALLAGHAN 1980 concerning differences in β-lactamase resistance of cephalosporin sulfoxides and sulfones, and compare modest improvements in β-lactamase resistance by manipulation of the 3-substituents, for example with cefotiam, discussed in Sect. C.II.3). Manipulation of the α-carbon of the 7β-side-chain on the cephalosporins can extend the staphylococcal β-lactamase resistance which these compounds have already to include resistance to the gram-negative β-lactamases. A second route to this goal is introduction of substituents on the 6(7)α-position. It will be seen later (Sect. D.I.1) that this latter method for inducing high resistance to β-lactamase inactivation is also applicable to β-lactams with fused five-membered rings (thienamycin) when the chemical system is activated sufficiently that a 6β-acylamino group is not required.

1. Cephalosporins with Moderate β-Lactamase Resistance

As indicated in Table 13, the generally lower intrinsic activity of the cephalosporins precludes incorporation of the side-chain α-carbon atom into a ring in order to increase steric bulk. Likewise multiple substitution of the α-carbon atom with alkyl and aryl groups, or the like, has a deleterious effect on activity. However, introduction of certain polar substituents on this carbon atom results in increased resistance to β-lactamases and generally broader in vitro activity against gram-negative bacteria. Cephalexin, with an α-amino substituent, exhibits modestly increased resistance to β-lactamases although this is not translated into a significantly broader spectrum of activity. An α-hydroxyl group is more efficacious in this respect. Cefamandole and cefonicid (Table 15B) exhibit increased resistance to chromosomally mediated type I cephalosporinases and as a consequence, in addition to the organisms listed earlier for the β-lactamase-sensitive cephalosporins, these agents exhibit activity against some *Enterobacter* sp., indole-positive *Proteus* sp., *H. Influenzae*, and *Bacteroides* sp. (see Table 27 for the MIC values of cefamandole).

A large number of β-lactamases of gram-negative origin have now been described (see Chap. 12; also RICHMOND and SYKES 1973; SYKES and MATTHEW 1976), but a smaller number occur with sufficient frequency to constitute major clinical significance (see, for example, SIMPSON et al. 1980). Table 28 compares the relative rates at which cefamandole and several other cephalosporins are hy-

Table 27. In vitro activities of cephalosporins moderately resistant to β–lactamases, and cefoxitin, versus the β–lactamase–susceptible standards cephalothin and cefazolin

	MIC (μg/ml)						
	Source	Cephalothin	Cefazolin	Cefamandole	SQ69013	Cefuroxime	Cefoxitin
S. aureus	a	–	0.78	0.39	6.3	0.78	1.56
H. influenzae	b	–	–	0.8	–	0.5	–
N. gonorrhoeae	b	–	–	1.6	–	0.005	–
E. coli	a	–	1.2	0.6	0.47	1.56	1.56
E. coli	c	400	–	1.6	–	12.5	3.1
K. pneumoniae	a	–	1.2	0.6	0.32	1.2	1.2
K. pneumoniae	c	400	–	1.6	–	3.2	3.1
S. schottmuelleri	a	–	1.2	0.39	0.12	0.78	1.2
P. mirabilis	c	400	–	0.8	–	25	3.1
P. rettgeri	a	–	>50	1.56	0.4	0.78	12.5
P. morganii	c	>400	–	12.5	–	50	12.5
E. cloacae	a	–	>50	4.7	0.6	6.25	>50
C. freundii	c	400	–	3.2	–	1.6	100
S. marcescens	a	–	>50	9.4	1.6	12.5	4.7
Providencia sp.	c	400	–	25	–	25	25
Ps. aeruginosa	a	–	>50	>50	>100	>50	>50
B. fragilis	c	200	–	50	–	200	3.1

Sources: [a)]Breuer et al. 1978. [b)]Actor et al. 1978. O'Callaghan 1975. [c)]Neu and Fu 1978b. Test conditions: [a)]broth dilution using 10^5 CFU; [b)], [c)]agar dilution using 10^5 CFU. See original articles for additional test conditions and description of bacterial strains.

drolyzed by five different β-lactamases that are believed to be representative of most of the enzymes produced by clinically important pathogens. The complexity of the β-lactamase susceptibility profiles vis-à-vis antibacterial spectrum of activity is underscored by comparison of the β-lactamase-susceptibility data contained in this table with the in vitro antibacterial spectra for the various analogs in the tables which follow. Resistance to β-lactamase inactivation may not correlate with protective effectiveness because of a number of factors. The structural manipulation which confers β-lactamase resistance may lower antibacterial activity as well (cephamycins). Unless resistance to the enzyme is virtually complete its net effect will depend not only on the level of resistance, but also on the relative degree of binding of the antibiotic to the enzyme and the amount and location of the β-lactamase that is produced by the strain under antibiotic attack. Nevertheless, these correlations are fairly predictive for moderately resistant analogs and more firmly so for the highly resistant analogs such as cefotaxime and moxalactam.

There are additional substituents which, when placed on the α-carbon of the acylamino side chain, lower susceptibility to β-lactamases. A number of 7β-ureidoacetyl cephalosporins (see Table 15B, SQ69613, SQ14359, and SQ81015) exhibit activity against bacteria which include β-lactamase-producing Enterobacteriaceae. This broad-spectrum activity is observed over a range of structural analogs with variation of the 7β-side-chain (phenyl, hydroxyphenyl, thienyl, furyl), and the 3′-substituent (acetoxy, 4-carbamoylpyridinium, various heterocyclic thio groupings), with and without a 7α-methoxy substituent. SQ69613 exhibits in vitro activ-

Table 28. Relative susceptibility of selected cephalosporins to five β–lactamases of clinical significance, expressed as V_{rel}[a]

	V_{rel}[a]				
	Plasmid	Chromosomal			
Classification of enzyme:	IIIa (TEM)	Ia (P99)	Id (Ps. 18H)	IVc (Kl)	B33
Producing organism:	Enterobacteriaceae (e.g., *E. coli*) *H. influenzae* *N. gonorrhoeae*	*E. cloacae* *P. morganii*	*Ps. aeruginosa*	*Klebsiella* sp.	*B. fragilis*
Specificity	PASE/CASE	CASE	CASE	PASE/CASE	CASE
Cephaloridine	100	100	100	100	100
Ampicillin	130	10	–	243	–
Cephalexin	0.5	12.5	70	0.5	–
Cefazolin	15–20	12–45	40–75	66–112	71
Cefamandole	20–60	0.1–3	0	20–60	16
Cefuroxime	0.1–0.75	0–0.1	0.9	11–13.7	64–107
Cefoxitin	0[b]	0	–	0	0
Cefotaxime	0.15	0.06	–	0.6	17
Moxalactam	<0.03[b]	<0.03	<0.03	<0.03	<0.03
Cefsulodin	<2	<0.2	<2	–	–

Sources: RICHMOND and WOTTON 1976; RICHMOND 1980a, b; O'CALLAGHAN 1980; KING et al. 1980. [a])Relative rate of hydrolysis compared to cephaloridine (=100). Consult original articles for indication of binding affinities and absolute hydrolysis rates. [b])The values O and <0.03 are probably not significanty different.

ity equivalent to that of cefamandole, except that it is less active against *S. aureus* (Table 27; BREUER et al. 1978). Contrary to usual experience the analogs with the L-configuration on the 7β-acylamino side-chain (7α-H series) are substantially more active than those with the D-configuration in vitro and in vivo particularly, but not exclusively, against Enterobacteriaceae that produce chromosomal cephalosporinases. For example, the D- and L-7β-(2-thienylureidoacetyl) analogs of SQ69613 bind primarily to the PBP3 of both *E. coli* and *E. cloacae* with equal affinity (I_{100} values (D/L): PBP1, 2/>30; PBP2, 30/>30; PBP3, 0.5/0.5 μg/ml). Yet the MIC values for the D and L isomers against an *E. cloacae* strain are 75 and 1.6 μg/ml, respectively (GEORGOPAPADAKOU et al. 1980). This unusual superiority of analogs with the L- over those with the D-side-chain configuration has been attributed to enhanced resistance to and inhibition of β-lactamases (GADEBUSCH et al. 1978). In addition to the cephalosporins with an unsubstituted α-ureido grouping just described, a growing number of analogs are appearing which carry a 7β-phenylglycine side-chain on which the amine is part of a substituted ureido group or is acylated with heterocyclic carboxylic acids (cefoperazone, Table 15B; analogs listed in Table 35). These β-lactamase-resistant broad-spectrum cephalosporins are included in Sect. C.IV.3.

Table 29. In vitro activities of some 7β(α–oxyiminoarylacetylamino) cephalosporanic acids

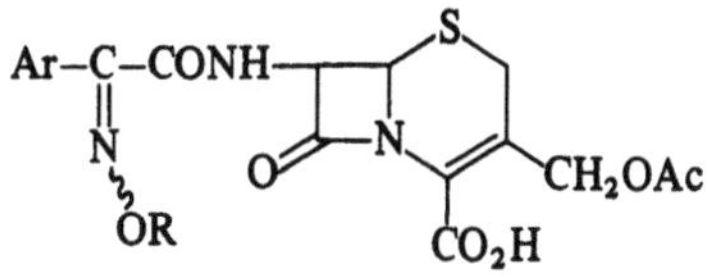

Ar	R	MIC (µg/ml) *S. aureus* (R)	*E. coli* (S)	*E. coli* (R)	*P. morgani*
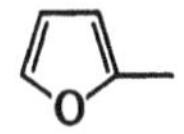	CH_3 (*syn*)	1	4	4	0.2
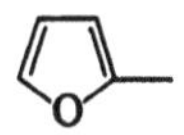	CH_3 (*anti*)	1	16	62	4
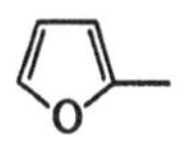	H (*syn*)	0.6	2	4	2
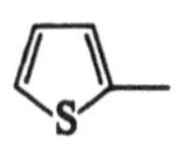	CH_3 (*syn*)	0.6	31	31	8
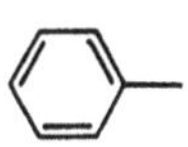	CH_3 (*syn*)	0.6	8	16	4

Source: WEBBER and OTT 1977.

The use of 7β-acyl side chains carrying on α-oxyimino carbon is currently one of the most effective routes to broad-spectrum cephalosporins. Introduction of an oxymino group results in a high level of β-lactamase resistance without the reduction in activity which accompanies incorporation of this carbon atom into an aromatic ring or multiple substitution. The selection of cefuroxime (Table 15B; O'CALLAGHAN et al. 1976; CHERRY et al. 1977) for clinical use is indicated by the structure–activity relationships of analogous cephalosporanic acid derivatives summarized in Table 29. The *syn* isomers are consistently more active against gram-negative bacteria than the *anti* isomers. The furyl ring provides an activity advantage over phenyl and thienyl. The methoxyimino grouping was selected over the hydroxy analog on the basis of pharmacokinetic behaviour (e.g., serum binding). Cefuroxime has a carbamoyloxy group at the 3′-position in place of the acetoxy group. As indicated later the oxyimino oxygen atom can be substituted with other alkyl groups with retention of activity.

As seen in Table 28 cefuroxime has increased stability toward β-lactamases, but it does not have the uniform resistance exhibited by the cephamycins and later "third generation" cephalosporins. Consequently, its spectrum of activity (Table 27) and clinical utility resemble most closely cefamandole. Both agents exhibit useful levels of activity against *H. influenzae*, and cefuroxime is especially active against *N. gonorrhoeae* and *N. meningitidis* (BRORSON and NORRBY 1978). The pharmacokinetic behavior of cefamandole is somewhat poorer than that of cephaloridine, and cefuroxime gives higher peak levels with about the same half-life (Table 22). Cefuroxime is also less bound by serum proteins.

Table 30. Effect of 7α–substitition on in vitro activity of cephalothin

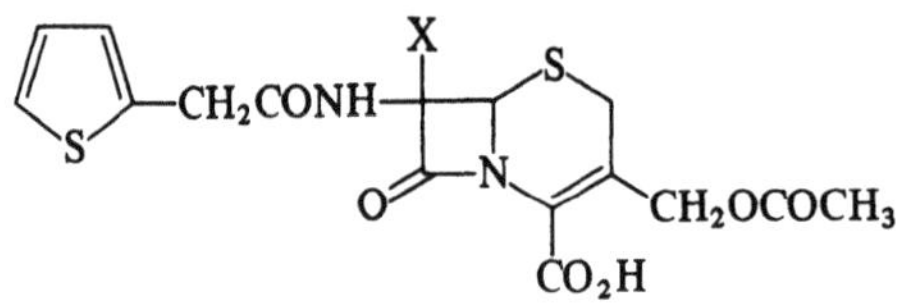

	MIC (μg/ml)					Destruction by *E. coli* β–lactamase (%)
	S. aureus	*E. coli* (S)	*E. coli* (R)	*P. mirabilis*	*P. vulgaris*	
Cephamycin C	>100	25	25	3.12	1.56	–
Cefoxitin	6.25	6.25	6.25	6.25	1.56	0
X						
–H	0.39	6.25	50	6.25	100	>99
$–OCH_3$	6.25	25	50	25	0.78	16
$–OCH_2CH_3$	50	>100	>100	>100	25	0
$–SCH_3$	50	>100	>100	>100	100	20
$–CH_2OH$	>100	>100	>100	>100	50	0
$–CH_2CH_3$	>100	>100	–	>100	>100	–

Source: STAPLEY et al. 1979a

2. Cephamycins

The discovery of the natural cephamycins provided access to an effective alternative method for protecting β-lactams from attack by β-lactamases. Indeed, the methoxy group and other substituents on the 6(7)α-position of the penicillins and cephalosporins protect the β-lactam ring from attack more efficiently than the structural changes on the 6(7)β-acyl group discussed to this point (however, see below). While cefuroxime and cefamandole remain at least partially susceptible to all of the β-lactamases listed in Table 28 and highly susceptible to some, cefoxitin exhibits essentially complete resistance to hydrolysis by all of the representative enzymes in this group. The high resistance of cefoxitin to inactivation has been demonstrated for many more β-lactamases than those listed in Table 28 (see for example, FU and NEU 1978b, 1979, 1980).

Although most of the β-lactamase resistance of these cephalosporins can be attributed to 7α-substitution, the nearly complete resistance to inactivation observed with cefoxitin is not solely due to this structural feature. Cephamycin C with the 7α-methoxy and 3-carbamoyloxymethyl substituents of cefoxitin, but with a 7β-D-aminoadipoylamino group, is hydrolyzed 174 times faster than cefoxitin by the β-lactamase of *E. cloacae* (V_{max}: 3.3×10^{-3} vs. 0.019×10^{-3} μ*M*/min per mg protein; Km: 2.4×10^{-2} vs. 0.6×10^{-2} μ*M*; STAPLEY et al. 1979b). Likewise, the 3′-acetoxy analog of cefoxitin (7α-methoxycephalothin) retains some sensitivity to β-lactamase from *E. coli* (see Table 30): and thus both the 7β-thienylacetylamino and the 4-carbamoyloxymethyl substituents appear to augment the 7α-methoxy group in providing the extreme β-lactamase resistance of cefoxitin.

The prevention of β-lactam-ring hydrolysis by this mechanism is not without cost in terms of in vitro activity. Introduction of the 7α-methoxy group on the cephalosporins generally lowers the activity relative to the corresponding unsubstituted analog (however, compare oxacephalosporins below), and the many other substituents that were placed synthetically on the 7α-position following the discovery of the cephamycins [see HOOVER and DUNN (1979) for a listing of substituents and access references] drastically lower the activity against both gram-positive and gram-negative bacteria. This is illustrated by Table 30.

Cefoxitin, with a 3′-carbamoyloxy grouping in place of acetoxy, has poor activity against gram-positive bacteria as compared with that of cephalothin (EICKHOFF and EHRET 1976), but its activity against gram-negative bacteria that do not produce β-lactamases [examples: *E. coli* (S), *P. mirabilis* in Table 30] is comparable to cephalothin rather than the less active α-methoxy analog of the latter. Cefoxitin retains this level of activity against the β-lactamase producers so that it exhibits clinically useful activity against most *E. coli*, *Klebsiella*, *Serratia*, and indole positive *Proteus* sp. (Table 27). It is less active than cefamandole against *Enterobacter* and *Haemophilus* sp. It is active against *Neisseria* sp., and it exhibits activity against anaerobes, including *B. fragilis*, superior to cefamandole and cefuroxime. Thus it can be seen from Table 27 that in spite of its higher resistance to β-lactamase inactivation, cefoxitin has an in vitro antibacterial spectrum that resembles those of cefamandole and cefuroxime.

Structure–activity studies that examine the effects of changes at both the 3- and 7-position have been reported (NAKAO et al. 1976; SHIMIZU et al. 1976) and reviewed (WEBBER and OTT 1977). Generally, these studies have introduced 7-acyl (thienylacetyl, tetrazoleacetyl, mandeloyl, phenylmalonyl, heterocyclic thioacetyl) and 3′-substituents (acetoxy, carbamoyloxy, azido, heterocyclic thio) widely used with the cephalosporins, with fairly predictable results. The newer cephamycin analogs that have been selected for further study (Table 15B: cefmetazole; cefotetan; SQ14359; 7β-CF_3SCH_2CONH, SK&F 73678) all have the methyltetrazolethiomethyl moiety at the 3-position. Except for cefotetan, these analogs exhibit antibacterial spectra that are similar to that of cefoxitin, but they are generally 2–4 times more potent. These in vitro antibacterial profiles are compared by O'CALLAGHAN (1979). Cefotetan (Table 15B) has an unusual 7β-acyl group for a cephalosporin. It is approximately half as active as cefoxitin against gram-positive bacteria, probably due to the acidic function on its 7β-acyl side chain, but activity against gram-negative organisms are from 3 to over 100 times that of cefoxitin based on MIC_{50} values from clinical isolates. (MIC_{50} values against gram-negative bacteria including *E. cloacae*, *Citrobacter freundii* and *S. marcescens:* 0.13–3.13 μg/ml for cefotetan versus 4.22–84.5 for cefoxitin; TODA 1980). Cefotetan exhibits a strong affinity for PBPs 3 and 1B. Using the ^{14}C-labeled antibiotic, four new membrane proteins (MW: 53,000–75,000) were bound that are not detected using ^{14}C-benzylpenicillin. Neither cefotetan nor any of the other cephamycins are active against *Ps. aeruginosa*.

The oxacephalosporin moxalactam also contains a 7α-methoxy group which contributes to protection of the molecule against enzymatic inactivation with little reduction in intrinsic activity. The structure–activity relationships that pertain to this antibiotic are examined in Sect. C.V following.

Table 31. Structure–activity relationships of 2–aminothiazol–4–yl cephalosporin analogs

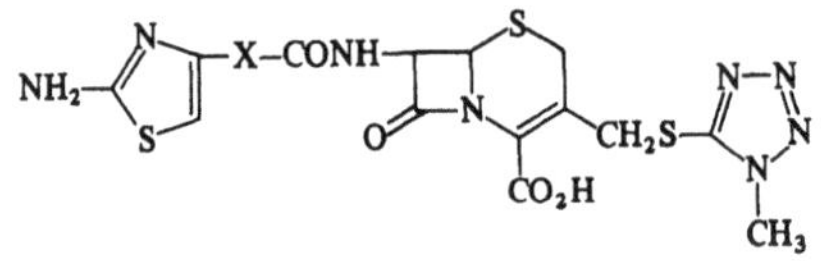

X	*S. aureus* (R) (1840)	*E. coli* (S) (JC2)	*E. coli* (R) (T7)	*P. vulgaris* sp.	*E. cloacae* (TN1282)	*S. marcescens* (TN24)
>CH_2	0.78	0.39	6.25	0.39	>100	>100
>$C(CH_3)_2$	50	–	>100	>100	>100	>100
>$CHCH_3$[a]	3.13	–	25	>100	100	12.5
>$CHNH_2$[a]	12.5	–	3.13	>100	25	50
>CHOH[a]	1.56	–	1.56	>100	6.25	25
>C=N–OH	–	0.05	0.78	6.25	6.25	0.39
>C=N–OCH_3[b]	3.13	0.10	0.78	0.39	1.56	0.20
>C=N–OCH_3(E)[c]	–	3.13	50	>100	50	3.13
>C=N–OC_2H_5	3.13	–	1.56	1.56	3.13	3.13
>C=N–OC_3H_7–i	3.13	–	6.25	12.5	6.25	3.13
>C=N–OCH_2COONa	50	–	0.39	0.025	0.78	0.78
	(Sa)	(TEM–)	(TEM+)	(P.v.)	(P99+)	(9782)
>$CHNHCONH_2$(L)[d]	6.3	<0.2	<0.2	>50	50	1.6

Sources: MORITA et al. 1980; NUMATA et al. 1977; OCHAI et al. 1977, 1980a,b,c, 1981; POLACEK and STARKE 1980. See original articles for description of organisms and test systems used. [a]Racemic side–chain. [b]Cefmenoxime [c]*Anti*–oxime, all others are *syn*–(Z). [d]SQ 81015

3. Cephalosporins with Significant β-Lactamase Resistance

The eight analogs listed in the right column of Table 15B represent a new group of cephalosporins that approach cefoxitin in their resistance to β-lactamase inactivation, without benefit of a 7α-methoxy substituent. As a group, they exhibit a level of activity against gram-negative bacteria never before encountered with β-lactam antibiotics. The 7β-(2-aminothiazol-4-yl)acetylamino side-chain occurs with high frequency on these analogs. The potential for achieving unusually high activity against gram-negative bacteria through the use of this heterocyclic substituent was illustrated in the structure–activity relationships, tabulated in Table 21, that led to cefotiam. Consistent with the structural requirements already discussed, the analogs in Table 21 (substituted on the α-carbon atom only by the aminothiazole ring) exhibit modest resistance to β-lactamase inactivation, at best. The effects of structural modifications involving the α-carbon of the side-chain follow a pattern predictable from other cephalosporin SAR experience, illustrated in Table 31.

Acquisition of β-lactamase resistance by incorporation of the α-carbon atom into a *syn*-oxyimino grouping is predicted by the structure–activity relationships of cefuroxime. However, the level of resistance achieved is significantly higher than with the furanylacetylamino side-chain (compare cefotaxime and cefuroxime, Table 28) and the increase in intrinsic gram-negative activity is unexpected (compare *E. coli* MIC values where X= CH_2 vs. X= C=$NOCH_3$(Z), Table 31). The increase in in vitro activity which accompanies the establishment of β-lactamase resistance in this case is remarkable not only in the level achieved but also by the fact that it is essentially independent of 3-substituent influence. Thus the in vitro ac-

Table 32. Structure–activity relationships of additional 2–aminothiazol–4–yl cephalosporin analogs

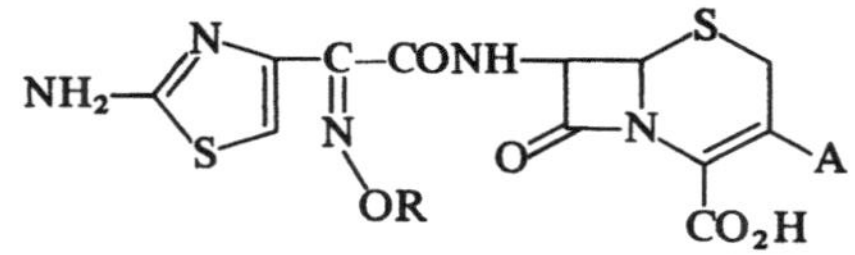

R	A	*S. aureus* (R)	*E. coli* (S) (ATCC11303)	*E. coli* (R) (T026) (B6)	*K. pneumoniae* (R2536)	*P. mirabilis* PI (A235)	*P. vulgaris* PI (A232)	*E. cloacae* (sp.)	*S. marcescens* (sp)
$-CH(CH_3)_2$	$-CH_2OAc$	3	0.5	1	10	0.5	0.5	–	2
$-C_2H_5$	$-CH_2OAc$	2	0.2	0.4	2	0.05	1	–	2
$-H$	$-CH_2OAc$	0.5	0.02	0.1	0.1	0.05	40	–	0.4
$-CH_3$	$-CH_2OAc$[a]	2	0.02	0.1	0.05	0.02	10	–	0.5
$-CH_2CO_2Et$	$-CH_2OAc$	3	0.5	0.1	2	0.2	1	–	5
$-CH_2CONH_2$	$-CH_2OAc$	5	0.05	0.1	0.5	0.1	5	–	2
$-CH_2CO_2H$	$-CH_2OAc$	20	0.05	0.1	0.1	0.02	0.1	–	1
		(663E)	(851E)	(1193E)	(1371E)	(431E)	(1352E)	(1083E)	(1324E)
$-C(CH_3)_2CO_2H$	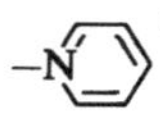 [b]	8	0.1	0.2	1	0.06	0.2	0.1	0.06
		(Newman)	JC2	28	(NCTC418)	(1)	(IAM1025)	(1)	–
$-CH_3$	$-H$[c]	1.56	0.05	0.2	⩽0.02	⩽0.02	0.05	12.5	–

Sources: Bucourt et al. 1980; O'Callaghan et al. 1980; Kamimura et al. 1979. Test conditions and laboratory strains used vary. Consult original articles for details. [a]Cefotaxime, [b]Ceftazidime, [c]Ceftizoxime.

Table 33. In vitro activity of cephalosporins highly resistant to β-lactamase against resistant β-lactamase-producing gram-negative bacteria

	MIC (μg/ml)			
	Cefoxitin	*Cefotaxime Ceftizoxime*	*Ceftriaxon*	*Moxalactam*
E. coli	12.5	0.1	0.05	0.4
K. pneumoniae	100	0.2–0.4	0.1	0.2
S. typhimurium	1.6	0.05–0.1	0.02	0.1
P. mirabilis	>400	1.6–3.1	0.05	0.1
P. vulgaris	3.1	0.1	0.05	0.8
P. rettgeri	100	0.05–0.1	0.05	0.1
E. aerogenes	>400	0.02–1.6	0.05	0.8
E. cloacae	>400	0.05–0.1	0.1	0.2
E. cloacae	>400	12.5	25	6.2
S. marcescens	>400	12.5–25	25	12.5
Ps. aeruginosa	>400	25	50	6.2
Ps. aeruginosa	>400	50–100	100	12.5
C. freundii	>100	0.4	0.8	0.4
B. fragilis	12.5	25	25	1.6

Source: Neu et al. 1981; β–Lactamase–producing strains resistant to cephalothin (⩾50 μg/ml) and carbenicillin (⩾200 μg/ml). The values for cefotaxime and ceftizoxime are virtually the same and fall within the ranges indicated.

tivities of the 3′-acetoxy (cefotaxime; Table 32) and the 3′-methyltetrazolethio (cefmenoxime; Table 31) analogs are virtually the same and, indeed, the analog with only hydrogen on the 3-position (ceftizoxime; Table 32) exhibits MIC values as good as, or better than those of cefotaxime – with potential advantages associated with the absence of the 3-acetoxymethyl group (Nakano 1981). In addition, the fourth methoxyimino analog ceftriaxon (see Sect. C.III.1) and the L-α-ureido analog SQ81015 (Table 15B) exhibit spectra of antibacterial activity that are essentially the same as that of cefotaxime (Neu et al. 1981; Breuer et al. 1980; Polacek and Starke 1980).

Table 33 illustrates the outstanding and closely parallel antibacterial activities of three of these analogs against β-lactamase-producing strains of gram-negative bacteria resistant to cephalothin and carbenicillin. These agents are active at clinically achievable serum concentrations against most gram-negative bacteria including *Enterobacter*, *Serratia*, and *Citrobacter* sp. and many strains of *Ps. aeruginosa*. As expected, cefotaxime has been found to have a very high affinity for the critical penicillin-binding proteins of *E. coli* K12 (Curtis et al. 1979; Table 14), especially for both PBP 1A and 3. This should be a contributing factor that helps account for the extraordinarily high in vitro activities of these cephalosporins. However, it should be noted that binding studies using ^{14}C-cefotaxime produced lower PBP 1 and 3 binding values than the competition studies using ^{14}C-benzylpenicillin and, as with cefotetan (Sect. C.IV.2), labeling of new proteins was observed (PBP 3′, 4′,

7, 8 and an additional protein with molecular weight higher than PBP 1A; Cefotaxime exhibited strong affinity for the high-molecular-weight protein; LABIA et al. 1980). Whether binding to these additional proteins contributes to the high level of activity of these cephalosporins remains to be seen. Pharmacokinetic properties of these cephalosporins were included in Table 22, and the prolonged serum levels of ceftriaxon were noted earlier.

While the unalkylated *syn*-oxyimino analogs exhibit good in vitro activities (Table 31) they are more highly bound by serum proteins and their pharmacokinetic properties are inferior to the *O*-alkylated derivatives. Activity declines with increase in the bulk of the alkyl group for some organisms, but there is a fairly broad structural latitude. This has permitted the introduction of alkyl groups carrying a carboxyl function (ceftazidime; Table 32). Somewhat analogously to carbenicillin, introduction of a carboxyl group on the 7β-side chain lowers the gram-positive activity, in this case rather significantly, but activity is increased against some gram-negative bacteria including *Ps. aeruginosa*. Thus ceftazidime is reported to exhibit better activity against clinical isolates of *Ps. aeruginosa* than cefotaxime, moxalactam, carbenicillin, and azlocillin (MIC_{50} values: 1 µg/ml vs. 8, 16, 43, and 4 µg/ml, respectively; $n=40$; 10^6 CFU; WISE et al. 1980c; compare VERBIST and VERHAEGEN 1980). This cephalosporin gives peak serum level and half-life values similar to those of cefotaxime (peak: 17.8 vs. 21.8 µg/ml with 500 mg dose, i.m.; $t_{1/2}$ 1.8 vs. 1.25 h; urinary recovery 82% vs. 60%–70%; HARDING et al. 1980; LUTHY et al. 1978). In mice this agent exhibits PD_{50} values against infections by the Enterobacteriaceae generally equal to or better than those of cefotaxime; protective effectiveness against *Pseudomonas* infections is significantly better and approximately equivalent to that of gentamicin [typically, ceftazidime/cefotaxime/gentamicin: 1.6/33.0/3.6 mg/kg (3×), s.c.; ACRED et al. 1980]. The implication of these structural changes on activity against a broader group of bacteria are presented in Table 34. This table also includes data on the compounds (cefsulodin, cefaperazone) which follow immediately in this discussion.

The parallel in the effect of side-chain structure on activity against *Ps. aeruginosa*, seen with ceftazidime and carbenicillin, extends to other analogs as well. Cefsulodin carries the 7-D-(α-sulfo)phenylacetamido side-chain of the broad-spectrum penicillin sulbenicillin and, like the latter, it exhibits significant activity against strains of *Ps. aeruginosa*. It resembles sulbenicillin in that the diastereomer with the D-configuration is significantly more active than the one with the L-side chain (NOMURA et al. 1974). However, it differs sharply from this penicillin, and other cephalosporins reported to be active against *Ps. aeruginosa* in its overall spectrum of activity. Cefsulodin has a very narrow spectrum of activity that is restricted essentially to *S. aureus* and *Ps. aeruginosa*. Table 34 illustrates the narrow range of activity of this agent. The MIC values against the Enterobacteriaceae range from 50 to 800 µg/ml whether or not the organism is a β-lactamase producer. This table also indicates the low susceptibility of cefsulodin to the β-lactamases of the bacteria which produce these enzymes. A rather plausible indication of the factors that contribute to the narrow spectrum of cefsulodin is provided by CURTIS et al. (1980b). The differences in MIC values (6.4 vs. 25 µg/ml) between the permeability mutant *E. coli* DC2 and its parent *E. coli* DC0 (Table 14) indicates that cefsulodin has difficulty in passing the permeability barrier of *E. coli* K12. But this is not the case

Table 34. β–Lactamase–resistant cephalosporins with activity against *Ps. aeruginosa*

	MIC (μg/ml)					
	Moxolactam[a]	*Cefotaxime*[b]	*Ceftazidime*[b]	*Cefoperazone*[c]	*Cefsulodin*[d]	*HR*
S. aureus	6.2	–	–	0.78	6.2	–
S. aureus	6.2	1	16	1.6	6.2*	<1
S. faecalis	>100	–	–	25	–	–
E. coli	0.1	<0.06	0.1	⩽0.1	100	–
E. coli	0.78*	0.06*	0.5*	–	800*	<1
Klebsiella sp.	0.1	–	–	⩽0.1	50	–
Klebsiella sp.	0.1*	62*	2*	–	400*	<1
Salmonella sp.	–	0.1	0.2	0.2	50	–
P. mirabilis	0.1	0.1	0.1	–	>100	–
P. morganii	0.2*	16*	4*	0.78	200	<1
P. vulgaris	0.2*	1*	1*	0.78	800*	31
Enterobacter sp.	0.2*	0.2	0.2	⩽0.1	–	–
E. cloacae	12.5*	16*	8*	0.78	800*	1
S. marcescens	0.2*	0.2*	0.1*	0.2	400	<1
Providencia sp.	–	62	8	–	–	–
Ps. aeruginosa	50*	31*	4*	1.6	1.56*	<1
Ps. aeruginosa	1.6	16	1	0.78	12.5*	<1
Ps. aeruginosa	6.2	16	2	0.78	25*	<1
Ps. aeruginosa	–	16	4.5	⩽0.1	6.2*	<1
C. freundii	0.2*	–	–	–	–	–
B. fragilis	0.78*	–	–	–	–	–

Sources: [a]Yoshida et al. 1978, 1980. [b]O'Callaghan et al. 1980; Acred et al. 1980. [c]Mitsuhashi et al. 1978. [d]Tsuchiya et al. 1978a. All agar dilution: [a, c]10^6 CFU; [b]10^7 CFU; [d]10^8 CFU. HR: β–lactamase hydrolysis rate (%) for cefsulodin *vs.* benzylpenicillin (100%). See original sources for test conditions and identity of strains.
* Reported β–lactamase–producer; enzyme activity of other organisms not reported.

for *Ps. aeruginosa* (1855AI$^-$) against which cefsulodin has an MIC value of 0.8 μg/ml. The permeability difference is further enhanced by a difference in pattern and level of binding to the PBPs of the two species (Tamaki et al. 1977). The behavior of cefsulodin has been discussed here only in the context of the 7β-acylamino side chain. The contribution of the 3′-substituent to activity and spectrum is also significant in this case, as indicated in the additional data contained in the cited studies (Curtis et al. 1980b; Nomura et al. 1974, 1976).

In still another parallel to penicillin structure–activity relationships, the spectrum of activity of 7β-phenylglycylcephalosporin analogs has been extended to the more resistant organisms, including *Ps. aeruginosa*, by appropriate acylation of the α-amino group. The phenylglycyl side-chain of piperacillin (Fig. 2) and the p-hydroxyphenylglycyl group of cefoperazone (Table 15B) carry the same ureido acyl group. Both antibiotics have a broad spectrum of activity which includes the common enteric bacteria and *Ps. aeruginosa*. Their relative antibacterial spectra can be

Table 35. Additional experimental cephalosporins with high resistance to β-lactamase

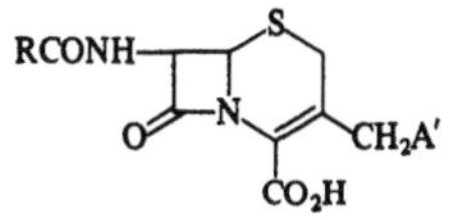

R	*Code*	*A'*	*Reference*
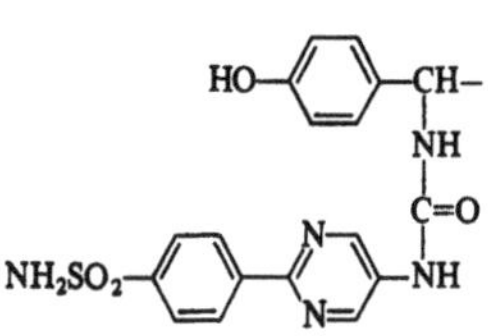	VX–YD–2	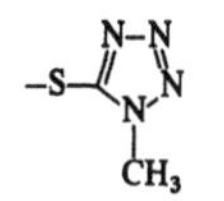	WETZEL et al. 1980
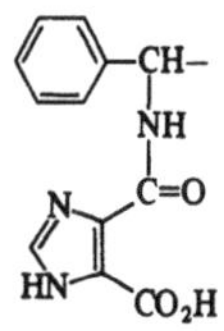	AC–1370	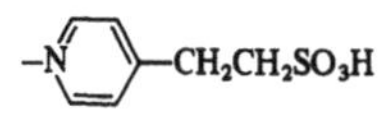	MURATA et al. 1980
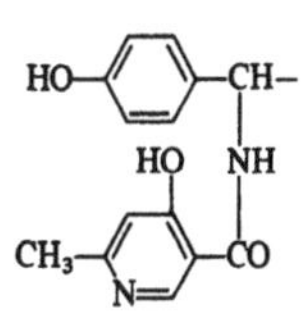	SM–1652	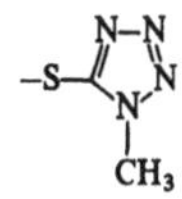	KOMATSU et al. 1980
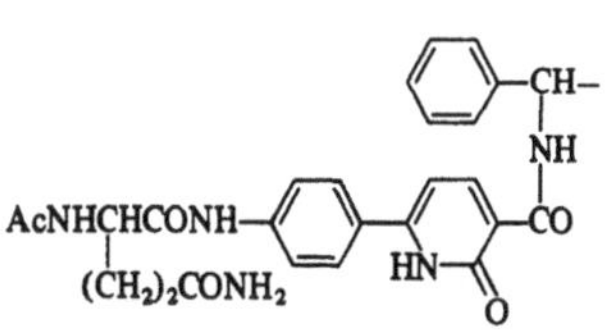	CN–92982 ($R=CH_3$) CN–106947 ($R=CH_2SO_3H$)	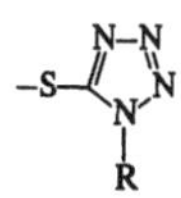	MICH et al. 1980a MICH et al. 1980b
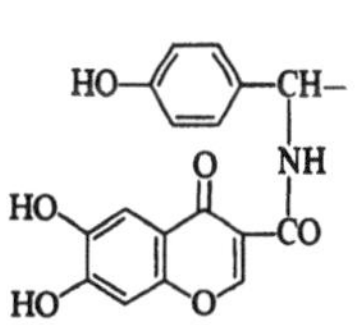	E 0702	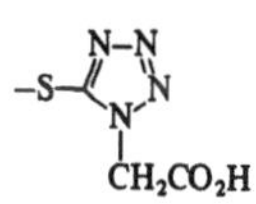	KATSU et al. 1981

compared in a general way by consulting Tables 5 (piperacillin) and 34 (cefoperazone), keeping in mind that the MIC values reported were obtained in different laboratories. The relative activities against clinical isolates reflect those reported here for the individual laboratory strains (HINKLE et al. 1980b; NEU et al. 1979). In general piperacillin is more active than cefoperazone against susceptible *S. aureus*, *S. pyogenes*, and especially *S. faecalis*, as expected. These analogs are about equal in activity against *Haemophilus*, *Salmonella*, and *Proteus* species, but cefoperazone is consistently more active against *Pseudomonas* sp. and significantly more so against *E. coli* and *Klebsiella* strains. Cefoperazone exhibits poor activity against *Bacteroides* and other anaerobes. Its minimum bactericidal concentrations are within one or two dilutions of its minimum inhibitory concentrations except for

S. aureus, where there is a substantial difference (e.g., 3.1 vs. 100 μg/ml). But, like the acylampicillins, cefoperazone undergoes a significant decrease in in vitro activity when the inoculum is increased from 10^5 to 10^7 CFU/ml. This inoculum effect is observed with other cephalosporins, for example, cefamandole.

In spite of what might appear to be an adequate number of cephalosporin analogs with activity profiles able to meet most future clinical needs, new candidates are disclosed regularly. In general, these new compounds utilize and extend the principles of structure–activity relationships that have led to the cephalosporins in Tables 15A and B. Some of the more recently described cephalosporins with broad-spectrum activity and high resistance to β-lactamases are listed with accessing references in Table 35.

V. Oxacephalosporins

Like most other positions on the penicillin and cephalosporin rings the sulfur atom at the 1-position has been a target for modification. Most of the structural changes involving this position on the penicillins and the cephalosporins have been unproductive in terms of improvement of biological activity. Thus removal of the sulfur atom completely, to give desthiopenicillin (see Sect. D.II), results in loss of bioactivity. Oxidation of the benzylpenicillin sulfur atom to the β-sulfoxide or sulfone lowers the activity against gram-positive and gram-negative bacteria (GUDDAL et al. 1962). These relationships are illustrated in Table 36 using *S. aureus* and *E. coli* MIC data from the different laboratories indicated. Interchange of the sulfur and carbon atoms at positions 1 and 2 also reduces activity, but less drastically (HUFFMAN et al. 1978). Variation of the cephalosporin structure in this way results in similar effects on the biological activity (Table 36; DEKONING et al. 1977; BRYAN et al. 1977).

However, it should be noted that the α-sulfoxides of cephalothin, and cephalexin, exhibit in vitro activity similar to that of the parent sulfides (DEKONING et al. 1977; Table 36). The *R*-sulfoxide of penicillin V has also been reported to be five times more active than the *S*-isomer against gram-positive bacteria (GORMAN and RYAN 1972). The effects of replacing the sulfur atom by carbon or oxygen are also suggested by the data in this table. An attempt to prepare carbapenam analogs of penicillins failed (LOWE and RIDLEY 1973), but the racemic 1-carbacephalosporin analog of cephalothin exhibits activity similar to its *thia*-counterpart (CAMA and CHRISTENSEN 1974). Recently several 1-carba analogs of cefotaxime were reported to exhibit in vitro activities very similar to those of cefotaxime itself (HIRATA et al. 1982). Replacement of the penicillin sulfur with oxygen is reported to lower gram-positive activity, but with retention of a low (63 μg/ml), but broad, level of activity against a number of gram-negative bacteria (WOLFE 1976). In contrast, introduction of oxygen into the cephalosporin structure elicits activity levels significantly higher than those exhibited by the sulfur-containing analogs (HAMASHIMA et al. 1978). While somewhat less so, this activity differential is retained when the hetero and carbon atoms are transposed on the 1- and 2-positions (DOUGLAS et al. 1978).

The replacement of the sulfur atom in cephalosporins by oxygen is an important development. The design of chemical procedures to permit the synthesis of

Table 36. Modifications involving the 1–position of penicillins and cephalosporins

Structure	X	Y	A	MIC (μg/ml) *S. aureus*	MIC (μg/ml) *E. coli*
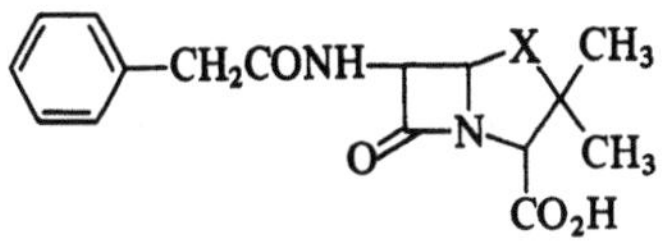	S[a]			0.01	30
	SO(β)			2.3[e]	>100
	SO_2			1.1[e]	>100
	O			16	63
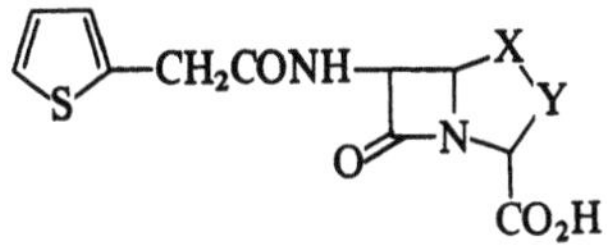	S	$C(CH_3)_2$[b]		0.2	12.5
	CH_2	S[f]		6.3	25
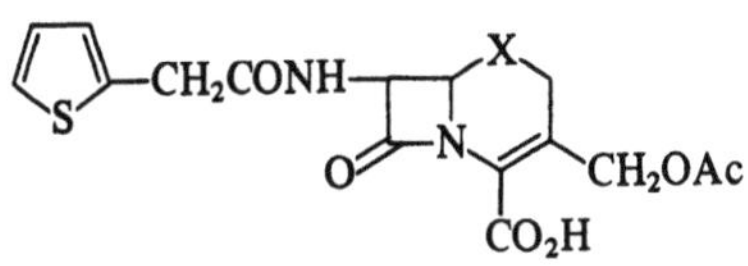	S[c]			0.05–0.5	3–6
	SO(β)			12	50
	SO(α)			0.7	12
	CH_2[f]			1.6	6
	O			0.1	0.8
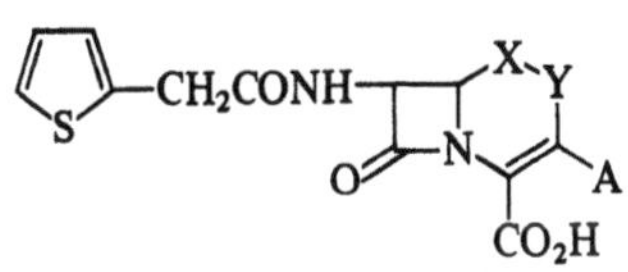	S	CH_2	H[d]	1.6	25
	CH_2	S	H	12.5	12.5
	S	CH_2	CH_2OAc[c]	1	16
	CH_2	O	CH_2OAc	0.25	4

Sources: GUDDAL et al. 1962; WOLFE 1976; HUFFMAN et al. 1978; DE KONING et al. 1977; CAMA et al. 1974; HAMASHIMA et al. 1978; BRYAN et al. 1977; DOUGLAS et al. 1978. Consult original articles for description of organisms and methods. Compare MIC values (from different laboratories) with standards: [a]benzylpenicillin; [b]thienylmethylpenicillin; [c]cephalothin; [d]deacetoxymethylcephalothin; [e]IC_{50} values; [f]racemic.

many analogs of this type and to provide promise of commercial applicability is a remarkable chemical accomplishment. This conversion generally results in increase in antibiotic activity. With a large variety of 7-acylamino substituents the improvement in activity was found to be more pronounced for gram-negative (up to 16-fold) than gram-positive organisms (1- to 4-fold; YOSHIDA 1980). Comparison of the six analogs listed in Table 37 indicates that the in vitro structure–activity relationships of the oxacephalosporins closely parallel those already demonstrated for the cephalosporins with respect to substituent variation at the 3-, 7β-,

Table 37. Comparative in vitro activity of some cephalosporins and their 1–oxa–analogs

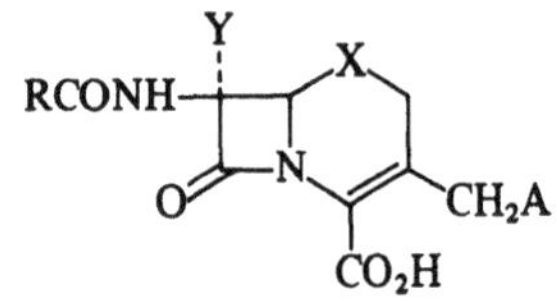

	MIC (μg/ml)					
R/Y/A =	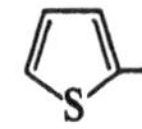–CH_2/H/OAc		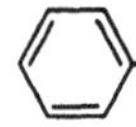–CH/H/SMTZ OH		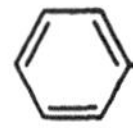–CH/OCH_3/SMTZ OH	
X =	S	O	S	O	S	O
S. aureus (S)	0.05	0.01	0.1	0.02	0.8	0.4
S. aureus (R)	0.2	0.1	0.4	0.4	3.1	0.4
E. coli	6.3	0.8	0.4	0.05	1.6	0.05
K. pneumoniae	0.8	0.2	0.4	0.05	0.8	0.1
K. pneumoniae	>100	>100	>100	100	0.8	0.1
P. mirabilis	3.1	0.4	0.8	0.1	1.6	0.2
P. vulgaris	50	50	0.8	0.1	0.8	0.2
E. cloacae	>100	100	3.1	0.4	12.5	3.1
S. marcescens	>100	>100	50	6.2	12.5	3.1

Source: HAMASHIMA et al. 1978; SMTZ: 1–methyltetrazol–5–ylthio.

Table 38. Comparative susceptibility of cephalosporins and their 1–oxa–analogs to β–lactamase hydrolysis

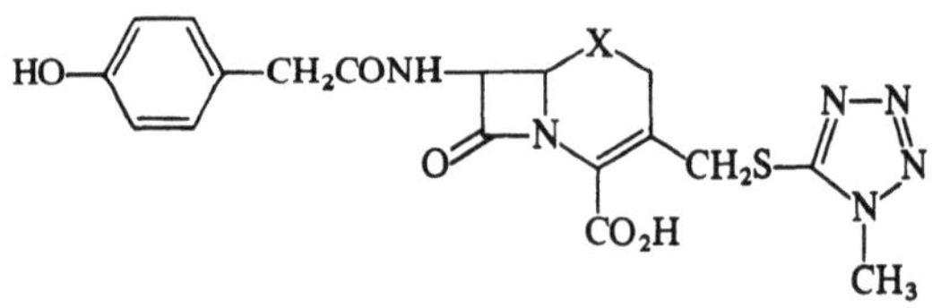

β–Lactamase	Class		V_{rel}[a]	
		X =	S	O
E. coli 6	Ib		80	840
E. cloacae 214	Ia		31	86
P. vulgaris 31	Ic		380	3600
E. coli W3110 R_{TEM}	III		13	240
E. cloacae 53	IV		7	56
Klebsiella sp. 363	IV		97	690

Source: YOSHIDA 1980. [a)]rate of hydrolysis relative to cephaloridine (=100).

Table 39. Effect of methoxy and carboxyl substituents on in vitro activity of 1-oxacephalosporins

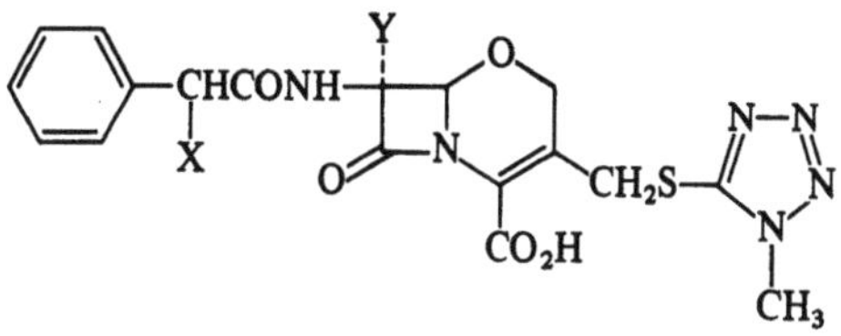

	MIC (μg/ml)			
X/Y =	H/H	H/OCH_3	COOH/H	COOH/OCH_3
E. coli	0.8	0.1	0.2	0.2
E. coli (R)	>100	0.8	50	0.4
Klebsiella sp. (R)	>100	0.2	100	0.1
P. vulgaris (R)	>100	1.6	12.5	0.4
E. cloacae	>100	100	0.4	0.2
S. marcescens	>100	6.3	0.8	0.4
P. aeruginosa	>100	>100	>100	12.5

Source: Yoshida 1980

and 7α-positions, with the important exception that when a methoxy group is introduced on the 7α-position the loss in activity is less than with the cephalosporins (Yoshida 1980). With the 7β-phenylmalonylamino analog variation of the 3-substituent results in a constant increase in gram-negative activity, and a nearly constant increase in gram-positive activity, in the series: CH_3, OCH_3, CH_2OCH_3, CH_2OCOCH_3, 2-methyl-1,3,4-thiadiazol-5-ylthiomethyl, 1-methyltetrazol-5-ylthiomethyl.

However, the 1-oxacephems are significantly more susceptible to β-lactamase inactivation than the corresponding cephalosporins (Table 38). Introduction of a 7α-methoxy group provides resistance to the penicillinase-type β-lactamase but does not effectively suppress the cephalosporinase type. However, a carboxyl group on the α-carbon of the 7-acyl side chain stabilizes the 1-oxacephalosporin to cephalosporinase-type β-lactamase (with little suppression of the penicillinase type). Conveniently, simultaneous introduction of both groups on the molecule provides broad protection against the β-lactamases of both types, with essentially no loss in in vitro activity. The resulting derivative is moxalactam (Table 15B). The effects on in vitro activity of adding the methoxy and carboxyl groups to the molecule are summarized in Table 39 (Yoshida 1980).

The in vitro spectrum of moxalactam is listed along with that of cefotaxime and other cephalosporins on Tables 33 and 34. Its spectrum and level of activity compare well with those of the cephalosporins listed. These data, obtained using laboratory strains, have been verified by an enormous number of studies using clinical isolates. Both moxalactam and cefotaxime exhibit MIC values against many strains of *Ps. aeruginosa* that are clinically achievable. However, the other cephalosporins listed on Table 34 appear to be more active in some cases. The pharmaco-

Table 40. Structure–activity relationships of some alkoxyimino–1–oxa–cephalosporins

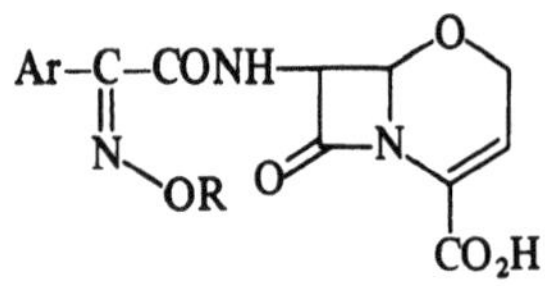

Ar	R	MIC (μg/ml) *S. aureus*	*E. coli*	*K. pneumoniae*	*P. mirabilis*	*Ps. aeruginosa*
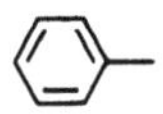	CH_3–	1.56	25	12.5	6.25	800
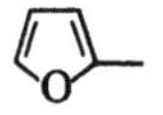	CH_3–	12.5	6.25	1.56	0.78	800
	CH_3–[a]	12.5	6.25	1.56	3.13	800
	CH_3–	25	0.2	0.78	0.2	800
	C_2H_5–	6.25	0.1	0.1	0.05	3.1
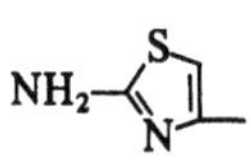	$(CH_3)_2CH$–	12.5	0.78	0.78	0.2	12.5
	C_4H_9–	12.5	0.78	3.13	0.78	12.5
	$CH_2{=}CHCH_2$–	6.25	3.13	1.56	0.1	50
	$CH{\equiv}CCH_2$–	12.5	1.56	0.2	0.1	400
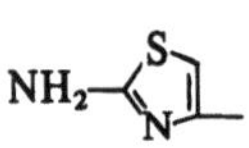	CH_3–(thia)[b]	6.25	0.05	0.05	0.025	25

Source: HAGIWARA et al. 1980. [a] *Anti*–oxime, all other oximino structures are *syn*.
[b] 1–thia–analog (O=S).

kinetic properties of moxalactam resemble those of cefotaxime with respect to serum peak levels, and level of serum binding; the serum half-life is slightly longer (Table 22). In contrast to cefotaxime, moxalactam is excreted unchanged in the urine with a high recovery rate.

While moxalactam appears to be an outstanding therapeutic agent, it may not be the final word in oxacephalosporin design. For example, a number of related 7β-oxyiminoacetyl analogs have recently been described (HAGIWARA et al. 1980). Some of the structure–activity relationships for this compound group are summarized on Table 40. This group illustrates a partial exception to a prior SAR statement. The *oxa*-derivative where *R* is methyl is not more active in vitro than its *thia*-analog, although the homologous ethoxyimino derivative compares well with the methoxyimino cephalosporin. The lack of significant differences between these analogs, which combine the effects of the aminothiazole acetyl side chain and the *oxa*-substitution for sulfur, may signal that this compound type is approaching the limits of antibiotic activity for the β-lactams. Synthetic approaches and structure–activity relationships that led to its selection for clinical evaluation have been reviewed along with the biological properties of moxalactam (OTSUKA et al. 1981).

D. Nonclassic β-Lactams

From 1940 to 1970 the known natural β-lactam antibiotics were produced by fungi. The penicillins and cephalosporins so obtained permitted extensive SAR-based modifications, but the ring system variations consisted essentially of the differences between the penams and cephems. Thus the concepts of the β-lactam structures that occur naturally and the structural requirements for good antibiotic activity conformed largely to the by then classic arrangement of the atoms in the penicillin and cephalosporin rings, the stereochemistry of the attachment of their substituents, and the appropriate lack of substituents on the 5(6)α- and 6(7)α-positions. In 1971 the cephamycins were described almost simultaneously by workers at Lilly and Merck (NAGARAJAN et al. 1971; STAPLEY et al. 1971). These substances introduced the important concept that 7α-methoxylation of the cephalosporin structure carries with it unexpected biological advantages; but this work also disclosed a second finding that has had broader repercussions. The cephamycins are produced by *Streptomyces* species rather than fungi. The versatility of the Actinomycetaceae in elaborating varied antibiotic structures is well documented. Investigation of the fermentation products obtained from microorganisms of this type has resulted in the discovery of the entirely new natural β-lactams discussed in the following sections. The natural occurrence of β-lactams has been shown to be still broader by the disclosure of the nonantibiotic β-lactam-containing substance tabtoxin (wildfire toxin), the later description of a structurally similar antibacterial (SCANNEL et al. 1975), and the recent disclosure of the sulfazecins and other monobactams, all produced by bacteria (Sect. D.III). The discovery of the cephamycins occurred at the time when many new ways were being found to dismantle and reconstruct the rings annelated to the β-lactam ring. Totally synthetic methods for constructing new β-lactam ring systems were also rapidly developing. All of this has resulted in many new so-called nonclassic β-lactams which differ sharply from the penicillins and cephalosporins in their ring systems, substituents, stereochemistry of substituent attachment, and biological properties. The major classes of these newer nonclassic β-lactams of potential clinical value are discussed in this section. The *oxa*-analogs of the cephalosporins, exemplified by moxalactam, were discussed in Sect. C.V.

I. Penems and Carbapenems

Among the most exciting of the recent β-lactams are those with an annelated five-membered ring containing a double bond. This type of structure, which combines the β-lactam-activating influences of the five-membered penicillin ring and the conjugated cephalosporin double bond, was long considered unlikely to exhibit sufficient stability to exist and to express antibacterial activity. However, the tangibility of such structures was demonstrated first by the isolation of carbapenems from natural sources (KAHAN et al. 1976; BROWN et al. 1976) and shortly afterwards by the synthesis of penems (WOODWARD 1977). The delicate balance of chemical reactivity and stability is epitomized in these structures. Because of the increased reactivity derived from the ring system itself, older rules concerning 6-substituent requirements that applied to the penicillins and cephalosporins become inoperative.

In fact the contribution of the 6-substituent to biological activity in the penicillins is reversed for the penems. The simple penam system is essentially inactive biologically, presumably because its chemical reactivity is below that required for antibiotic expression in most cases. (The influence of the 6-acylamino substituent on the chemical reactivity of the β-lactam ring was noted earlier; WOODWARD 1949 and 1980.) However, the 6-unsubstituted penems and carbapenems, and those with 6-substituents that would be excluded under the old rules, exhibit surprisingly good antibiotic activities while 6-acylaminopenems are less active than expected. Woodward suggested that in the latter case the side-chain raises the reactivity of the already activated β-lactam system to an unacceptable level. However, studies by SHIH and RATCLIFFE (1981; cf. SCHMITT et al. 1980a), indicate that the potent antibacterial activity of the carbapenems is dependent on the double activating influence of ring strain and the electronic effects of the adjacent double bond. The peripheral substituents (e.g., hydroxyethyl, aminoethylthio) described in the next section provide binding sites to the target enzymes, impart β-lactamase stability, and alter lipophilicity resulting in agents which resemble the third generation cephalosporins in their ability to reach their targets and bind to them with great efficiency. This is reflected in the PBP binding values listed for thienamycin in Table 14 (obtained before PBP 1 was found to be separable into the 1 A and 1 B components).

1. Carbapenems: Thienamycins, Olivanic Acids, and Related Structures

At least 28 carbapenems have now been isolated from fermentation broths. Their nomenclature has been complicated by the use of two generic designations (thienamycins/epithienamycins and olivanic acids) and various specific names or codes depending on the investigators who isolated them. The structures and their designations are listed in Table 41. All are 1-carbapen-2-em 3-carboxylic acids with substituents at the 2- and 6-positions. The stereochemistry at the bridgehead carbon (C-5) is *R* and, in correlation with the penems (WOODWARD 1980) and the penicillins (KUKOLJA 1971; BUSSON and VANDERHAEGHE 1976), the *S* enantiomers in racemic mixtures obtained by total synthesis of analogs are essentially inactive (SCHMITT et al. 1980b). The 2-substituents are structurally derived from cysteamine with or without a *trans* double bond; in some of the unsaturated analogs the sulfur atom exists as the sulfoxide. In nearly all cases the amino group is acylated, except for thienamycin, northienamycin and NS-5, which occur as the free amine. The side chain at the 6-position is optically inactive in twelve natural analogs discovered so far (carpetimycins A and B, NS-5, PS-5, 6, 7, 8, northienamycin, the asparenomycins), but attachment can be α or β when these analogs have an SP^3 car-

Table 41. Naturally occurring carbapenems

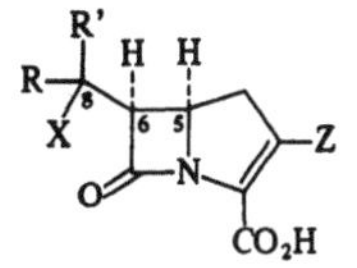

I

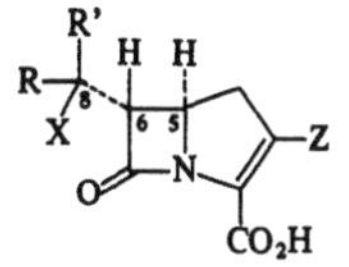

II

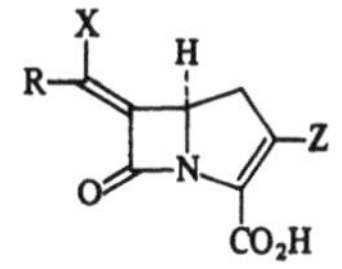

III

	$R(R'=CH_3)$	X	Z[a]	5, 6–*cis* (I)	5, 6–*trans* (II)
8*R*	H	OH	$SCH_2CH_2NH_2$	–	Thienamycin
	H	OH	SCH_2CH_2NHAc	–	*N*–Acetylthienamycin
	H	OH	SCH=CHNAc	–	*N*–Acetyldehydrothienamycin
8*S*	H	OH	SCH_2CH_2NHAc	Epithienamycin A MM22380	Epithienamycin C MM22381, $17927A_1$
	H	OSO_3H	SCH_2CH_2NHAc	890A10 MM17880	–
	H	OH	SCH=CHNHAc	Epithienamycin B MM22382	Epithienamycin D MM22383, $17927A_2$
	H	OH	SOCH=CHNHAc	$C–19393E_5$	–
	H	OSO_3H	SCH=CHNHAc	890A9 MM13902	–
	H	OSO_3H	SOCH=CHNHAc	MC696–SY2–A MM4550	–
8–Opt.	H	H	$SCH_2CH_2NH_2$	–	NS–5
Inact.	H	H	SCH_2CH_2NHAc	–	PS–5
	H	H	SCH=CHNHAc	–	PS–7
	CH_3	H	SCH_2CH_2NHAc	–	PS–6
	CH_3	H	SCH=CHNHAc	–	PS–8
	CH_3	OH	SOCH=CHNHAc	Carpetimycin A $C19393H_2$	–
	CH_3	OSO_3H	SOCH=CHNHAc	Carpetimycin B $C19393S_2$	–
	R(R'=H)	**X**	**Z**	**5, 6–*cis* (I)**	**5, 6–*trans* (II)**
	H	OH	$SCH_2CH_2NH_2$	–	Northienamycin
	R	**X**	**Z**		**Structure III**
	CH_3	CH_2OH	SOCH=CHNHAc	–	Asparenomycin A
	CH_3	CH_2OH	$SOCH_2CH_2NHAc$	–	Asparenomycin B
	CH_3	CH_2OH	SCH=CHNHAc	–	Asparenomycin C
	CH_3	CH_2OH	SCH_2CH_2NHAc	–	6643–X

[a] Terminal N–acyl groups, in addition to –Ac, include $CH_3CH_2CO–$(MM27696) and $HOCH_2C(CH_3)_2CH(OH)CONHCHCH_2CO–$(OA–6129A, B_1, B_2, C).

bon at the 6-position. The remaining analogs, with optically active side chains, can occur as epimers involving both the 6- and 8-carbon atoms. All are represented except for the 5,6-*cis*-8*R* disastereomer. Analogs having this configuration have been synthesized but their biological properties were not yet described at the time of this writing.

The carbapenems are extremely potent antibiotics active against a broad range of gram-positive and gram-negative bacteria, including species of *Serratia*, *Enterobacter*, in some cases *Pseudomonas*, and anaerobes such as *Bacteroides* sp. that are normally resistant to many of the earlier β-lactam antibiotics (Tables 42 and 43). In addition, some of these agents are also powerful β-lactamase inhibitors. The olivanic acids were originally discovered on the basis of this activity (BROWN et al.

Table 42. In vitro activities (MIC, μg/ml) of olivanic acids and thienamycins

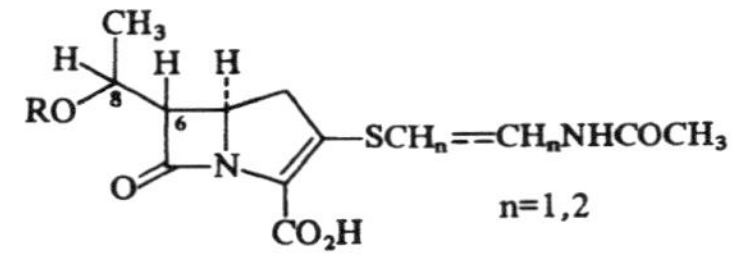

	8S								8R	
	5, 6–*cis* (6*R*)					5, 6–*trans* (6*S*)			5, 6–*trans* (6*S*)	
	8–OSO_3H			8–OH		8–OH			8–OH	
	SOC=C (MM4550)	SC=C (MM13902)	SC–C (MM17880)	SC=C Epi–THM B (MM22382)	SC–C Epi–THM A (MM22380)	SC=C Epi–THM D (MM22383)	SC–C Epi–THM C (MM22381)	Strain	SC–C *N*–Acetyl THM	SC–C Thienamycin (NH_2)
S. pyogenes	6.2	0.2	0.1(0.1)	0.05	0.1(0.05)	1.6	0.8(0.8)	CN10	(0.05)	(0.01)
S. faecalis	50	6.2	6.2(6.2)	1.6	1.6(1.6)	50	25(25)	I	(6.2)	(1.6)
S. aureus (S)	25	1.6	1.6(1.6)	0.4	0.4(0.4)	6.2	3.1(3.1)	Russell	(0.2)	(0.04)
S. aureus (R)	50	1.6	1.6	0.4	0.8	6.2	3.1		–	–
S. aureus (MR)	100	12.5	12.5	6.2	6.2	100	100		–	–
H. influenzae (S)	6.2	0.1	0.2	0.1	0.2	6.2	6.2		–	–
H. influenzae (R)	6.2	0.1	0.2	0.5	1.0	6.2	6.2		–	–
E. coli (S)	12.5	0.2	0.2(0.2)	0.2	0.2(0.2)	12.5	6.2(6.2)	0111	(0.8)	(0.2)
E. coli (R)	25	1.6	1.6(1.6)	25	25(25)	12.5	6.2(6.2)	JT39	(0.8)	(0.4)
K. aerogenes (S)	12.5	0.4	0.4(0.4)	0.4	0.8(0.8)	6.2	6.2(6.2)	A	(0.4)	(0.4)
K. aerogenes (R)	50	3.1	3.1(3.1)	100	50(50)	12.5	6.2(6.2)	VA2	(0.8)	(0.4)
P. mirabilis (S/R)	12.5	0.2	0.4(0.4)	0.2	0.8(0.8)	12.5	12.5(12.5)	977/889	(3.1)	(3.1)
P. morgani	25	0.4	0.4	0.8	1.6	25	12.5		–	–
P. rettgeri	25	0.4	0.8(0.8)	1.6	3.1(1.6)	12.5	12.5(12.5)	WM16	(3.1)	(3.1)
P. vulgaris	12.5	0.4	0.8	0.8	1.6	6.2	6.2		–	–
E. aerogenes	25	3.1	3.1(3.1)	1.6	1.6(1.6)	12.5	6.2(6.2)	T728	(3.1)	(1.6)
E. cloacae	100	12.5	6.2	3.1	3.1	25	12.5	N1	–	–
S. marcescens	25	3.1	3.1(3.1)	3.1	3.1(3.1)	12.5	12.5(12.5)	US20	(3.1)	(1.6)
Ps. aeruginosa	>100	25–50	100(>100)	>100	>100(>100)	>100	>100(>100)	10662	(25)	(3.1)
B. fragilis	3.1	0.4	0.4(0.4)	0.4	0.4(0.4)	3.1	3.1(3.1)	BC–16	–	(0.4)

Source: Basker et al. 1980; MICs (*vs.* 10^6CFU/ml in appropriate broth using microtiter, see reference for conditions) without parentheses to left of strain column are median values from 10 clinical isolates in each case. Those in parentheses and MICs of THM and *N*–acetyl THM, for comparison, are single-strain values for the laboratory strains indicated.

Table 43. In vitro activities (MIC, μg/ml) of natural carbapenems with optically inactive 6-substituents

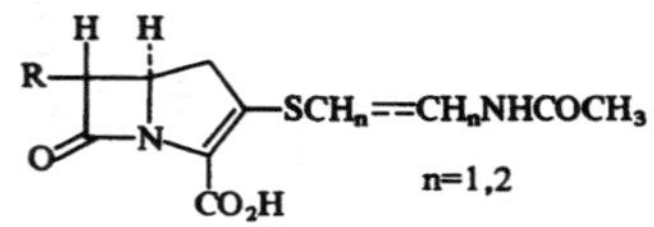

	5, 6-*cis*				5, 6-*trans*						
	R = Strain	$(CH_3)_2COH$ SOC=C (CPT-A)	$(CH_3)_2COSO_3H$[a] SOC=C (CPT-B)	CFX	Strain	CH_3CH_2 SC-C (PS-5)	CH_3CH_2 SC=C (PS-7)	$(CH_3)_2CH$[c] SC-C (PS-6)	CFX	CEZ	AMP
S. pyogenes	Cook	0.39	6.25	0.78	NY5	0.08	–	–	0.63	–	–
S. faecalis	–	–	–	–	–	0.39	–	–	0.78	–	–
S. aureus (S)	209P	0.39	6.25	1.56	209P	0.20	0.39	0.10	–	0.10	<0.01
S. aureus (R)	47	6.25	50	12.5	Russell	0.20	0.39	0.20	–	0.20	25
H. influenzae (S)	Km-1	0.78	6.25	6.25	–	–	–	–	–	–	–
E. coli (S)	JC-2	0.05	1.56	6.25	K12	3.13	0.78	6.25	–	1.56	3.13
E. coli (R)	59	0.05	1.56	6.25	RGN823	3.13	1.56	6.25	–	200	>400
K. pneumoniae (S)	PCI602	0.2	6.25	0.78	K2	3.13	–	–	6.25	–	–
K. pneumoniae (R)	32	3.1	12.5	>100	K13	6.25	3.13	25	–	400	>400
P. mirabilis[b]	21100	1.56	>25	–	P6	12.5	6.25	12.5	–	6.25	3.13
P. morganii	03168	0.39	12.5	6.25	–	–	–	–	–	–	–
P. rettegeri	013501	1.56	50	1.56	P7	12.5	1.56	6.25	–	>400	>400
P. vulgaris	IID874	0.39	12.5	6.25	GN76	25	12.5	12.5	–	>400	>400
E. aerogenes	D972	0.1	3.1	>100	E19	6.25	–	–	>100	–	–
E. cloacae	3	3.1	12.5	>100	–	6.25	3.13	25	–	>400	>400
S. marcescens (S)	NHL	0.2	6.2	12.5	–	–	–	–	–	–	–
S. marcescens (R)	4R	3.1	25	50	S18	6.25	3.13	25	–	>400	200
Ps. aeruginosa	10490	6.2	25	>100	10490	25	6.25	50	–	>400	>400
B. fragilis	–	3.1	50	25	–	–	–	–	–	–	–

Sources: [a]Mori et al. 1980, Nakayama et al. 1980 (except: [b]Imada et al. 1980); [c]Sakamoto et al. 1979, 1980. MICs by agar dilution, 10^6–10^8 CFU. CFX=cefoxitin; CEZ=cefazolin; AMP=ampicillin.

1976). The role of the carbapenems as β-lactamase inhibitors is developed in a later section on this subject. In this section the discussion of these agents is restricted primarily to their potential use as broad-spectrum antibiotics.

Tables 42 and 43 illustrate some of the biological consequences of the structural variations among the natural carbapenems in terms of in vitro activities. Although several of the analogs are exceptionally active against a broad spectrum of bacteria, thienamycin ranks the highest when activity against *Ps. aeruginosa* is included. The contribution of the basic free amino group to activity against this organism is seen in the lower MIC value for thienamycin than for its closest analog, *N*-acetylthienamycin. This will be examined further later on. In other respects the natural 2-substituents do not appear to have strict structural requirements critical to the activity. The activities of otherwise equivalent analogs with or without a double bond in this side chain are essentially the same (e.g., MM 13902 vs. MM 17880, MM 22382 vs. MM 22380, and MM 22383 vs. MM 22381). Analogs (6-unsubstituted) have been synthesized with the side-chain double bond *cis* as well as *trans*. Both are reported to exhibit activity against a wide range of bacteria with the *trans* isomer slightly, but not significantly, more active than the *cis* isomer (Baxter et al. 1980; Basker et al. 1981). In fact, replacement of this side chain by hydrogen or phenyl results in derivatives with activities equivalent to the natural analogs with nonbasic (*N*-acetylated) side chains (Table 47). The combination of oxidation of the sulfur atom to the sulfoxide and an 8-sulfonic acid group does reduce gram-positive and gram-negative activity, markedly for the olivanic acid MM 4550 (Table 42) and somewhat less so for carpetimycin B (Table 43). However, the lower activity of the sulfoxide (MM 4550) as compared to that of the analogous sulfide (MM 13902) (Table 42) has been attributed to its relatively poor chemical stability ($t_{1/2}$, 2 and 12 h, respectively) under the conditions (37°, 18 h) used to determine the MIC values (Basker et al. 1980). However, this lack of chemical stability does not appear to account for the differences in activity between carpetimycin A and B (M. J. Basker, personal communication). The OA-6129 analogs which carry the pantetheinyl-containing acyl group are less active than their *N*-acetyl counterparts (Sakomoto et al. 1982).

The 6-substituents play a much greater role in determining the level and the profile of antibiotic activity that these analogs display. The configuration of the optically active side-chains (8*R*, 8*S*) influences intrinsic activity; the stereochemistry of their attachment (5,6-*cis*, *trans*) also influences the level of activity but, in addition, it largely determines the behaviour of the analog toward β-lactamases. Thus, among the 8*S* analogs, the *cis* isomers (Table 42: MM 22382, MM 22380) are generally more active than the corresponding *trans* isomers (MM 22393, MM 22381) against normally susceptible bacteria. However, when the side chain has the 8*R* configuration (thienamycin/*N*-acetylthienamycin) activities comparable to those of the *cis* isomers are observed even though the configuration of side-chain attachment is *trans*. Both the 8*R* and 8*S* isomers with the *trans* attachment at the 6-position exhibit broad activity against β-lactamase producers (for example, compare susceptible and resistant strains of *E. coli* and *Klebsiella*, Table 42). The reduced activity of the *cis* isomers against the resistant strains of *E. coli* and *K. aerogenes* and the undiminished activity of the *trans* isomers correlates with the instability and resistance of the *cis* and *trans* isomers, respectively, to the R_{TEM} β-lactamase produced by these bacteria (BASKER et al. 1980). Further correlation of β-lactamase resistance with in vitro activity is given in the discussion of thienamycin and its analogs. The observation of good β-lactamase resistance for the *trans* isomers is not very surprising since they have the bulky 1-hydroxyethyl group on the α-side of the ring system analogously to the α-methoxy group of the cephamycins. It is remarkable that the effect of the bulky α-substituent in reducing the in vitro activity can be reversed by the inversion of the 8-carbon atom to the *R* configuration (thienamycin).

The presence of a sulfate moiety on the 8-carbon also appears to enhance resistance to β-lactamase, although the effect is less striking than the *cis–trans* relationship discussed above. For example, the β-lactamase-producing and the β-lactamase-free strains of *E. coli* and *K. aerogenes* exhibit less differences in susceptibility to the *cis* olivanic acids with a sulfate ester group on the side chain than the corresponding 8-hydroxyl analogs (MM 12902, MM 17880 vs. MM 32382, MM 22380, respectively). Again the MIC values correlate with the demonstration of greater stability for MM 17880 toward isolated R_{TEM} β-lactamase (BASKER et al. 1980).

For the asparenomycins, side chain attachment at the 6-position is through a double bond (Table 41). Nevertheless, analogously to carbapenems having an SP^3 carbon at the 6-position, these analogs exhibit broad-spectrum antibacterial activities in vitro, including activity against β-lactamase-producers (KIMURA et al. 1982). Like the olivanic acids (e.g., MM 4550), inhibition (e.g., by asparenomycin B) of a broad spectrum of β-lactamases, and synergy with other β-lactams (e.g., ampicillin) can be demonstrated (e.g., with asparenomycin B).

Among the naturally occurring carbapenems, thienamycin possesses the optimal combination of substituents and stereochemistry (5*R*, 5,6-*trans*, 8*R*) for attaining a high level of in vitro activity against the broadest spectrum of bacteria, both gram-positive and gram-negative. In expanded studies using clinical isolates, thienamycin was as active as gentamicin against *E. coli* and *Klebsiella*, and it retained effectiveness against *Pseudomonas* species that were resistant to gentamicin (KROPP et al. 1976). A more recent comparison of the effectiveness of thienamycin vs. gentamicin, carbenicillin, and two cephalosporins using laboratory strains is summarized in Table 44 (KROPP et al. 1980a). These data support the earlier findings. In addition, activity of thienamycin against anaerobes including *B. fragilis*, other *Bacteroides* spp. and *Clostridium* spp. was slightly better than that of clindamycin and distinctly better than of penicillin G (TALLY et al. 1978; KROPP et al. 1976). In spite of its chemical instability, thienamycin compares favorably with other antibiotics such as cephalothin, ampicillin, cefazolin and gentamicin when tested for in vivo protective effectiveness in laboratory animals. Typical subcutaneous PD_{50} values for thienamycin compared with those for cephalothin and cefoxitin are included in Table 44. The in vivo effectiveness of thienamycin vs. gentamicin against *Ps. aeruginosa* was reported in the earlier study: *Ps. aeruginosa* (S), 2.4 versus 9.4 mg/kg (×3); *Ps. aeruginosa* (R), 4.1 versus >200 mg/kg (×3) (KROPP et al. 1976).

The free amino group in thienamycin contributes to its considerable concentration-related chemical instability which precludes its use per se in clinical applications. In dilute solution (30 mg/ml) the stability profile of thienamycin resembles

Table 44. In vitro and in vitro activity of MK0787 and thienamycin compared with gentamicin, carbenicillin, cefazolin, cefoxitin and cefotaxime

	MIC (μg/ml) *vs.* laboratory strains ED_{50} (mg/kg, dose x2 or 3) in parentheses[a]							MIC (μg/ml) *vs.* β–lactamase–producing multiply resistant bacteria[b]			
Organism	Strain	MK0787	THM	GEN	CAB	CEF	CFX	CFX	CTX	THM	β–Lactamase
S. aureus	2985	0.01(0.06)	0.02(0.26)	0.32	0.63	0.2(5.0)	3.2	–	–	–	
S. aureus	2867	0.02	0.04	0.63	20	0.8	6.3	>50	12.5	3.1	Pase
S. aureus	4428	20.0	40.0	5.0	80	>100	>100	–	–	–	
E. coli	2884	0.08(2.5)	0.16(4.2)	1.3	5.0	6.3(60)	6.3	–	–	–	
E. coli	2891	0.16(0.65)	0.16(1.6)	2.5	40	>100(>500)	50(31.2)	3.1	0.05	0.8	IIIB/V
K. pneumoniae	2921	0.63	0.63	1.3	>80	12.5	6.3	1.6	0.1	1.6	
K. pneumoniae	2888	0.63(0.64)	1.3(1.6)	1.3	10	>100(>500)	>100(250)	25	0.2	3.1	IV
P. mirabilis	3125	5.0(1.0)	10.0(11.1)	5.0	1.3	6.3(3.0)	3.2	>50	0.1	3.1	
P. morganii	2833	5.0(0.94)	5.0(6.25)	2.5	>80	>100(>500)	12.5	6.2	1.6	25	
E. cloacae	2647	0.16	0.32	1.3	20	12.5	12.5	>400	>50	6.3	Ib
E. cloacae	2646	0.63(0.65)	0.63(4.9)	1.3	>80	>100(>2000)	>100	>400	12.5	6.3	
Serratia sp.	2855	0.63	2.5	1.3	>80	>100	12.5	–	–	–	
Providencia sp.	2851	1.3	2.5	0.63	1.3	>100	1.6	6.3	0.8	6.3	
Ps. aeruginosa	40	1.6(0.74)	3.1(1.56)	50(85)	50	–	–	>400	>100	0.8	Id
Ps. aeruginosa	3350	10(1.2)	20(2.5)	>20(>200)	>80	–	–	>400	>100	25	
Ps. aeruginosa	4294	12.5(1.9)	50	25(50)	100	–	–	–	–		
P. rettgeri	–	–	–	–	–	–	–	6.3	0.05	12.5	
P. rettgeri	–	–	–	–	–	–	–	>50	3.1	25	

Sources: [a]Kropp et al. 1980a; [b]Romagnoli et al. 1980. MICs versus cephalothin: all >400 μg/ml; versus cefamandole: >400 μg/ml except *K. pneumoniae*, 50 μg/ml; *P. rettgeri, Providencia stuartii*, 6.3 μg/ml. THM=thienamycin, GEN=gentamicin, CAB=carbenicillin, CEF=cephalothin, CFX=cefoxitin, CTX=cefotaxime.

that of benzylpenicillin, but the half-life is about one-tenth of that of penicillin G. At higher concentrations self-inactivation occurs ($t_{1/2}$ at pH 7.0 and 25 °C: 1 mg/ml, 100 h; 57 mg/ml, 6 h). A search for derivatives of thienamycin which retain its broad-spectrum activity and which have better stability characteristics has led the Merck group to investigate several hundred analogs with varied functionalizations on the 2-aminoethylthio, the 8-hydroxyl, and the 3-carboxyl groupings. In general, carboxyl group esterification results in a lower level of stability, and alkylation or esterification of the hydroxyl group lowers the activity against gram-positive and gram-negative bacteria. While it contributes to the molecule's instability, the basic character of the amino group appears to enhance the moderate activity of the *N*-acetylated carbapenem analogs against *Ps. aeruginosa* to a level that represents clinical usefulness. An indication of this is seen in the MIC values of 3.1 μg/ml for thienamycin compared with 25 μg/ml for *N*-acetylthienamycin and 25–>100 μg/ml for the other analogs listed in Table 42. Thus, much of the derivatization of thienamycin has centered on the amino group. Alkylation lowers activity generally and conventional acylation tends to lower the activity against the gram-positive bacteria as well as *Ps. aeruginosa*, although improving in vitro activity against gram-negative bacteria such as *E. coli*. From a large number of *N*-alkyl and *N*-acyl derivatives, *N*-formimidoyl thienamycin (MK 0787; Table 45) has been selected for clinical development. The amidino group improves stability, with retention of overall potency, and for several important genera such as *Pseudomonas*, *Bacteroides*, and *Enterococcus* the activity becomes at least twofold superior to that of thienamycin. This can be seen in the MIC values for MK 0787 and thienamycin against the laboratory strains listed in Table 44. The relative in vitro effectiveness of both thienamycin and MK 0787 against anaerobes can be judged by the following comparison of MIC value ranges for 29 strains of *B. fragilis* (Kropp et al. 1980 a): MK 0787, 0.13–1.0 μg/ml; thienamycin, 0.25–2.0 μg/ml; clindamycin <0.06–4.0 μg/ml; cefoxitin 8–>32 μg/ml. Since activity against *Ps. aeruginosa* is an important consideration for the third-generation cephalosporins and the antipseudomonal penicillins, as well as the thienamycins, in vitro (MIC) and in vivo (PD_{50}) data from a side-by-side comparison of MK 0787, thienamycin, carbenicillin, moxalactam, cefotaxime, and piperacillin by the Merck invstigators are included in Table 45.

Like thienamycin, MK 0787 exhibits little or no inoculum effect against *S. aureus* (R) and several gram-negative bacteria at intermediate levels (10^3 vs. 10^5 CFU per microtiter well). The MIC values increased about fourfold at 10^7 CFU, a very modest rise (Kropp et al. 1980 a). The minimum bactericidal concentrations were generally the same as, or within one dilution of, the MICs. This experience has been verified by other workers. The relatively small difference in MBC values compared to MIC values for MK 0787 is shared by piperacillin and the third-generation cephalosporins (e.g., moxalactam, cefotaxime, cefoperazone). However, the very modest inoculum effect on MK 0787 contrasts with pronounced effects of inoculum size on the antipseudomonal acylampicillins and these new cephalosporins. These differences are illustrated by the comparison of the influence of inoculum size on MIC values for typical β-lactams given in Table 46.

The in vivo effectiveness of MK 0787 in protecting the mouse against acute experimental infections is outstanding, as seen by the selected ED_{50} values given in

Table 45. Comparison of in vitro effectiveness of six new β–lactams against *Ps. aeruginosa*

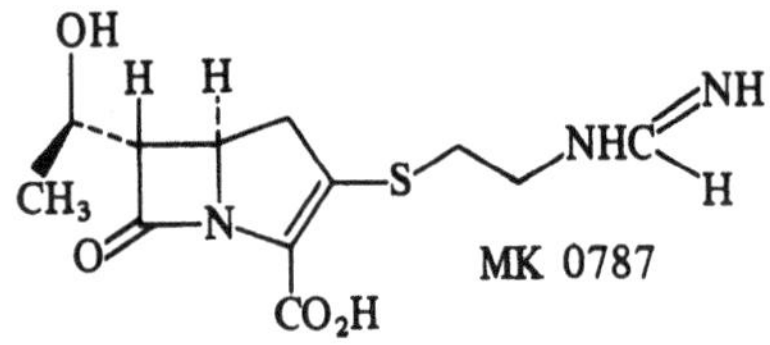
MK 0787

	MIC (ED_{50}) Individual isolates				MIC Range Thirteen Clinical Isolates
	40	3286	4293	4294	
MK0787	1.6(0.74)	2.5(0.95)	6.3(0.78)	12.5(1.9)	0.8–12.5
Thienamycin	3.1(1.56)	10(4.65)	25	50	1.6–50
Carbenicillin	50(133)	80(334)	100	100	50–>400
Moxalactam	12.5(13.2)	50(33.4)	25	25	12.5–>50
Cefotaxime	12.5(118)	25(>500)	25	25	12.5–>100
Piperacillin	3.1(29.4)	6.3(245)	6.3	6.3	3.1–>100

Source: KROPP et al. 1980b. Clinical isolates; MICs (μg/ml) done by agar dilution using 10^5 CFU/ml; ED_{50} (mg/kg/dose) given in parentheses. Regimen: 3 doses s.c 0, 2 and 4 hr. post challenge; see reference for description of tests, isolates and challenge dosages.

Table 46. Influence of inoculum size on in vitro activity (MIC, MBC) of five new β–lactams and gentamicin against *Ps. aeruginosa*

		Range[a]		MIC_{50} and MBC_{50}[a]	
		5x10^3[b]	5x10^7	5x10^3	5x10^7
Gentamicin	MIC	0.06–64	0.5–128	0.25	1
	MBC	0.06–128	0.5–128	0.5	2
MK0787	MIC	0.06–8	0.5–16	0.5	4
	MBC	0.25–8	1.0–16	1	4
Moxalactam	MIC	0.5–32	16–>128	4	128
	MBC	0.5–64	16–>128	8	>128
Cefotaxime	MIC	1–64	16–>128	4	>128
	MBC	1–128	64–>128	8	>128
Cefoperazone	MIC	0.5–16	16–>128	2	>128
	MBC	0.5–32	32–>128	2	>128
Piperacillin	MIC	0.5–16	32–>128	2	>128
	MBC	1–16	64–>128	2	>128

Source: CORRADO et al. 1980. [a])From 40 susceptible isolates. [b])Inoculum size in CFU/ml.

parentheses in Tables 44 and 45. These values were obtained by parenteral treatment since, like thienamycin, MK 0787 exhibits poor oral activity. They predict a high level of effectiveness in man. Ironically, while MK 0787 is resistant to practically all bacterial β-lactamases, it has been found to be rapidly degraded with opening of the β-lactam ring by the *mammalian* renal dipeptidase, dehydropeptidase I (E.C.3.4.13.11). This renal enzyme appears to be broadly distributed; porcine and human preparations were found to hydrolyze thienamycin. The enzyme hydrolyzes nonbasic *N*-acylated thienamycin analogs and the natural *N*-acetylated epithienamycins and olivanic acids 4–50 times faster than thienamycin (KROPP et al. 1980b). This explains, in part, low protective effectiveness observed for some of these latter agents in experimental infections.

Since this metabolic susceptibility raises serious questions about the clinical potential for the carbapenems, the possibility of specifically inhibiting the renal dipeptidase has been investigated (ASHTON et al. 1980). Various 3-substituted-Z-2-acylamino propenoates have been found to effectively protect thienamycin and MK 0787 when coadministered with the antibiotic. The most promising analog was the compound where the acyl group is *S*-2,2-dimethylcyclopropyl carboxy and the 3-substituent is L-$(CH_2)_4$-*S*-$CH_2CH(NH_2)COOH$:

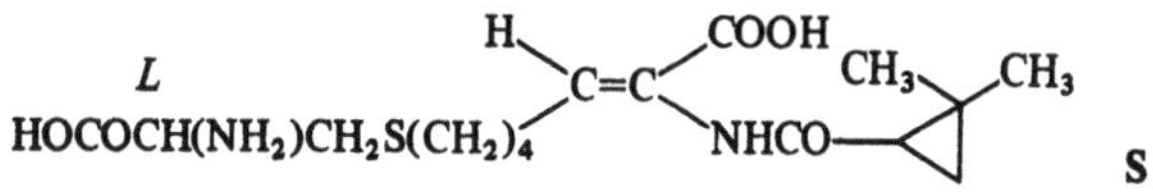

A recent comparison of the in vitro activities of thienamycin with those of cefoxitin and cefotaxime using bacteria uniformly resistant to cephalothin (MICs >400 μg/ml) and, in most cases, to cefamandole is summarized on the right side of Table 44 (ROMAGNOLI et al. 1980). These results indicate fewer advantages than expected for the thienamycins to offset the disadvantages of the instability inherent in this structural type and their unexpected susceptibility to mammalian renal dipeptidases. Thus, while thienamycin is active against bacteria producing β-lactamases of each of the major classes (last column), and it is superior to cefotaxime and similar new cephalosporins against benzylpenicillin-resistant *S. aureus* (as well as *S. faecalis* and *B. fragilis*) it was found to be only as active, or less active, against indole-positive *Proteus*, cefamandole-resistant *P. mirabilis*, *Enterobacter*, and *Providencia* sp.

The suspectibility of thienamycin, MK 0787 and other carbapenems to renal dipeptidase (DHP-1) has led to a further broad search for derivatives which are resistant to inactivation by this enzyme while retaining the spectrum and potency of MK 0787. This appears to have been accomplished synthetically through the construction of analogs of MK 0787 with the amidine group attached to the side chain through the carbon rather than the nitrogen atom in structures such as the following, for example, where $R = CH_3$ and $R' = H$ or CH_3:

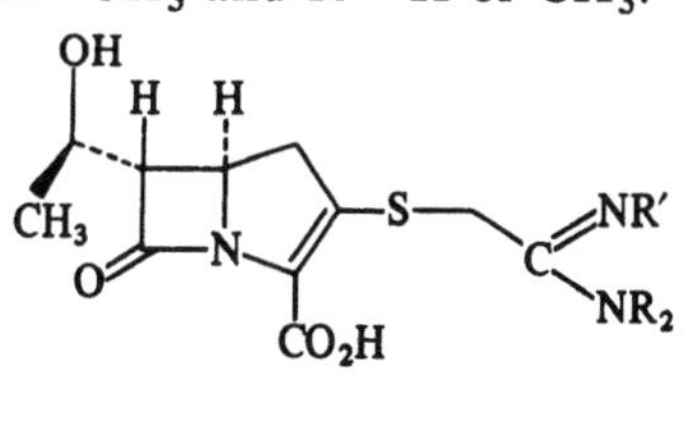

Table 47. Effects of modifications of the thienamycin structure on in vitro activity

	Cmpd	Disc content (nM)	Inhibitory zone diameters (mm) *S. aureus* 2985	*S. aureus* 2314	*E. coli* 2482	*E. coli* 2964	*E. cloacae* 2647	*E. cloacae* 2646	*Ps. aeruginosa* 3835	*Ps. aeruginosa* 3350
Ampicillin		28	33	13	20	0	18	0	–	–
Carbenicillin		118	34	18	24	0	22	16	21	0
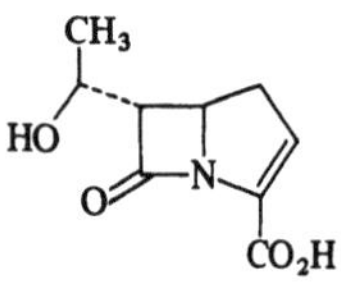 *I*	*I*	117	40	38	31	33	31	30	23	20
	THM	92	41	40	28	29	26	26	26	24
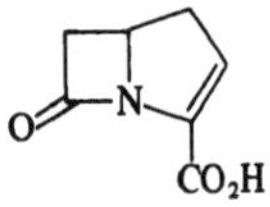 *II*	*II*	54[a]	20	0	20	0	21	16	–	–
	THM	23	38	38	25	25	22	22	–	–
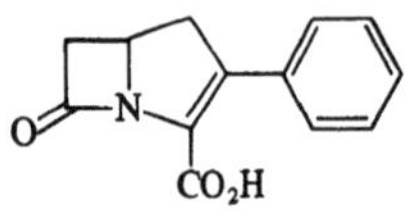 *III*	*III*	49[a]	30	24	29	0	25	9	–	–
	THM	23	38	38	25	25	22	22	–	–

Additional analogs with broad spectrum activity:

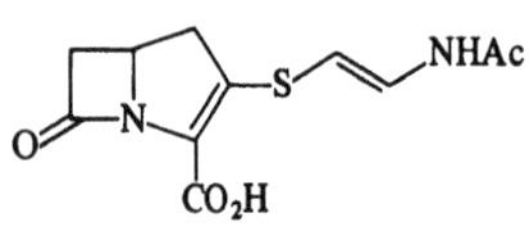

IV

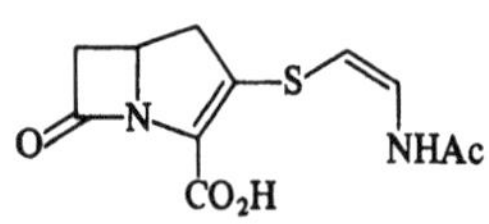

V

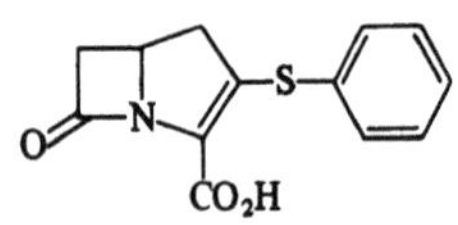

VI

Analogs inactive or with low activity:

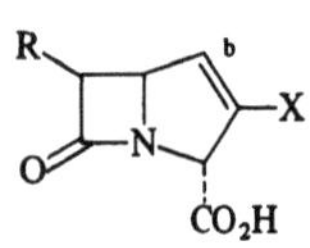

VII

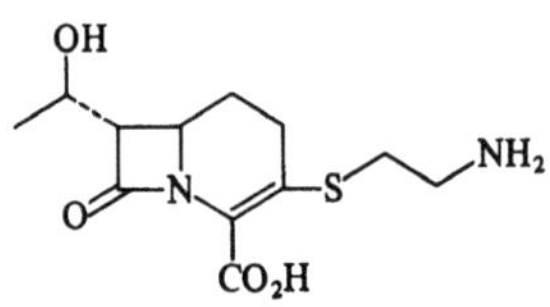

VIII

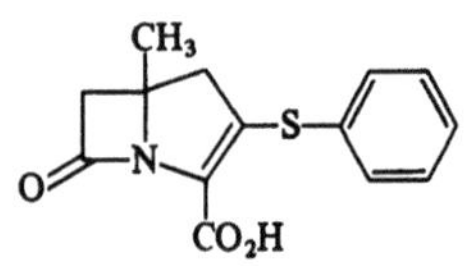

IX

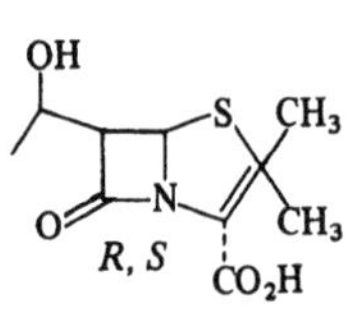

X

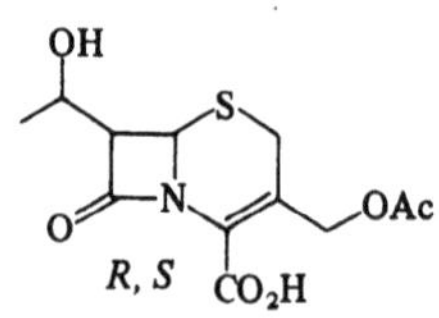

XI

Sources and test descriptions: see text. [a]Racemic. [b]R=H, CH_3CHOH, X=H, SC_6H_5, $SCH_2CH_2NH_2$

More extensive modifications around the thienamycin structure than those just described have been accomplished by semi- and total synthesis. The most definitive work in terms of structure–activity relationships has been carried out by the Merck investigators. So far the data generated by these studies tend to verify the conclusions arrived at from investigators of the naturally occuring carbapenems. Some of these results are presented in Table 47. The effects of structural changes on in vitro activity were observed by comparing inhibitory zone diameters (agar disc diffusion technique) produced by approximately equimolar amounts of the analog and thienamycin (SHIH et al. 1978; CAMA and CHRISTENSEN 1978a, 1980). With racemic mixtures one isomer is assumed to be inactive. The comparison was done using pairs of resistant (β-lactamase mediated) and sensitive *S. aureus* and gram-negative strains. The sensitivity profiles of the test organisms can be inferred from the zone diameters produced with ampicillin and carbenicillin at the top of the table. A 3-mm increase in zone diameter represents an approximate doubling of the activity. As predicted on the basis of ring strain considerations discussed earlier, the unsubstituted carbapenem ring system itself (compound II) possesses antibacterial activity. The level of activity is significantly below that of thienamycin and activity against β-lactamase producers is absent or diminished. Introduction of 2-substituents analogous to the natural carbapenems (structures IV and V) has been reported, but quantitative data regarding the effect of this change on in vitro activity were not included (BAXTER et al. 1980). Placing a phenyl group on the 2-position (compound III) results in improvement of activity against the sensitive strains and, interestingly, moderate activity against the resistant *S. aureus* strain is now observed. This is not unexpected in light of the generally equal activities of the natural *cis* carbapenems against the sensitive and resistant strains of *S. aureus* in Table 42. Decysteaminylthienamycin (compound I) exhibits lower (approximately 50%) activity against *Ps. aeruginosa*, but its profile against *S. aureus* and the Enterobacteriaceae generally equals or exceeds that of thienamycin. This finding is congruent with the earlier premise that a basic moiety on the side-chain at the 2-position contributes to the antipseudomonal activity.

Several inactive or poorly active analogs of thienamycin have been reported (Table 47). As might be expected, homothienamycin (VIII) and the penam (X) and cephem (XI) analogs with a 6(7)-hydroxyethyl group are inactive or exhibit a low level of antibacterial activity (SALZMANN et al. 1980; DININNO et al. 1977). Likewise, while 2-phenylthio carbapenem (VI) has broad spectrum activity its analog with a methyl group on the 5-bridgehead position (IX) has only weak activity (PONSFORD et al. 1979). The inactivity of carbapen-1-em-3-carboxylic acid (VII) was discussed in the introduction to this section. These compounds serve to underscore the argument advanced there that the β-lactam ring reactivity must be confined within an optimal range for expression of antibiotic activity.

2. Penems

It is convenient to examine penem SAR in the context of the data that pertain to the carbapenems since, even though the penems were probably conceived (WOODWARD 1977; ERNST et al. 1978) before the discovery of the natural carbapenems was disclosed, delineation of their structure–activity relationships has followed that of the latter. The early SAR data reported by WOODWARD et al. are summarized in

Table 48. In vitro activities (MIC, μg/ml) of penems

			S. aureus		*E. coli*		*S. typhimurium*	*P. rettgeri*	*E. cloacae*	*Ps. aeruginosa*
		Source	Smith	2999	205	205 RTEM	277	K856	P99	K1118[e]
Penicillin V		a	0.05	64	128	–	64	>128	–	>128
Cephalexin		a	1	8	8	–	4	128	–	>128
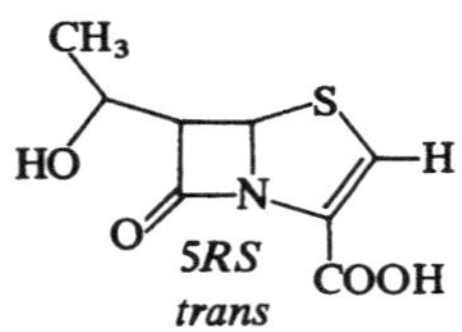	erythro	a	64	64	128	128	64	–	>128	(>128)
	threo	a	1	1	8	8	4	–	8	(64)
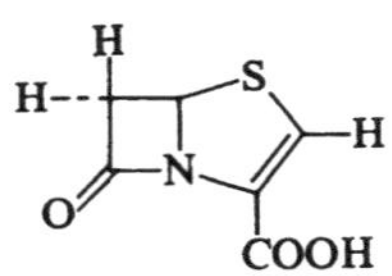	*5RS*	a	8	8	4	32	4	–	>128	(16)
	5S	b	in	in	in	–	–	–	–	(in)
	5R	b	4	2	2	–	–	–	–	(4)
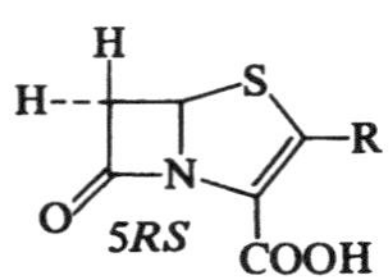	$-CH_3$	c	1	1	8	–	8	4	–	8
	$-C_5H_{11}$	c	0.2	2	32	–	18	32	–	64
	$-C_6H_5$	c	1	4	8	–	8	4	–	–
	$-SCH_2CH_3$	d	1	2	0.5	–	0.5	2	–	–
	$-S(CH_2)_2NHAc$	d	4	32	2	–	2	>128	–	–

Sources: [a] PFAENDLER et al. 1980; [b] PFAENDLER et al. 1979; [c] LANG et al. 1979; [d] LANG et al. 1980. [e] *Ps. aeruginosa* 12055 in parentheses.

Table 48. Thse data tend in large part to reiterate relationships observed with the carbapenems. For example, as with other β-lactam systems, the configuration of the bridgehead carbon must be *R*, the corresponding 5-*S* epimers are inactive (Table 48). In parallel with the carbapenems, the substituent at the 6-position plays a decisive role in controlling the level of activity and in providing stability towards the β-lactamases of the gram-negative bacteria. The 5-*R*,*S*-5,6-*trans* penem analogs with a 6-hydroxyethyl group exhibit the striking differences in intrinsic activity (*threo* versus *erythro* isomers; Table 48) observed with thienamycin (8*R*-5,6-*trans;* Table 42) and epithienamycin C (8*S*-5,6-*trans;* MM 22381). In addition, these analogs with a 6α-substituent (*erythro* and *threo*) are equally active against *E. coli* 205 and its β-lactamase-producing mutant *E. coli* 205 R_{TEM}, while the 6α-unsubstituted nucleus is less active against the R_{REM} strain (MIC = 32 μg/ml) than the parent (MIC 4 μg/ml).

Several reports now describe more extensive studies on the structure–activity relationships of the penems (FRANCHESCHI et al. 1980; OIDA et al. 1980a; BANVILLE et al. 1981; GIRIJAVALLABHAN et al. 1981; MCCOMBIE et al. 1981). Tables 49 and 50 present a synopsis of these studies. The MIC values listed in Table 49 were obtained in part from various laboratory strains (MIC) and in part from multiple clinical isolates (MIC_{50}) of the species listed. The original sources, which list strains and test condiditons that were used, should be consulted for a more accurate and complete assessment of the SAR that are presented here. In general these data support and extend the conclusions just drawn. Penems without a substituent on the 6-position resemble ampicillin in their activity against gram-positive bacteria and they lack resistance to gram-negative β-lactamases (compare MIC values of susceptible and resistant *E. coli* strains). The analogs that are included in Table 49 illustrate that the acetoxymethyl and tetrazolethiomethyl substituents, which provide good leaving groups for the cephalosporins, are not particularly efficacious on the penem structure. In fact, as with the carbapenems, variation of the 2-substituent exerts only a modest effect on in vitro activity. For example, 21 of 24 such variations by OIDA et al. (1980a) produced analogs with MIC values which fall within the relatively narrow ranges listed in Table 49 where the 2-substituent is indicated by −SR (21). These substituents are listed in Table 50. The wider variations of the MIC values of the three remaining analogs (see footnote b, Table 49) appear to reflect the effect of those substituents on the lipophilicity of the molecule, as seen with penicillins (also compare the $-CH_3$ and $-C_5H_{11}$ analogs in Table 48). Similar trends are observed with variation of the 2-substituents on analogs studied by BANVILLE et al. (1981), some of which are also listed in Table 50. The numbers which accompany these analogs indicate the averaged log 2 changes in activity against 13 gram-negative bacteria (*E. coli*, 2; *Klebsiella*, 2; *Proteus*, 4; *Serratia*, 1; *Enterobacter*, 2; *Ps. aeruginosa*, 2), relative to the activity of 2-methylpenem against the same organisms (see Tables 48 and 49 for representative MIC values of this standard). Most of the changes from the 2-methyl group produce moderate loss (0 to −1.4) or improvement (0 to +2.6) of averaged gram-negative activity; a few polar groups (CF_3, $CONH_2$, CH_2S-tetrazole) produce significant activity loss (−4, −5).

6-Substituent variations have been described for penems having a methyl (BANVILLE et al. 1981), ethyl (FOXTON et al. 1981) or ethylthio group (MCCOMBIE et al.

Table 49. In vitro activities of some additional penems

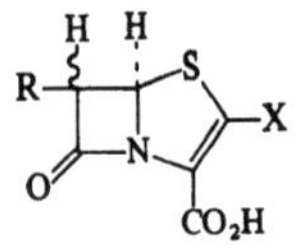

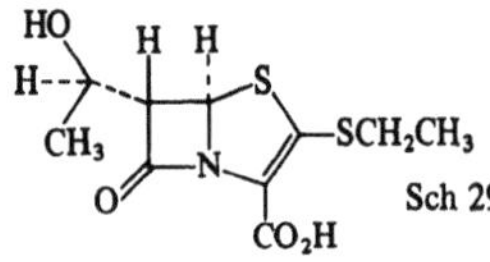

Sch 29482

R	X	Ref.	*S. aureus* (S)	*S. aureus* (R)	*E. coli* (S)	*E. coli* (R)	*Klebsiella*	*Proteus*	*Enterobacter*	*Ps. aeruginosa*
			MIC (μg/ml)							
H	CH_2OAc	a	<0.2	1.6	1.6	>100	–	3	12	>100
H	CH_2SMTZ	a	0.4	0.8	0.8	–	–	6	>100	>100
Ampicillin		a	<0.2	1.6	1.6	>100	–	1.6	>100	>100
H	SR(21)	b	<0.1–0.8	0.4–3	0.4–6	50–>100	0.8–12	6–25	–	50–>100
Ampicillin		b	≤0.1	1.5	3	>100	50	1.5	–	>100
H	CH_3	c	–	–	8	–	8	4–16	16	63
CH_3CHOH	CH_3									
cis–8–S		c	0.25	–	1	–	4	2	2	16
cis–8–R		c	1	–	2	–	16	8	16	63
trans–8–S		c	125	–	–	–	–	–	–	–
trans–8–R[f]		c	0.13	–	2	–	4	4	4	125
			MIC_{50} (μg/ml)							
H	SCH_2CH_3	d	2.4	–	4	–	24	>32	8	>32
$(CH_3)_2COH$	SCH_2CH_3	d	>64	–	>64	–	>64	>64	>64	>64
CH_3CHF	SCH_2CH_3	d	10	–	>64	–	>64	>64	>64	>64
CH_2OCH_3	SCH_2CH_3	d	3	–	24	–	48	56	64	64
CH_2OH	SCH_2CH_3	d	0.8	–	1.2	–	1.2	6	6	>64
CH_3CHOH	SCH_2CH_3									
cis–8–S		d	0.8	–	1.8	–	6	5	10	>16
cis–8–R		d	10	–	10	–	14	>16	>16	>16
trans–8–S		d	>16	–	>16	–	>16	>16	>16	>16
trans–8–R[f]		d	0.2	–	0.6	–	0.8	2.5	3	28
CH_3CHOH	$SCH_2CH_2NH_2$									
trans–8–R		d	0.2	–	6	–	4	24	5	32
Sch 29482		e	0.06	–	0.5	–	0.5	1.4	1	>128

Sources: [a]Franchesci et al. 1980; SMTZ=1–methyltetrazol–5–ylthiomethyl. [b]Oida et al. 1980a; see table 50 for examples of SR(21); SR(22–24)=$SCH_2CH_2SCSN{=}(CH_2)_4$, $SCH_2C_6H_5$, $SCH_2CH_2CO_2H$. [c]Banville et al. 1981; see table 50 for additional 2– and 6–substituted analogs of racemic 3–methyl penem. [d]Mccombie et al. 1981; MIC_{50} values calculated from graphic presentation of data obtained on racemic analogs. [e]Reeves et al. 1981. [f]Racemic Sch 29482.

1981) on the 2-position. Here, the 2-cysteamine residue does not produce the improvement in spectrum over the 2-ethylthio group (Table 49) predicted by the thienamycin relationships. With both the 2-methyl and 2-ethylthio substituents, most of the structural changes at the 6-position are accompanied by a general lowering of in vitro activity (see Tables 49 and 50). Exceptions are 6-hydroxymethyl- and 6-hydroxyethylpenems (Table 49). The effect of the side-chain configuration (*R*,*S*) of the hydroxyethyl group and the stereochemistry of its attachment (*cis*, *trans*) appears less striking for the 2-methyl analogs than the 2-ethylthiopenems. While the MIC values of many of these penem analogs are better than those for penicillin V, they are not very different from the MIC values of ampicillin. However, the re-

Table 50. Additional penem analogs

Active:

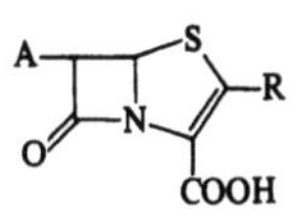

R(A=H)
CH_3 (0)
$(CH_2)_3CH_3$ (−1)
$CH_2C(CH_3)_3$ (−1.2)
$CH_2C_6H_5$ (0)
Cyclopropyl (+0.5)
$CH{=}CH_2$ (+0.8)
$CH_2CH_2CH{=}CH_2$ (+1.3)
$(CH_2)_3Cl$ (+1.3)
CH_2SCH_3 (+2.1)
$CH_2CH_2SCH_3$ (+2.1)
$CH_2CH_2SOCH_3$ (+2.2)
$CH_2CH_2SO_2CH_3$ (+1.9)
$(CH_2)_3CN$ (+2.3)
SCH_2CH_3 (+2.5)

R(A=H)
CH_2OH (−0.7)
CH_2OCH_3 (+1.5)
CH_2OCH_2Ph (−0.9)
CH_2OAc (−1.8)
CH_2NH_2 (+2.6)
$(CH_2)_2NH_2$ (+1.5)
$(CH_2)_3NH_2$ (+1.5)
$(CH_2)_4NH_2$ (+2.6)
$(CH_2)_5NH_2$ (+1.1)
CH_2F (−1.3)
CF_3 (−4)
CH_2STZ (−5)
$CH_2CH_2CO_2H$ (+1)
$CH{=}CHCO_2H$ (−1.4)
$CH_2CH_2CONH_2$ (+1)
$CH_2CH_2CON(CH_3)_2$ (+1.3)
$CONH_2$ (−4)
Phenyl (−0.5)
3–Pyridyl (+0.6)
2–Furyl (0)
4–Thiazolyl (−1)
CH_2–2–Furyl (+0.5)
CH_2–4–Thiazolyl (−4)

R(A=H) (SR21)
$-SCH_3$
$-SCH_2CH_2CH_3$
$-SCH_2CH_2OH$
$-SCH_2CH_2CH_2OH$
$-SCH_2CH_2OCOCH_3$
$-SCH_2CH_2CH_2OCOCH_3$
$-SCH_2CH_2OSO_2CH_3$
$-SCH_2CH_2OCOCOOCH_3$
$-SCH_2CH_2OCH_2CH_3$
$-SCH_2CH_2SCH_3$
$-SCH_2CH_2SCSNH_2$
$-SCH_2CH_2COOC_2H_5$
$-SCH_2CH_2N_3$
$-SCH_2CH_2NH_2$
$-SCH_2CH_2CH_2NH_2$
$-SCH_2CH_2NHCOCH_3$
$-SCH_2CH_2CH_2NHCOCH_3$
$-SCH_2CH_2NHCOCH_2C_6H_5$
$-SCH_2CH_2NHCOCH(NH_2)C_6H_4$–p–OH
$-SCH_2CH_2NHCON\langle CO{-}CO \rangle NC_2H_5$
$-SCH_2CH_2NHCOC(=NOCH_3)CH_3$

A($R=CH_3$)
H (0)
C_2H_5 (*cis*) (−3.8)
C_2H_5 (*trans*) (−2.1)
C_3H_7 (−3)
CH_2Ph (−5)
$CH_2CH{=}CH_2$ (−4)
$CH_2CH{=}NOCH_3$ (−4)
OCH_3 (*cis*) (−1.3)
SCH_3 (−3)
CH_2OH (−2)
CH_2OAc (−1.8)
CH_2NHCHO (−1.5)
CH_2CO_2Et (−3)
$(CH_3)_2CHOH$ (*cis*) (−4)
$(CH_3)_2CHOH$ (*trans*) (−2.2)
CH_3CHX-
H (−1.9)
CH_3 (+0.9)
C_2H_5 (−4)
$(CH_2)_4CH_3$ (+2.9)
CH_2Cl (−4)
CO_2Et (−4)
N_3 (−0.5)
NH_2 (−4)
OMe (−0.5)
OAc (−4)
OH (+0.7)

Inactive or with reduced activity:

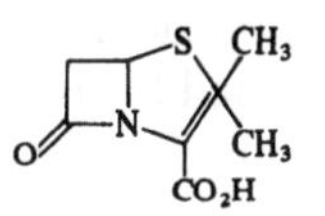

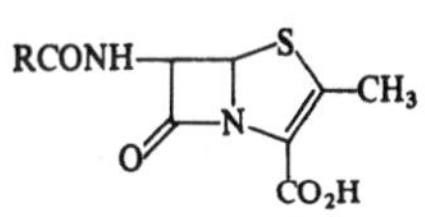

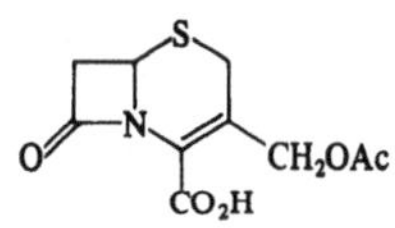

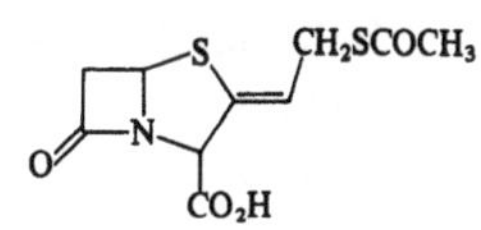

Sources: Woodward 1980; Ernst et al. 1978; Cherry et al. 1979, 1980; Banville et al. 1981; Oida et al. 1980a. Values in parentheses, see text.

markable superiority of activity of 8*R*-6-(1-hydroxyethyl)-2-ethylthiopenem-3-carboxylic acid (Sch 29482, Table 49) has led to its selection for clinical evaluation.

The excellent in vitro activity of Sch 29482 against gram-positive organisms and a large number of non-*Pseudomonas* gram-negative bacteria provide the basis for its evaluation as a potential clinical agent (Gural et al. 1981). The broad spectrum of activity indicated by its MIC values on Table 49 extends to *Citrobacter*, *Serratia*, *Providencia*, and other aerobic gram-negative species. This agent also exhibits good activity against *H. influenzae* and *Neisseria* sp., as well as *B. fragilis* and other anaerobes (Reeves 1981; Neu 1981). The activity is minimally altered by changes in pH, medium, and inoculum size. Its MBC values are close to the MIC (Neu 1981; Hare et al. 1981). The protective effectiveness of the compound (subcutaneously and orally) in mice is congruent with its MIC values against the infect-

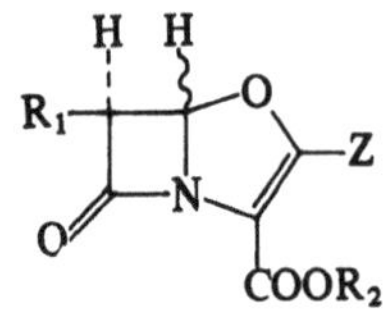

R_1	Z	R_2
H	$-CH=CH_2$	$CH_2C_6H_5$
H	$-CH_3$	CH_3
H	$-CH_2CH_3$	$CH_2C_6H_4NO_2$
H	$-CH_2CH_3$	H
$(C_6H_5)_3CNH$	$-CH_3$	CH_3
$(CH_3CH_2)_2N$	$SCH_2CH_2NH_2$	H

Fig. 4. Disclosed 1-oxa-2-penems (source: see text)

ing organisms (LOEBENBERG 1981). Sch 29482 is rapidly absorbed on oral administration, and it is well tolerated in humans (serum peak with 1 g dose: 20–24 μg/ml; half-life: 0.9–1.4 h; GURAL et al. 1981). Urinary recovery (24 h) of the drug is only 3%. Low urinary recovery in laboratory animals has been reported for other penems (OIDA et al. 1980 a). Sch 29482 is highly bound (>95%) by serum proteins and the addition of serum lowers its in vitro activity significantly (HARE et al. 1981).

3. Oxapenems

The 1-oxa-2-penem structure is a logical extension of the penems and carbapenems. Clavulanic acid is, of course, an *exo*-double-bond isomer of this chemical system, and it provides facile access to the 1-oxa-2-penem ring system (CORBETT et al. 1977; CHERRY et al. 1978). One patent and several literature articles describe methods of preparing oxapenems by semi- and total syntheses (CHRISTENSEN and DININNO 1979; EGLINGTON 1977; BENTLEY et al. 1977). The oxapenems described in these publications are listed in Fig. 4. It has been reported that 2-ethyl-1-oxa-2-penem 3-carboxylic acid is a more powerful *β*-lactamase inhibitor than clavulanic acid (CHERRY et al. 1978; see Sect. D.III.2, Fig. 4) but the 6-tritylamino-2-methyl methyl ester analog has only weak activity probably because of chemical instability (EGLINGTON 1977). Otherwise, the biological properties of these interesting substances have not been described.

Table 51. Naturally occurring nocardicins

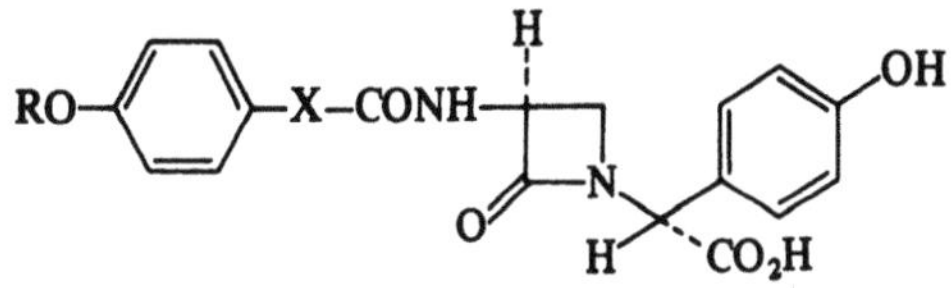

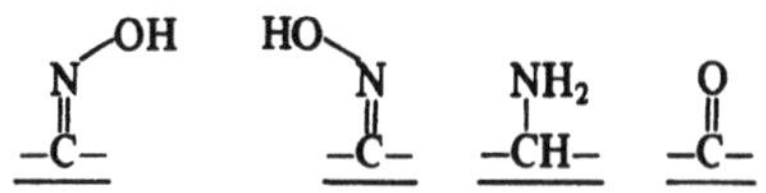

R	X =			
D–$HO_2CCH(NH_2)CH_2CH_2$–	A	B	C	D
H	E	F	G	–

	Minimum inhibitory concentration (μg/ml)			
	S. aureus	*E. coli*	*P. vulgaris*	*Ps. aeruginosa*
	209P	JC–2	IAM 1025	10490
Nocardicin A	>800	100	3.1	2.5
Nocardicin C	>800	400	400	50
Nocardicin D	>800	50	12.5	800

Source: KAMIYA 1977; HOSODA et al. 1977. MIC values for nocardicins E, F and G were >400 μg/ml for organisms listed except *Ps. aeruginosa*: E, 12.5 μg/ml; F, 100 μg/ml; G, 400 μg/ml.

II. Monocyclic β-Lactams

An early reaction used to characterize benzylpenicillin involved the mild removal of the sulfur atom from the thazolidine ring by treatment with Raney nickel to give desthiobenzylpenicillin (KACZKA and FOLKERS 1949). This monocyclic lactam was found to be devoid of antibacterial activity. In light of this finding, and the arguments advanced earlier which relate biological activity to β-lactam reactivity, the antibiotic activities exhibited by the nocardicins and the monobactams represent an anomaly.

1. Nocardicins

The structures and comparative in vitro activities of the seven nocardicins (A–G) that have been isolated from fermentation broths are summarized in Table 51 (KAMIYA 1977; HOSODA et al. 1977). As indicated in Sect. A.I, the stereochemical configurations of the attachment of the acyl-amino group to the β-lactam ring and the attachment of the carboxyl group to the bridging carbon are congruent with the stereochemistry of the corresponding positions of the penicillins. Of the naturally occurring analogs, nocardicin A is the most active. It contains an oximino group

Table 52. Antimicrobial spectrum of nocardicin A versus carbenicillin

	Strain	MIC (μg/ml)	
		Nocardicin A	*Carbenicillin*
S. pyogenes	S23	200	0.2
S. aureus	209P	800	0.78
S. faecalis	6733	>800	25
C. diphtheriae	PW8	12.5	0.05
E. coli	CJ2	100	12.5
E. coli	1341–18	100	>800
K. pneumoniae	NCTC418	200	50
Sh. sonnei	IEW33	12.5	0.78
S. typhi	0–901	100	1.56
S. typhimurium	1406	25	0.78
P. mirabilis	1437–75	1.56	0.78
P. vulgaris	IAM1025	1.56	0.39
P. rettgeri	1434–3	3.13	>800
P. morganii	1433–2	200	3.13
E. aerogenes	1402–10	200	6.25
E. cloacae	1401–4	800	12.5
Ps. aeruginosa	1101–75	12.5	50
Ps. aeruginosa	67	50	>800
Ps. aeruginosa	139	100	>800
S. marcescens	1421–4	800	12.5
N. gonorrhoeae	–	1.56	–

Source: Nishida et al. 1977. Agar dilution using 10^6 cells/ml in special media. See source reference and KOJO et al. (1977) for description of test restrictions and interfering constituents.

in the *syn* configuration and a D-3-amino-3-carboxypropyl side chain. Analogs without the oximino group but with the D-homoserine side chain are less active. Those without this side chain (nocardicins E, F, G) are essentially inactive (see below). The antimicrobial spectrum of nocardicin A against a larger group of laboratory strains of bacteria is compared with that of carbenicillin in Table 52 (Nishida et al. 1977). Nocardicin A does not exhibit significant activity against most gram-positive and many gram-negative bacteria. Activity is observed against the narrow group of gram-negative bacteria consisting essentially of *Ps. aeruginosa*, *Proteus* sp. (except *P. morganii*), and *Neisseria* species. Even these activities are difficult to demonstrate in vitro since the degree of inhibition is influenced by inoculum size and the presence of certain constituents found in most assay media, including sodium chloride, some amino acids, sugars and divalent cations (Kojo et al. 1977). Nocardicin A is bactericidal to *Ps. aeruginosa* at approximately double its MIC. Surprisingly, in spite of its fastidious requirements in order to demonstrate activity in vitro, this antibiotic exhibits increased activity against *Ps. aeru-*

Table 53. In vitro activity of nocardicin A versus protective activity in mice

		MIC (μg/ml)			ED_{50} (mg/kg)			
Organism	*Strain*	*Nocardicin A*	*AMP*	*CAB*	LD_{50}	*Nocardicin A*	*AMP*	*CAB*
S. pyogenes	S–23	400	0.1	–	15	>870	0.4	–
S. aureus	2005	>400	6.25	–	10	>4900	400	–
K. pneumoniae	282	100	50	–	30	85.1	740	–
E. coli	312	100	–	12.5	10	96	–	48.5
P. mirabilis	545	12.5	–	1.56	200	13.9	–	61.5
P. vulgaris	629	12.5	–	1.56	200	9.6	–	117.1
S. marcescens	112	25	–	>400	15	18.2	–	>952
Ps. aeruginosa	704	25	–	200	20	11.1	–	188.0
Ps. aeruginosa[a]	708	12.5	–	12.5	40	2.6	–	14.1
Ps. aeruginosa[b]	708	12.5	–	6.2	–	6.6	–	100
Ps. aeruginosa[b]	720	50	–	50	–	4.4	–	200

Sources: [a]) MINE et al. 1977a; selected data; ED_{50} in mice challenged i.p. and dosed s.c. (x 1).
[b]) COOPER 1978; AMP=ampicillin, CAB=carbenicillin.

ginosa in the presence of serum – in contrast to many other antibiotics (human serum binding, 23%; NISHIDA et al. 1977); and although it has only weak activity against *E. coli*, its activity is also increased in the presence of polymorphonuclear leukocytes (NISHIDA et al. 1977). Thus, in spite of the poor in vitro activity in most media, nocardicin A exhibits PD_{50} values in mice that are significantly better than those obtained for carbenicillin and cefazolin, not only against *Ps. aeruginosa* and sensitive *Proteus* species, but also against *E. coli* species that are essentially insensitive to the antibiotic in vitro (MINE et al. 1977). This rather remarkable phenomenon is not seen with gram-positive bacteria, where the MIC prediction of inactivity in vivo is observed. Selected examples of this unexpected in vitro/in vivo relationship are included in Table 53.

Several syntheses of nocardicin A and its analogs have been described and the activities of a few analogs have been reported (COOPER 1980; HAKIMELAHI and JUST 1979a, b). In general, the structural changes described (amino group alkylation, acylation variation of the oximino moiety, fusion of β-lactam to six-membered ring) have resulted in reduction of in vitro activity.

The structure of the nocardicins encourages the tacit assumption that these antibiotics have a mechanism of action in common with the other β-lactams. The data now available do not provide a clear answer to this question. AOKI et al. (1976) observed protoplast or spheroplast formation with a sensitive *Ps. aeruginosa* isolate at lethal concentrations of nocardicin A in high osmotic media. Nocardicin only partially inhibited the binding of benzylpenicillin to the PBPs 1, 2, and 3 of *B. subtilis* at 1 m*M* concentration, while essentially complete inhibition was seen with ampicillin at 0.01 m*M* (HORIKAWA and OGAWARA 1980). The MIC of nocardicin A against this strain of *B. subtilis* was > 100 μg/ml while ampicillin inhibited the bacterium at <1 μg/ml. Similar PBP binding and MIC ratios have been observed for *S. faecalis* (COYETTE et al. 1980). Unfortunately, the level and distribution of binding of nocardicin A to the PBPs of sensitive bacteria such as *Ps. aeruginosa* have not been described.

2. Monobactams

Although the antibacterial monocyclic β-lactam-1-sulfonic acids – initially called sulfazecins, later given the generic designation monobactams – were first disclosed in 1981 (IMADA et al. 1981; SYKES et al. 1981 a), a large number of their structure–activity relationships have been described (CIMARUSTI et al. 1981 a, b; BREUER et al. 1981; SCHWIND et al. 1981). In fact, the SAR studies, which have drawn heavily on prior knowledge of the penicillins and cephalosporins, have already produced a monobactam, azthreonam, which has been selected for evaluation as a potential clinically useful antibiotic (Table 56). In contrast to the penicillins, cephalosporins, and carbapenems, the natural monobactams are obtained from bacteria. The simplicity of structure lends itself to total synthesis and the structure of azthreonam incorporates features (acyl group, 4α-methyl) not found in the naturally occuring analogs. Structures of commonly encountered natural monobactams are listed in Table 54 along with an indication of the in vitro activities of the sulfazecin members of this group. MIC values for SQ 26 180 are included in Table 55. While these naturally occuring antibiotics are poorly active against gram-positive bacteria, the activity of sulfazecin against the Enterobacteriaceae is relatively good. The stereochemistry of the attachment of the acylamino and methoxy substituents corresponds with that of the classic β-lactams (IMADA et al. 1981), and this is a requirement for activity. The *R* enantiomer of the desmethyl analog of azthreonam was found to be inactive, for example, against a strain of *P. rettgeri* that is highly sensitive to the *S* enantiomer (MIC, >100 vs. <0.05 μg/ml; CIMARUSTI et al. 1981 a). Changes in cell morphology (*E. coli:* formation of filaments at bacteriostatic concentrations and ghosts at bactericidal concentrations) and PBP-binding patterns of sulfazecin [^{14}C-benzylpenicillin-binding I_{50} values using *E. coli* LD2 PBPs (in μg/ml): 1A, 11; 1B, 270; 2, >500; 3, 180; 4, 2.2; 5 and 6, 1.6; IMADA et al. 1981] and other natural and synthetic monobactam analogs (GEORGOPAPADAKOU et al. 1981 a; compare the profile of azthreonam below) indicate a cell-wall-related mechanism of antibacterial action analogous to that of classic fused-ring β-lactams. The correspondence between the monobactams and, especially, the cephalosporins in structure–activity trends with acyl group variation reinforces this assumption. Thus the most surprising aspects of the monobactams are the presence of the sulfamic acid grouping, rarely encountered in nature, and the ability to achieve good antibacterial activity by a structure not obviously equipped (fused ring) to produce a relatively high level of β-lactam-ring reactivity. Presumably the strong electronegativity of the sulfamate moiety is sufficient to activate the β-lactam ring in lieu of the ring strain effects. This capability is not limited to the natural sulfamate group. Synthetic alternatives now include phosphonates [$-OP(OCH_3)OH$, less effective], *N*-aminosulfonyl amides ($-CO\bar{N}SONR_2$, effective) and O-sulfates ($-OSO_3H$, very effective). Analogs with a carboxyl group on the ring nitrogen are unstable.

Table 54. Structures of commonly encountered naturally occurring monobactams and in vitro activity of sulfazecin and isosulfazecin

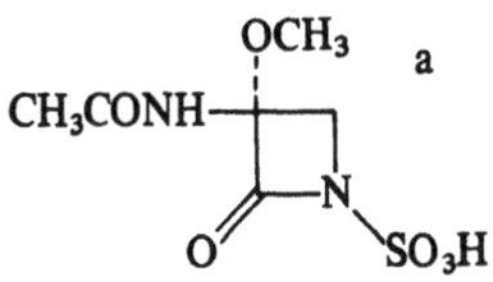

SQ26180

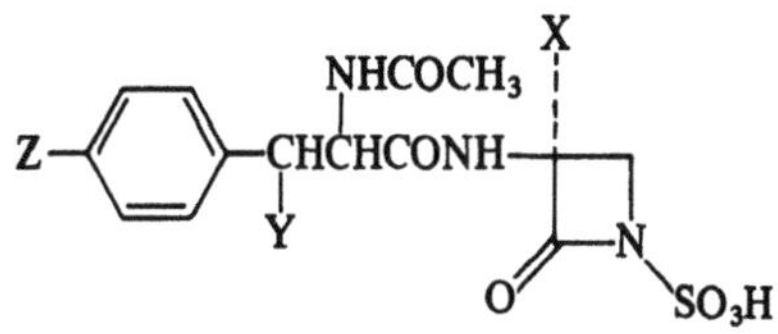

X=H, OCH_3 ; Y, Z=H, OH, OSO_3Na
(SQ26700, 26812, 26823, 26875, 26970)

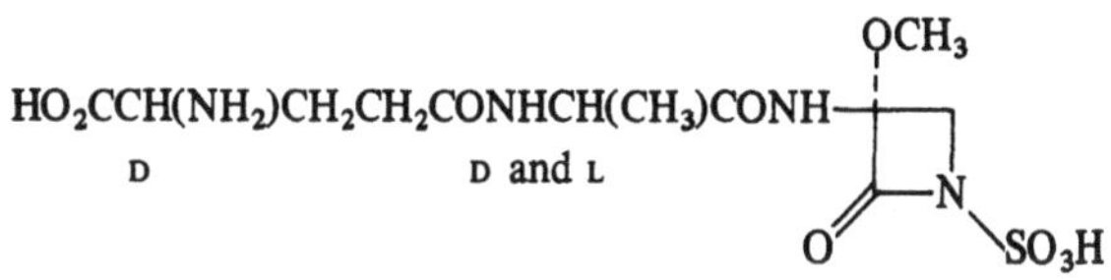

(iso) sulfazecins; SQ26445(D)

	MIC (μg/ml)	
Organism	*Sulfazecin* (D)	*Isosulfazecin* (L)
S. aureus 209P	200	200
A. faecalis IF01311	25	25
E. coli MIHSJC2	100	12.5
K. pneumoniae IF03318	400	25
S. typhimurium IF012529	100	6.2
P. mirabilis ATCC21100	100	3.1
P. vulgaris IF03988	100	6.2
Ps. aeruginosa IF03080	1600	800
S. marcescens IF012648	100	25
Fungi	>800	>800

Source: IMADA et al. 1981; CIMARUSTI et al. 1981a. [a]in vitro activity: see compound 1, table 55.

Some of the structure–activity relationships of the monobactams are illustrated in Table 55. Lack of susceptibility of natural monobactams to many lactamases provides an approach to structures with very broad β-lactamase resistance (e.g. azthreonam). The inherent lack of susceptibility to staphylococcal penicillinase is implied in the relatively equivalent MIC values against the PENase−(2399) and PENase+(2400) strains of *S. aureus*. The same is true for the TEM β-lactamase of *E. coli* [compare MIC values of the TEM−(10439) and TEM+(10404) strains], but not the K-1 β-lactamase of *Klebsiella* (10440 vs. 10436). Resistance of natural monobactams (SQ 26 180, and sulfazecin, Table 54) to PC-1, TEM-2, and the P-99 β-lactamase from *Enterobacter*, has been verified using isolated enzyme preparations. This study also documented the resistance of azthreonam to inactivation by

Table 55. In vitro activities of representative monobactams

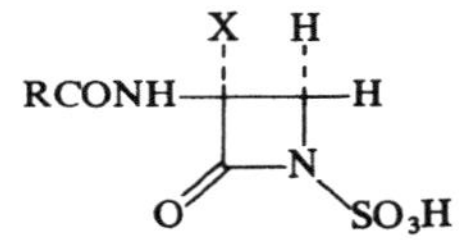

R	X	MIC (μg/ml) S. aureus 2399	S. aureus 2400	E. coli 10439	E. coli 10404	K. aerogenes 10440	K. aerogenes 10436	Proteus rettgeri[a]	Proteus vulgaris[b]	E. cloacae 8236	S. marcescens 9783	Ps. aeruginosa 8329
1. CH_3	OCH_3	(*S. pyogenes*>100)		50	50	3.2	>100	>100	–	25	3.1	100
2. 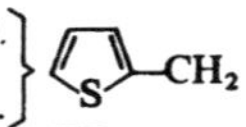	OCH_3	(*S. pyogenes*>100)		12.5	6.3	6.3	25	25	–	12.5	25	25
3.	H	3.1	3.1	50	50	100	>100	–	–	100	–	>100
4. 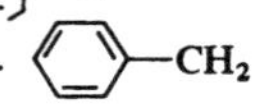	H	3.1	6.3	12.5	50	50	>100	–	–	>100	–	>100
5. 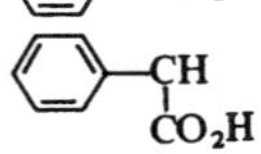	H	100	100	>100	>100	>100	>100	–	–	100	–	50
6. 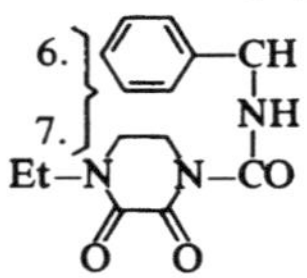	OCH_3	6.3[c]	12.5	3.1	6.3	6.3	–	–	<0.05	3.1	3.1	25
7.	H	1.6[c]	1.6	0.4	0.8	1.6	–	–	<0.05	0.8	3.1	3.1
8. 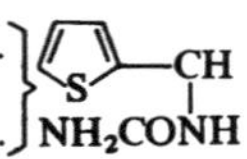	OCH_3	0.3[c]	6.3	3.1	3.1	3.1	–	–	3.1	12.5	6.3	12.5
9.	H	12.5[c]	12.5	50	100	100	–	–	50	100	25	>100
10. 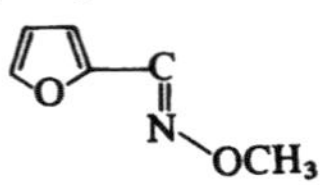	H	3.1	6.3	25	>100	25	>100	12.5	–	12.5	–	100
11. 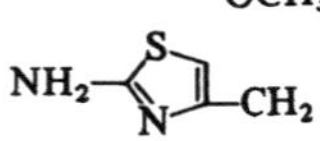	H	12.5[c]	12.5	>100[d]	>100[e]	>100	–	–	>100	>100	6.3	50[f]

Table 55. In vitro activities of representative monobactams (cont'd.)

R	X	MIC (μg/ml)										
		S. aureus		*E. coli*		*K. aerogenes*		*Proteus*		*E. cloacae*	*S. marcescens*	*Ps. aeruginosa*
		2399	2400	10439	10404	10440	10436	*rettgeri*[a]	*vulgaris*[b]	8236	9783	8329
12. 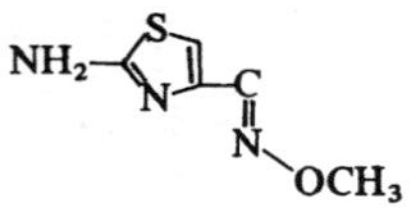	H	6.3	6.3	0.8 / 0.8[d]	6.3 / 0.4[e]	0.8	>100	<0.05	0.8	0.8	25	12.5 / 16[f]
13. (4α–CH_3)–12	H	–	50	0.1[d]	<0.05[e]	0.2	–	<0.05	<0.05	0.2	0.8	0.8[f]
14. (4β–CH_3)–12	H	–	25	0.1[d]	<0.05[e]	0.2	–	<0.05	<0.05	0.1	0.2	0.4[f]
15. (4di–CH_3)–12	H	–	>100	25[d]	3.1[e]	50	–	–	6.3	50	50	>100[f]
16. 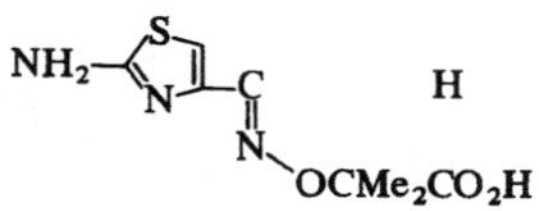	H	>100	>100	0.4	3.1	0.2	>100	<0.05	–	0.4	–	3.1
17. Azthreonam[g]		>100	>100	0.2	0.1	<0.05	50	–	–	–	–	3.1
18. Benzylpenicillin		<0.05	3.1	12.5	>100	12.5	>100	3.1	–	>100	–	>100
19. Carbenicillin		0.2	6.3	12.5	>100	12.5	>100	0.4	–	12.5	–	50
20. Piperacillin		0.4	3.1	3.1	>100	3.1	>100	0.1	–	1.6	–	3.1
21. Cephalothin		0.1	0.2	1.6	6.3	3.1	>100	0.1	–	>100	–	>100
22. Cefotaxime		0.8	0.8	<0.05	<0.05	<0.05	1.6	<0.05	–	0.4	–	12.5

Sources: Cimarusi et al. 1981a, b; Breuer et al. 1981; Schwind et al. 1981. MIC values obtained by agar dilution; inoculum size, 10^4 CFU; 35°, 18 h. Strains as indicated except: [a]8479, [b]9416, [c]1267, [d]8294, [e]10857, [f]9545. [g]see Table 56.

a large variety of plasmid- and chromosomally mediated β-lactamases (BUSH et al. 1981). The 3α-methoxy group enhances β-lactamase resistance (ibid).

In general, the influence of the acylamino side-chain on the in vitro activity of monobactams largely recapitulates penicillin and cephalosporin SAR. Thus, analogs 2 and 3, with the thienylacetyl and phenylacetyl side chains, are less active than benzylpenicillin against penicillin-susceptible *S. aureus*, but they exhibit in vitro spectra which otherwise resemble that of the latter. Reduction of activity when the polarity of the molecule is increased is observed with the carbenicillin- and SQ69613-type analogs (compounds 5 and 9), and even more so with the sulfonic acid (sulbenicillin)–type analog (SCHWIND et al. 1981). A number of the *N*-acyl arylglycine monobactam analogs (azlocillin, mezlocillin, piperacillin type) exhibit good broad-spectrum in vitro activity (BREUER et al. 1981). This is exemplified by analog 7 which carries the acyl side chain of piperacillin. Surprisingly, introduction of the α-methoxyiminofuranylacetyl and the aminothiazolylacetyl side chains on the monobactam structure (analogs 10 and 11) results in unimpressive in vitro activity. However, the α-oximino-2-aminothiazol-4-ylacetyl–type side chain, the mainstay of the third-generation cephalosporins, confers a high level of activity, especially against gram-negative bacteria (compare analogs 12–18).

The biological consequences of substitution of the 4-position by methyl and variation of the oximino moiety over a broad range of alkyl and aliphatic acid groups, have been described (CIMARUSTI et al. 1981 b). A few of these relationships are summarized in Table 55. As indicated by the MIC value for the analogs listed, introduction of a single methyl group (α or β) at the 4-position of the ring and a dimethylacetic acid moiety on the α-oximino grouping of the side chain results in optimization of broad-spectrum activity against gram-negative bacteria and resistance to β-lactamases produced by these organisms, at the expense of gram-positive activity. The resulting product, azthreonam, has an in vitro spectrum of activity closely resembling that of the analogous cephalosporin, ceftazidime.

The structure and some biological properties of azthreonam are listed in Table 56. Azthreonam does not inhibit gram-positive or anaerobic bacteria at therapeutically effective concentrations. However, in studies using 600 clinical isolates it was found to inhibit 90% of the *E. coli*, *Klebsiella*, *Salmonella*, *Providencia*, *Shigella*, *Citrobacter*, and *Morganella* strains tested at concentrations (≦0.4 μg/ml) equivalent to or better than those required for cefotaxime and moxalactam. This agent is equivalent to moxalactam and cefotaxime against *Serratia* sp., *E. cloacae*, and *E. aerogenes* and it inhibits strains of *Ps. aeruginosa* resistant to cefoperazone, cefsulodin, ceftazidime, and tobramycin at ≦25 μg/ml (75% at 6.3 μg/ml). It is highly active against *H. influenzae* and *N. gonorrheae* (Table 56). Its activity is not significantly altered by pH or medium test conditions. It exhibits a high level of stability toward most gram-negative plasmid and chromosomal β-lactamases (e.g., TEM-1, 2, SHV-1, OXA-2,3, P-99 and PSE-1,2,3,4 types). In most cases, the effects of inoculum size (10^2 vs. 10^6 CFU) on MIC values were minimal, similar to the inoculum effects exhibited by cefotaxime and ceftazidime (NEU and LABTHAVIKUL 1981; SYKES et al. 1981 b). Except for the P-99 cephalosporinase (Ki, 7.2 n*M*), azthreonam is poorly bound by β-lactamases (Km, 0.3–8.0 *M*), and it is generally not an inhibitor of these enzymes (BUSH et al. 1981). In contrast to most β-lactam antibiotics, induction of β-lactamases by azthreonam is extremely low

Table 56. Structure and biological properties of azthreonam

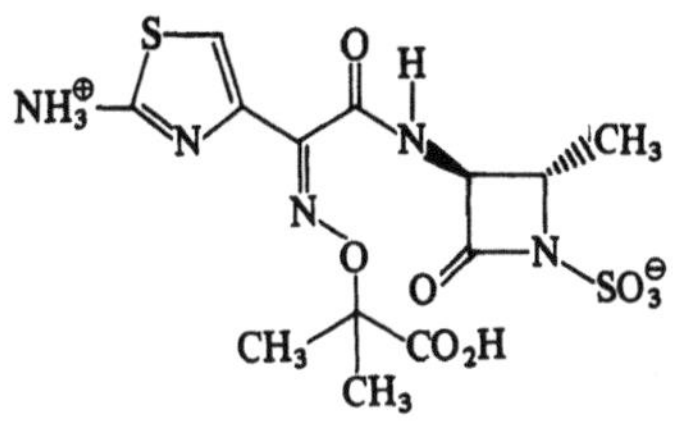

SQ 26,776

	In vitro activity			Protective effectiveness[c]			
	(N>400)[a]	Laboratory strains[b]		Azthreonam		Cefotaxime	
	MIC$_{50}$ (μg/ml)	Strain	MIC (μg/ml)	MIC (μg/ml)	ED$_{50}$ (mg/kg)	MIC (μg/ml)	ED$_{50}$ (mg/kg)
Streptococci	14–>100	*pyogenes*	>100	–	–	–	–
Staphylococci	>100	*aureus* 2400	>100	–	–	–	–
Streptococcus	–	*faecalis* 2811	>100	–	–	–	–
Escherichia	0.06	*coli* 10439 *coli* 10404	0.2 0.4	0.4	0.4	0.1	0.2
Klebsiella	0.09	*pneumoniae* 11066 *aerogenes* 10440 *aerogenes* 10436	0.4 <0.05 50	0.1	0.4	>0.05	0.2
Proteus (Indole –)	0.007		–	–	–	–	–
Proteus (Indole +)	0.01	*rettgeri* 8217 *vulgaris* 10851B	<0.05 <0.05	<0.05	0.6	<0.06	0.3
Enterobacter	0.08	*cloacae* 10441 *cloacae* 10435	0.1 12.5	0.1	3.7	0.1	24.4
Serratia	0.10	*marcescens* 9782	1.6	0.4	0.5	0.8	1.1
Citrobacter	0.17	*freundi* 10204	0.1	0.1	0.9	0.1	3.1
Pseudomonas	5.75	*aeruginosa* 8329 9545	3.1 0.4	3.1 6.3	24.7 59.6	12.5 12.5	480 >200
Nisseria	0.09	*gonorrhea*	–	–	–	–	–
Hemophilus	0.06	*influenzae*	–	<0.05	0.4	<0.05	<0.1
Bacteroides	39.2	*fragilis* 11834	25	–	–	–	–

Sources: [a]EICKHOFF and EHRET 1981. Clinical isolates, broth, 10^5 CFU. [b]CIMARUSTI et al. 1981a, b. Agar, 10^4 CFU. [c]FERNANDES et al. 1981. MIC: 10^5 CFU; ED$_{50}$: In mice at +1 and +5 h post–infection with >100 LD$_{50}$ of pathogen.

(e.g., relative β-lactamase activities after induction by cefotaxime versus azthreonam: *Proteus*, 34/<0.1; *Providencia*, 3.4/1.1; *Enterobacter* sp., 0.9/<0.1, 338/1.3; *Serratia* 1.1/<0.2. No inducer: 1, SYKES et al. 1981 b). Azthreonam is highly efficacious in mouse protection tests (Table 56). It is well tolerated on injection in humans, and produces good serum levels (1-g dose i.m.: serum peak, approx 50 μg/ml; $t_{1/2}\beta$, 1.7 h). Urinary recovery after 24 h is approximately 68% (unmetabolized; SWABB et al. 1981).

Azthreonam induces filament formation in *E. coli* and it binds specifically to the PBP 3 of this organism (concentration in μg/ml to completely inhibit binding of benzylpenicillin: azthreonam: 1A, 10: 1B, ≧100; 2, >100; 3, 0.1; 4, 100; 5/6, 100; MIC, 0.1 μg/ml. Cephalothin: 1A, 0.5; 1B, 100; 2, 100; 3, 2.0; 4, 100; 516, >100; MIC, 1.6 μg/ml). These data have led to the conclusion that the antibacterial activity of azthreonam is probably due exclusively to inhibition of septation in susceptible organisms. (GEORGOPAPADAKOU et al. 1981 b). The properties of azthreonam and associated monobactam analogs have been reviewed (SYKES and PHILLIPS 1981). This collection of papers provides ready access to much of the data discussed here.

III. β-Lactamase Inhibitors

Protection of β-lactam antibiotics from inactivation by β-lactamases can be achieved by incorporation of structural features which decrease susceptibility – the major thrust in β-lactam discovery and design – or by the use of β-lactamase inhibitors. Random-based searches for such inhibitors and studies designed to locate the active site of these enzymes have turned up many nonspecific inactivators such as p-chloromercuribenzoate, iodine, tetranitromethane, carbodiimide, papain, β-lactamase antisera, and the like (for compilations see: COLE 1979 a; FISHER et al. 1980). This list includes structures with inhibitory activity that indicate specificity for the active site. Three examples of such inhibitors without a β-lactam ring are xylocaine (VACZI and URI 1954), phenylpropynal (SCHENKEIN and PRATT 1980) and the macrolide, izumenolide (LIU et al. 1980; BUSH et al. 1980 a, b). However, the β-lactamase inhibitors which have held out the promise of practical use in the clinical context generally contain a β-lactam ring. They comprise two types: the first are penicillins and cephalosporins which bind, at least to some extent reversibly, to the enzyme and subsequently are converted via the normal hydrolytic sequence to penicilloic or cephalosporic acids and their further decomposition products – usually at a very slow rate. The second type are the more recently discovered "suicide" β-lactams (clavulanic acid, olivanic acids, penicillanic acid sulfones, etc.) which in the course of the normal hydrolytic reaction sequence undergo, to a variable extent, secondary reactions which stabilize the enzyme-substrate intermediate, resulting in progressive irreversible inhibition of the β-lactamase. Agents of the first type tend to be competitive inhibitors with high affinity for the enzymes and a suitably low V_{max}; but high concentrations are required for effective protection of the susceptible β-lactam which provides the antibiotic activity, and biological effectiveness can be variable. The second type can exhibit impressive synergistic effects when combined with β-lactamase-susceptible antibiotics, the most promising of such to date being the 2:1 mixture of amoxicillin and clavulanic acid now marketed for clinical use under the trade name Augmentin.

1. Penicillins and Cephalosporins as Inhibitors

The inhibition of β-lactamases was first demonstrated for cephalosporin C (ABRAHAM and NEWTON 1956) and methicillin (ROLINSON et al. 1960). Subsequent screening of penicillins and cephalosporins produced a small group of analogs which exhibit a tantalizingly marginal level of inhibitory activity, primarily against plasmid- and chromosomally mediated lactamases of gram-negative bacteria (COLE et al.

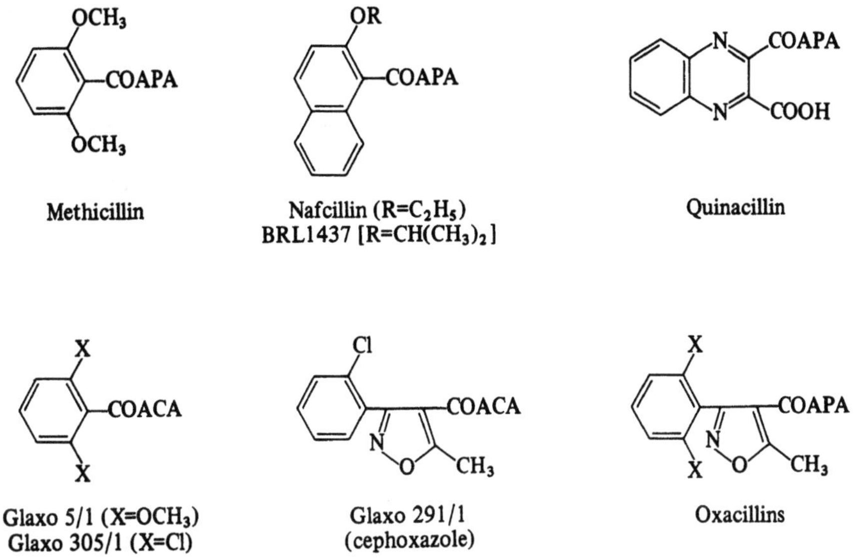

Fig. 5. Penicillins and cephalosporins studied extensively as β-lactamase inhibitors

1972; O'CALLAGHAN et al. 1967; O'CALLAGHAN and MORRIS 1972). Staphylococcal penicillinase was found to be inhibited at reasonably low concentrations by cephalothin, less so by other cephalosporins, and very little by penicillins (see references in COLE 1979a). Analogs found to have activity levels against the gram-negative β-lactamases sufficient to encourage extensive evaluations are listed in Fig. 5. For the most part, they are penicillins resistant to staphylococcal penicillinase (methicillin, nafcillin, quinacillin, cloxacillin), or analogs with similar side chains (BRL 1437), or with these side-chains on the cephalosporin nucleus (cephoxazole, Glaxo 5/1, Glaxo 305/1). Carbenicillin and ticarcillin have also been found to exhibit selective inhibitory activity against gram-negative β-lactamases (see references in COLE 1979a), but not staphylococcal penicillinase. Although marked enhancement of activity of β-lactamase-sensitive penicillins or cephalosporins is possible in some instances by addition of these inhibitors, the number of different β-lactamases inhibited is usually relatively low and the concentration of inhibitor required for effectiveness is higher than desired (e.g., MIC values for *E. cloacae* P99: cephaloridine, 2,000 μg/ml; cloxacillin, >1,000 μg/ml; cephaloridine plus cloxacillin, 50+50 μg/ml; O'CALLAGHAN and MORRIS 1972). In addition, since inhibition depends on competitive binding to the enzyme, with some hydrolytic susceptibility on the part of the inhibitor, the effect is transient – the more effective inhibitors morely prolonging the time required for regrowth of seemingly lysed bacterial cultures, in vitro and in vivo (GREENWOOD and O'GRADY 1975). The significant differences in level and breadth of the β-lactamase inhibitory activity of the agents described next as compared to these penicillins and cephalosporins are apparent in the listing of I_{50} values for these agents and for clavulanic acid given in Table 57.

The numerous studies of the inhibition of β-lactamases by these penicillin and cephalosporin analogs have been extensively tabulated in recent reviews (COLE

Table 57. Comparison of representative inhibition profiles of penicillins and cephlosporins with that of clavulanic acid

	I_{50} Value for β-lactamase of strain indicated (μg/ml)[a]						
	E. coli	*E. coli*	*P. mirabilis*	*K. aerogenes*	*E. cloacae*	*Ps. aeruginosa*	*S. aureus*
Inhibitor	K12 R_{TEM}	JT414 (chromosomal)	C889	ATCC 15380	10005	A	MB9
Carbenicillin	in[b]	0.6	in	in	2.1	10	in
Methicillin	24	18	–	2.5	–	7.5	in
Cloxacillin	–	0.14	–	–	2.5	2.2	in[c]
BRL–1437	0.21	16	13	0.88	4	14	>40
Cephalothin	–	–	–	–	–	–	10
Cefoxazole	in	4	in	11	0.9	0.4	in
Cefoxitin	–	24	–	–	–	40	–
Cefuroxime	in	2.3	–	–	4.3	5.0	–
Clavulanic acid	0.08	50	0.01	0.1	50	>50	0.02

Source: Cole 1979a. [a] I_{50} value determined for benzylpenicillin (1 mg/ml) added as substrate 15 min after inhibitor, velocity determined by hydroxylamine assay after 30 min, pH7, 37°C. [b] Inactive based on 0% inhibition using 40 μg/ml of inhibitor under conditions described. [c] 2% inhibition.

1979a, b). It is not surprising that the new cephalosporins that bind β-lactamases tightly are found to function as inhibitors since they are highly resistant to hydrolysis by these enzymes. Recent reports include cefotaxime, cefoxitin (Fu and Neu 1978b, 1979), cefonicid, and cefuroxime (Newman et al. 1980; Mehta et al. 1981) and other members of the cephamycin family in addition to cefoxitin: cefmetazole, cefotetan, and moxalactam (Toda et al., 1981).

2. Progressive β-Lactamase Inhibitors

Progressive β-lactamase inhibitors include clavulanic acid, certain carbapenems, and several semisynthetic β-lactam derivatives. These agents are listed in Fig. 6. They appear to represent a diversity of structures. However, similarities in structural characteristics can be attributed to many of these substances which would account for inactivation of β-lactamases along related chemical pathways (Fisher et al. 1978, 1980; Charnas et al. 1978; Cartwright and Coulson 1979; Reading and Hepburn 1979; Fisher et al. 1981; Charnas and Knowles 1981).

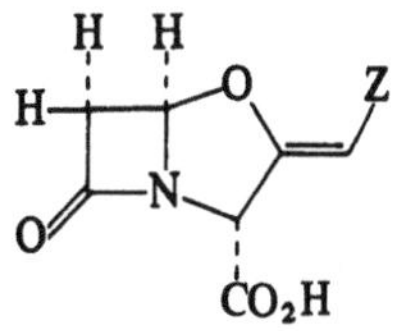

Clavulanates

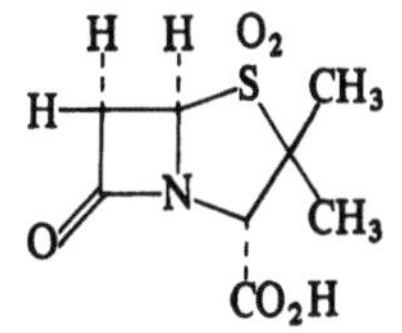

Penicillanic acid sulfone (sulbactam)

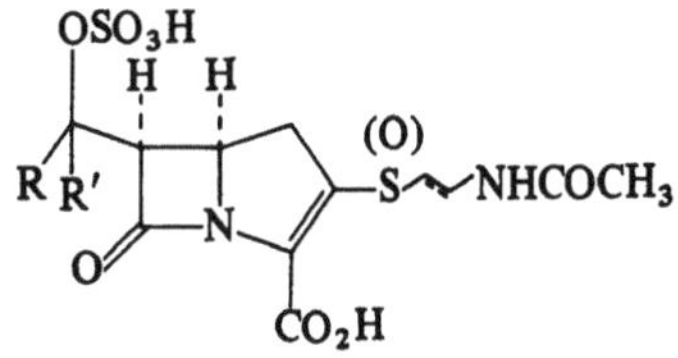

5,6–*cis* Carbapenems

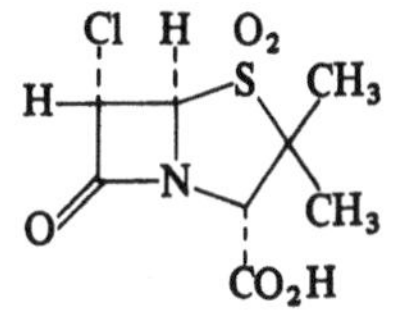

6α–Choropenicillanic acid sulfone

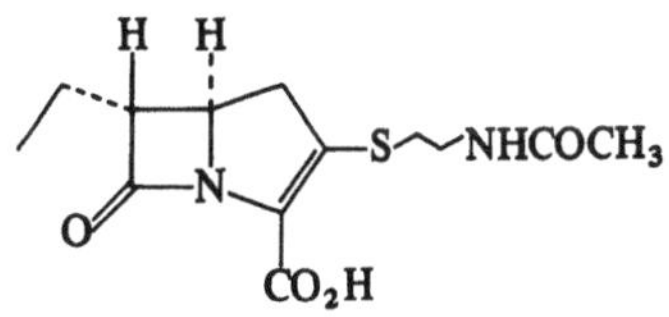

PS–5

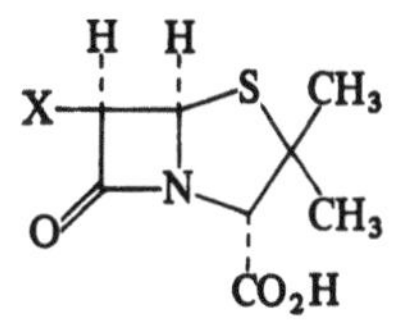

6β–Halopenicillanic acids (X = Br, I)

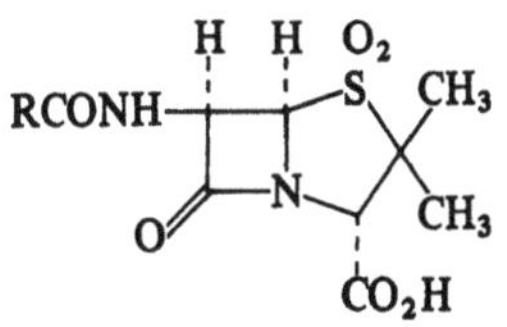

Methicillin and quinacillin sulfones

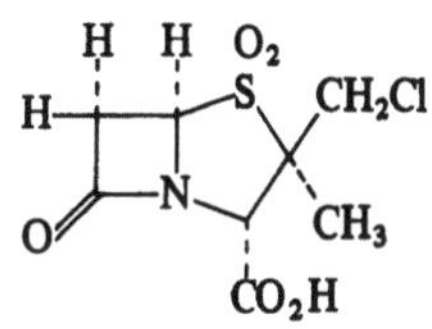

BL–P 2013

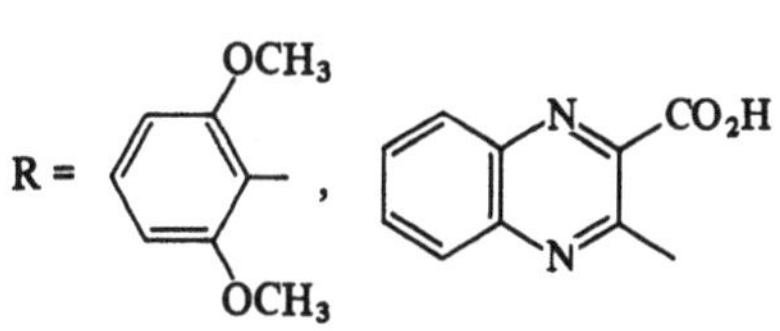

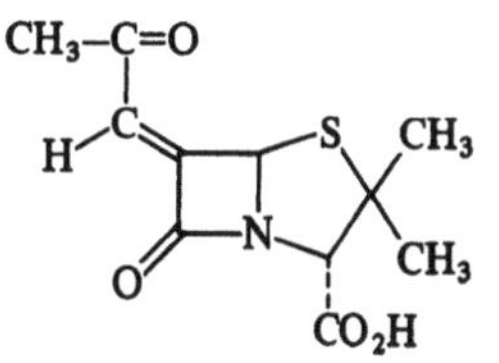

RO15–1903

Fig. 6. Progressive inhibitors of β-lactamases

A plausible explanation of the sequence of chemical events which lead to inactivation can be applied to those members of this group which meet three basic criteria: (1) a β-lactam ring which can undergo normal enzyme attack to form an acyl-enzyme intermediate which hydrolyzes at a relatively slow rate; (2) a sufficiently acidic 6α-proton to participate in facile elimination with formation of a double bond; and (3) a good leaving group β- to the acidic 6-proton which can

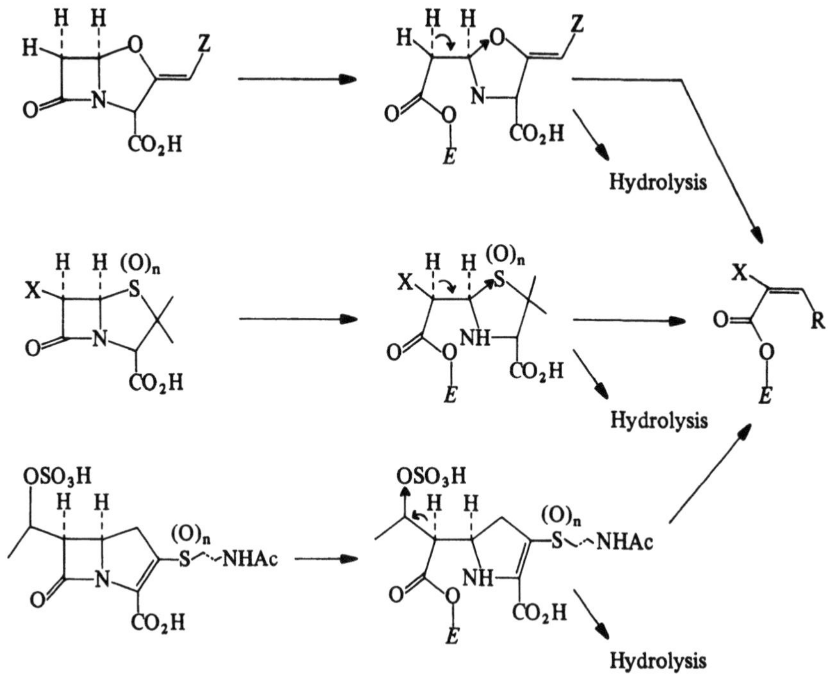

R = NHCH(COOH)COCH$_2$OH, NHCH(COOH)C(CH$_3$)$_2$S(O)$_n$H, CH$_3$, etc.

X = H, Br, Cl, 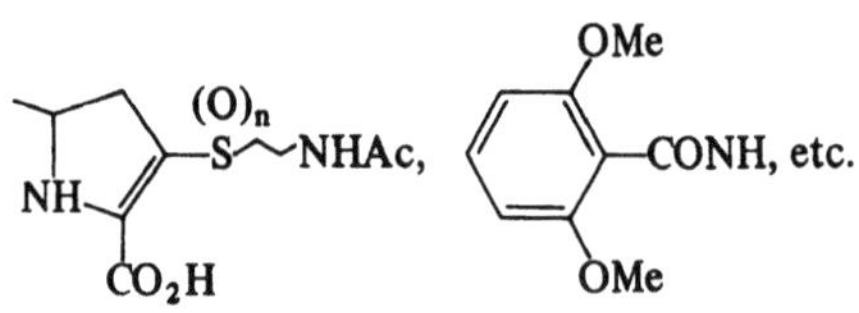

E = Enzyme; Z = CH$_2$OH, CH$_3$, etc.; n = 0,1

Scheme A. Possible inactivation pathways for progressive β-lactamase inhibitors

undergo *anti*-elimination to form the double bond. The unsaturated acyl enzyme complexes which result may be sufficiently stable per se to permit nearly irreversible inactivation, or they may undergo double-bond migration and/or secondary Michael addition to the double bond (including internal cyclization) to give appropriately stabilized acyl-enzyme complexes (Cohen and Pratt 1980). These reaction sequences are summarized in Scheme A. This inactivating sequence occurs parallel to and simultaneously with the normal hydrolytic β-lactam ring-opening reactions involved in β-lactamase activity (Chap. 12). Consequently the most efficient inactivators of this type are those which are sensitive to the β-lactamase, but for which the V_{max} is relatively poor for the normal enzyme function, viz, hydrolysis and release of the β-lactam-opened product. A poor substrate should have longer residence time in the normal transient acyl-enzyme stage to permit loss of the 6-hydrogen and *anti*-elimination to the more stable crotonate structure. From struc-

Table 58. Progressive effect of MM4550 and clavulanic acid on β–lactamases

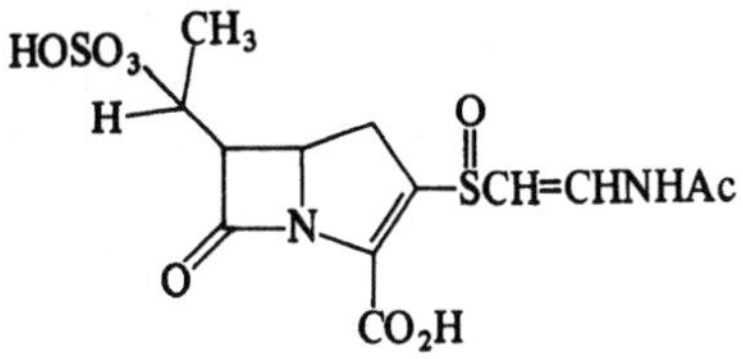

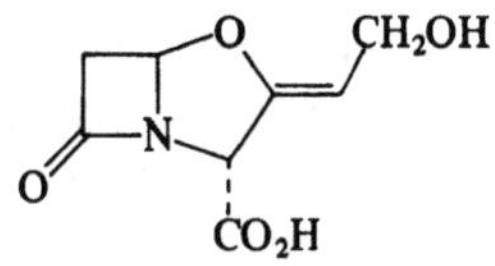

	I_{50} (μg/ml)			
	MM4550[a]		Clavulanic acid[b]	
β–Lactamase source	With substrate	15 min before substrate	With substrate	15 min before substrate
S. aureus MB9	0.016	0.0037	0.84	0.02
E. coli K12 R_{TEM}	0.0014	0.00046	0.56	0.08
K. aerogenes A	0.002	0.0008	0.11	0.01
P. mirabilis C889	0.00063	0.00035	0.69	0.01

Source: COLE 1980. [a]Substrate: benzylpenicillin. [b]Substrate: amoxycillin (1 mg/ml).

tural and kinetic considerations FISHER et al. (1978, 1980) have estimated hydrolytic to inactivation turnover ratios of the following orders: clavulanic acid, 115; penicillanic acid sulfone, 4,500; methicillin sulfone, 22,500; quinacillin sulfone, 400. Reference to these agents as irreversible inhibitors is not completely accurate since partial recovery of activity (around 35%) has been accomplished by treatment of the inactivated enzymes with hydroxylamine (CHARNAS et al. 1978) and staphylococcal β-lactamase inhibited by clavulanic acid has been observed to regenerate, slowly, at pH 7 (50% recovery in 50 min) and more rapidly at acid pHs (50% recovery in 10 min at pH 4) when the enzyme is freed of excess clavulanic acid (READING and HEPBURN 1979). However, at clavulanate:enzyme ratios above 350 no regeneration is seen (FISHER et al. 1978). This mechanism also does not provide an universal explanation for the activity of these agents. The carbapenem PS-5 does not have the requisite structural characteristics, yet it is reported to function as a progressive inhibitor, accompanied by slow hydrolysis and following a brief period of competive inhibition. Its mechanism of inactivation has been attributed to a probable conformational change of the enzyme resulting from the formation of a relatively stable secondary complex of unknown structure between PS-5 and the β-lactamase (OKAMURA et al. 1980). Slow but complete recovery of activity is observed upon depletion of the inhibitor implying reversal of the conformational change. The progressive action of these inhibitors is illustrated by the difference in I_{50} values when the inhibitor is added at the same time as the substrate or 15 min before. Table 58 compares these effects for MM4550, which is a good competitive inhibitor showing high initial activity, and clavulanic acid, with lower initial binding levels.

Of the various progressive inhibitors that have been reported, clavulanic acid and penicillanic acid sulfone (CP45889; sulbactam) have been investigated most thoroughly. Clavulanic acid inhibits a number of clinically important β-lactamases from both gram-positive and gram-negative bacteria including straphylococcal penicillinase PC 1, most of the plasmid mediated penicillinases including type III R_{TEM} found in many Enterobacteriacae and *H. influenzae* and some, but not all, of the chromosally mediated cephalosporinases. The type IV enzyme K 1 of *Klebsiella* is inhibited (O'CALLAGHAN 1980; cf. Table 57). Typically I_{50} values below 0.3 μg/ml are observed with benzylpenicillin- or ampicillin-hydrolyzing β-lactamases that are obtained from organisms that includes *S. aureus* (Russell), *H. influenzae* (4482), *E. coli* (JT4, JY20), *K. aerogenes* (E70, Ba 95), *P. mirabilis* (C889), *Ps. aeruginosa* (Dalgleish, 1822). *S. marcescens* (U39), and *B. fragilis* (COLE 1980; HUNTER and READING 1976). Inhibition at this level is also seen with a few enzymes which efficiently hydrolyze cephalosporins principally of the R_{TEM} type (e.g., from *E. coli*, *P. mirabilis*) but generally the cephalosporinases are more resistant with IC_{50} values in the range of 10–40 μg/ml. This is true for enzymes from *E. cloacae* (P99, type Ia), *E. coli* (JT410, Type Ib), *Ps. aeruginosa* (A, Sabath, Type Id), *P. morganii* G, and the like. The expected synergistic effect of this inhibitory activity on the in vitro antibiotic activity of β-lactams against antibiotic-resistant β-lactamase-producing bacteria has been demonstrated for benzylpenicillin, ampicillin, amoxicillin, cephalothin, cephaloridine, mezlocillin, carbenicillin, ticarcillin, piperacillin, cefoperazone, and others. The relationship of IC_{50} to synergistic activity for ampicillin and cephaloridine is illustrated in Table 59 using a selected group of bacteria (READING and COLE 1977). A plethora of additional examples have been published.

Sulbactam (penicillanic acid sulfone) has been shown to have a similar but somewhat different spectrum of inhibition of β-lactamases than that of clavulanic acid (ENGLISH et al. 1978). Side-by-side comparisons of clavulanic acid and penicillanic acid sulfone indicate that, while both compounds are synergistic within the constraints just described, in most cases clavulanic acid is more effective on an equivalent weight basis. The reverse is true in a few cases, notably with certain strains of *Enterobacter*, *Serratia*, and indole-positive *Proteus* (WISE et al. 1980b; HUNTER and WEBB 1980). Likewise the synergistic effects reported for PS-5 (OKAMURA et al. 1979) appear less striking than those for clavulanic acid.

Penicillanic acid sulfone (sulbactam) is well tolerated in man when given intravenously and intramuscularly in single doses up to 1,000 mg. The intramuscular dose produces serum peak levels of approximately 30 μg/ml with a $t_{1/2}$ of about 1 h. Its pharmacokinetic behavior is similar to that of ampicillin or amoxicillin. However, single oral doses of 500 mg produce peak serum concentrations of only about 1.4 μg/ml (FOULDS et al. 1980). This has resulted in the testing of the pivaloyloxymethyl ester of penicillinanic acid sulfone (CP47904; Fig. 7). Orally, a single dose of this pro-drug equivalent to 250 mg sulbactam produces mean peak serum concentrations of 4.9 mg of the latter per milliliter. Two intriguing additional prodrugs of sulbactam have been described (BALTZER et al. 1980). These are the mixed oxymethyleneoxy esters of penicillanic acid sulfone with ampicillin (VD1827) and

Table 59. Correlation of β–lactamase inhibition with synergistic effect of clavulanic acid with penicillins and cephalosporins

Organism (lactamase type)	β–Lactamase inhibition		Minimum inhibitory concentrations (μg/ml)						
			Clavulanic acid	*Ampicillin plus CA*[a]			*Cephaloridine plus CA*		
	Substrate	I_{50} (μg/ml)		0	1	5	0	1	5
S. aureus Russel	PNG	0.06	15	500	0.8	0.02	0.6	0.15	0.06
E. coli JT39 (R Factor)	PNG	0.08	31	>2000	31	4	62	4	2
E. coli JT410 (chromosomal)	CER	56	31	250	250	250	62	62	62
K. aerogenes NCTC418	PNG	0.03	31	250	0.4	0.1	–	–	–
P. mirabilis C889	PNG	0.03	62–125	>2000	62	8	62	8	4
Ps. aeruginosa Dalgleish	PNG	0.1	250	>2000	2000	500	–	–	–

Source: Reading and Cole 1977. [a]Clavulanic acid added: 0, 1 and 5 μg/ml; PNG=benzylpenicillin, CER=cephaloridine.

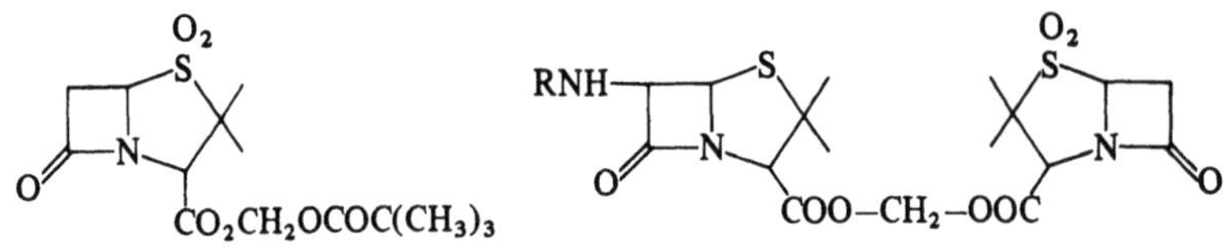

CP47904

VD 1827 [R = $C_6H_5CH(NH_2)CO$–]
VD 1825 [R = $(CH_2)_6N$=CH–]

Fig. 7. Pro-drugs of CP45899

mecillinam (VD1825) illustrated in Fig. 7. These mutual pro-drugs are absorbed on oral administration and cleaved to give serum concentration curves in which the penicillin (ampicillin, mecillinam) and the penicillanic acid sulfone closely match each other. The mean serum peak levels (approximately 1 h) in man are 11 µg/ml with a 475-mg oral dose of VD1827 and approximately 4.2 µg/ml with a 260-mg dose of VD1825.

In contrast to sulbactam, clavulanic acid is well absorbed when given orally. A 125-mg dose produces peak serum concentrations (1 h) in the range of 2.5–3.0 µg/ml and urine concentrations over 100 µg/ml are maintained for 4 h (COLE 1980). The pharmacokinetic properties of clavulanic acid parallel those of amoxicillin. Results such as these have led to the introduction of a 2:1 mixture of amoxicillin and clavulanic acid into clinical practice under the name of Augmentin. The in vitro activities of this mixture as compared to those of its components against various bacteria are given in Table 60 (COMBER et al. 1980). This table also illustrates the relative performance of Augmentin against 570 β-lactamase-producing clinical isolates with high levels of resistance to ampicillin and amoxicillin (VAN LANDUYT et al. 1981). The in vivo effectiveness of this combination is demonstrated by the protective effectiveness of Augmentin reflected in the PD_{50} values of Table 61 (COMBER et al. 1980).

There are far fewer biological data for the other β-lactamase inhibitors listed in Fig. 6, or for the many clavams that have now been synthesized. The reports describing the chemistry of clavulanic acid and its analogs are now quite numerous but most of the biological data concerning these compounds are still contained in patents. A recent review of the status of clavulanic acid research incorporates much of the patent data (COOPER 1980) and a few of these results are included herein. The review cited should be consulted for a more complete coverage of activity trends among these analogs.

The sulfones of methicillin and quinacillin were designed to fit the criteria outlined at the beginning of this section. The success of this design is reflected by $t_{1/2}$ inactivation rates for *E. coli* R_{TEM} β-lactamase of about 1 min for both derivatives compared to 44 min for penicillanic acid sulfone (FISHER et al. 1980). Parallel reasoning has led to the finding that 6α-chloropenicillanic acid sulfone efficiently and irreversibly inactivates extracellular penicillinase from *S. aureus* (CARTWRIGHT and COULSON 1979). Since this molecule has a 6α-chloro-substituent, facile epimerization at the 6-position would be expected to play a role in the inactivation process. In contrast to clavams, which can exhibit activity without the 3-carboxyl group, penam sulfones on which the carboxyl group has been replaced by hydroxyl or

Table 60. Typical antibacterial spectra of Augmentin and its components

Organism	MIC (μg/ml)[a]			Clinical isolates (% Strains inhibited)[b]	
	Augmentin	Amoxicillin	Clavulanic acid	n	%
S. aureus	0.1	0.05	25	–	–
S. aureus	2.5	125	25	102	93
S. pyogenes	0.01	0.01	25	–	–
S. pneumoniae	0.02	0.02	12.5	–	–
S. faecalis	0.5	0.5	250	–	–
N. gonorrhoeae	0.01	0.005	1.25	–	–
N. gonorrhoeae	1.25	>10	5.0	–	–
H. influenzae	0.25	0.25	12.5	–	–
H. influenzae	1.25	>50	>50	40	95
E. coli	5.0	5.0	50	–	–
E. coli	25	>500	50	163	27
K. aerogenes	2.5	125	50	–	–
K. pneumoniae	–	–	–	117	73
P. mirabilis	1.25	1.25	125	–	–
P. mirabilis	12.5	>500	125	20	80
P. morganii	250	500	125	44	0
P. rettgeri	–	–	–	1	0
P. vulgaris	5.0	>500	125	26	100
E. cloacae	125	>500	125	–	–
Enterobacter sp.	–	–	–	29	3
Ps. aeruginosa	250	>500	125	–	–
Providencia stuartii	–	–	–	5	0
S. marcescens	125	125	125	15	0
Citrobacter sp.	–	–	–	8	38
B. fragilis	1.25	25	50	–	–

Sources: [a]COMBER et al. 1980. [b]VAN LANDUYT et al. 1981. Percent of numbers (n) of β-lactamase-producing strains (clinical isolates) inhibited by 2 μg/ml for *S. aureus* and *Hemophilus* sp. and 8 μg/ml for Enterobacteriaceae isolates. Percent of strains inhibited by ampicillin or amoxicillin alone was 0 except: *S. aureus*, 8% and 9% and *Hemophilus* sp. 12.5% and 7.5% respectively.

Table 61. Protective effectiveness in mice of Augmentin compared with its components

	PD_{50} (mg/kg)		
	Augmentin	Amoxicillin	Clavulanic acid
S. aureus Smith	0.35	0.23	96
E. coli 8	25	25	>200
E. coli JT39	114	>1000	340
K. aerogenes T767	84	>2000	>2000
K. pneumoniae 62	400	>3200	>3200
P. mirabilis 889	280	>1000	>1000
P. vulgaris E	120	>1000	>1000

Source: COMBER et al. 1980. Inoculum: 10–100 LD_{50} intraperitonally; Dosages: p.o. 1 and 5 h post–infection.

acetoxy (Fig. 8, I) are reported to be poor inhibitors of β-lactamases (SHEEHAN et al. 1980).

Most of the studies on 6β-bromopenicillanic acid have been carried out on epimeric mixtures containing initially 6%–28% of the thermodynamically less stable β-isomers (equilibrium mixture: 12% 6β-epimer). The 6α-epimer, which can be obtained pure, has no effect on β-lactamases from *B. cereus* and *E. coli* (LOOSEMORE and PRATT 1978). As expected, the activity of the 6β-epimer varies depending on the β-lactamase source (PRATT and LOOSEMORE 1978). For example, enzymes incubated with 10:1 and 100:1 molar ratios, respectively, of inhibitor to enzyme retained the following percentages (in parentheses) of original activities after 1 h: *B. cereus* I (0, 0); *B. cereus* II (95, 95); *S. aureus* (68, 0), *E. coli* (90, 20), and *B. licheniformis* (0, 0). This agent is of interest in that it binds irreversibly; activity is not restored on treatment with hydroxylamine or imidazole, or by exhaustive dialysis. The stability of the bound enzyme complex makes it a promising tool for active site studies. It has been reported to react with the serine at position 44 of the β-lactamase I of *B. cereus* (KNOTT-HUNZTKER et al. 1979; ORLEK et al. 1980). 6β-Iodopenicillanic acid has also been reported to be an inhibitor of β-lactamases (KEMP et al. 1980). Both 6β-bromo- and 6β-iodopenicillanic acids have been shown to exhibit synergistic activity with ampicillin comparable to that of clavulanic acid and greater than that of sulbactam (WISE et al. 1981). Similarly, BL-P 2013 (Fig. 6) was

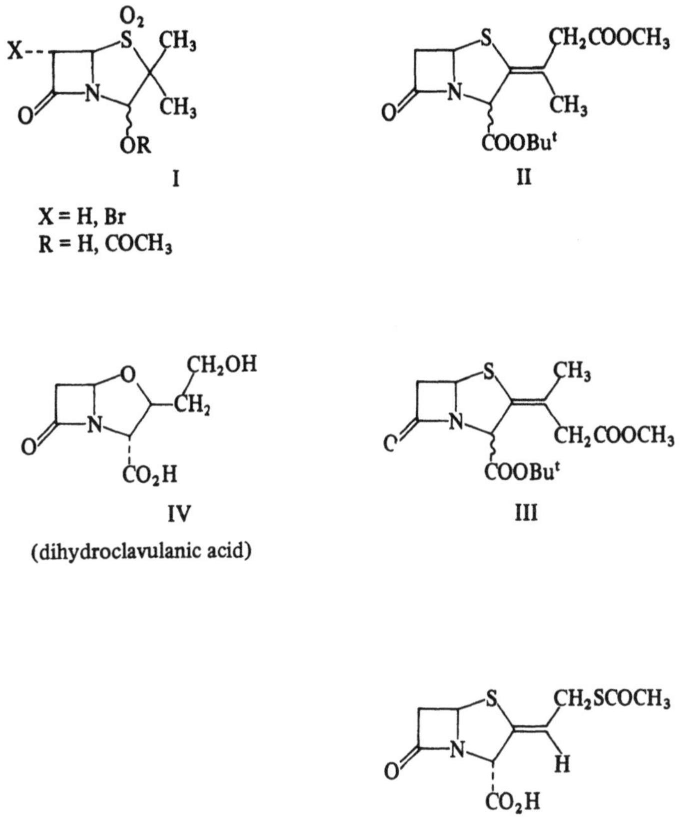

Fig. 8. Analogs of β-lactamase inihibitors, inactive or with lowered activity

found to be comparable to sulbactam in inhibiting β-lactamase from *B. fragilis* and Type IIIa (TEM) β-lactamase from *E. coli*. It was more effective than sulbactam against the type IIa and Va and staphylococcal β-lactamases, and it inhibited type and Ib β-lactamases which are refractory to sulbactam and clavulanic acid (PURSIANO et al. 1981) Likewise, the carpetimycins C19393 S_2 and H_2 have been reported to exhibit better I_{50} values than those of clavulanic acid against a range of β-lactamases (OKONOGI et al. 1981).

For clavulanic acid, the data that have been published indicate that activity can be retained across rather extensive structural variations. β-Lactamase inhibition is not appreciably affected by esterification. The methyl and benzyl esters exhibit synergy with ampicillin similarly to clavulanic acid (COLE et al. 1979). Many modifications of the allylic hydroxymethyl substituent result in retention or improvement of inhibitory activity. Replacement of the hydroxyl group by an amino function, whether free, or acylated in a variety of ways, results in a higher level of β-lactamasee inhibition (Table 62). Both the primary 9-amino analog (p.o. and s.c.) and the 9-benzylamino derivative (s.c.) have been reported in the patent literature (HABRIDGE 1978) to exhibit better synergistic activity with amoxicillin than clavulanic acid in protecting mice infected with *E. coli* JT39. In addition to improved in vitro activity, 9-aminoclavulanic acid was found to provide higher and longer serum

Table 62. Effects of replacement of hydroxyl group of clavulanic acid on β-lactamase inhibitory activity

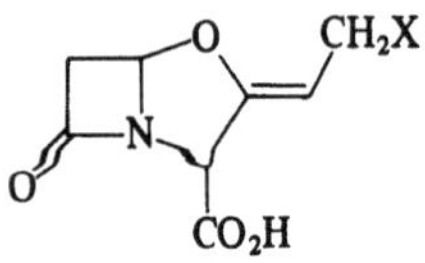

X	I_{50} (μg/ml)		
	PASE	Type III	Type IV
–OH(CA)[a]	8.2	1.35	0.62
$-NH_2$	0.85	0.08	0.25
–NHCHO	0.04	0.01	0.6
$-NHCOCH_3$	0.15	0.3	0.4
$-NHCOC_6H_5$	0.83	–	0.72
$-NHCONHC_6H_5$	0.12	0.06	0.11
$-NHSO_2CH_3$	1.15	0.33	0.64
$-CH(COCH_3)_2$	0.6	0.3	1.2
$-SCH_2CH_2OH$	1.7	0.05	0.66
$-SCH_2CH_2NH_2$	0.23	0.05	1.5
$-SCH_2CH_2CO_2H$	0.6	0.6	1.9
$-SCSNH_2$	3.8	0.08	1.3

X	I_{50} (μg/ml)		
	PASE	Type III	Type IV
$-OCH_3$	5.8	0.17	0.28
$-SCH_2$	1.6	1.1	3.8
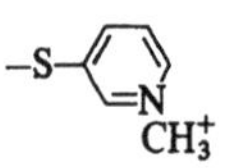	0.09	0.08	0.23

X	PASE[c]	Type IIIa R_{TEM}[d]	Type IV[e]
–OH(CA)[b]	0.06	0.07	0.03
–H	0.12	0.09	–
$-OCOCH_3$	0.04	–	–
$-OCONHCH_3$	1.5	2.5	–
$-OCH_3$	0.05	0.18	0.01
$-OCH_2C_6H_5$	0.005	0.1	0.02
$-SCH_3$	0.11	0.04	0.01
$-N(CH_2C_6H_5)_2$	0.002	0.04	0.01

Sources: [a]NEWALL et al. 1978. [b]BROWN 1981. Procedures differ, compare relative values with clavulanic acid (CA) in each case. [c]From *S. aureus* Russel. [d]From *E. coli*. [e]From *P. mirabilis* C889.

Table 63. Additional analogs of clavulanic acid

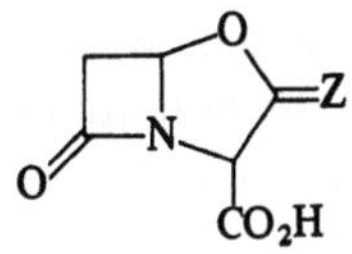

Z	Inhibition[a] *S. aureus* Russell	Inhibition[a] *E. coli* JT4/JT39	Z	Inhibition[a] *S. aureus* Russell	Inhibition[a] *E. coli* JT4/JT39
CH_2OH	0.05	0.07	CH_2NHR[b]	Syn	Syn
C_6H_5	<0.08	0.2			
$CH_2OCH_2OCH_3$	Syn	Syn	CH_2OH	0.6	–
$CH_2OCH(CH_3)OC_4H_9$	Syn	Syn	CH_3	Syn	–
CH_2OSO_3H	–	3.4	$COOCH_3$	0.11	0.18

Inactive[c]	Active[c]		
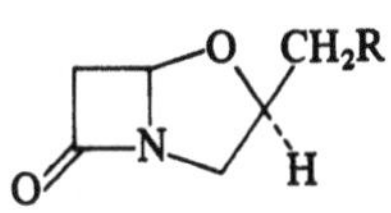	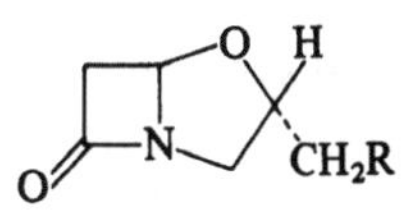		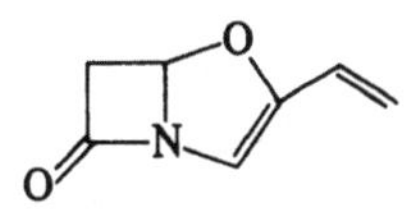
R	R		
–Br	–Br	$-OC_6H_4NO_2$	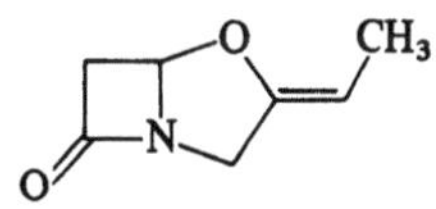
$-OCH_2C_6H_5$	$-OCH_2C_6H_5$	$-O_2CC_6H_4NO_2$	
–OCHO	–OCHO	$-SO_2C_6H_5$	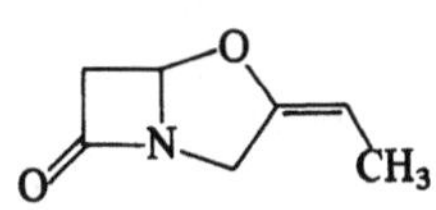
	–OH	$-SOC_6H_5$	
	–I	$-OCONHC_6H_5$	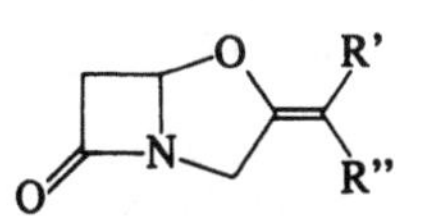
	$-SC_6H_5$	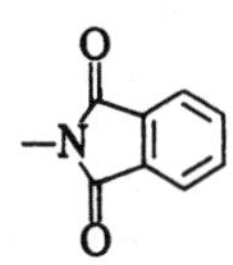	R', R''= $COOCH_3$, H; H, $COOCH_3$; $COOCH_3$, Cl; H, OH; H, OCH_3; OH, H; OCH_3, H

Sources: Cole 1980; Cooper 1980; Hunt et al. 1977; Bentley and Hunt 1978; Hunt 1979, 1981.
[a]Inhibitory activity indicated by I_{50} listed or by demonstration of synergy (Syn) with appropriate penicillin or cephalosporin. [b]R=CH_2CH_2OH, C_6H_5, $CH_2C_6H_5$, $CH_2C_6H_4F$, $CH_2C_6H_4OCH_3$, $CH_2C_6H_4NHCOCH_3$. [c]Inhibitors of β–lactamase from *S. aureus*.

levels than clavulanic acid. The relatively high tolerance for structural variation with retention of inhibitory activity is seen for the other 9-position substituents listed in Table 63. The analogs in Table 62 with phenylureido and the quaternized pyridinium substituents emphasize the potential to increase the level of β-lactamase inhibition activity over that of clavulanic acid with appropriate modifications of this side-chain. The latitude for structural variations of the clavams is also underscored by the activity, at least against penicillinase, reported for the analogs which carry no carboxyl group (Hunt et al. 1977; Bentley and Hunt 1978; Hunt 1979, 1981), also listed in Table 63, and the high activity exhibited especially against type I β-lactamases by the 2-ethyl oxapenem analog of clavulanic acid with an endocyclic double bond (Cherry et al. 1978).

E. Other Structure–Activity Relationships

The scope of the structure–activity relationships that have now been described for the β-lactams has required that the data selected for inclusion in this review focus on structural manipulations and biological properties that have led to clinically useful agents or major trends in biological activity that were important in achieving this end. Many other structural changes have been carried out have been less successful in this respect. Several reviews examine this aspect of β-lactam SAR. Hoover and Dunn (1979) summarize much of the systematic manipulation carried out on the penicillin and cephalosporin ring systems. Jung et al. (1980) similarly review direct manipulation of the penicillin and cephalosporin structures, and also include structures obtained by semi- and total syntheses directed at these ring systems. Much of the exploratory chemistry associated with the nonclassic β-lactams (clavulanic acid, 1-oxacephalosporin, carbapenems, nocardicins) is reviewed in detail by Cooper (1980).

References

Abraham EP, Newton GGF (1956) Comparison of the action of penicillinase on benzylpenicillin and cephalosporin N and the competitive inhibition of penicillinase by cephalosporin C. Biochem J 63:628–634

Acocella G, Baroni GC, Nicolis FB (1965) Adsorption and excretion of a new semisynthetic penicillin (betacin) in man. Curr Ther Res 7:226–234

Acred P, Brown DM, Knudsen ET, Rolinson GN, Sutherland R (1967) New semisynthetic penicillin active against *Pseudomonas pyocyanea*. Nature 215:25–30

Acred P, Hunter PA, Migen L, Rolinson GN (1971) α-Carboxy-3-thienylmethyl penicillin (BRL 2288), a new semisynthetic penicillin: in vivo evaluation. Antimicrob Agents Chemother – 1970, pp 396–401

Acred P, Ryan DM, Harding SM, Muggleton PW (1980) In vivo properties of GR20263. In: Nelson JD, Grassi C (eds) Current chemotherapy and infectious disease, vol 1. American Society of Microbiology, Washington DC, pp 271–273

Actor P, Pitkin DH, Lucyszyn G, Weisbach J, Bran JL (1976a) A new parenteral cephalosporin, SK & F 59962: Serum levels and urinary recovery in man. Chemotherapy (Tokyo) 5:253–257

Actor P, Pitkin DH, Lucyszyn G, Weisbach J, Bran JL (1976b) Cefatrizine (SK & F 60771) a new oral cephalosporin: Serum levels and urinary recovery in humans after oral or intramuscular administration – comparative study with cephalexin and cefazolin. Antimicrob Agents Chemother 9:800–803

Actor P, Uri JP, Zajac IH, Guarini JR, Phillips L, Pitkin D, Berges DH, Dunn GL, Hoover JRE, Weisbach J (1978) SK & F 75073, a new parenteral broad-spectrum cephalosporin with high and prolonged serum levels. Antimicrob Agents Chemother 13:784–790

Anonymous (1979) Sarmoxicillin, BL-91780, a new antibiotic. Drugs Future 4:672–674

Aoki H, Saki H, Kohsaka M, Konomi T, Hosoda J, Kubochi Y, Iguchi E, Imanaka H (1976) Nocardicin A, a new monocyclic β-lactam antibiotic I. Discovery, isolation and characterization. J Antibiot 29:492–500

Asawapokee N, Asawapokee P, Fu KP, Neu HC (1978) In vitro activity and beta-lactamase stability of BL-S786 compared with those of other cephalosporins. Antimicrob Agents Chemother 14:1–5

Ashton WT, Barash L, Brown JE, Brown RD, Canning LF, Chen A, Graham DW, Kahan FM, Kropp H, Sundelof JG, Rogers EF (1980) Z-2-Acylamino-3-substituted propenoates. Inhibitors of the renal dipeptidase (Dehydropeptidase-I) responsible for thienamycin metabolism. In: 20th intersci conf antimicrob agents chemother, New Orleans, Abstract 271

Baltzer B, Lund F, Rustrup-Andersen N (1979) Degredation of mecillinam in aqueous solution. J Pharm Sci 68:1207–1215

Baltzer B, Binderup E, Von Doehne W, Godtfredsen WU, Hansen K, Nillsen B, Sorensen H, Vangedal S (1980) Mutual pro-drugs of β-lactam antibiotics and β-lactamase inhibitors. J Antibiot 33:1183–1192

Banville J, Belleau B, Dextraze P, Douglas JL, Leitner F, Martel A, Menard M, Saintonge R, Veda Y (1981) Synthesis and structure-activity relationships in the penem series. 182nd ACS national meeting, New York, Abstract MEDCHEM 3

Barker BM, Prescott F (1973) Antimicrobial agents in medicine. Blackwell, London

Barza M, Berman H, Michaeli D, Molavi A, Weinstein L (1971) In vitro studies of BL-P1462, a new semisynthetic penicillin with antipseudomonas activity. Antimicrob Agents Chemother – 1970, pp 341–345

Basker MJ, Boon RJ, Hunter PA (1980) Comparative antibacterial properties in vitro of seven olivanic acid derivatives: MM 4550, MM 13902, MM 17880, MM 22380, MM 22381, MM 22382 and MM 22383. J Antibiot 33:878–884

Basker MJ, Bateson JH, Baxter AJG, Ponsford RJ, Roberts PM, Southgate R, Smale TC, Smith J (1981) Synthesis of 6-unsubstituted olivanic acid analogues and their antibacterial activities. J Antibiot 34:1224–1226

Bax RP, White LO, Holt A, Bywater M, Reeves DS (1981) Metabolism of β-lactam antibiotics. N Engl J Med 304:734–735

Baxter AJG, Ponsford RJ, Southgate R (1980) Synthesis of olivanic acid analogues. Preparation of 7-oxo-1-azabicyclo[3.2.0]hept-2-ene-2 carboxylates containing the 3-(2-acetamidoethenylthio) side chain. J Chem Soc Chem Commun: 429–431

Bentley PH, Brooks G, Gilpin ML, Hunt E (1977) Total synthesis of clavulanic acid analogues via isomerization of 7-oxo-4-oxa-1-azabicyclo[3.20]hep-2-enes. J Chem Soc Chem Commun: 905–906

Bentley PH, Hunt E (1978) Total synthesis of β-lactamase inhibitors based on the 4-oxa-1-azabicyclo[3.2.0]hept-7-one ring system. J Chem Soc [Perkin I]: 2222–2227

Bergan T (1978) Penicillins. In: Shoenfeld (ed) Antibiotics and chemotherapy, vol 25. Karger, Basel, pp 1–122

Berges DA (1975) 3-Acyloxymethyl-7-(2-thienylacetamido-3-cephem-4-carboxylic acids, an improved synthesis and biological properties. J Med Chem 18:1264–1265

Berges DA, Dunn GL, Hoover JRE, Schmidt SJ, Chan GW, Taggart JJ, Kinzig CM, Pfeiffer FR, Actor P, Sachs CS, Uri JR, Weisbach JA (1976) Preliminary studies on parenteral 3-tetrazolethiomethyl cephalosporins with high serum levels. In: 16th intersci conf antimicrob agents chemother, Chicago, abstract 87

Binderup ET (1980) Derivatives of penicillanic acid. U.S. Patent 4229443, assigned to Leo Pharmaceutical Products Ltd.

Binderup ET, Godtfredsen WO, Roholt K (1971) Orally active cephaloglycin esters. J Antibiot 24:767–773

Bodey GP, Deerake B (1971) In vitro studies of α-carboxyl-3-thienylmethyl penicillin, a new semisynthetic penicillin. Appl Microbiol 21:61–65

Bodey GP, LeBlanc B (1978) Pipericillin: in vitro evaluation. Antimicrob Agents Chemother 14:78–87
Bodey GP, Weaver S, Pan T (1978) PC904, a new semisynthetic penicillin. Antimicrob Agents Chemother 13:14–18
Boyd DB, Lunn WH (1979) Theoretical criteria for predicting biological activity of cephalosporin antibiotics. J Antibiot 32:855–856
Boyd DB, Herron DK, Lunn WHW, Spitzer WA (1980) Parabolic relationships between antibacterial activity of cephalosporins and β-lactam reactivity predicted from molecular orbital calculations. J Am Chem Soc 102:1812–1814
Brain EG, Doyle FP, Hardy K, Long AAW, Mehta MD, Miller D, Nayler JHC, Soulal MJ, Stove ER, Thomas GR (1962) Derivatives of 6-aminopenicillanic acid. Part II. Trisubstituted acetyl derivatives. J Chem Soc: 1445–1453
Brain EG, Doyle FP, Mehta MD, Miller D, Nayler JHC, Stove ER (1963) Derivatives of 6-aminopenicillanic acid. Part IV. Analogues of 7,6-dimethoxypenicillin in the naphthalene and quinoline series. J Chem Soc: 491–497
Breuer H, Treuner UD, Schneider HJ, Young MG, Bosch HI (1978) Diastereomeric 7-ureidoacetyl cephalosporins I. Superiority of 7α-H-L-isomers over D-isomers. J Antibiot 31:546–560
Breuer H, Lindner KR, Treuner UD (1980) Diastereomeric 7α-ureidoacetyl cephalosporins: preparation and antibacterial activity in vitro of 7-(α-ureido-2-amino-4-thiazolylacetyl)-cephalosporins. In: Nelson JD, Grassi C (eds) Current chemotherapy and infectious disease, vol 1. American Society of Microbiology, Washington DC, pp 282–285
Breuer H, Treuner UD, Denzel T, Applegate HE, Bonner DP, Bush K, Cimurusti CM, Koster WE, Siusarchyk WA, Sykes RB, Young M (1981) Monocyclic β-lactam antibiotics. Activity relationships with α-acylamino derivatives. In: 21st intersci conf antimicrob agents chemother, Chicago, abstract 878
Brorson JE, Norrby R (1978) Comparative in vitro activity of cefamandole, cefoxitin, cefuroxime, and cephalothin. Scand J Infect Dis [Suppl] 13:88–93
Broughall JM, Bywater MJ, Holt HA, Reeves DS (1979) Stabilization of cephalosporins in serum and plasma. J Antimicrob Chemother 5:471–472
Brown AG (1981) New naturally occurring β-lactam antibiotics and related compounds. J Antimicrob Chemother 7:15–48
Brown AG, Butterworth D, Cole M, Hanscomb G, Hood JD, Reading C, Rolinson GN (1976) Naturally occurring β-lactamase inhibitors with antibacterial activity. J Antibiot 29:668–669
Bryan DB, Hall RF, Holden KG, Huffman WF, Gleason JG (1977) Nuclear analogs of β-lactam antibiotics 2. The total synthesis of 8-oxo-4-thia-1-azabicyclo[4.2.0]-oct-2-ene-2-carboxylic acids. J Am Chem Soc 99:2353–2355
Bucourt R, Heymes R, Lutz A, Penasse L, Perronnet J (1980) New very efficient antibiotics in the field of cephalosporin derivatives. Philos Trans R Soc London B289:361–363
Bush K, Bonner DP, Sykes RB (1980a) Izumenolide – a novel β-lactamase inhibitor produced by *Micromonospora* II. Biological properties. J Antibiot 33:1267–1269
Bush K, Freudenberger J, Sykes RB (1980b) Inhibition of *Escherichia coli* TEM-2 β-lactamase by the sulfated compounds izumenolide, panosialin and sodium dodecyl sulfate. J Antibiot 33:1560–1562
Bush K, Freudenberger JS, Pilkiewicz FG, Remsburg BJ, Sykes RB (1981) Interaction of the monobactam SQ20776 with β-lactamases. In: 21st intersci conf antimicrob agents chemother, Chicago, abstract 488
Busson R, Vanderhaeghe H (1976) Preparation and isomerization of 5-epibenzylpenicillins. J Org Chem 41:2561–2565
Bustrack JA, Lawson LA, Bauer LA, Wilson HD, Foster TS (1980) A comparative pharmacokinetic and safety study of an investigational oral cephalosporin RMI 19592. Curr Ther Res 28:208–217
Cama LD, Christensen BG (1974) Total synthesis of β-lactam antibiotics VII. Total synthesis of (±)-1-oxacephalothin. J Am Chem Soc 96:7582–7584
Cama LD, Christensen BG (1978a) Total synthesis of thienamycin analogues 1. Synthesis of the thienamycin nucleus and dl-descysteaminylthienamycin. J Am Chem Soc 100:8006–8007

Cama LD, Christensen BG (1978b) Structure activity relationships of non-classical β-lactam antibiotics. In: Clarke FH (ed) Annual reports in medicinal chemistry – 13, Academic Press, New York, Chap. 16

Cama LD, Christensen BG (1980) Total synthesis of thienamycin analogs II. Synthesis of 2-alkyl and 2-aryl thienamycin nuclei. Tetrahedron Lett 21:2013–2016

Cartwright SJ, Coulson AFW (1979) A semisynthetic penicillanase inactivator. Nature 278:360–361

Charnas RL, Fisher J, Knowles JR (1978) Chemical studies on the inactivation of *Escherichia coli* RTEM β-lactamase by clavulanic acid. Biochemistry 17:2185–2189

Charnas RL, Knowles JR (1981) Inhibition of the RTEM β-lactamase from Escherichia coli. Interaction of enzyme with derivatives of olivanic acid. Biochemistry 20:2732–2737

Chauvette RR, Flynn EH, Jackson BG, Lavagnino ER, Morin RB, Mueller RA, Pioch RP, Roeske RW, Ryan CW, Spencer JL, van Heyningen E (1963) Structure-activity relationships among 7-acylamidocephalosporanic acids. Antimicrob Agents Chemother – 1962, pp 687–694

Cherry PC, Cook MC, Foxton MW, Gregson M, Gregory GI, Webb GB (1977) 7 α-(α-Hydroxyiminoarylacetamido)cephalosporanic acids and related compounds. In: Elks J (ed) Recent advances in the chemistry of β-lactam antibiotics. Chemical Society, London, Chap. 15

Cherry PC, Newall CE, Watson NS (1978) Preparation of the 7-oxo-4-oxa-1-azabicyclo[3.2.0]hept-2-ene system and the reversible cleavage of its oxazoline ring. J Chem Soc Chem Commun: 469–470

Cherry PC, Newall CE, Watson NS (1979) Synthesis of antibacterial pen-2-em-3-carboxylic acids from clavulanic acid. J Chem Soc Chem Commun: 663–664

Cherry PC, Evans DN, Newall CE, Watson NS (1980) Conversion of clavulanic acid into thiadeoxa nuclear analogues. Tetrahedron Lett 21:561–564

Chow AW, Hall NM, Hoover JRE, Dolan MM, Ferlauto RJ (1966) Semisynthetic penicillins III. Heterocyclic penicillins. J Med Chem 9:551–555

Christensen BG, Dininno FP (1979) 6-(1′-Hydroxyethyl)-2-aminoethylthio-oxapen-2-em-3-carboxylic acid. U.S. Patent 4172895, assigned to Merck & Co., Inc.

Cimarusti CM, Sykes RB, Applegate HE, Bonner DP, Breuer H, Chang HW, Denzel T, Floyd DM, Fritz A, Koster WH, Liu W, Parker WL, Rathnum ML, Slusarchyk WA, Treuner U, Young M (1981a) Monobactams – monocyclic β-lactam antibiotics produced by bacteria. 182nd Am chem soc natl mtg, New York, abstract MEDI 4

Cimarusti CM, Breuer H, Denzel T, Kronenthal DK, Treuner UD, Bonner DP, Sykes RB (1981b) Monobactams – monocyclic β-lactam antibiotics. Structure-activity relationships with α-oximino acyl derivatives. 21st intersci conf antimicrob agents chemother, Chicago, abstract 487

Clarke HT, Johnson JR, Robinson R (eds) (1949) The chemistry of penicillin. Princeton University Press, Princeton NJ

Clayton JP, Cole M, Elson SW, Hardy KD, Mizen LW, Sutherland R (1975) Preparation, hydrolysis and oral absorption of α-carboxy esters of carbenicillin. J Med Chem 18:172–177

Cohen SA, Pratt RF (1980) Inactivation of *Bacillus cereus* β-lactamase I by 6β-bromopenicillanic acid: Mechanism. Biochemistry 19:3996–4003

Cole M (1979a) Inhibition of β-lactamases. In: Hamilton-Miller JMT, Smith JT (eds) β-Lactamases. Academic Press, New York, pp 205–289

Cole M (1979b) Inhibitors of antibiotic-inactivating enzymes. In: Williams JD (ed) Antibiotic interactions. Academic Press, London, pp 99–135

Cole M (1980) β-lactams as β-lactamase inhibitors. Philos Trans R Soc London B289:207–223

Cole M, Elson S, Fullbrook PD (1972) Inhibition of the β-lactamase of *Escherichia coli* and *Klebsiella aerogenes* by semi-synthetic penicillins. Biochem J 127:295–308

Cole M, Howarth TT, Reading C (1979) Antibacterial clavulanic acid and its salts. U.S. Patent 4110165, assigned to Beecham Group Ltd

Comber KR, Horton R, Mizen L, White AR, Sutherland R (1980) Activity of amoxicillin/clavulanic acid (2:1) [BRL 25000, Augmentin] in vitro and in vivo. In: Nelson JD, Grassi

C (eds) Current chemotherapy and infectious disease, vol 1. American Society Microbiology, Washington DC, pp 343–344
Cooper RDG (1978) Chiral synthesis of a new β-lactam antibiotic. 176th natl mtg Am chem soc, Miami Beach, abstract MEDI 16
Cooper RDG (1980) New β-lactam antibiotics. In: Sammes PG (ed) Topics in antibiotic chemistry, vol 3. Ellis Horwood, Chichester, pp 39–199
Corbett DF, Howorth TT, Stirling I (1977) Oxidation of clavulanic acid and a ready synthesis of the 7-oxo-4-oxa-1-azalicyclo[3.2.0]hept-2-ene ring system. J Chem Soc Chem Commun: 808
Corrado ML, Landesman SH, Cherubin CE (1980) Influence of inoculum size on activity of cefoperazone, cefotaxime, moxalactam, piperacillin, and N-formimidoyl thienamycin (MK0787) against *Pseudomonas aeruginosa*. Antimicrob Agents Chemother 18:893–896
Coyette J, Ghuysen JM, Fontana R (1980) The penicillin-binding proteins in *Streptococcus faecalis*, ATCC 9790. Eur J Biochem 110:445–456
Curtis NAC, Orr D, Ross GW, Boulton MG (1979) Affinities of penicillins and cephalosporins for penicillin binding proteins of *Escherichia coli* K12 and their antibacterial activity. Antimicrob Agents Chemother 16:533–539
Curtis NAC, Orr DC, Boulton MG (1980a) The action of some β-lactam antibiotics on the penicillin-binding proteins of gram-negative bacteria. Philos Trans R Soc London B289:368–370
Curtis NAC, Boulton MG, Orr D, Ross GW (1980b) The competition of α-sulfocephalosporins for the penicillin binding proteins of *Escherichia coli* K12 and *Pseudomonas aeruginosa* – Comparison with effects upon morphology. J Antimicrob Chemother 6:189–196
Dash CH (1975) Penicillin allergy and cephalosporins. J Antimicrob Chemother [Suppl] 1:107–118
DeKoning JJ, Marx AF, Poot MM, Smid PM, Verweij J (1977) Stereo-specific synthesis of biologically active cephalosporin R-sulphoxides. In: Elks J (ed) Recent advances in the chemistry of β-lactam antibiotics. Chemical Society, London, pp 161–166
Dininno F, Beattie TR, Christensen BG (1977) Aldol condensation of regiospecific penicillinate and cephalosporanate enolates. Hydroxyethylation at C-6 and C-7. J Org Chem 42:2960–2963
Dolan MM, Bondi A, Hoover JRE, Tumilowicz R, Stewart RC, Ferlauto RJ (1962) A new semisynthetic penicillin, SK&F 12141 I. Microbiological studies. Antimicrob Agents Chemother – 1961, pp 648–654
Dolfini JE, Applegate HE, Bach G, Basch H, Bernstein J, Schwartz J, Weisenborn FL (1971) A new class of semisynthetic penicillins and cephalosporins derived from D-2-(1,4-cyclohexadienyl)-glycine. J Med Chem 14:117–119
Douglas JL, Doyle TW, Conway TT, Menard M, Belleau B, Misiek M (1978) Synthesis and structure activity relationships of nuclear analogs of cephalosporins. 176th natl mtg Am chem soc, Miami Beach, Abstract MEDI 11
Doyle FP, Nayler JHC (1966) 6-(α,α,α-Trisubstituted-acetamido) penicillanic acids and salts thereof. U.S. Patent 3245983, assigned to Beecham Group, Ltd
Doyle FP, Nayler JHC, Smith H, Stove ER (1961a) Some novel acid stable penicillins. Nature 191:1091–1092
Doyle FP, Long AAW, Nayler JHC, Stove ER (1961b) A new penicillin stable towards both acid and penicillinase. Nature 192:1183–1184
Doyle FP, Hardy K, Nayler JHC, Soulal MJ, Stone ER, Waddington HRJ (1962a) Derivatives of 6-aminopenicillanic acid, part III. 2,6-Dialkoxybenzoyl derivatives. J Chem Soc: 1453–1458
Doyle FP, Fosker GR, Nayler JHC, Smith H (1962b) Derivatives of 6-aminopenicillanic acid, part I. α-Aminobenzylpenicillin and some related compounds. J Chem Soc: 1440–1444
Doyle FP, Nayler JHC (1964) Penicillins and related structures. In: Harper NJ, Simmonds AB (eds) Advances in drug research, vol 1. Academic Press, New York, pp 1–69

Doyle FP, Hanson JC, Long AAW, Nayler JHC (1963 a) Derivatives of 6-aminopenicillanic acid, part VII. Further 3,5-disubstituted isoxazole-4-carboxylic acid derivatives. J Chem Soc: 5845–5854
Doyle FP, Hanson JC, Long AAW, Nayler JHC, Stove ER (1963 b) Derivatives of 6-aminopenicillanic acid, part VI. Penicillins from 3- and 5-phenylisoxazole-4-carboxylic acids and their alkyl and halogen derivatives. J Chem Soc: 5838–5845
Dunn GL, Hoover JRE, Berges DA, Taggart JJ, Davis LD, Dietz EM, Jakas DR, Yim N, Actor P, Uri JV, Weisbach JA (1976) Orally active 7-phenylglycyl cephalosporins. Structure-activity studies related to cefatrizine (SK&F 60771). J Antibiot 29:65–80
Eglington AJ (1977) Syntheses based on 1,2-secopenicillins; the synthesis of the 1-oxadethiapenem ring system. J Chem Soc Chem Commun: 720
Eickhoff TC, Ehret JM (1976) In vitro comparison of cefoxitin, cefamandole, cephalexin, and cephalothin. Antimicrob Agents Chemother 9:994–999
Eickhoff TC, Ehret JM (1981) In vitro evaluation of SQ26726. 21st intersci conf antimicrob agents chemother, Chicago, Abstract 497
Ekstrom B, Gomez-Revilla A, Mollberg R, Thelin H, Sjoberg B (1965) Semisynthetic penicillins III. Aminopenicillins via azidopenicillins. Acta Chem Scand 19:281–299
English AR, Retsema JA, Ray VA, Lynch JE (1972) Carbenicillin indanyl sodium, an orally active derivative of carbenicillin. Antimicrob Agents Chemother 1:185–191
English AR, Retsema JA, Girard AE, Lynch JE, Barth WE (1978) CP45889, a beta-lactamase inhibitor that extends the antibacterial spectrum of β-lactams: Initial bateriological characterization. Antimicrob Agents Chemother 14:414–419
Ernst I, Gosteli J, Greengrass CW, Hollich W, Jackman DE, Pfaendler HR, Woodward RB (1978) The penems, a new class of β-lactam antibiotics: 6-Acylaminopenem-3-carboxylic acids. J Am Chem Soc 100:8214–8222
Essery JM (1969) Preparation and antibacterial activity of α-(5-tetrazolyl)benzylpenicillin. J Med Chem 12:703–705
Fernandes PB, Bonner DP, Whitney RR, Miller BH, Baughn CO, Sykes RB (1981) SQ26776: Efficacy in experimental infections. 21st intersci conf antimicrob agents chemother, Chicago, Abstract 490
Fillastre JP, Leroy A, Godin M, Oksenhendler G, Humbert G (1978) Pharmacokinetics of cefoxitin sodium in normal subjects and in uremic patients. J Antimicrob Chemother [Suppl B] 4:79–83
Fisher J, Charnas RL, Knowles JR (1978) Kinetic studies on the inactivation of *Escherichia coli* RTEM β-lactamase by clavulanic acid. Biochemistry 17:2180–2184
Fisher J, Belasco JG, Charnas RL, Khosla S, Knowles JR (1980) β-Lactamase inactivation by mechanism-based reagents. Philos Trans R Soc London B289:309–319
Fisher J, Charnas RL, Bradley SM, Knowles JR (1981) Inactivation of the RTEM β-lactamase from *Escherichia coli*. Interaction of penam sulfones with enzyme. Biochemistry 20:2726–2731
Florey HW, Chain E, Heatley MG, Jennings MA, Saunders AG, Abraham EP, Florey ME (1949) Antibiotics, vol 2. Oxford University Press, London
Foord RD (1976) Cefuroxime: Human pharmacokinetics. Antimicrob Agents Chemother 9:741–747
Foulds G, Barth WE, Bianchine JR, English AR, Girard D, Hayes SL, O'Brien MM, Somani P (1980) Pharmacokinetics of CP45899 and prodrug CP47904 in animals and humans. In: Nelson JD, Grassi C (eds) Current chemotherapy and infectious disease, vol 1. American Society Microbiology, Washington DC, p 353
Foxton MW, Newall CE, Ward P (1981) Total synthesis of 6-Substituted pen-2-em-3-carboxylic acids. In: Gregory GI (ed) Recent advances in the chemistry of β-lactam antibiotics. The Royal Society of Chemistry, London, pp 281–290
Francheschi G, Foglio M, Arcamone F (1980) Antibacterial activity of novel broad-spectrum (5R)-penem derivatives. J Antibiot 33:453–454
Fu KP, Neu HC (1978 a) Piperacillin, a new penicillin active against many bacteria resistant to other penicillins. Antimicrob Agents Chemother 13:358–367
Fu KP, Neu HC (1978 b) β-Lactamase stability of HR 756, a novel cephalosporin compared to that of cefuroxime and cefoxitin. Antimicrob Agents Chemother 14:322–326

Fu KP, Neu HC (1979) The comparative β-lactamase resistance and inhibitory activity of 1-oxacephalosporin, cefoxitin, and cefotaxime. J Antibiot 32:909–913
Fu KP, Neu HC (1980) Comparative β-lactamase resistance and inhibitory activity of 1-oxacephalosporin, cefoxitin, and cefotaxime. In: Nelson JD, Grassi C (eds) Current chemotherapy and infectious disease, vol 1. American Society of Microbiology, Washington DC, pp 73–74
Fuchs PC, Thornsberry C, Barry AL, Gavan TL, Gerlach EH, Jones RN (1977) Ticarcillin, carbenicillin, and BL-P1908. In vitro comparison of three antipseudomonal semisynthetic penicillins. J Antibiot 30:1098–1106
Gadebusch HH, Miraglia GJ, Basch HI, Goodwin C, Pan S, Renz K (1972) Cephradine – a new orally absorbed cephalosporin antibiotic. In: Hejzlar M, Semonsky M, Masak S (eds) Advances in antimicrobial and antineoplastic chemotherapy, vol I/2. University Park Press, New York, pp 1059–1062
Gadebusch HH, Basch HI, Lukaszow P, Remsburg B, Schwind R (1978) Diastereomeric 7-ureidoacetyl cephalosporins III. Contribution of D- and L-isomers to the growth inhibiting activities of 7α-H and 7α-OCH_3 derivatives for gram-positive and gram-negative bacteria. J Antibiot 31:570–579
Gambertoglio JG, Barriere SL, Lin ET, Conte JE (1980) Pharmacokinetics of mecillinam in healthy subjects. Antimicrob Agents Chemother 18:952–956
Geddes AM, Wise R (eds) (1977) Mecillinam. J Antimicrob Chemother 3 [Suppl B] 1–160
Georgopapadakou NH, Lin FY, Andetti MA (1980) Comparison of D and L isomers in 7-substituted cephalosporins. In: Nelson JD, Grassi C (eds) Current chemotherapy and infectious disease, vol 1. American Society Microbiology, Washington DC, pp 284–285
Georgopapadakou NH, Smith SA, Cimarusti CM, Sykes RB (1981a) Binding of monobactams to penicillin binding proteins of *Escherichia coli* and *Staphylococcus aureus*. Relation to antibacterial activity. 21st intersci conf antimicrob agents chemother, Chicago, Abstract 881
Georgopapadakou NH, Smith SA, Sykes RB (1981b) Mode of action of the monobactam SQ26776. 21st intersci conf antimicrob agents chemother, Chicago, Abstract 880
Girijavallabhan VM, Ganguly AK, McCombie SW, Pinto P, Rizvi R (1981) Chiral synthesis of Sch29482. 21st intersci conf antimicrob agents chemother, Chicago, Abstract 829
Gorman M, Ryan CW (1972) Structure-activity relationships of β-lactam antibiotics. In: Flynn EH (ed) Cephalosporins and penicillins. Academic Press, New York, pp 532–582
Gottschlich R, Rudolph V, Wahlig H, Poetsch E (1980) EMD39734 and related pyridylurediopenicillins: Structure-activity relationships of a new class of ureidopenicillins. 20th intersci conf antimicrob agents chemother, New Orleans, Abstract 146
Gottstein WJ, Kaplan MA, Cooper JA, Silver VH, Nachfolger SJ, Granatek AP (1976) 7-(2-Aminomethylphenylacetamido)-3-(1-carboxymethyltetrazol-5-yl-thiomethyl)-3-cephem-4-carboxylic acid. J Antibiot 29:1226–1229
Grant MS, Pain DL, Slack R (1965) Isothiazoles, part VI. Phenylisothiazoles. J Chem Soc: 3842–3845
Grappel SH, Phillips L, Actor P, Weisbach JA (1980) Comparison of cefonicid with cefamandole and cefoxitin as prophylactic agents in mouse protection tests. In: Nelson JD, Grassi C (eds) Current chemotherapy and infectious disease, vol 1. American Society Microbiology, Washington DC, pp 249–250
Greenwood D, O'Grady F (1973) FL1060: A new beta-lactam antibiotic with novel properties. J Clin Pathol 26:1–6
Greenwood D, O'Grady F (1975) Potent combinations of β-lactam antibiotics using the β-lactamase inhibition principle. Chemotherapy (Basel) 21:330–341
Gregory GI (ed) (1981) Recent advances in the chemistry of β-lactam antibiotics. The Royal Society of Chemistry, London
Grunberg E, Cleeland R, Beskid G, DeLorenzo WF (1976) In vivo synergy between β-amidinopenicillanic acid derivatives and other antibiotics. Antimicrob Agents Chemother 9:589–594
Guddal E, Morch P, Tybring L (1962) Penicillin oxides. Tetrahedron Lett 3:381–385
Gural RP, Oden E, Lin C, Brick I, Darragh A, Digiore C (1981) Oral absorption and tolerance of a new penem antibiotic, Sch 29482. 21st intersci conf antimicrob agents chemother, Chicago, Abstract 836

Habridge JB (1978) Clavulanic acid derivatives. German patent 2818309, assigned to Beecham Group Ltd
Hagiwara D, Takeno H, Aratini M, Hemmi K, Hashimoto M (1980) Synthesis and antibacterial activity of new 1-oxa-1-dethiacephalosporins. J Med Chem 23:1108–1113
Hakimelahi GH, Just G (1979a) β-Lactams V. The synthesis of D,L-4-hydroxymethylnocardicin A (17N), D,L-4-hydroxymethyl-N-phenylacetylnocardicinic acid (8N-f), and their α-epimers 17U and 8U-f. Can J Chem 57:1932–1938
Hakimelahi GH, Just G (1979b) β-Lactams VI. The synthesis of homocycloanalogs of nocardicin A. Can J Chem 57:1939–1944
Hamashima Y, Narisada M, Yoshida M, Uyeo S, Tsuji T, Kikkawa I, Nagata W (1978) Efficient synthesis of 1-oxacephalosporins from penicillins. 176th natl mtg Am chem Soc, Miami Beach, Abstract MEDI 14
Hannah J, Johnson CR, Wagner AF, Watson E (1982) Quaternary heterocyclylamino β-lactams: A generic alternative to the classical acylamino side chain. J Med Chem 25:457–469
Hansch C, Steward AR (1964) The use of substituent constants in the analysis of structure-activity relationships in penicillin derivatives. J Med Chem 7:691–694
Hanson JC, Nayler JHC, Taylor T, Gore PH (1965) Derivatives of 6-aminopenicillanic acids, part IX. 2,4-Di- and 2,4,5-trisubstituted-3-furylpenicillins. J Chem Soc: 5984–5988
Harding SM, Ayrton J, Thornton JE, Munro AJ, Hogg MIJ (1980) Cephalosporin GR 20263: Pharmacokinetics in normal subjects. 20th intersci conf antimicrob agents chemother, New Orleans, Abstr 93
Hare RS, Miller GH, Naples L, Sabatelli F, Loebenberg D, Waitz JA (1981) Sch 29482, a new penem antibiotic: Evaluation of in vitro activity and effect of test conditions. 21st intersci conf antimicrob agents chemother, Chicago, Abstr 831
Harvengt C, Meunier H, Lang F (1977) Pharmacokinetic study of cefazaflur compared to cephalothin and cefazolin. J Clin Pharmacol 17:128–133
Hatanaka M, Ishimaru T (1973) Synthetic penicillins. Heterocyclic analogs of ampicillin. Structure-activity relationships. J Med Chem 16:978–984
Heatley NG, Florey HW (1953) A comparison of the biological properties of cephalosporin N and penicillin. Brit J Pharmacol 8:252–258
Hinkle AM, Bodey GP (1980) In vitro evaluation of Ro 13-9904. Antimicrob Agents Chemother 18:574–578
Hinkle AM, LeBlanc B, Bodey GP (1980) In vitro evaluation of cefoperazone. Antimicrob Agents Chemother 17:423–427
Hirata T, Ogasa T, Saito H, Kobayashi S, Sato A, Ono Y, Hashimoto Y, Takasawa S, Sato K, Mineura K (1982) Antimicrobial activity of carbacephem compounds, novel cephalosporin-like β-lactams. 22nd intersci cont antimicrob agents chemother, Miami Beach, Abstr 557
Hoover JRE, Dunn GL (1979) The β-lactam antibiotics. In: Wolff M (ed) Burgers medicinal chemistry, 4th edn, part II. Wiley, New York, pp 83–172
Hoover JRE, Chow AW, Stedman RJ, Hall NM, Greenberg HS, Dolan MM, Ferlauto RJ (1964) Semisynthetic penicillins I. 2-Biphenylpenicillins. J Med Chem 7:245–251
Horikawa S, Ogawara H (1980) Penicillin binding proteins in *Bacillus subtilis*. The effects of penicillin binding proteins and the antibacterial activities of β-lactams. J Antibiot 33:614–619
Hosoda J, Konomi T, Tani N, Aoki H, Imanaka H (1977) Isolation of new nocardicins from *Nocardia uniformis* subsp. *tsuyamanensis*. Agric Biol Chem 41:2013–2020
Huffman WF, Hall RF, Grant JA, Holden KG (1978) Nuclear analogs of β-lactam antibiotics 4. Total synthesis of bisnorisopenicillins from antibacterially active monocyclic β-lactam precursors. J Med Chem 21:413–415
Hunt E (1979) Dehydrative decarboxylation of clavulanic acid. A ready synthesis of 7-oxo-3-vinyl-4-oxa-1-azabicyclo[3.2.0]hept-2-ene. J Chem Soc Chem Commun: 686–687
Hunt E (1981) Decarboxylation of clavulanic acid and its 9-methyl ester. J Chem Res (S): 64
Hunt E, Bentley PH, Brooks G, Gilpin M (1977) Total synthesis of β-lactamase inhibitors related to clavulanic acid. J Chem Soc Chem Commun: 906–907

Hunter PA, Reading C (1976) Sodium clavulanate, a novel and potent β-lactamase inhibitor. 16th intersci conf antimicrob agents chemother, Chicago, Abstract 211
Hunter PA, Webb JR (1980) Comparative in vitro activity of two novel β-lactamase inhibitors – clavulanic acid and CP 45899. In: Nelson JD, Grassi C (eds) Current chemotherapy and infectious disease, vol 1. American Society Microbiology, Washington DC, pp 340–342
Imada A, Nozaki Y, Kintaka K, Okonogi K, Kitano K, Harada S (1980) C-19393S_2 and H_2, new carbapenem antibiotics I. Taxonomy of the producing strain, fermentation and antibacterial properties. J Antibiotics 33:1417–1424
Imada A, Kitano K, Kitaka K, Muroi M, Asai M (1981) Sulfazecin and isosulfazecin, novel β-lactam antibiotics of bacterial origins. Nature 289:590–591
Indelicato JM, Norvilas TT, Pfeiffer RR, Wheeler WJ, Wilham WL (1974) Substituent effects on the base hydrolysis of penicillins and cephalosporins. Competitive intramolecular nucleophilic amino attack in cephalosporins. J Med Chem 17:523–527
Indelicato JM, Dinner A, Peters LR, Wilham WL (1977) Hydrolysis of 3-chloro-3-cephems. Intramolecular nucleophilic attack in cefaclor. J Med Chem 20:961–963
Jung FA, Pilgrim WR, Poyser JP, Siret PJ (1980) The chemistry and antimicrobial activity of new synthetic β-lactam antibiotics. In: Sammes PG (ed) Topics in antibiotic chemistry, vol 4. Ellis Horwood, Chichester, pp 10–273
Kaczka E, Folkers K (1949) Desthiobenzylpenicillin and other hydrogenolysis products of benzylpenicillin. In: Clarke HT, Johnson JR, Robins R (eds) The chemistry of penicillin. Princeton University Press, Princeton, pp 243–268
Kahan FM, Goegelman R, Currie SA, Jackson M, Stapley EO, Miller TW, Miller AK, Hendlin D, Mochales S, Hernandez S, Woodruff HB (1976) Thienamycin. A new β-lactam antibiotic. 16th intersci conf antimicrob agents chemother, Chicago, Abstract 227
Kamimura T, Matsumoto Y, Okada N, Mine Y, Nishida M, Goto S, Kuwahara S (1979) Ceftizoxime (FK 749), a new parenteral cephalosporin: in vitro and in vivo antibacterial activities. Antimicrob Agents Chemother 16:540–548
Kamiya T (1977) Studies on the new monocyclic β-lactam antibiotics, nocardicins. In: Elks J (ed) Recent advances in chemistry of β-lactam antibiotics. Chemical Society, London, pp 281–294
Katsu K, Inoue M, Ohya Y, Kitoh K, Mitsuhashi S (1981) In vitro and in vivo antibacterial activities of E-0702, a new parenteral cephalosporin. 21st intersci conf antimicrob agents chemother, Chicago, Abstract 119
Kemp JEG, Closier MD, Naryana S, Stefania MH (1980) Nucleophilic S_N2 displacements of penicillin-6-triflates and cephalosporin 7-triflates. 6β-Iodopenicillanic acid, a new β-lactamase inhibitor. Tetrahedron Lett 21:2991–2994
Kimura T, Endo H, Yoshikawa M, Muranishi S, Sezaki H (1978) Carrier mediated transport systems for aminopenicillins in rat small intestine. J Pharmacobio-Dyn 1:262–267
Kimura Y, Motokawa K, Nagata H, Kameda Y, Matsuura S, Myama M, Yoshida T (1982) Asparenomycins A, B and C, new carbapenem antibiotics IV. Antibacterial activity. J Antibiot 35:32–38
King A, Shannon K, Phillips I (1980) In vitro antibacterial activity and susceptibility of cefsulodin, an antipseudomonal cephalosporin, to β-lactamases. Antimicrob Agents Chemother 17:165–169
Kirby WMM (chairman) (1970) Symposium on carbenicillin. J Infect Dis 122 [Suppl]: S1–S116 (16 articles)
Knott-Hunziker V, Waley SG, Orlek BS, Sammes PG (1979) Penicillinase active sites: Labelling of serine-44 in β-lactamase I by 6β-bromopenicillanic acid. FEBS Lett 99:59–61
Koczka I, Feher O, Vargha L (1970) Pirazlocillin: A new semisynthetic penicillin. In: Progress in antimicrobial agents and chemotherapy. Proc of the 6th int congress of chemotherapy, vol 1. University Park Press, Baltimore, pp 44–55
Koe BK, Seto TA, English AR, McBride TJ (1963) Preparation and antibiotic properties of some phosphinylaminopenicillanic acids and phosphinothiolaminopenicillanic acids. J Med Chem 6:653–658
Koenig HB, Metzger KG, Offe HA, Schroeck W (1977) Antibacterial activity and structural constants of acylureidomethylpenicillins. In: Elks J (ed) Recent advances in the chemistry of β-lactam antibiotics. Chemical Society, London, pp 78–91

Kojo H, Mine Y, Nishida M, Yokota T (1977) Nocardicin A, a new monocyclic β-lactam antibiotic IV. Factors influencing the in vitro activity of nocardicin A. J Antibiot 30:926–931

Komatsu T, Okuda T, Noguchi H, Fukasawa M, Yano K, Kato M, Mitsuhashi S (1980) SM-1652, a new parenterally active cephalosporin: microbiological studies. In: Nelson JD, Grassi C (eds) Current chemotherapy and infectious disease, vol 1. American Society of Microbiology, Washington DC, pp 275–278

Koupal LR, Weissberger B, Shungu DL, Weinberg E, Gadebusch HH (1983) Quaternary heterocyclamino β-lactams II. The in vitro antibacterial properties of L-640, 876, a new type of β-lactam antibiotic. J Antibiot 36:47–53

Kropp H, Kahan JS, Kahan FM, Sundelof J, Darland G, Birnbaum J (1976) Thienamycin. A new β-lactam antibiotic II. In vitro and in vivo evaluation. 16th intersci conf antimicrob agents chemother, Chicago, Abstract 228

Kropp H, Sundelof JG, Kahan JS, Kahan FM, Birnbaum J (1980a) MK 0787 (N-formimidoyl thienamycin): evaluation of in vitro and in vivo activities. Antimicrob Agents Chemother 17:993–1000

Kropp H, Sundelof JG, Hajdu R, Kahan FM (1980b) Metabolism of thienamycin and related carbapenem antibiotics by the renal dipeptidase: Dehydropeptidase-I. 20th intersci conf antimicrob agents chemother, New Orleans, Abstract 272

Kucers K, Bennett N McK (1975) The use of Antibiotics, 2nd edn, Heinemann, London

Kuck NA, Redin GS (1978) In vitro and in vivo activity of piperacillin, a new broad-spectrum semisynthetic penicillin. J Antibiot 30:1175–1182

Kukolja S (1971) A stereoselective synthesis of 6-phthalimido-5-epipenicillanates. J Am Chem Soc 93:6269

Kurita M, Teraji T, Saito Y, Hadara H, Hattori K, Kamiya T, Nishida M, Takano T (1972) Structure-activity studies in semisynthetic cephalosporins. In: Hejzlar M, Semonsky M, Masak S (eds) Advances in antimicrobial and antineoplastic chemotherapy, vol I/2. University Park Press, New York, pp 1055–1057

Kurtz S, Holmes K, Turck M (1975) Disparity between inhibitory and killing effects of BL-P1654. Antimicrob Agents Chemother 7:215–218

Labia R, Kuzmierczak A, Guionie M, Masson JM (1980) Some bacterial proteins with affinity for cefotaxime. J Antimicrob Chemother 6 [Suppl A]: 19–23

Lamb SW, Foglesong MA (1976) Cefaclor stability in blood. 16th intersci conf antimicrob agents chemother, Chicago, Abstract 355

Lang M, Prasad K, Halick W, Gosteli J, Ernst I, Woodward RB (1979) The penems, a new class of β-lactam antibiotics 2. Total synthesis of racemic 6-unsubstituted representatives. J Am Chem Soc 101:6296–6301

Lang M, Prasad K, Gosteli J, Woodward RB (1980) The penems, a new class of β-lactam antibiotics 6. Synthesis of 2-alkylthiopenem carboxylic acids. Helv Chem Acta 63:1093–1097

Leitner F, Misiek M, Pursiano TA, Buck RE, Chisholm DR, DeRegis RG, Tsai YH, Price KE (1976) Laboratory evaluation of BL-S786, a cephalosporin with broad spectrum antibacterial activity. Antimicrob Agents Chemother 10:426–435

Liu WC, Astle G, Wells JS, Trejo WH, Principe PA, Rathnum ML, Parker WL, Kocy OR, Sykes RB (1980) Izumenolide – a novel β-lactamase inhibitor produced by *Micromonospora* I. Detection, isolation and characterization. J Antibiot 33:1256–1261

Loebenberg D, Miller GH, Moss EL, Oden E, Hare RS, Chung M, Waitz JA (1981) Sch 29482, a new penem antibiotic. Relationship between in vitro activity, in vivo potency and pharmacokinetics. 21st intersci conf antimicrob agents chemother, Chicago, Abstract 835

Long AAW, Nayler JHC (1972) p-Hydroxyampicillin and salts thereof. U.S. Patent 3674776, assigned to Beecham Group Ltd

Loosemore MJ, Pratt RF (1978) On the epimerization of 6α-bromopenicillanic acid and the preparation of 6β-bromopenicillanic acid. J Org Chem 43:3611–3613

Lowe G, Ridley DD (1973) Synthesis of β-lactams by photolytic Wolff rearrangement. J Chem Soc Perkin Trans I: 2024–2029

Lund FJ (1977) 6β-Amidinopenicillanic acids – synthesis and antibacterial properties. In: Elks J (ed) Recent advances in the chemistry of β-lactam antibiotics. Chemical society, London, pp 25–45

Lund F, Tybring L (1971) 6-β-Amidinopenicillanic acids – a new group of antibiotics. Nature 236:135–137

Luthy R, Bhend HJ, Munch R, Seigenthaler W (1978) Clinical pharmacology of HR 756, a new cephalosporin. 18th intersci antimicrob agents chemother, Atlanta, Abstract 83

Lynn B (1965) The semisynthetic penicillins. Antibiot Chemother 13:125–226

Mandell GL (1979) Cephalosporins. In: Mandel GL, Douglas RG, Bennett JE (eds) Principles and practice of infectious diseases. Wiley, New York, pp 238–248

Martin WJ (1967) The penicillins. Lancet 87:79–88

Matsumoto K, Ishigami J, Shimizu K, Ooka T (1980) SCE 1365 – a newly developed parenteral cephalosporin: Its antimicrobial activity on clinical isolates, human pharmacokinetics and clinical experience. 20th intersci conf antimicrob agents chemother, New Orleans, Abstract 152

McCarthy CG, Finland M (1960) Absorption and excretion of four penicillins: penicillin G, penicillin V, phenethicillin and phenylmercaptomethyl penicillin. New Engl J Med 263:315–326

McCombie SW, Ganguly AK, Girisavallabhan VM, Hare R, Jeffrey P, Lin S, Loebenberg D, Miller G (1981) 2,6-Disubstituted penem antibacterial agents related to Sch 29482. 21st intersci conf antimicrob agents chemother, Chicago, Abstract 830

Mehta RJ, Newman DJ, Bowie BA, Nash CH, Actor P (1981) Cefonicid: a stable β-lactamase inhibitor. J Antibiot 34:202–205

Micetich RG, Raap R (1968) Penicillins from 3- and 5-phenylisothiazole-4-carboxylic acids and alkoxy derivatives. J Med Chem 11:159–160

Mich TF, Huang GG, Woo PWK, Sanchez JP, Heifetz CL, Schweiss D, Kroll U, Hutt MP, Culbertson TP, Haskell TH (1980a) Synthesis and biological activity of a new semisynthetic cephalosporin, CN 92 982. J Antibiot 33:1352–1356

Mich TF, Huang GG, Schweiss D, Sanchez JP, Hutt MP, Kaltenbronn JS, Culbertson TP, Heifetz CL, Haskell TH (1980b) Synthesis and comparative biological activities of a new series of semisynthetic cephalosporins. 20th intersci conf antimicrob agents chemother, New Orleans, Abstract 148

Mine Y, Nonoyama S, Koja H, Fukada S, Nishida M (1977) Nocardicin A, a new monocyclic β-lactam antibiotic V. In vivo evaluation. J Antibiot 30:932–937

Mitsuhashi S, Matsubara N, Minami S, Muraoka T, Yasuda T, Saikawa I (1978) Antibacterial activities of a new semisynthetic cephalosporin, T-1551. 18th intersci conf antimicrob agents chemother, Atlanta, Abstract 153

Mori T, Nakayama M, Iwasaki A, Kimura S, Mizoguchi T, Tanabe S, Murakami A, Watanabe I, Okuchi M, Itoh H, Saino Y, Kobayashi F (1980) Carpetimycins A and B. New β-lactam antibiotics. 20th intersci conf antimicrob agents chemother, New Orleans, Abstract 165

Morimoto S, Nomura H, Ishiguro T, Fugono T, Maeda K (1972) Semisynthetic β-lactam antibiotics 1-acylation of 6-aminopenicillanic acid with activated derivatives of α-sulfophenylacetic acid. J Med Chem 15:1105–1111

Morin RB, Gorman M (eds) (1982) Chemistry and biology of β-lactam antibiotics, vols 1, 2, 3. Academic Press, New York

Morin RB, Jackson BG, Mueller RA, Lavagnino ER, Scanlon WB, Andrews SL (1969) Chemistry of cephalosporin antibiotics XV. Transformation of penicillin sulfoxide, a synthesis of cephalosporin compounds. J Am Chem Soc 91:1401–1407

Morita K, Nomura H, Numata M, Ochiai M, Yoneda M (1980) An approach to broad-spectrum cephalosporins. Philos Trans R Soc London B289:181–190

Moyer AJ, Coghill RD (1946) Penicillin X. The effect of phenylacetic acid on penicillin production. J Bacteriol 53:329–341

Muggleton PW, O'Callaghan CH, Foord RD, Kirby SM, Ryan DM (1969) Laboratory appraisal of cephalexin. Antimicrob Agents Chemother – 1968, pp 353–360

Murakawa T, Sakamoto H, Fukada S, Nakamoto S, Hirose T, Ito N, Nishida M (1980) Pharmacokinetics of ceftizoxime (FK 749) in animals after parenteral dosing. In: Nel-

son JD, Grassi C (eds) Current chemotherapy and infectious disease, vol 1. American Society of Microbiology, Washington DC, pp 257–259
Murata T, Yasuda N, Hirose Y, Inoue M, Mitsuhashi S (1980) In vitro and in vivo antibacterial activities of AC-1370, a new parenterally active cephalosporin. 20th intersci conf antimicrob agents chemother, New Orleans, Abstract 150
Murray B, Moellering R (1979) The cephalosporin and cephamycin antibiotics: A status report. Clin Ther 2:155–172
Nagarajan R, Boeck LD, Gorman M, Hamill RL, Higgens CE, Hoehn MM, Stark WM, Whitney JG (1971) β-Lactam antibiotics from *Streptomyces.* J Am Chem Soc 99:2308–2310
Naito T, Nakagawa S, Okumura J, Konishi M, Kawaguchi H (1965) Synthesis of 6-aminopenicillanic acid derivatives I. 6-(Acylureido) penicillanates and some related compounds. J Antibiot Ser A 18:145–157
Naito T, Nakagawa S, Takahashi K, Fujisawa K, Kawaguchi H (1968) Synthesis of 6-aminopenicillanic acid derivatives IV. 6-(Sydnone-3-acetamido)penicillanates and 7-(sydnone-3-acetamido)cephalosporanates. J Antibiot 21:300–305
Naito T, Okumura J, Kasai K, Masuko K, Hoshi H, Kamachi H, Kawaguchi H (1977a) Cephalosporins I. Cephaloglycin analogs with six-membered heterocycles in the C-3 side chain. J Antibiot 30:691–697
Naito T, Okumura J, Kasai K, Masuko K, Hoshi H, Kamachi H, Kawaguchi H (1977b) Cephalosporins II. 7-(o-Aminomethylphenylacetamido)-cephalosporanic acids with six-membered heterocycles in the C-3 side chain. J Antibiot 30:698–704
Naito T, Okumura J, Kamachi H, Hoshi H, Kawaguchi H (1977c) Cephalosporins III. 7-(o-Aminomethylphenylacetamido)cephalosporanic acids with bicyclic heteroaromatics in the C-3 side chain. J Antibiot 30:705–713
Nakano H (1981) Structure-activity relationships related to ceftizoxime (FK 749). Med Res Rev 1:127–157
Nakao H, Yanagisawa H, Shimizo B, Kaneko M, Nagano M, Sugawara S (1976) A new semisynthetic 7α-methoxycephalosporin, CS-1170: 7β[[(cyanomethyl)thio]acetamido]-7α-methoxy-3[[(1-methyl-1H-tetrazol-5-yl)thio]methyl]-3-cephem-4-carboxylic acid. J Antibiot 29:554–558
Nakagawa K, Kido Y, Ito Y, Komiya K, Kikuchi Y, Tachibana A, Yano K (1980) YM 09330, a new parenteral cephamycin: pharmacokinetics in humans. 20th intersci conf antimicrob agents chemother, New Orleans, Abstract 160
Nakayama I, Iwamoto H, Iwai S, Kawabe T, Mizuashi H, Ishiyama S (1977) A new cephalosporin antibiotic SCE-963; absorption, distribution and metabolism. 17th intersci conf antimicrob agents chemother, New York, Abstract 46
Nakayama M, Iwasaki A, Kimura S, Mizoguchi T, Tanabe S, Murakami A, Watanabe I, Okuchi M, Itoh H, Saino Y, Kobayshi F, Mori T (1980) Carpetimycins A & B, new β-lactam antibiotics. J Antibiot 33:1388–1389
Nannino G, Perrone E, Severino D, Bedeschi A, Baisoli G, Mainardi G, Bianchi A (1981) Cephalosporins. II Synthesis and structure activity relationships of new 7-vinylenethioacetamido and thioacrylamido cephalosporins. J Antibiot 34:412–426
Nayler JHC (1973) Advances in penicillin research. In: Harper NJ, Simmonds AB (eds) Advances in drug research, vol 7. Academic Press, New York, pp 1–105
Neu HC (1975) Aminopenicillins – clinical pharmacology and use in disease states. Int J Clin Pharmacol Biopharm 11:132–144
Neu HC (1979) Penicillins. In: Mandell GL, Douglas RG, Bennett JE (eds) Principles and practice of infectious diseases. Wiley, New York, pp 218–238
Neu HC (1981) The in vitro activity and β-lactamase stability of Sch 29482, an oral penem, compared to that of β-lactams, aminoglycosides and trimethoprim. 21st intersci conf antimicrob agents chemother, Chicago, Abstract 839
Neu HC, Fu KP (1978a) Cefaclor: in vitro spectrum of activity and β-lactamase stability. Antimicrob Agents Chemother 13:584–588
Neu HC, Fu KP (1978b) A beta-lactamase-resistant cephalosporin with a broad spectrum of gram-positive and -negative activity. Antimicrob Agents Chemother 13:657–664

Neu HC, Labthavikul P (1981) The in vitro activity and β-lactamase stability of SQ20776, a novel monocyclic β-lactam agent compared to other agents. 21st intersci conf antimicrob agents chemother, Chicago, Abstract 494
Neu HC, Winshell EB (1971 a) In vitro antimicrobial activity of 6[D(−)α-amino-p-hydroxyphenylacetamido]penicillanic acid, a new semisynthetic penicillin. Antimicrob Agents Chemother – 1970, pp 407–410 (and four following articles)
Neu HC, Winshell EB (1971 b) Semisynthetic penicillin 6-[D(−)α-carboxy-3-thienylacetamido]penicillanic acid active against *Pseudomonas* in vitro. Appl Microbiol 21:66–70
Neu HC, Fu KP, Aswapokee N, Aswapokee P, Kung K (1979) Comparative activity and β-lactamase stability of cefoperazone, a piperazine cephalosporin. Antimicrob Agents Chemother 16:150–157
Neu HC, Meropol NJ, Fu KP (1981) Antibacterial activity of ceftriaxon (Ro 13-9904), a β-lactamase-stable cephalosporin. Antimicrob Agents Chemother 19:414–423
Newall CE, Cherry PC, Gregory GI, Tonge AP, Ward P, Watson NS (1978) Clavulanic acid derivatives with improved biological activity. 176th natl meeting, Am Chem Soc, Miami Beach, Abstract MEDI 15
Newman DJ, Mehta RJ, Bowie BA, Nash CH, Actor P (1980) Cefuroxime inhibition of cephalothin hydrolysis by the constitutive β-lactamase from *E. cloacae* P 99. J Antibiot 33:1202–1203
Newton GGF, Abraham EP (1954) Degradation, structure and some derivatives of cephalosporin N. Biochem J 58:103–111
Nishida M, Mine Y, Nonoyama S, Kojo H (1977) Nocardicin A, a new monocyclic β-lactam antibiotic III. In vitro evaluation. J Antibiot 30:917–925
Nomura H, Fugono T, Hitaka T, Minami I, Azuma T, Morimoto S, Mosuda T (1974) Semisynthetic β-lactam antibiotics 6. Sulfocephalosporins and their antipseudomonal activities. J Med Chem 17:1312–1315
Nomura H, Fugono T, Hitaka T, Minami I, Azuma T, Morimoto S, Mosuda T (1975) Antipseudomonal β-lactam antibiotics with sulfoacyl side chains. 170th natl mtg, Amer Chem Soc, Chicago, Abstract MEDI 2
Nomura H, Minami I, Hitaka T, Fugono T (1976) Semisynthetic β-lactam antibiotics 8. Structure-activity relationships of α sulfocephalosporins. J Antibiot 29:928–936
Nozaki Y, Imada A, Yoneda M (1979) SCE-963, a new potent cephalosporin with high affinity for penicillin-binding proteins 1 and 3 of *Escherichia coli*. Antimicrob Agents Chemother 15:20–27
Nozaki Y, Kawashima F, Imada A (1981) C-19393S_2 and H_2, new carbapenem antibiotics III. Mode of action. J Antibiot 34:206–211
Numata M, Minamida I, Tsushima S, Nishimura T, Yamaoka M, Matsumoto N (1977) Synthesis of new cephalosporins with potent antibacterial activities. Chem Pharm Bull 25:3117–3119
Numata M, Minamida I, Yamaoka M, Shiraishi M, Miyawaki T, Akimoto H, Naito K, Kida M (1978) A new cephalosporin. SCE-963: 7-[2-(2-Aminothiazol-4-yl)acetamido]3-[[[1-(2-dimethylaminoethyl)-1H-tetrazol-5-yl]thio]methyl]ceph-3-em-4-carboxylic acid. J Antibiot 31:1262–1271
O'Callaghan CH (1975) Classification of cephalosporins by their antibacterial activity and pharmacokinetic properties. J Antimicrob Chemother 1 [Suppl]:1–12
O'Callaghan CH (1978) Irreversible effects of serum proteins on β-lactam antibiotics. Antimicrob Agents Chemother 13:628–633
O'Callaghan CH (1979) Description and classification of the newer cephalosporins and their relationships with established compounds. J Antimicrob Chemother 5:635–671
O'Callaghan CH (1980) Structure-activity relations and β-lactamase resistance. Philos Trans R Soc London B289:197–205
O'Callaghan CH, Morris A (1972) Inhibition of β-lactamases by β-lactam antibiotics. Antimicrob Agents Chemother 2:442–448
O'Callaghan CH, Muggleton PW, Kirby SM, Ryan DM (1967) Inhibition of β-lactamase decomposition of cephaloridine and cephalothin by other cephalosporins. Antimicrob Agents Chemother – 1966, pp 337–343
O'Callaghan CH, Sykes RB, Griffith A, Thornton JE (1976) Cefuroxime, a new cephalosporin antibiotic: activity in vitro. Antimicrob Agents Chemother 9:511–519

O'Callaghan CH, Acred P, Harper PB, Ryan DM, Kirby S, Harding SM (1980) GR 20263 a new broad-spectrum cephalosporin and antipseudomonal activity. Antimicrob Agents Chemother 17:876–883
Ochiai M, Aki O, Morimoto A, Okada T, Matsushita Y (1977) New cephalosporin derivatives with high antibacterial activities. Chem Pharm Bull 25:3115–3117
Ochiai M, Morimoto A, Matsushita Y, Kaneko T, Kida M (1980a) Synthesis and structure-activity relationships of 7β-[2-(2-aminothiazol-4yl)acetamido]cephalosporin derivatives. J Antibiot 33:1005–1013
Ochiai M, Morimoto A, Matsushita Y, Kida M (1980b) Synthesis and structure-activity relationships of 7β-[2-(2-aminothiazol-4-yl)acetamido]cephalosporin derivatives. J Antibiot 33:1014–1021
Ochiai M, Morimoto A, Okada T, Matsushita Y, Yamamoto H, Aki O, Kida M (1980c) Synthesis and structure-activity relationships of 7β-[2-(2-aminothiazol-4-yl)acetamido]cephalosporin derivatives. J Antibiot 33:1022–1030
Ochiai M, Morimoto A, Miyawaki T, Matsushita Y, Okada T, Natsugari H, Kida M (1981) Synthesis and structure-activity relationships of 7β-[2-(2-aminothiazol-4-yl)acetamido]cephalosporin derivatives. J Antibiot 34:171–185
Oida S, Yoshida A, Hayashi T, Takeda N, Nishimura T, Ohki E (1980a) Synthesis of penems and their antibacterial activities. J Antibiot 33:107–109
Oida S, Yoshida A, Ohki E (1980b) Synthetic approach directed at 1-carbapenems and 1-carbapenams. Chem Pharm Bull 28:3494–3500
Okamura K, Sakomoto M, Fukagawa Y, Ishikura T (1979) PS-5 – a new β-lactam antibiotic III. Synergistic effects and inhibitory activity against a β-lactamase. J Antibiot 32:280–286
Okamura K, Sakamoto M, Ishikura T (1980) PS-5, inhibition of a β-lactamase from *Proteus vulgaris*. J Antibiot 33:293–302
Okonogi K, Nozaki Y, Imada A, Kuno M (1981) C-19393S_2 and H_2, new carbapanem antibiotics IV. Inhibitory activity against β-lactamases. J Antibiot 34:212–217
Orlek BS, Sammes PG, Knott-Hunziker V, Waley SG (1980) On the chemistry of β-lactamase inhibition by 6β-bromopenicillanic acid. J Chem Soc, Perkin Trans I: 2322–2329
Otsuka H, Nagata W, Yoshioka M, Narisada M, Yoshida T, Harada Y, Yamada H (1981) Discovery and development of moxalactam (6059S): the chemistry and biology of 1-oxacephems. Med Res Rev 1:217–248
Pala G, Coppi G, Mantegano A, Crescanzi E (1969) Bacteriological and pharmacological properties of 6-(4-sydnone carboxamido) penicillanic acids. Chim Ther 4:26–30
Park JT (1966) Some observations on murein synthesis and the action of penicillin. In: Newton BA, Reynolds PE (eds) Biochemical studies of antimicrobiol drugs. Cambridge University Press, Cambridge, pp 70–81
Park JT, Burman L (1973) FL-1060: A new penicillin with a unique mode of action. Biochem Biophys Res Comm 51:863–868
Perron YG, Minor WF, Holdrege CT, Babel W, Cheney LC (1960) Derivatives of 6-aminopenicillanic acid I. Partially synthetic penicillins prepared from α-aryloxyalkanoic acids. J Am Chem Soc 82:3934–3938
Perron YG, Minor WF, Crast LB, Cheney LC (1961) Derivatives of 6-aminopenicillanic acid II. Reactions with isocyanates, isothiocyanates and cyclic anhydrides. J Org Chem 26:3365–3373
Perron YG, Minor WF, Crast WB, Gourevitch A, Lein J, Cheney LC (1962) Derivatives of 6-aminopenicillanic acid III. Reactions with N-substituted phthalamic acids. J Med Pharm Chem 5:1016–1025
Pfaendler HR, Gosteli J, Woodward RB (1979) The penems, a new class of β-lactam antibiotics 4. Synthesis of racemic and enantiomeric penem carboxylic acids. J Am Chem Soc 101:6306–6310
Pfaendler HR, Gosteli J, Woodward RB (1980) The penems, a new class of β-lactam antibiotics 5. Total synthesis of racemic 6α-hydroxyethylpenemcarboxylic acids. J Am Chem Soc 102:2039–2043
Pitkin DH, Actor P, Alexander F, Dubb S, Stote R, Weisbach JA (1980) Cefonicid (SK & F 75073). Serum levels and urinary recovery after intramuscular and intravenous ad-

ministration. In: Nelson JD, Grassi C (eds) Current chemotherapy and infectious disease, vol 1. American Society of Microbiology, Washington DC, pp 252–254
Pitt J, Siasoco R, Kaplan K, Weinstein L (1968) Antimicrobial activity and pharmacological behavior of cephaloglycine. Antimicrob Agents Chemother – 1967, pp 630–635
Polacek I, Starke B (1980) Diastereomeric 7α-ureidoacetyl cephalosporins V. Antimicrobial activity, β-lactamase stability and pharmacokinetics of 7-(α-ureido-2-amino-4-thiazolylacetyl)-cephalosporins. J Antibiot 33:1031–1036
Ponsford RJ, Roberts PM, Southgate R (1979) Intramolecular Wittig reactions with thioesters: The synthesis of 7-oxo-phenylthio-1-azabicyclo[3.2.0]hept-2-ene-2-carboxylates. J Chem Soc Chem Commun: 847–848
Pratt RF, Loosemore MJ (1978) 6β-Bromopenicillanic acid, a potent β-lactamase inhibitor. Proc Natl Acad Sci USA 75:4145–4149
Price KE (1970) Structure-activity relationships of semisynthetic penicillins. Adv Appl Microbiol 11:17–75 (Reprinted in: Perlman D (ed) SAR among the semisynthetic antibiotics. Academic Press, New York, 1977, pp 1–60)
Price KE (1977) Structure-activity relationships of semisynthetic penicillins (Supplement). In: Perlman D (ed) SAR among the semisynthetic antibiotics. Academic Press, New York, pp 61–86
Price KE, Bach JA, Chisholm DR, Misiek M, Gourevitch A (1969a) Preliminary microbiological and pharmacological evaluation of 6-(R-α-amino-3-thienylacetamido)penicillanic acid (BL-P875). J Antibiot 22:1–11
Price KE, Chisholm DR, Leitner F, Misiek M, Gourevitch A (1969b) Antipseudomonal activity of α-sulfaminopenicillins. Appl Environ Microbiol 17:881–887
Pursiano TA, Buck RE, Randolph JA, Misiek M, Price KE, Leitner F (1981) In vitro evaluation of BL-P 2013, a new β-lactamase inhibitor. 21st intersci conf antimicrob agents chemother, Chicago, Abstract 435
Quay JF (1972) Transport interaction of glycine and cephalexin in rat jejunum. Physiologist 15:241
Raap R (1971) Synthesis and antibacterial activities of penicillins from (+) and (−)-α-amino-4-isothiazolylacetic acids. J Antibiot 24:695–703
Raap R, Micetich RG (1968) Penicillins and cephalosporins from isothiazolylacetic acids. J Med Chem 11:70–74
Reading C, Cole M (1977) Clavulanic acid: a β-lactamase inhibiting β-lactam from *Streptomyces clavuligerus*. Antimicrob Agents Chemother 11:852–857
Reading C, Hepburn P (1979) The inhibition of β-lactamase by clavulanic acid. Biochem J 179:67–76
Reeves DS, Bywater MJ, Holt HA, White LO, Davis AJ, Elliot PJ, Foulds G (1980) Pharmacokinetics of cefoperazone in man. 20th intersci conf antimicrob agents chemother, New Orleans, Abstract 13
Reeves DS, Bywater MJ, Holt HA (1981) Comparative in vitro activity of Sch 29482. 21st intersci conf antimicrob agents chemother, Chicago, abstract 744
Reiner R, Weiss U, Brombacher U, Lenz P, Montavon M, Furlenmeier A, Angehrn P, Probst PJ (1980) R 13-9904/001, a novel potent and long-acting parenteral cephalosporin. J Antibiot 33:783–786
Retsema JA, English AR, Lynch JE (1976) Laboratory studies with a new broad-spectrum penicillin, pirbenicillin. Antimicrob Agents Chemother 9:975–982
Richmond MH (1980a) The β-lactamase stability of a novel β-lactam antibiotic containing a 7α-methoxyoxacephem nucleus. J Antimicrob Chemother 6:445–453
Richmond MH (1980b) β-lactamase activity of cefotaxime. J Antimicrob Chemother 6 [Suppl]:13–17
Richmond MH, Sykes RB (1973) The β-lactamases of gram-negative bacteria and their possible physiological role. Adv Microb Physiol 2:31–88
Richmond MH, Wotton S (1976) Comparative study of seven cephalosporins: Susceptibility to β-lactamases and ability to penetrate the surface layers of *Escherichia coli*. Antimicrob Agents Chemother 10:219–222
Roholt K, Nielson B, Kristensen E (1975) Pharmacokinetic studies with mecillinam and pivmecillinam. Chemotherapy 2:146–166

Rolinson GN, Sutherland R (1973) Semisynthetic penicillins. Adv Pharmacol Chemother 11:151–220
Rolinson GN, Stevens S, Batchelor FR, Cameron-Wood J, Chain EB (1960) Bacterological studies on a new penicillin – BRL 1241. Lancet ii:564–567
Romagnoli MF, Fu KP, Neu HC (1980) The antibacterial activity of thienamycin against multiresistant bacteria – comparison with β-lactamase stable compounds. J Antimicrob Chemother 6:601–606
Rosenman SB, Warren GH (1962) In vitro evaluation of semisynthetic penicillins WY-3206 and WY-3277. Antimicrob Agents Chemother – 1961, pp 611–619 (and two following articles)
Rosenman SB, Weber LS, Owen G, Warren GH (1968) Antimicrobial activity and pharmacological distribution of WY-4508, an aminoalicyclic penicillin. Antimicrob Agents Chemother – 1967, pp 590–596 (and references cited therein)
Ryan DM, Monsey D (1981) Bacterial filamentation and in vivo efficacy: A comparison of several cephalosporins. J Antimicrob Chemother 7:57–63
Sabath LD, Wilcox C, Garner C, Finland M (1973) In vitro activity of cefazolin against recent clinical bacterial isolates. J Infect Dis 128 [Suppl]:S320–S326
Sakamoto M, Iguchi H, Okamura K, Hori S, Fukagawa Y, Ishikura T, Lein J (1979) PS-5, a new β-lactam antibiotic II. Antimicrobial activity. J Antibiot 32:272–279
Sakamoto M, Shibamoto N, Iguchi H, Okamura K, Hori S, Fukagawa Y, Ishikura T (1980) PS-6 and PS-7, new β-lactam antibiotics in vitro and in vivo evaluation. J Antibiot 33:1138–1145
Sakamoto M, Kojima I, Okabe M, Fukagawa Y, Ishikura T (1982) Studies on the OA-6121 group of antibiotics, new carbapenem compounds II. In vitro evaluation. J Antibiot 35:1264–1270
Salzmann TN, Ratcliffe RW, Christensen BG (1980) Total synthesis of (−)-homothienamycin. Tetrahedron Lett 21:1193–1196
Sanders C (1977) In vitro studies with cefaclor, a new oral cephalosporin. Antimicrob Agents Chemother 12:490–497
Sassiver ML, Lewis A (1970) Structure activity relationships among semisynthetic cephalosporins. Adv Appl Microbiol 13:163–236 (Reprinted in: Perlman D (ed) SAR among the semisynthetic antibiotics. Academic Press, New York, 1977, pp 87–160)
Scannel JP, Preuss DL, Blount JF, Ax HA, Kellett M, Weiss F, Demny TC, Williams TH, Stempel A (1975) Antimetabolites produced by microorganisms XII. (S)-alanyl-3[α-(S)-chloro-3-hydroxy-2-oxo-3-azetidinylmethyl]-(S)-alanine, a new β-lactam-containing natural product. J Antibiot 28:1–6
Schaeder RW, Warren G (1980) Effect of cyclacillin and ampicillin on the gut flora of mice. Chemotherapy 26:289–296
Schenkein DP, Pratt RF (1980) Phenylpropynal, a specific, irreversible, non-β-lactam inhibitor of β-lactamases. J Biol Chem 255:45–48
Schmitt SM, Johnston DBR, Christensen BG (1980a) Thienamycin total synthesis 2. Model studies – Synthesis of a simple 2-(alkylthio) carbapen-2-em. J Org Chem 45:1135–1142
Schmitt SM, Johnston DBR, Christensen BG (1980b) Thienamycin total synthesis 3. Total synthesis of (±)-thienamycin and (±)-8-epithienamycin. J Org Chem 45:1142–1148
Schwind RA, Bonner DP, Minassian BF, Froggatt LM, Sykes RB (1981) Monobactams: relationship to homologous penicillins and cephalosporins. 21st intersci conf antimicrob agents chemother, Chicago, Abstract 879
Scully B, Neu HC (1981) The human pharmacology of ceftriaxon. 21st intersci conf antimicrob agents chemother. Chicago, abstract 805
Seddon M, Wise R, Gillett AP, Livingston R (1980) Pharmacokinetics of Ro 13-9904, a broad spectrum cephalosporin. Antimicrob Agents Chemother 18:240–242
Selwyn S (1979) Microbiological and clinical implications of the pharmacokinetics of cephalosporins. Int Congr Ser-Exerpta Medica 477:147–157
Shannon K, King A, Warren C, Phillips I (1980) The in vitro antibacterial activity and susceptibility of the cephalosporin Ro 13-9904 to β-lactamases. Antimicrob Agents Chemother 18:292–298
Sheehan JC, Hoff DR (1957) The synthesis of substituted penicillins and simpler structural analogs XII. 6-Benzenesulfonamidopenicillanic acid. J Am Chem Soc 79:237–240

Sheehan JC, Shibahara S, Chacko E (1980) Simple β-lactam compounds derived from 6-aminopenicillanic acid. J Med Chem 23:809–811
Shih DH, Ratcliff RW (1981) Preparation and antibacterial activity of Δ^1-thienamycin. J Med Chem 24:639–643
Shih DH, Hannah J, Christensen BG (1978) Descysteaminylthienamycin. J Am Chem Soc 100:8004–8006
Shimizu B, Kaneko M, Kimura M, Sugawara S (1976) Synthesis of 7α-methoxy-7-[2-(substituted thio)acetamido]cephalosporin derivatives and their antibacterial activities. Chem Pharm Bull (Tokyo) 24:2629–2636
Shiobara Y, Tachibana A, Sasaki H, Watanabe T, Sado T (1974) Phthalidyl D-α-aminobenzylpenicillanate hydrochloride (PC183), a new orally active ampicillin ester I. Absorption, excretion and metabolism of PC-183 and ampicillin. J Antibiot 37:665–673
Simpson IN, Harper PB, O'Callaghan CH (1980) Principal β-lactamases responsible for resistance to β-lactam antibiotics in urinary tract infections. Antimicrob Agents Chemother 17:929–936
Sjovall J, Magni L, Bergan T (1978) Pharmacokinetics of bacampicillin compared with those of ampicillin, pivampicillin, and amoxicillin. Antimicrob Agents Chemother 13:90–96
Slocombe B, Basker MJ, Bentley PH, Clayton JP, Cole M, Comber KR, Dixon RA, Edmonson RA, Jackson D, Merriken DJ, Sutherland R (1981) BRL 17421, a novel β-lactam antibiotic, highly resistant to β-lactamases, giving high and prolonged serum levels in humans. Antimicrob Agents Chemother 20:38–46
Soper QF, Whitehead CW, Behrens OK, Course JJ, Jones RG (1948) Biosynthesis of penicillins VII. Oxy and mercaptoacetic acids. J Am Chem Soc 70:2849–2855
Spencer JL, Siu FY, Flynn EH, Jackson BG, Sigal MV, Higgins HM, Chauvette RR, Andrews SL, Bloch DE (1967) Synthesis and structure-activity relationships of cephaloridine analogues. Antimicrob Agents Chemother – 1966, pp 573–580
Spratt BG (1977) Properties of the penicillin-binding proteins of *Escherichia coli* K 12. Eur J Biochem 72:341–352
Spratt BG (1978) *Escherichia coli* resistance to β-lactam antibiotics through a decrease in the affinity of a target for lethality. Nature 274:713–715
Spratt BG (1980) Biochemical and genetical approaches to the mechanism of action of penicillin. Philos Trans R Soc London B289:273–283
Spratt BG, Jobanputra V, Zimmerman W (1977) Binding of thienamycin and clavulanic acid to the penicillin binding proteins of *Escherchia coli* K 12. Antimicrob Agents Chemother 12:406–409
Srinivasom S, Neu HC (1980) The pharmacology of ceftizoxime compared with that of cefamandole in normal individuals. 20th intersci conf antimicrob agents chemother, New Orleans, Abstract 157
Stapley EO, Hendlin D, Hernandez S, Jackson M, Mater JH, Miller AK, Woodruff HB, Miller TW, Albers-Schonberg G, Arison BH, Smith JL (1971) Cephamycins: Production by actinomycetes, biological characteristics and chemical characterization. 11th intersci conf antimicrob agents chemother, Atlantic City, Abstract 15
Stapley ED, Daoust DR, Hendlin D, Miller AK, Zimmerman SB, Birnbaum J, Cama LD, Christensen BG (1979a) Cefoxitin: mechanism of activity against cephalosporin-resistant bacteria. In: Mitsuhaski S (ed) Microbiol drug resistance, vol 2. Japan Scientific Societies Press, Tokyo; Univ Park Press, Baltimore, pp 405–417
Stapley ED, Birnbaum J, Miller AK, Wallick H, Hendlin D, Woodruff HB (1979b) Cefoxitin and cephamycins: microbiological studies. Rev Inf Dis 1:73–89
Stedman RJ, Hoover JRE, Chow AW, Dolan MM, Hall NM, Ferlauto RJ (1964) Semisynthetic penicillins II. Structure-activity studies on the 2-biphenylyl side chain. J Med Chem 7:251–255
Stewart D, Bodey GP (1977) Azlocillin: in vitro studies of a new semisynthetic penicillin. Antimicrob Agents Chemother 11:865–870
Stewart GT (1965) The penicillin group of drugs. Elsevier, New York
Strominger JL, Tipper DJ (1965) Bacterial cell wall synthesis and structure in relation to the mechanism of action of penicillins and other antibacterial agents. Am J Med 39:708–721

Swabb EA, Sugerman AA, Platt TB, Pilkiewicz FG (1981) Pharmacokinetics of SQ26776, a monocyclic beta-lactam antimicrobial agent, in healthy subjects. 21st intersci conf antimicrob agents chemother, Chicago, Abstract 493

Sweet RM, Dahl LF (1970) Molecular architecture of the cephalosporins. Insights into biological activity based on structural investigations. J Am Chem Soc 92:5489–5507

Sykes RB, Phillips I (eds) (1981) Azthreonam, a synthetic monobactam. J Antimicrob Chemother 8 [Suppl E]:1–147

Sykes RB, Matthew M (1976) The β-lactamases of gram-negative bacteria and their role in resistance to β-lactam antibiotics. J Antimicrob Chemother 2:115–157

Sykes RB, Cimarusti CM, Bonner DP, Bush K, Floyd DM, Georgopapadakou NH, Koster WH, Liu WC, Parker WL, Principe PA, Rathnum ML, Slwsarchyk WA, Trejo WH, Wells TS (1981a) Monocyclic β-lactam antibiotics produced by bacteria Nature 291:489–491

Sykes RB, Bush K, Freudenberger JS (1981b) Interaction of SQ26776 and third generation cephalosporins with β-lactamases and β-lactamase-producing gram-negative rods. 21st intersci conf antimicrob agents chemother, Chicago, Abstract 489

Tachibana A, Komiya M, Kikuchi Y, Yano K, Mashimo K (1980) Pharmacological studies on YM 09330, a new parenteral cephamycin derivative. In: Nelson JD, Grassi C (eds) Current chemotherapy and infectious disease, vol 1. American Society Microbiology, Washington DC, pp 273–275

Takaya T, Kamimura T, Koso H, Matsumoto Y, Nishida M (1982) Antibacterial activity of FR 17027, a new oral cephalosporin. 22nd intersci conf antimicrob agents chemother, Miami Beach, Abstract 621

Tally FP, Jacobus NV, Gorbach SL (1978) In vitro activity of thienamycin. Antimicrob Agents Chemother 14:436–438

Tamaki S, Nakajima S, Matsuhashi M (1977) Thermosensitive mutation in *Escherichia coli* simultaneously causing defects in penicillin binding proteins 1Bs and in enzyme activity for peptidoglycan synthesis in vitro. Proc Natl Acad Sci USA 74:5472–5476

Toda M, Saito T, Yano K, Suzaki K, Saito M, Mitsuhashi S (1980) In vitro and in vivo antibacterial activities of YM 09330, a new cephamycin derivative. In: Nelson JD, Grassi C (eds) Current chemotherapy and infectious disease, vol 1. American Society Microbiology, Washington DC, pp 280–281

Toda M, Ikeuchi T, Tajima M, Inoue M, Mitsuhashi S (1981) Comparative inhibition of β-lactamases by cephamycin antibiotics. J Antibiot 34:114–117

Tsuchiya K, Oishi T, Iwagishi C, Iwahi T (1971) In vitro antibacterial activity of disodium α-sulfobenzylpenicillin. J Antibiot 24:607–619

Tsuchiya K, Kondo M, Nagatomo H (1978a) SCE-129, antipseudomonal cephalosporin: in vitro and in vivo antibacterial activities. Antimicrob Agents Chemother 13:137–145

Tsuchiya K, Makoto K, Kondo M, Ono H, Takeuchi M, Nishi T (1978b) SCE-963, a new broad-spectrum cephalosporin. In vitro and in vivo antibacterial activities. Antimicrob Agents Chemother 14:551–568

Tsuji A, Nakashima E, Asano T, Nakashima R, Yamana T (1979) Saturable absorption of aminocephalosporins by the rat intestine. J Pharm Pharmacol 31:718–720

Tybring L, Melchior NH (1975) Mecillinam (FL 1060) a 6β-amidinopenicillanic acid derivative: bactericidal action and synergy in vitro. Antimicrob Agents Chemother 8:271–278

Vaczi L, Uri J (1954) Studies on the enzyme penicillinase. Acta Microbiol Acad Sci Hung 2:167–177

Vanderhaeghe H, Van Dijck P, Claesen M, DeSomer P (1962) Preparation and properties of 3,4-dichloro-α-methoxybenzylpenicillin. Antimicrob Agents Chemother – 1961, pp 581–587

Van Heyningen E (1967) Cephalosporins. In: Harper NJ, Simmonds AB (eds) Advances in drug research, vol 4. Academic Press, New York, pp 1–70

Van Landuyt HW, Pyckavet M, Lambert AM (1981) Comparative activity of BRL 25000 with amoxycillin against resistant clinical isolates. J Antimicrob Chemother 7:65–70

Verbist L (1978) In vitro activity of piperacillin, a new semisynthetic penicillin with an unusually broad spectrum of activity. Antimicrob Agents Chemother 13:349–357

Verbist L (1979) Comparison of the activities of the new ureidopenicillins, piperacillin, mezlocillin, azlocillin and Bay K 4999 against gram-negative organisms. Antimicrob Agents Chemother 16:115–119
Verbist L, Verhaegen J (1980) GR-20263: A new aminothiazolyl cephalosporin with high activity against Pseudomonas and Enterobacteriaceae. Antimicrob Agents Chemother 17:807–812
Wallace JF, Atlas E, Bear DM, Brown NK, Clark H, Turck M (1971) Evaluation of an indanyl ester of carbenicillin. Antimicrob Agents Chemother – 1970, pp 223–226
Weaver SS, Bodey GP (1980) CI-867, a new semisynthetic penicillin. In vitro studies. Antimicrob Agents Chemother 18:939–943
Webber JA, Ott JL (1977) Structure-activity relationships in the cephalosporins II. Recent developments. In: Perlman D (ed) SAR among the semisynthetic antibiotics. Academic Press, New York, pp 161–237
Webber JA, Huffman GW, Koehler RE, Murphy CF, Ryan CW, Van Heyningen EM, Vasileff RT (1971) Chemistry of cephalosporin antibiotics 22. Chemistry and biological activity of 3-alkoxymethyl cephalosporins. J Med Chem 14:113–116
Wetzel B, Woitun E, Reuter W, Maier R, Lechner U, Werner R, Goeth H (1980) Pyrimidinylureido-cephalosporins. Synthesis and structure-activity relationships. 20th intersci conf antimicrob agents chemother, New Orleans, Abstract 147
Wheeler WJ, Wright WE, Line VD, Frogge JA (1977) Orally active esters of cephalosporin antibiotics. Synthesis and biological properties of acyloxymethyl esters of 7-(D-2-amino-2-phenylacetamido)-3-[5-methyl-(1,3,4-thiadiazol-2-yl)-thiomethyl-3-cephem-4-carboxylic acid. J Med Chem 20:1159–1164
Wick WE (1966) In vitro and in vivo laboratory comparison of cephalothin and desacetylcephalothin. Antimicrob Agents Chemother – 1965, pp 870–875
Williamson GM, Morrison JK, Stevens KJ (1961) A new semisynthetic penicillin PA 248. Lancet i:847–850
Wise R, Andrews JM, Bedford KA (1978) Comparison of the in vitro activity of Bay K 4999 and pipericillin, two new antipseudomonal broad spectrum penicillins, with other β-lactam drugs. Antimicrob Agents Chemother 14:549–552
Wise R, Wills PJ, Andrews JM, Bedford KA (1980a) Activity of the cefotaxime (HR 756) desacetyl metabolite compared with those of cefotaxime and other cephalosporins. Antimicrob Agents Chemother 17:84–86
Wise R, Gillett AP, Andrews JM, Bedford KA (1980b) Ro 139904: A new cephalosporin with a high degree of activity and broad spectrum antibiotic activity: an in vitro comparative study. J Antimicrob Chemother 6:595–600
Wise R, Andrews JM, Bedford KA (1980c) Comparison of in vitro activity of GR 20263, a novel cephalosporin derivative with activities of other β-lactam compounds. Antimicrob Agents Chemother 17:884–889
Wise R, Andrews JM, Bedford KA (1980d) Clavulanic acid and CP 45899: a comparison of their in vitro activity in combination with penicillins. J Antimicrob Chemother 6:197–206
Wise R, Andrews JM, Patel N (1981) 6-β-Bromo- and 6-β-iodo penicillanic acid, two novel β-lactamase inhibitors. J Antimicrob Chemother 7:531–536
Wolfe S (1976) 2,2-Dimethyl-3R-carboxy-6S-amino-1-oxa-5R-bicyclo[3.2.0]heptan-7-one. US Patent 3948927, assigned to Queens University, Kingston, Ont
Woodward RB (1949) The constitution of the penicillins. In: Clark HT, Johnson JR, Robins R (eds) The chemistry of penicillin. Princeton University Press, Princeton, pp 440–454
Woodward RB (1977) Recent advances in the chemistry of β-lactam antibiotics. In: Recent advances in the chemistry of β-lactam antibiotics. Chemical Society, London, pp 167–180
Woodward RB (1980) Penems and related substances. Philos Trans R Soc London B289:239–250
Wright RB, Makover SD, Telep E (1981) Ro 13-9904: Affinity for penicillin binding proteins and effect on cell wall synthesis. J Antibiot 34:590–595
Yamazaki T, Tsuchiya K (1971) In vivo antibacterial activity of disodium α-sulfobenzylpenicillins. J Antibiot 24:620–625
Yamazaki T, Tsuchiya K (1976) 3-Deacetoxy-7-(α-aminocyclohexenylacetamido)cephalosporic acid (SCE 100), a new semisynthetic cephalosporin. J Antibiot 29:559–578

Yasuda K, Kurashige S, Mitsuhashi S (1980) Cefroxadine (CGP-9000), an orally active cephalosporin. Antimicrob Agents Chemother 18:105–110

Yoshida T (1980) Structural requirements for antibacterial activity and β-lactamase stability of 7β-acylmalonylamino-7α-methoxy-1-oxacephalosporins. Philos Trans R Soc London B289:231–237

Yoshida T, Narisada M, Matsuura S, Nagata W, Kuwahara S (1978) 6059-S, a new parenterally active 1-oxacephalosporin (1) microbiological studies. 18th intersci conf antimicrob agents chemother, Atlanta, Abstract 151

Yoshida T, Matsuura S, Mayama M, Kameda Y, Kuwahara S (1980) Moxalactam (6059-S), a novel 1-oxa-β-lactam with an expanded antibacterial spectrum: laboratory evaluation. Antimicrob Agents Chemother 17:302–312

Yoshikawa TT, Shibata SA, Herbert P, Oill PA (1980) In vitro activity of Ro 13-9904, cefuroxime, cefoxitin and ampicillin against *Neisseria gonorrhoeae*. Antimicrob Agents Chemother 18:355–356

Zajac I, Bartus H, Actor P, Weisbach J (1980) Comparative in vitro activity of cefonicid and other selected cephalosporins against *Neisseria gonorrhoeae*. In: Nelson JD, Grassi C (eds) Current chemotherapy and infectious disease, vol 1. American Society of Microbiology, Washington DC, pp 250–252

Zimmerman W (1980) Penetration of β-lactam antibiotics into their target enzymes in *Pseudomonas aeruginosa:* comparison of a highly sensitive mutant with its parent strain. Antimicrob Agents Chemother 18:94–100

CHAPTER 15

Pharmacokinetics of β-Lactam Antibiotics

K. C. KWAN and J. D. ROGERS

A. Introduction

An attempt has been made to review the absorption, distribution, biotransformation, and excretion characteristics of β-lactam antibiotics. With the exception of organ and tissue distribution data, which are derived primarily from experimental animals, emphasis is on human pharmacokinetics, including the effects of disease.

Wherever possible, the kinetics of drug elimination is described in terms of its serum clearance, which is the sum of all net losses by urinary excretion, biliary secretion, biotransformation, etc. Thus, for example, the ratio of renal to serum clearance should be equal to the fraction of an intravenous dose recovered in the urine unchanged. Serum half-life, on the other hand, is a function of drug distribution as well as elimination. Therefore, it may not change in direct proportion to changes in drug elimination. Nevertheless, serum half-life is a useful indicator of a drug's potential to accumulate. The amount absorbed by nonvascular routes is estimated by comparing serum concentration and/or urinary excretion data with those following an intravenous dose. In this context, the term bioavailability is often used to exclude the effects of biotransformation during the process of absorption, such as in transit through the gut wall or first passage through the liver.

For completeness and other perspectives on the kinetic and metabolic disposition of β-lactam antibiotics, recent reviews by PRICE (1977a, b), SASSIVER and LEWIS (1977), WEBBER and OTT (1977), ROLINSON and SUTHERLAND (1973), BERGAN (1978c), BROGARD et al. (1978), MOELLERING and SWARTZ (1976), ANDRIOLE (1978), MURRAY and MOELLERING (1979), BARZA and MIAO (1977), WEINSTEIN (1980), and NIGHTINGALE et al. (1975b) should be consulted. There is surprisingly little information on the biotransformation of this important class of therapeutic agents. Much of the available evidence is circumstantial and qualitative. In concert with recent advances in separation and quantitation techniques, deficiencies in this area appear to be on the mend. In anticipation of this kind of information on established agents and the current proliferation of novel structures, a further update on this subject is probably needed before long.

B. Penicillins

For most penicillins, renal excretion is the major route of elimination. With few exceptions, renal clearance tends to exceed glomerular filtration rate. In all cases studied, there is evidence of active renal tubular secretion in that the coadministration of probenecid invariably causes a decrease in renal clearance, an increase in serum concentrations, and/or a prolongation in serum-life. By the same token, renal dysfunction has a profound effect on elimination rate, serum levels, and drug accumulation. While hemodialysis or peritoneal dialysis can be effective in some patients with end-stage renal failure, the rate of drug removal is not simply related to serum protein binding.

Even though antimicrobial activity in bile is usually high compared to that in serum, bilary excretion contributes only insignificantly to the elimination of most penicillins. Notable exceptions are metampicillin, nafcillin, and the ureidopenicillins.

β-Lactam cleavage appears to be a common metabolic pathway among penicillins. Penicilloic acid formation, while variable, may represent as much as 50% of total clearance of a given agent. Part of this may occur in the gastrointestinal lumen or during initial transit through the gut wall and liver following oral administration. Although there is evidence of *N*-deacylation for some penicillins, only traces of 6-aminopenicillanic acid or penicic acid are found in human urine.

Pharmacokinetic interpretation should be attempted with caution in situations where antimicrobial activity includes unknown contributions from active metabolites or diastereomers whose disposition is stereospecific. In either case, the various chemical species are not likely to be equipotent against a particular test organism. Therefore, apparent concentrations will also differ depending on the assay. Finally, heterogeneities attendant to samples obtained by gastrointestinal aspiration and by heel and finger punctures should also be weighed accordingly.

I. Benzylpenicillin (Penicillin G)

Elimination of benzylpenicillin is rapid and primarily by urinary excretion. Following intravenous administration in man, serum antimicrobial activity declines in a biexponential manner with a terminal half-life of about 42 min (DITTERT et al. 1969). Clearance rate from serum is estimated to be 550 ml/min while renal clearance is 433 ml/min. Thus, about 79% of the activity is recovered in the urine. Biliary excretion is negligible in man. In cholecystectomized patients with T-tube drainage, biliary clearance is 0.6 ml/min or 0.1% of total clearance (BROGARD et al. 1979c).

Probable routes of biotransformation are shown in Fig. 1; apparent conflicts exist in the literature. After intramuscular injections in man, COLE et al. (1973) recovered 82% of the dose in urine as either benzylpenicillin or its penicilloic acid, which represents about 19% of the total. This ratio appears to fit nicely with the urinary excretion pattern after intravenous administration. The presence of penicilloic acid in rat urine was also shown by WALKENSTEIN et al. (1954a, b). In contrast, INGOLD (1976) failed to detect any benzylpenicilloic acid in the urine of healthy volunteers after 300-mg injections intramuscularly. However, the same investigator found large quantities of penicilloic acid in the urine of healthy volunteers and in patients who ingested the drug orally. A possible explanation for the difference may be assay sensitivity and/or specificity. Whereas INGOLD (1976) relied on color formation attendant to the reduction of arsenomolybdic acid, COLE et al. (1973) used a modification of the iodometric assay of ALICINO (1946) for the determination of penicilloic acid. Differences between patients and healthy volun-

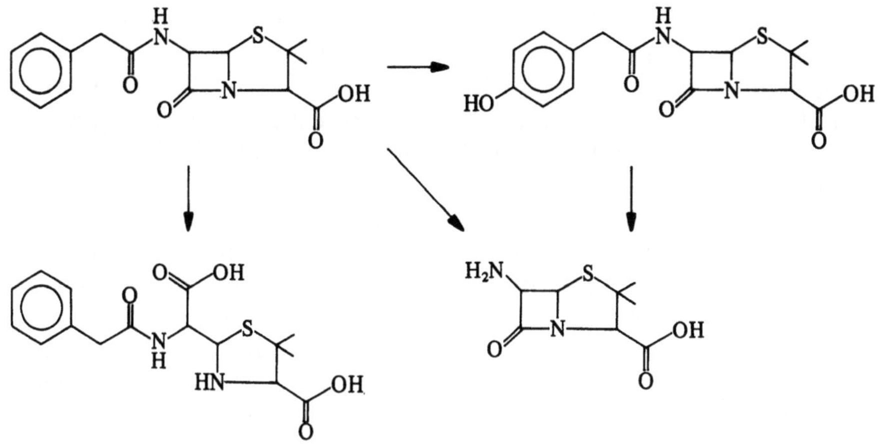

Fig. 1. Biotransformation of benzylpenicillin

teers are not surprising in that the therapeutic levels of benzylpenicillin are promptly negated by a single injection of penicillinase (WESTERMAN et al. 1964). An active metabolite, more polar than benzylpenicillin, is present in human urine. ROLINSON and BATCHELOR (1962) made no attempt at structural identification but estimated its presence to be less than 5% of the total antimicrobial activity in urine against *Bacillus subtilis*. Based on chromatographic behavior, ENGLISH et al. (1960) suggested p-hydroxybenzylpenicillin as a possibility. Unknown quantities of 6-aminopenicillanic acid have been detected in the urine of mice, rats, monkeys, rabbits, and man following oral doses of benzylpenicillin. Since acylase activity was found only in intestinal contents and not in tissue homogenates, ENGLISH et al. (1960) concluded that this particular biotransformation may be mediated by the gut flora. These observations were not confirmed by COLE et al. (1973) who did not find 6-aminopenicillanic acid in the urine of healthy volunteers after oral doses of benzylpenicillin. On balance, the experimental evidence suggests that benzylpenicilloic acid is the major metabolite, the origin of which is probably systemic as well as gastrointestinal; that p-hydroxybenzylpenicillin is tentatively the minor but active metabolite; and that 6-aminopenicillanic acid may be formed in trace amounts.

Benzylpenicillin is poorly bioavailable by the enteral routes (RAMMELKAMP and KEEFER 1943; VAN DIJCK et al. 1962; WAGNER et al. 1969). In man, only 2%–19% of the dose is recovered in the urine after oral or rectal administration as the sodium salt. Probable causes are inherently poor permeability with efficient absorption limited mainly to the duodenum, acid lability, and inactivation by bacterial enzymes (ABRAHAM and CHAIN 1940). Better absorption and more prolonged serum levels are achieved with penamecillin, the acetoxymethyl ester, which confers greater lipophilicity for transport and releases benzylpenicillin on hydrolysis by nonspecific acetylesterases in serum and tissues (AGERSBORG et al. 1966).

Absorption is efficient following intramuscular or subcutaneous injection; up to 80% of the administered activity can be recovered in human urine (RAMMELKAMP and KEEFER 1943; LEVY 1967). In order to extend the duration of therapeutic serum concentration per injection, sparingly soluble salts and esters have been used to create a depot effect at the site of administration. Notable examples of these are procaine penicillin (SULLIVAN et al. 1948), benzathine penicillin (ELIAS et al. 1951; SZABO et al. 1951), and the hydroiodide salt of the β-diethylaminoethyl ester of benzylpenicillin (JENSEN et al. 1951; HEATHCOTE and NASSAU 1951; FLIPPIN et al. 1952). Urinary recoveries and the duration of therapeutic levels seem to be affected by the physical activity of the patient (LUKASH and FRANK 1963; BALLARD 1966; LEVY 1967).

Within the therapeutic concentration range, benzylpenicillin is about 52%–66% bound to serum proteins, depending on the method of determination (KUNIN 1965, 1966b; ROLINSON and SUTHERLAND 1965; MOSKOWITZ et al. 1973; BIRD and MARSHALL 1967; PETERSON et al. 1977). At drug concentrations of 500 μg/ml and above, the bound fraction decreases rapidly (PETERSON et al. 1977). CRAIG and SUH (1978) recorded a 30% decrease in protein binding in uremic patients as compared to healthy subjects. They postulated the existence of an endogenous binding inhibitor that accumulates in renal impairement.

In vitro and in vivo studies indicate that benzylpenicillin migrates into and out of human erythrocytes (KORNGUTH and KUNIN 1976a). Benzylpenicillin is bound to hemoglobin and heme-free globin and is inactivated by human erythrocyte lysates (KORNGUTH and KUNIN 1976b). WAGNER et al. (1977) showed that benzylpenicillin is metabolized within human erythrocytes. Unlike the parent, the resulting penicilloic acid does not permeate the cell wall despite exhaustive dialysis.

Cerebrospinal fluid (CSF) levels of benzylpenicillin are normally 0.5%–2.0% those in serum but rise to 6% in meningitis (BARZA and WEINSTEIN 1976). Unlike procaine penicillin (McCRACKEN et al. 1973), CSF levels after benzathine penicillin are considered inadequate in the treatment of congenital syphilis in the neonate (SPEER et al. 1977). Significant antimicrobial activities are achieved in middle-ear effusions after single intramuscular injections in patients with suppurative and secretory otitis media (SILVERSTEIN et al. 1966). After an intravenous injection, antibiotic concentrations in blister fluid reached a maximum at 30 min and were consistently higher than those in serum after 1.5 h (SCHREINGER et al. 1978). At steady state, lymph concentrations in the dog are about 73% of those in plasma (VERWAY and WILLIAMS 1962). Negligible amounts of benzylpenicillin are excreted in the milk of lactating ewes (ZIV and SULMAN 1974).

The effect of probenecid is primarily to inhibit renal tubular secretion (BEYER et al. 1951) and secondarily to block the active transport of penicillin by the choroid plexus (SPECTOR and LORENZO 1974). Both effects tend to elevate and maintain higher serum concentrations. In patients with nearly normal renal function, the serum clearance of benzylpenicillin is decreased by about 60% and serum half-life is increased by 30% when pretreated with 1 g probenecid 8 h and 1 h before the penicillin (GIBALDI et al. 1970; JUSKO and GIBALDI 1972). Therefore, with chronic probenecid administration, antibiotic concentrations at steady state may be tripled. Prolongation of penicillin half-life has also been noted after repeated daily doses of phenylbutazone, sulfapyrazone, acetylsalicylic acid, sulfaphenazole, and indomethacin (KAMPMANN et al. 1972). In rats, liver and kidney uptake of radioactivity following ^{14}C-benzylpenicillin is reduced with concomitant administration of probenecid (BERGHOLZ et al. 1980).

Renal handling in children (3–12 years) is similar to that in adults. Renal clearance in both populations is about 4 times that of inulin. In newborn infants, how-

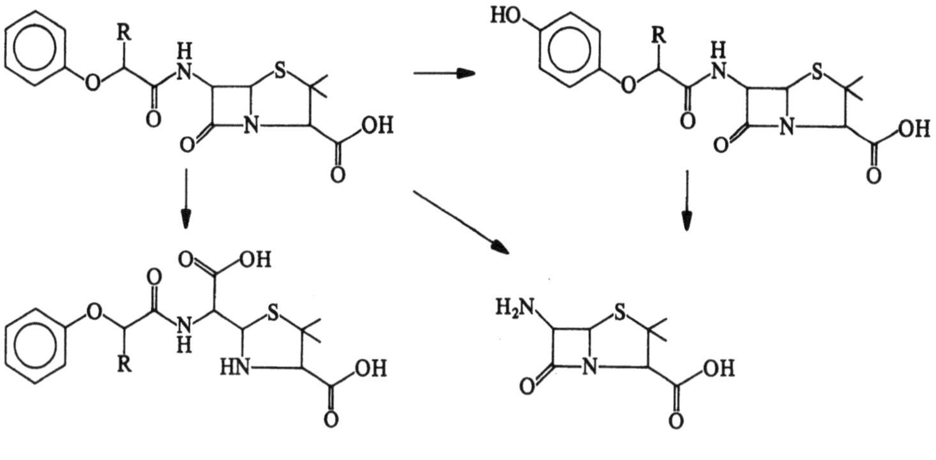

R: H Penicillin V
CH_3 Pheneticillin
CH_3CH_2 Propicillin
C_6H_5 Phenbenicillin

Fig. 2. Biotransformation of phenoxyalkylpenicillins

ever, renal clearance of benzylpenicillin is only twice that of inulin, which is inherently low compared to the adult (BARNETT et al. 1949). Immature renal function is said to be one of the factors in the more sustained therapeutic levels following oral doses of penicillin G in infants (HUSSON 1947). On the other hand, renal clearance of benzylpenicillin in diabetic children is about twice that in normal children (MAD'ACSY et al. 1975).

In azotemic patients PLAUT et al. (1969) found an inverse logarithmic relationship between serum half-life and inulin or p-aminohippurate clearance rate.

II. Phenoxyalkylpenicillins

Two basic characteristics of this family of penicillins preclude rigorous pharmacokinetic interpretation of their fate. Except for phenoxymethylpenicillin, an additional chiral center is present in the acyl side-chain. There are strong indications that the D- and L-isomers differ in potency against a variety of microorganisms and that their physiological disposition is stereospecific. Therefore, the relative abundance of the isomers in serum and urine changes continuously with time following the administration of a diastereomeric mixture of the two. Besides, active metabolites are known to be formed in varying amounts. Without prior separation, microbiological assays of biological specimens would not discern the contributions of the disastereomeric parents and metabolite(s). The metabolic scheme given in Fig. 2 is generally applicable to phenoxyalkylpenicillins; hydroxylation has been inferred but not characterized in most cases.

1. Phenoxymethylpenicillin (Penicillin V)

Following an intravenous injection in healthy subjects, serum antimicrobial activity declines more or less biexponentially with a terminal half-life of about 27 min

(SIMON et al. 1976a). Fifty percent of the administered activity is recovered in the urine. Serum and renal clearance rates are 800 and 400 ml/min, respectively. On the basis of relative areas under the serum curves in the same panel of subjects, the bioavailability of orally administered potassium phenoxymethylpenicillin is approximately 57%.

After oral doses of potassium ^{35}S-phenoxymethylpenicillin, 49% of the radioactivity appeared in the urine while another 32% was recovered in the stool. HELLSTRÖM et al. (1974b) estimated that about 30% of the administered dose was excreted in the urine as unchanged phenoxymethylpenicillin. Similarly, COLE et al. (1973) and BOND et al. (1963) each recovered 26% of the administered antimicrobial activity in urine. Thus, there is good agreement among investigators on the absorption and excretion of potassium phenoxymethylpenicillin.

Hydrolytic cleavage of the β-lactam ring is the major route of phenoxymethylpenicillin biotransformation in man. The presence of phenoxymethylpenicilloic acid in urine has been identified by direct iodometric assay (COLE et al. 1973), and by spectrophotometric (BIRNER 1970) or radiometric (HELLSTRÖM et al. 1974b) assays following chromatographic separation. COLE et al. (1973) estimated that 57% of the drug-related substances is urine is the penicilloic acid. Comparing the composition of gastric and intestinal aspirates following oral doses of ^{35}S-phenoxymethylpenicillin and ^{35}S-phenoxymethylpenicilloate, HELLSTRÖM et al. (1974b) concluded that part of the penicilloic acid is formed in the gastrointestinal tract, although its subsequent absorption is relatively slow and incomplete. There is no evidence of biliary excretion for the drug or metabolite.

The presence of an active metabolite was first noted by ROLINSON and BATCHELOR (1962) and subsequently identified as p-hydroxyphenoxymethylpenicillin by VANDERHAEGHE et al. (1963). According to HELLSTRÖM et al. (1974b), this metabolite represents less than 5% of the radioactivity in urine. Thus, a bias of up to 10% may be inherent in serum and urine levels based on microbiological assay and pharmacokinetic parameters derived therefrom.

Chromatographic evidence indicates that a second active metabolite, more polar than the p-hydroxy analog, is present in the urine of some people. VANDERHAEGHE et al. (1963) suggested that it may be the dihydroxy derivative, but a bioautographically labile conjugate of phenoxymethylpenicillin or its p-hydroxy metabolite is equally compatible with the evidence. Finally, traces of 6-aminopenicillanic acid have been detected in urine after oral doses of phenoxymethylpenicillin (COLE et al. 1973).

At concentrations up to 200 μg/ml, binding of penicillin V to serum proteins ranges from 78.5% to 83.4% depending on the method of determination (KUNIN 1965, 1966b; BIRD and MARSHALL 1967; ROLINSON and SUTHERLAND 1965; BOND et al. 1963).

In patients recovering from myringotomy, therapeutic concentrations in middle-ear effusions can be achieved with oral doses of penicillin V (SILVERSTEIN et al. 1966). At steady state, lymph to plasma concentration ratio in the dog is 0.63 (VERWAY and WILLIAMS 1962). In the rat, the ratio of tissue to blood concentrations are 0.1 in muscles, 0.2 in the heart, spleen, and liver, 1.9 in the gut wall, and 6.6 in the kidney (TSUJI et al. 1979). When ^{3}H-phenoxymethylpenicillin was incubated with rat liver slices, a steady-state level of unchanged drug was achieved within 15 min. However, the uptake of radioactivity continues to increase with time, presumably because of metabolite formation and binding (RYRFELDT 1973).

Several types of pharmaceutical dosage forms of phenoxymethylpenicillin are used orally in the clinic. In general, tablets of the potassium or calcium salt are comparable to aqueous solutions of the potassium salt while tablets of the benzathine salt and oil suspensions of the calcium or benzathine salt are more slowly and incompletely absorbed (BOLME and ERIKSSON 1976, 1978; BERGAN et al. 1976; PALATSI and KAIPAINEN 1971; ROLLAG et al. 1975). Infants younger than 6 months tend to produce higher serum levels than older children and adults after a comparable dose, presumably because absorption is enhanced while excretion may be delayed (BOLME and ERIKSSON 1978; SIMON et al. 1972). Absorption is reduced in patients with coeliac disease (BOLME et al. 1977; DAVIS and PIROLA 1968).

While available for use, the intramuscular forms of penicillin V offer no obvious advantage over that of benzylpenicillin in view of the former's higher clearance rate and more extensive binding to serum proteins.

2. Pheneticillin

Pheneticillin is a mixture composed of about 66% of the L-isomer and 34% of the D-isomer of α-phenoxyethylpenicillin (ENGLISH and MCBRIDE 1961). In various tests of antimicrobial activity in vitro and in vivo, the L-isomer is at least comparable, but often superior, to the D-isomer. With minor exceptions, the anticipated difference in potency between the L-isomer and pheneticillin prevails (ENGLISH and MCBRIDE 1961; WICK et al. 1961). Apparent inconsistencies can be rationalized on the basis of stereoselectivity in the absorption or disposition in vivo.

After oral administration in man, 22% of the dose appears in the urine as the penicilloic acid(s) and small quantities of 6-aminopenicillanic acid (COLE et al. 1973). Also present in urine is another metabolite that is biologically active, more polar than the parent, and thought to be hydroxylated pheneticillin (ROLINSON and BATCHELOR 1962; VANDERHAEGHE et al. 1963).

Absorption of orally administered potassium pheneticillin appears to be incomplete and highly variable. Urinary recovery of microbiological activity ranges from 19% to 50% of the dose (MCCARTHY and FINLAND 1960; BOND et al. 1963; SIMON et al. 1976a; COLE et al. 1973). Aqueous solutions of the potassium salt are better absorbed than oily suspensions of the potassium and benzathine salts (MARTY and HERSEY 1975).

Pheneticillin is bound to human serum proteins to the extent of 75%–82% (BOND et al. 1963; ROLINSON and SUTHERLAND 1965; BIRD and MARSHALL 1967). In the dog, lymph concentrations are 63% of those in plasma at steady state (VERWAY and WILLIAMS 1962).

3. Propicillin

Commercially available propicillin is a mixture of the diastereoisomers. Against most microorganisms studied, the L-isomer is more potent than either the D-isomer or the mixture (WICK et al. 1961). Stereospecific absorption and elimination has been demonstrated by LEE and ANDERSON (1961). After oral and intravenous administration of individual epimers to the dog, differences were observed in serum

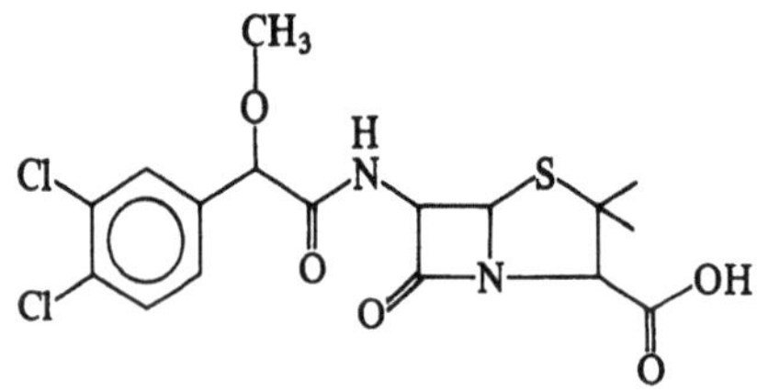

Fig. 3. Structure of clometocillin

half-life, renal clearance, plasma protein binding, amount absorbed, and amounts excreted after an oral and an intravenous dose.

In man, 50%–53% of the administered activity is recovered in the urine after gradated oral doses; 82% after an intravenous injection (SIMON et al. 1976a). BOND et al. (1963), on the other hand, recovered only 27% in the urine after a 250-mg oral dose. An unidentified, active metabolite, more polar than the parents, is found in human urine (ROLINSON and BATCHELOR 1962). Propicillin is 86%–89% bound to human serum (BOND et al. 1963; BIRD and MARSHALL 1967).

4. Phenbenicillin

Following oral doses of DL-α-phenoxybenzylpenicillin in man, 20%–23% of the administered activity is recovered in the urine (BOND et al. 1963; ROLLO et al. 1962). ROLINSON and BATCHELOR (1962) showed one active metabolite by bioautography against *Bacillus subtilis* while ROLLO et al. (1962) reported two metabolites accounting for 20% of the urinary activity against *Sarcina lutea*.

Phenbenicillin is 97% bound to serum proteins (BIRD and MARSHALL 1967; BOND et al. 1963). Thus, even though higher serum concentrations of antimicrobial activity are attained with phenbenicillin than with comparable oral doses of other phenoxyalkylpenicillins, corresponding unbound concentrations are pheneticillin > phenoxymethylpenicillin > propicillin > phenbenicillin (BOND et al. 1963; ROLLO et al. 1962; CARTER and BRUMFITT 1962).

III. Clometocillin

Like most phenoxyalkylpenicillins, clometocillin (Fig. 3) has an assymmetric carbon on the acyl side-chain and is administered as a mixture of the diastereoisomers. Against a few test organisms the D-isomer appears to be the more potent (VANDERHAEGHE et al. 1961). There is also bioautographic evidence of two active metabolites in human urine; their combined zones of inhibition are at least comparable to that of the parent(s) (VANDERHAEGHE et al. 1961; ROLINSON and BATCHELOR 1962).

Antimicrobial activity in human serum tends to be higher and more sustained after clometocillin than after the same oral dose of phenoxymethylpenicillin (pheneticillin) or the same intramuscular dose of benzylpenicillin. Peak serum activity is similar after oral and intramuscular doses. About 46% of the orally administered activity is renally excreted (VANDERHAEGHE et al. 1961; VAN DIJCK et al. 1962).

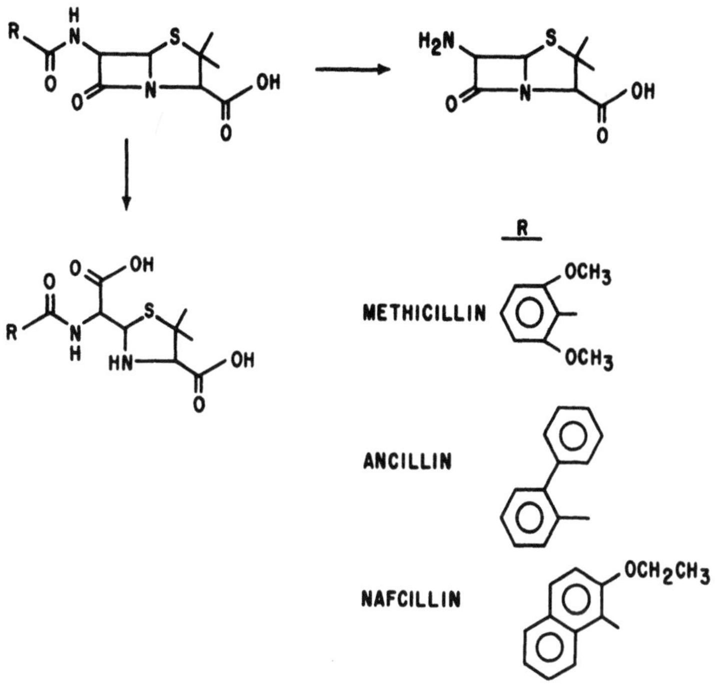

Fig. 4. Biotransformation of methicillin, ancillin, and nafcillin

The slow disappearance of serum activity can be explained in part by the fact that clometocillin is 92% bound to serum proteins (BIRD and MARSHALL 1967). Other contributing factors include active metabolite formation and enterohepatic circulation (VANDERHAEGHE et al. 1961).

IV. Methicillin

Methicillin is the first of the semisynthetic penicillins in which resistance to β-lactamase activity is conferred mainly by steric hindrance (Fig. 4). At doses of penicillinase activity which would completely destroy benzylpenicillin, serum concentrations of methicillin appear to be minimally affected (WESTERMAN et al. 1964). In human urine, about 7% of an intramuscular dose is recovered as the penicilloic acid (COLE et al. 1973), and there is no evidence of active metabolites being excreted (ROLINSON and BATCHELOR 1962).

Serum concentrations of methicillin decline biexponentially with time after an intravenous injection in healthy subjects. DITTERT et al. (1969) reported a mean serum clearance of 567 ml/min, half-life of 30 min, and urinary recovery of 61% after a 250-mg dose. Somewhat different estimates of 449 ml/min, 51 min, and 88%, respectively, were reported by YAFFE et al. (1977) after a dose of 15 mg/kg. Although therapeutic concentrations are achieved in bile, total biliary excretion is negligibly small, i.e., <0.01% (HENEGAR et al. 1961). In the absence of other known routes of elimination, the higher estimate of methicillin in urine appears more consistent with the observed recovery of the penicilloic acid.

Orally administered methicillin is poorly absorbed; less than 3% of the dose is recovered in the urine (SABATH et al. 1962). In contrast, 70%–75% of the dose is excreted in the urine after an intramuscular injection (COLE et al. 1973; KUNIN 1966a).

Values ranging from 37% to 62% have been reported for the serum protein binding of methicillin (KUNIN 1965; ROLINSON and SUTHERLAND 1965; BIRD and MARSHALL 1967; BENNETT and KIRBY 1965). In patients undergoing hip arthroplasty, methicillin levels in cortical bone samples 1 h after an intravenous dose averages 3.3 μg/g, which is twice that in synovial tissue and one-sixth of that in serum (FITZGERALD et al. 1978). On average fetal and maternal serum concentrations tend to be similar, although wide variations exist within individual mother-child pairs (DEPP et al. 1970; MACAULEY et al. 1973). After a single intravenous dose to the mother, amniotic fluid concentrations of methicillin rise and fall gradually with time. Detectable amounts of methicillin are present in CSF (BUNN et al. 1960; BARTOLOZZI et al. 1967). Methicillin does not penetrate into the aqueous humor of human eyes except when the blood–aqueous barrier has been altered by disease or local inflammatory processes (RECORDS 1966). In the dog, the lymph to plasma concentration ratio is 0.96 at steady state (VERWAY and WILLIAMS 1962).

The elimination rate of methicillin is slow in the newborn infant (3.3-h half-life) and changes rapidly during the first month of life. Further reductions in elimination rate are seen in the premature. Thus, serum half-lives in 1-month-old premature infants are similar to those in 4- to 5-day-old term infants (BOE et al. 1967). This inverse relationship between age and serum levels has also been reported by BARTOLOZZI et al. (1967), who noted a similar trend with respect to body weight, and by AXLINE et al. (1967), whose estimates of serum half-lives were probably too high because samples had been taken by heel punctures.

In patients with cystic fibrosis, the elimination rate of methicillin is enhanced. Compared to healthy subjects, serum clearance is higher by about 20%, all of which has been attributed to an increase in renal tubular secretion (YAFFE et al. 1977).

V. Ancillin

Like methicillin, ancillin is penicillinase-resistant. Unlike methicillin, it has a spectrum of activity similar to that of benzylpenicillin and is orally active.

Following oral and intramuscular doses to the dog, the ratio of tissue to serum activity ranges from about 0.05 in CSF to 570 in bile, while those in erythrocytes, kidney, liver, lung, and heart are in between (DOLAN et al. 1961). The lymph-to-plasma concentration ratio at steady state is 0.58 (VERWAY and WILLIAMS 1962).

In man, absorption after intramuscular injections appears to be uniform and reproducible. In the dose range of 250–1,000 mg, about 35% of the administered activity is excreted in the urine. On the other hand, absorption of orally administered ancillin is highly variable and adversely affected by food. In the best of circumstances, however, urinary recoveries after oral administration are comparable to those after intramuscular dosage (FARQUHAR et al. 1961; SABATH et al. 1963).

In the presence of probenecid, the area under the serum activity vs. time curve after an intramuscular dose of ancillin is essentially doubled while urinary recovery is halved, and serum half-life is increased by 17% (SABATH et al. 1963; GIBALDI and SCHWARTZ 1968). Thus, the effect of concomitant probenecid administration orally, 500 mg q.i.d., is to reduce serum clearance to one-half and renal clearance to one-quarter of their normal values.

Ancillin is 90%–91% bound to human serum proteins (BIRD and MARSHALL 1967; KUNIN 1966b).

The biotransformation of ancillin has not been reported (Fig. 4). However, judging from the reproducibility and the lack of dose dependence in the urinary recovery after intramuscular injections, two-thirds of the dose must have been eliminated extrarenally. Biliary excretion is not likely to be a significant factor since it is not dramatically different from methicillin or penicillin V in the dog and, more importantly, it can be efficiently absorbed from the gastrointestinal tract. Thus, chemical or biochemical transformation to inactive or weakly active species appears to be the primary means of ancillin elimination.

VI. Nafcillin

Steady-state serum concentrations of nafcillin are only transiently decreased by an intramuscular dose of penicillinase. By this criterion, its resistance to penicillinase is between those of methicillin and benzylpenicillin (WESTERMAN et al. 1964). Its spectrum of antimicrobial activity is not as limited as that of methicillin or as broad as that of ancillin.

After oral and intramuscular doses of side-chain carboxy-labeled ^{14}C-nafcillin to dogs, 72% of the radioactivity can be accounted for in urine and feces when plasma radioactivity remains substantial at 0.5–1.5 μg/ml nafcillin equivalents. At least three inactive metabolites have been separated by radioautography, accounting for 50% of the radioactivity in the 0- to 6-h urine. None of the metabolites have been identified although the absence of ^{14}C-ethoxynaphthoic acid and its metabolites rules out the possibility of 6-aminopenicillanic acid as a primary metabolite (Fig. 4). The remaining 50% has been identified as unchanged nafcillin. A somewhat higher percentage of the radioactivity in bile samples through 6 h is attributed to nafcillin while less than 20% is unchanged drug in plasma. By 24 h, little if any of the radioactivity in plasma, urine, and bile is nafcillin (WALKENSTEIN et al. 1963).

In healthy subjects, plasma concentrations of nafcillin after an intravenous injection decline rapidly with a terminal half-life of 33 min. Plasma and renal clearances are estimated to be 410 and 160 ml/min per 1.73 m^2, consistent with the urinary recovery of 38% (KIND et al. 1970). About 8% of an intravenous dose is recovered in the bile of a patient with an exteriorized cannula (NUNES et al. 1964). After intramuscular injections, KLEIN and FINLAND (1963b) recovered 31% of the dose in urine while FOLTZ et al. (1961) reported 49%. Absorption of orally administered nafcillin is incomplete and somewhat dependent on the formulation. On the basis of urinary recoveries, tablets of the sodium salt are about one-third as bioavailable as an intramuscular injection. Mean urinary recoveries of 7.4%, 12.1%, and 16.0% obtained following administration of the sodium salt, the sodium salt buffered with calcium carbonate, and the free acid, respectively. In whatever form, concomitant administration with food further decreases the bioavailability of nafcillin given orally KLEIN and FINLAND 1963b: WATANAKUNAKORN 1977).

Nafcillin in 89.5% bound to human serum proteins (BIRD and MARSHALL 1967; KUNIN 1965; BENNETT and KIRBY 1965). The distribution of nafcillin and related substances is ubiquitous in all tissues examined. In rats, the highest concentrations of radioactivity during the first 2 h are found in the liver and bladder, at later times, in the cecal wall (WALKENSTEIN et al. 1963). In patients undergoing major surgery, NUNES et al. (1964) reported antimicrobial activity in all tissues examined with the highest concentrations being in bile, gall bladder, and liver. Nafcillin given to pregnant women within 4 h before delivery is readily detectable in infants 1 h after birth (O'CONNOR et al. 1965). After intravenous injections of nafcillin, CSF concentrations rose to a peak at 2 h and declined slowly (FOSSIECK et al. 1977). Therapeutic levels of nafcillin are achievable in synovial fluids of the knee following single, 1,500-mg, intramuscular injections and are potentiated by the concomitant administration of probenecid (VIEK 1962).

The effect of intermittent, repeated oral doses of probenecid is to increase serum concentrations by a factor of more than 2 (KLEIN and FINLAND 1963b). Change of this magnitude cannot be explained solely on the basis of probenecid's effect on renal tubular secretion. Thus, even in patients without renal function, plasma clearance is 253 ml/min per 1.73 m^2 compared to 410 ml/min per 1.73 m^2 in healthy subjects (KIND and TUPASI 1970). On the other hand, the hepatobiliary system has a significant role in nafcillin elimination. MARSHALL et al. (1977) showed that plasma clearance of nafcillin is approximately halved in patients with alcohol-induced cirrhosis and approaches normal renal clearance in patients with extrahepatic biliary obstruction. These changes represent respectively 67% and 80% reductions in hepatic clearance. Finally, the kinetics of nafcillin disposition in patients with renal failure is little influenced by hemodialysis (DIAZ et al. 1977).

Serum concentrations in the newborn tend to be higher and more sustained than in older children. The difference is particularly noticeable during the first month and further exaggerated in the premature (GROSSMAN and TICKNOR 1965; O'CONNOR et al. 1964; FELDMAN et al. 1978; BANNER et al. 1980).

VII. Isoxazolylpenicillins

Penicilloic acid formation and hydroxylation of the 5-methyl substituent on the isoxazole ring are the only known routes of isoxazolylpenicillin biotransformation (Fig. 5). In relation to the parent, the 5-hydroxymethyl metabolites have antibacterial spectrums that are similar and potencies that are within a factor of two (COLE et al. 1973; THIJSSEN and MATTIE 1976; THIJSSEN 1979). Against *Sarcina lutea*, 21% of the 0- to 8-h activity in human urine following orally administered oxacillin may be attributed to the active metabolite, about 15% after cloxacillin and dicloxacillin, and 10% following flucloxacillin. Limited data on serum suggest that active metabolite contribution may be similar except in the presence of renal impairment (ROLINSON and BATCHELOR 1962; THIJSSEN and MATTIE 1976). Thus, pharmacokinetic parameters derived from serum and urinary antimicrobial activity should be interpreted with due caution.

1. Oxacillin

Following intravenous doses of oxacillin in man, estimates of serum and renal clearance of antimicrobial activity are similar among laboratories (ROSENBLATT et

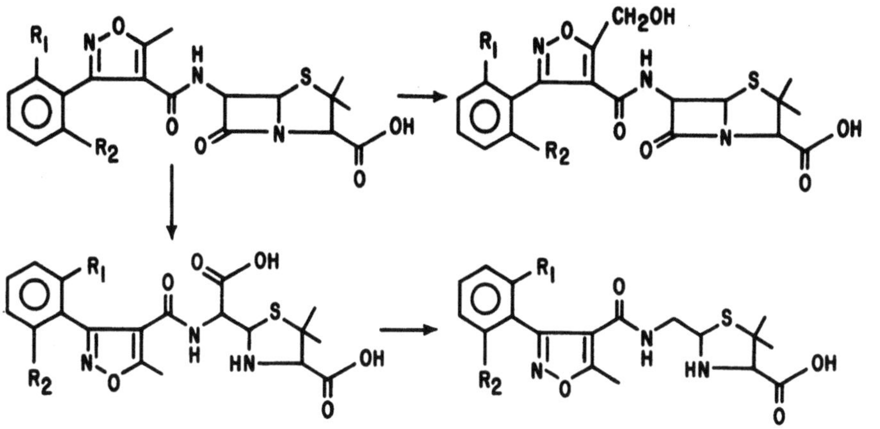

	R_1	R_2
OXACILLIN	H	H
CLOXACILLIN	Cl	H
DICLOXACILLIN	Cl	Cl
FLUCLOXACILLIN	Cl	F

Fig. 5. Biotransformation of isoxazolylpenicillins

al. 1969; DITTERT et al. 1969; KIND et al. 1970). The ratio of renal clearance, estimated during the 3rd h of a constant infusion, to serum clearance agrees nicely with the fractional urinary recovery of antimicrobial activity (KIND et al. 1970). The proximity between observed (0.47) and predicted (0.50) ratios strongly suggests that the relative abundance of active metabolite to drug is similar in serum (and urine) at corresponding times. These events are most likely to occur simultaneously if the elimination of the 5-hydroxymethyl metabolite is fast relative to its rate of formation. Based on observations that the metabolite is one-half as active as oxacillin when estimated with *S. lutea*, that 80% of the urinary activity is attributed to unchanged drug, and that a similar ratio obtains in serum (THIJSSEN and MATTIE 1976; ROLINSON and BATCHELOR 1962), it is estimated that on average 38% of an intravenous dose is excreted in urine as oxacillin and 19% as 5-hydroxymethyloxacillin, while serum and renal clearances of oxacillin are 475 and 180 ml/min per 1.73 m^2 respectively.

Sixteen percent of an oral dose of oxacillin is excreted in the urine as the penicilloic acid with no evidence of 6-aminopenicillanic acid (COLE et al. 1973; GRABER et al. 1976). Another 17%–21% is recovered as oxacillin equivalents of antimicrobial activity as determined by *S. lutea* (PRIGOT et al. 1962; KUNIN 1966a; COLE et al. 1973). Using chromatography and the UV chromophore of the penicillenic acid, GRABER et al. (1976) estimated that 27% of an oral dose is excreted in urine as oxacillin. Preliminary results by high performance liquid chromatography suggest that oxacillin and 5-hydroxymethyloxacillin are present in urine in about equal amounts after an oral dose (MURAI et al. 1980).

After intramuscular injections, 19%–44% of the activity is excreted in the urine. Recoveries are halved after concomitant administration of probenecid (PRIGOT et al. 1962; KUNIN 1966a).

Oxacillin is 92%–95% bound to human serum proteins (KUNIN 1965; BENNETT and KIRBY 1965). Unbound concentrations double on concomitant administration of sulfamethoxypyridine or sulfaethylthiadiazole, while areas under the serum level curve (free plus bound) are lowered by as much as 60% (KUNIN 1966b). Probenecid reduces serum protein binding and enhances oxacillin penetration into fibrin clots in vitro (LEE et al. 1975). After intravenous injections to pregnant women therapeutic levels are achieved in amniotic fluid, albeit slowly (BASTERT et al. 1975). After oral administration, detectable levels are present in the milk of nursing mothers; substantial levels are found in bile (PRIGOT et al. 1962). Oxacillin will penetrate into osseous and synovial tissues of the hip (FITZGERALD et al. 1978), but will not cross the blood–aqueous barrier in the eye (RECORDS 1967). Lung tissue levels are approximately one-quarter of those in serum (KISS et al. 1974). At steady state, lymph concentrations in the dog are 60% of those in plasma (VERWAY and WILLIAMS 1962).

In patients with chronic renal failure requiring hemodialysis, serum clearance of apparent oxacillin activity is about one-third of normal (KIND et al. 1970). In premature infants, the efficiency of elimination improves with age (BURNS et al. 1964; AXLINE et al. 1967).

2. Cloxacillin

HELLSTRÖM et al. (1974a) studied the disposition of ^{35}S-labeled cloxacillin and its penicilloic acid in man. After an intravenous dose of ^{35}S-cloxacillin, 82% of the radioactivity is excreted in the urine and 11% in the feces. The corresponding values after oral or intrajejunal administration are 54% and 33%. Metabolite patterns are similar regardless of the route of administration. Biologically inactive metabolite(s) constitutes 30% of the serum radioactivity at 60 min, >50% at 120 min. About 90% of the radioactivity in urine after 90 min is unchanged drug, 40%–80% thereafter. Small quantities are excreted in bile mainly as inactive metabolite(s). Except in highly acidic samples, most of the radioactivity in gastric aspirates is unchanged drug, which represents only 20% of the intestinal aspirates at later times. Penicilloic and/or penilloic acid accounts for most of the inactive metabolites in urine, bile, and gastrointestinal aspirates. Following oral administration of the ^{35}S-labeled penicilloic acid, gastrointestinal aspirates taken as a function of time contain increasing contributions from an unknown metabolite which is not penicic or the penilloic acid.

Two minor metabolites have been detected in rat urine (NAYLER et al. 1962). 5-Hydroxymethylcloxacillin has been identified as an active metabolite in rat urine (THIJSSEN 1979). An active metabolite, presumably the 5-hydroxy analog and equipotent to the parent against *S. lutea*, accounts for 10%–14% of the antimicrobial activity in human serum and urine (THIJSSEN and MATTIE 1976; ROLINSON and BATCHELOR 1962; NAYLER et al. 1962). Eleven percent of an oral dose of cloxacillin is recovered in the urine as the penicilloic acid (COLE et al. 1973).

In healthy subjects, 62%–76% of an intravenous dose is recovered in the urine as cloxacillin equivalents. Adjusting for the presence of the active metabolite, serum clearance of unchanged cloxacillin is about 174 ml/min. By direct measurement, THIJSSEN and MATTIE (1976) reported renal clearances of 110 ml/min for cloxacillin and 270 ml/min for the active metabolite. Orally administered cloxacillin is about 50% absorbed on the basis of urinary recoveries in relation to those after an intravenous dose (COLE et al. 1973; NAUTA and MATTIE, 1975, 1976; NAUTA et al., 1973; ROSENBLATT et al. 1968).

Cloxacillin is 94%–96% bound in human serum proteins (BENNETT and KIRBY 1965; ROLINSON and SUTHERLAND 1965; KUNIN 1965). A threefold increase in free fraction is seen in uremic sera (CRAIG and SUH 1978). Cloxacillin can displace bilirubin from neonatal serum, but only at concentrations far in excess of therapeutic (FRIEDMAN and LEWIS 1980). Protein binding has been suggested as an explanation for the relatively high concentration ratio of serum to synovial fluid, even though cloxacillin diffuses readily across the synovial membrane (HOWELL et al. 1972). Therapeutic concentrations in the aqueous humor can be attained after subconjunctival injections, but not after intramuscular doses (UWAYDAH et al. 1976). Detectable, but negligible amounts are secreted in the milk of lactating ewes (ZIV and SULMAN 1974), while 11% of an intravenous dose is excreted in rat bile (RYRFELDT 1971).

In patients with chronic renal failure, serum clearance of cloxacillin-like activity is reduced to about 40% of normal and apparently unaffected by hemodialysis. Attempts to estimate oral absorption in this population on the basis of area ratios of serum activity are probably not justified because of apparent difference in drug and active metabolite disposition (NAUTA and MATTIE 1975, 1976; NAUTA et al. 1973). After an oral dose, the contribution of the active metabolite to the serum activity at 1 h is 15% but increases rapidly to 44% at 4 h (THIJSSEN and MATTIE 1976).

3. Dicloxacillin

The 5-hydroxymethyl metabolite of dicloxacillin has been identified in the urine of rats, dogs, and man (VAN HARKEN et al. 1970; THIJSSEN 1979). This metabolite is 50% as active as dicloxacillin as determined with *S. lutea* and contributes 15% to the total activity recovered in human urine after an intravenous or oral dose of dicloxacillin (THIJSSEN and MATTIE 1976). Four percent of an intramuscular dose is excreted in the urine as the penicilloic acid (COLE et al. 1973).

Following a 2-min intravenous infusion, serum activity declines biexponentially. Apparent pharmacokinetic parameters derived from serum data accurately predict the time course of urinary excretion (DITTERT et al. 1969). This would be possible if the renal clearance of cloxacillin and 5-hydroxymethyldicloxacillin were each incrementally constant over time; renal clearance value for the two species need not be the same, however. Since the relative abundance of dicloxacillin in serum is not known, no estimate can be made of its true clearance. In the light of the foregoing, the ratio of total urinary recoveries should be a more reliable index of bioavailability than that of areas of serum activity.

From 56% to 73% of an intravenous dose is excreted in the urine as dicloxacillin-like activity, of which 85% can be attributed to unchanged drug while another 30% is the active metabolite (ROSENBLATT et al. 1968; NAUTA and MATTIE 1976; DITTERT et al. 1969). Urinary recoveries after oral and intramuscular doses are similar and range from 28% to 48% (DEFELICE 1967; DOLUISIO et al. 1969; KUNIN 1966a; COLE et al. 1973). In subjects who also received an intravenous dose, the bioavailability of orally administered dicloxacillin is estimated to be 74% (NAUTA and MATTIE 1976).

Dicloxacillin is 96%–98% bound to normal human serum proteins (KUNIN 1965; BENNETT and KIRBY 1965) and 90% bound in uremic sera (CRAIG and SUH 1978). Dicloxacillin is readily taken up by human red blood cells, is bound to hemoglobin and heme-free globin, and is inactivated by erythrocyte lysates (KORNGUTH and KUNIN 1976a, b). Dicloxacillin is poorly transported across the human placenta; concentrations in fetal serum and amniotic fluid, while detectable, are low relative to maternal serum (MACAULEY et al. 1968; DEPP et al. 1970). A substantial quantity of radioactivity is excreted in the bile after ^{35}S-dicloxacillin is administered in rats; 10% of it is identified as unchanged drug, another 20% as the 5-hydroxymethyl metabolite, while the remainder is unknown and inactive (VAN HARKEN et al. 1970).

Renal clearance of antimicrobial activity is tripled while unbound fraction in serum is doubled in patients with cystic fibrosis (JUSKO et al. 1975). In patients with renal dysfunction and requiring hemodialysis, apparent serum clearance is about 60% of normal (NAUTA and MATTIE 1976).

4. Flucloxacillin

The active metabolite of flucloxacillin contributes 10% to the recovered activity in human urine, is also present in human serum, and is equipotent to the parent drug against *S. lutea*. While 5-hydroxymethylflucloxacillin has been identified in rat urine (THIJSSEN 1978, 1979), it has not been confirmed in human urine (MURAI et al. 1980). About 4% of an oral dose in man is excreted in the urine as the penicilloic acid (COLE et al. 1973).

Seventy-four percent of an intravenous dose is excreted in the urine as flucloxacillin-like activity. Orally administered flucloxacillin is about 54% bioavailable on the basis of urinary recovery (NAUTA and MATTIE 1975). Thus, about 83% of an intravenous dose can be accounted for as unchanged drug (67%), active metabolite (7%), and the penicilloic acid (9%). Serum antimicrobial activity is similar to those following comparable doses of cloxacillin and dicloxacillin (BODEY et al. 1972). However, unbound concentrations are highest after intramuscular injections of flucloxacillin (SUTHERLAND et al. 1970b).

Flucloxacillin penetrates synovial and osseous tissues poorly and is not efficiently dialyzable, presumably because it is 93%–95% bound to serum proteins (SUTHERLAND et al. 1970b; BODEY et al. 1972). At therapeutic concentrations, flucloxacillin has no effect on the binding of bilirubin by neonatal serum (FRIEDMAN and LEWIS 1980). In patients undergoing total hip replacement, therapeutic levels of antibacterial activity are not achieved consistently in bone, synovial capsule, or synovial fluid (POLLARD et al. 1979). Antimicrobial activity in cantherides-induced blister fluids is about one-sixth that in serum while unbound concentration ratio of same is approximately one-third (WISE et al. 1980e).

The clearance rate of flucloxacillin from blood undergoing hemodialysis in vitro is 6.9 ml/min (VERHOEF et al. 1973), which contributes negligibly to drug removal in vivo (OE et al. 1973). In patients with chronic renal failure, clearance of apparent serum activity is about 40% of normal and little affected by hemodialysis (NAUTA and MATTIE 1975).

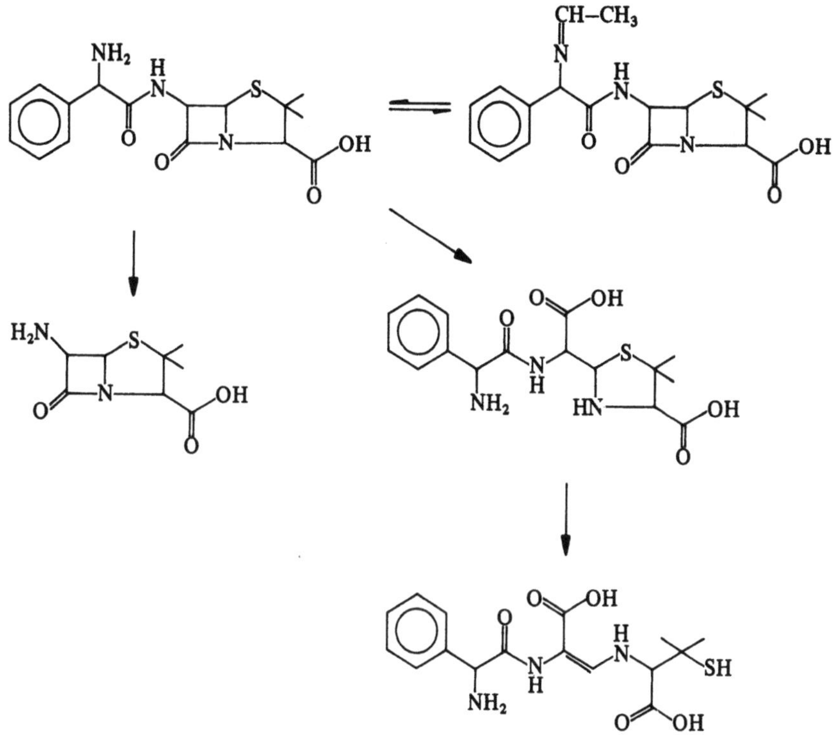

Fig. 6. Biotransformation of ampicillin

VIII. Ampicillin

Known products of ampicillin biotransformation are summarized in Fig. 6. About 10% of an oral dose is excreted in the urine as the penicilloic acid (COLE et al. 1973; SWAHN 1975; GRABER et al. 1976). While α-aminobenzylpenamaldic acid has been tentatively identified as a urinary metabolite in man (MASADE et al. 1979), it may also be the result of tautomerization ex vivo. Traces of 6-aminopenicillanic acid have been noted by some workers but not by others. ROLINSON and BATCHELOR (1962) did not find any evidence of active metabolite formation, but others have shown small quantities of a less polar substance in human urine by bioautography (ULLMANN and WURST 1979; GRABER et al. 1976; NISHIDA et al. 1971). This substance has been identified by MURAKAWA et al. (1972) as the Schiff base of ampicillin and acetaldehyde, which is present in small quantities in kidney, liver, serum, and urine. Since this adduct can be formed in vitro by incubation with appropriate tissues and is readily reversible, the observed microbiological activity may not be due to the adduct per se but to ampicillin formed in situ. Finally, there is no evidence of active metabolite formation as a result of hydroxylation (COLE and RIDLEY 1978).

Serum antimicrobial activity declines biexponentially with a terminal half-life of 1.0–1.5 h after intravenous administration of ampicillin in man. There is good agreement among laboratories that serum clearance is about 350 ml/min and that about 85% of the dose is excreted in the urine (EICKHOFF et al. 1965; TUANO et al.

1966a; DITTERT et al. 1969; MODR and DVORACEK 1970; KIRBY and KIND 1967; JUSKO and LEWIS 1973; JUSKO et al. 1973; LOO et al. 1974). The amount of ampicillin excreted in bile is negligible (BROGARD et al. 1977c; SWAHN 1975).

Ampicillin can be efficiently absorbed after intramuscular injection. LOO et al. (1974) estimated that 87% of a dose of sodium ampicillin is absorbed, most of it during the first 3 h. A somewhat lower estimate was reported by DOLUISIO et al. (1971) who used pharmacokinetic parameters derived from a separate panel of subjects. Absorption efficiency is diminished when ampicillin is injected as a suspension. Thus, the bioavailability of ampicillin trihydrate in suspension is 87% of that of an intramuscular injection of the sodium salt, while that of the benzathine salt is further reduced to about 33% (DOLUISIO et al. 1971; BERTE et al. 1972). Serum half-lives of ampicillin following an intramuscular dose tend to be longer than those after intravenous administration, probably because of continuing absorption. For example, apparent half-lives of 10.4 h have been reported after benzathine ampicillin.

Absorption of orally administered ampicillin is incomplete (32%–53%) and variable. Some of the variability can be directly attributed to differences in dosage forms administered (KLEIN and FINLAND 1963a; LOO et al. 1974; POOLE et al. 1968; HITZENBERGER and JASCHEK 1974; JUSKO and LEWIS 1973; LODE et al. 1974). Whereas absorption efficiency appears to be independent of dose up to 1,000 mg (KNUDSEN et al. 1961), food appears to delay the onset and reduce the total amount absorbed (WELLING et al. 1977; ESHELMAN and SPYKER 1978; NEUVONEN et al. 1977).

Absorption from the human lung was investigated by MADDOCKS (1975). Following intratracheal injections, serum concentrations increase in a dose-related manner. Up to 25% of the dose is excreted in the urine after 2 h.

Ampicillin is 18%–29% bound to human serum proteins (KUNIN 1965; ROLINSON and SUTHERLAND 1965; BIRD and MARSHALL 1967). It does not penetrate and is not bound to human erythrocytes (EHRNEBO 1978). Although little is excreted in bile, biliary concentrations of ampicillin are comparable to those in serum, even in the presence of probenecid (STEWART and HARRISON 1961; AYLIFFE and DAVIES 1965; LUND et al. 1974; KAMPMANN et al. 1973; BROGARD et al. 1977c). The area under the interstitial fluid level curve is comparable to that for serum and appears unaffected by lipopolysaccharide-induced inflammation (TAN et al. 1974; BARZA and WEINSTEIN 1974; TAN and SALSTROM 1979; SCHREINGER et al. 1978). Ampicillin readily crosses the synovial membrane with joint fluid concentrations approximating those in serum (HOWELL et al. 1972). Ratios of tissue to serum concentrations are <0.01 in saliva and tears, about 0.05 in bronchial secretions, 0.1 in nasal secretions, and 0.1–0.4 in CSF (BERGOGNE-BEREZIN et al. 1978; SIMON et al. 1978a; GIEBEL et al. 1978; CLUMECK et al. 1978). After an intraventricular injection, ampicillin concentrations in CSF are persistently high for 24 h or more (STEWART et al. 1961). Renal tissue concentrations range between one-half and twice those in serum and appear to be uniformly distributed among the cortex, medulla, and papilla (WHELTON et al. 1972; BIRO et al. 1972). From postmortem specimens of a patient who died of meningitis while under treatment with ampicillin, the highest concentrations were found in the kidney and, in decreasing order, the lung, spleen, CSF, adrenals, liver, and brain (EICKHOFF et al. 1965). Ampicillin levels in human milk lag behind, but reach 10%–30% of those in serum at 6 h (CECCARELLI and CIAMPINI 1979).

Ampicillin serum levels in pregnant women are approximately one-half those in nonpregnant women after a comparable dose but urinary recoveries appear similar (ASSAEL et al. 1979; PHILIPSON 1978). Therefore, renal clearance rate is doubled during pregnancy. Ampicillin levels in the placenta and umbilical blood are the same as those in maternal serum. In interrupted pregnancies, concentrations in amniotic fluid and fetal heart, lung, liver, kidney, bile, and CSF range from 10% to 50% of those in maternal serum and may be considerably higher in fetal plasma and urine (BOREUS 1971; ELEK et al. 1972).

Serum clearance in the newborn is about one-half to two-thirds that of an adult with normal kidney function. Serum half-life is about 2.2 h in infants 2–5 days old, 3.4 h in those under 1 day, and 1.1 h in those older than 4 months (YOSHIOKA et al. 1974; COLBURN et al. 1976; BOE et al. 1967; GINSBURG et al. 1979). A similar trend of decreasing half-life with age is also seen in premature infants during the first month of life (AXLINE et al. 1967).

In the anephric patient, serum clearance is about 15% of normal. JUSKO et al. (1973) reported a mean clearance of 12 ml/min and half-life of 20 h in 4 patients. Even though a 4-fold increase in elimination rate can be effected during hemodialysis, the absolute value is still small. Hence, therapeutic concentrations of ampicillin may be achieved with a dosing rate about one-tenth that of normal.

Concomitant probenecid administration effectively reduces the renal clearance of ampicillin to that of glomerular filtration rate (TUANO et al. 1966a). The net effect is to increase mean serum concentrations by a factor of 2 and to decrease urinary recovery by 18% (KLEIN and FINLAND 1963a). Concomitant administration of oxacillin or cimetidine has no effect on ampicillin absorption, biotransformation, or excretion (GRABER et al. 1976; ROGERS et al. 1980).

In cirrhotic patients, ampicillin levels in ascitic fluids are low, and serum half-lives are prolonged but unrelated to the degree of hepatic dysfunction (CHALAS et al. 1980).

A number of prodrugs of ampicillin have been made in attempts to improve its aqueous solubility, chemical stability, and/or oral absorbability (Fig. 7). All of these precursors are themselves devoid of antimicrobial activity and rely solely on the formation of ampicillin for effect. Pharmacokinetic considerations will, therefore, concentrate mainly on the rate and the completeness of bioactivation. To the extent that ampicillin is available to the systemic circulation, its subsequent disposition is identical to that following intravenously administered ampicillin.

1. Hetacillin

This is a condensation product of acetone and ampicillin. Following an intravenous dose, detectable levels of hetacillin are found only during the first hour in serum; little, if any, in urine. Hetacillin has a serum half-life of about 11 min and an estimated clearance rate of 7.5 liters/min. Mean area under the ampicillin serum concentration curve is the same as that following an equivalent intravenous dose of ampicillin, indicating that bioconversion is essentially quantitative (JUSKO and LEWIS 1972, 1973).

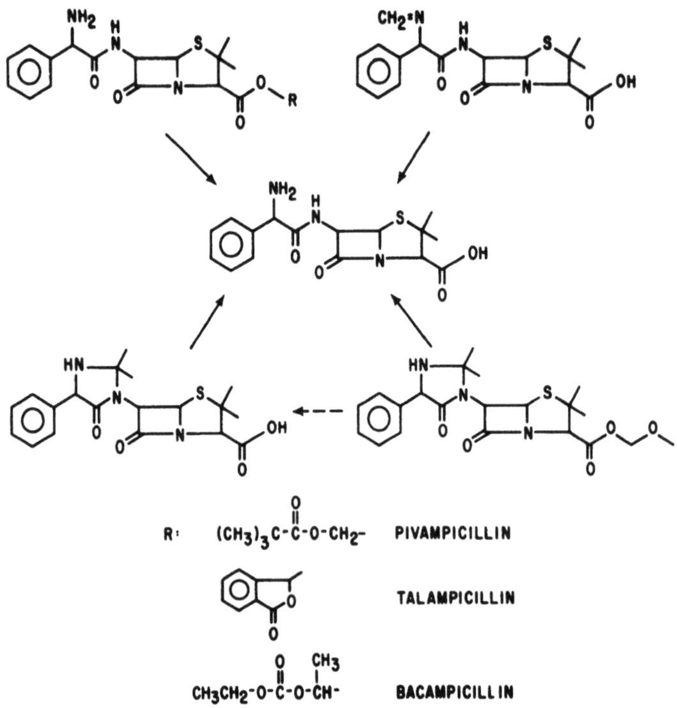

Fig. 7. Prodrugs of ampicillin (*center*): pivampicillin, talampicillin, and bacampicillin (*upper left*); metampicillin (*upper right*); hetacillin (*lower left*); and the methoxymethyl ester of hetacillin (*lower right*)

Within 10 min of an intramuscular injection, 68% of the apparent serum antibacterial activity is attributed to ampicillin; at 60 min, 90%. Peak concentrations of ampicillin are attained in about 1 h (Brown et al. 1969). These observations strongly suggest that most of the administered dose is absorbed into the systemic circulation as unchanged hetacillin.

In contrast, most, if not all, of the orally administered hetacillin must have been hydrolyzed in the gastrointestinal lumen. Except for a slight delay in onset, serum concentrations and urinary recoveries of total antimicrobial activity are the same as those after an equivalent oral dose of ampicillin (Kirby and Kind 1967; Modr and Dvoracek 1970). The bioavailability of ampicillin following an oral dose of hetacillin has been estimated to be 38%, but unlike ampicillin may be slightly enhanced when taken with a meal (Jusko and Lewis 1973).

There are no substantive pharmacokinetic properties which distinguish hetacillin from ampicillin. The only advantage appears to be that of better chemical stability following reconstitution for parenteral use (Schwartz and Hayton 1972).

2. Pivampicillin

The bioavailability of ampicillin following oral doses of pivampicillin has been estimated to be 82%–92% (Loo et al. 1974; Ehrnebo et al. 1979). It is the pivaloyloxymethyl ester which readily hydrolyzes to ampicillin, formaldehyde, and pivalic acid in the presence of nonspecific esterases. Half-life for hydrolysis in homogenates of human gastric and intestinal mucosa is about 5 min (VON DAEHNE et al. 1971). In vivo, concentrations of pivampicillin in the portal and the systemic circulation are always less than 1% those of ampicillin (LUND et al. 1976a). Thus, unlike hetacillin, most of the hydrolysis occurs in transit across the gastrointestinal wall.

Because of the difference in bioavailability, serum activity after pivampicillin tends to be 2–3 times higher that after an equivalent oral dose of ampicillin, while urinary recoveries tend to approach those following a parenteral dose of ampicillin (MODR et al. 1975; HULTBERG and BACKELIN 1972). Depending on the type of meal, most studies appear to show no significant effect of food on bioavailability (JORDAN et al. 1970; VON DAEHNE et al. 1970; FOLTZ et al. 1970; LITTLE and PEDDIE 1974; VERBIST 1974; NEUVONEN et al. 1977; MAGNI and SJOVALL 1972; FERNANDEZ et al. 1973).

The expected effects of probenecid on the serum concentration and urinary excretion of ampicillin are clearly evident following repeated doses of the probenecid salt of pivampicillin when the daily dose is equivalent to 800 mg probenecid (KAMPFFMEYER et al. 1975).

Pivampicillin and other esters of ampicillin are not given parenterally.

3. Bacampicillin

Bacampicillin is the ethylcarbonyloxyethyl ester of ampicillin. Like pivampicillin, orally administered bacampicillin is essentially completely bioavailable as ampicillin (EHRNEBO et al. 1979; BERGAN 1978a). Urinary recovery approximates to that after an intravenous dose of ampicillin (FERRARA and ZANON 1979). Even though an additional chiral center is introduced in the ester side-chain, the hydrolysis rates of both epimers are so facile that there is no practical distinction between them (BODIN et al. 1975). Liver dysfunction has no apparent effect on bioavailability (PARADISI and CIOFFI 1979).

In all respect, the pharmacokinetics of bacampicillin are indistinguishable from those of pivampicillin (SJOVALL et al. 1978). The absorption and elimination of ampicillin following bacampicillin appear similar in infants and in adults (BERGAN et al. 1978a).

4. Talampicillin

The phthalidyl ester of ampicillin is administered orally as the diastereoisomeric mixture. Although hydrolysis rates in human blood, liver, and intestine homogenates are clearly stereoselective, serum levels and urinary recoveries in man following the individual epimers and their 1:1 mixture are practically the same (CLAYTON et al. 1976). Besides ampicillin, the major metabolite in human urine is 2-hydroxymethylbenzoic acid, which accounts for at least 55% of the dose after 24 h (SHIOBARA et al. 1974; JEFFREY et al. 1978). Ninety-eight percent of the radioactivity is recovered in the urine 144 h after an oral dose of talampicillin-phthalidyl-^{14}C.

About 68% of an oral dose is excreted in the urine as ampicillin; another 25%–30% as α-aminobenzylpenicilloic acid (JONES et al. 1978; VERBIST 1976;

HAMILTON-MILLER and BRUMFITT 1979). On the basis of urinary recoveries, it would appear that talampicillin is less bioavailable than either pivampicillin or bacampicillin in delivering ampicillin to the systemic circulation. More extensive hydrolysis in the gastrointestinal lumen appears to be a likely cause since penicilloic acid formation is comparable to that following oral ampicillin (COLE et al. 1973) and it is more labile than pivampicillin in buffer and tissue homogenates (CLAYTON et al. 1974).

5. Metampicillin

Metampicillin is a Schiff base of ampicillin and formaldehyde that may exist in a hydrated form (GRANETEK 1963). Because it is more labile in an acidic environment than in the physiological pH range of serum or culture media, care should be exercised in interpreting data derived from microbiological assays using metampicillin, rather than ampicillin, as the standard (FRANCHI and PERRARO 1967). The parent compound is not unlike the acetaldehyde metabolite of ampicillin (MURAKAWA et al. 1972), the presence of which has not been reported following metampicillin.

After an oral dose of metampicillin, ampicillin serum profiles and urinary recoveries are similar to those following an oral dose of ampicillin. No unchanged metampicillin is found in serum or urine. Detectable levels of the adduct are found in serum after an intramuscular dose (SUTHERLAND et al. 1972). Thus, orally administered metampicillin appears to behave just like ampicillin, presumably because of rapid hydrolysis in transit through the stomach. On the other hand, hydrolysis at the site of an intramuscular injection appears to be less than quantitative.

Biliary excretion rate of metampicillin is unique in that it is by far the highest among penicillins studied (BROGARD et al. 1979c).

6. Methoxymethyl Ester of Hetacillin

Transport of methoxymethyl ester of hetacillin into the prostates and the CNS of dogs and rabbits is said to be enhanced because of its lipophilicity (KJAER et al. 1977; BODINE et al. 1976). Negligible excretion of ampicillin following ester administration would also indicate that hydrolysis in vivo is sluggish.

IX. Amoxicillin

The only known route of amoxicillin metabolism is penicilloic formation (Fig. 8), which represents 35% of the drug-related substances recovered in the urine (COLE et al. 1973; GRABER et al. 1976). Bioautographic studies failed to reveal the existence of active metabolites (ULLMANN and WURST 1979; COLE and RIDLEY 1978).

After an intravenous dose, serum concentrations decline biexponentially with a terminal half-life of 1.0–1.5 h. Serum clearance rate is about 5.5 ml/min per kilogram. On average, 80%–90% of orally and intramuscularly administered doses is absorbed as amoxicillin. Bioavailability is independent of dose between 250 and 1,000 mg (SPYKER et al. 1977). Urinary recovery of amoxicillin after oral and parenteral dose ranges from 50% to 70% and appears to be independent of the route

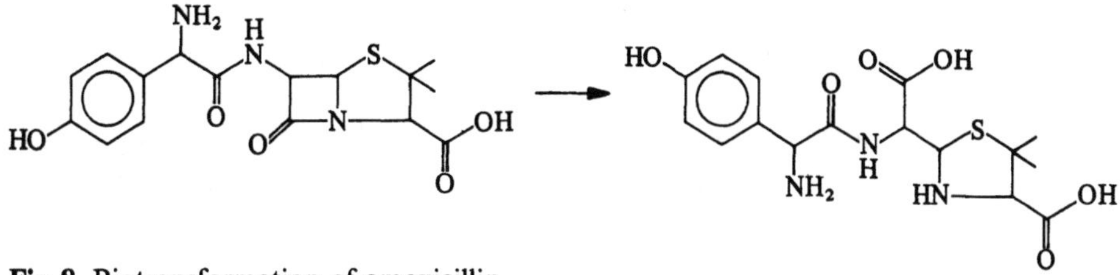

Fig. 8. Biotransformation of amoxicillin

of administration (ROLINSON 1974; NEU 1974; GORDON et al. 1972; PHILIPSON et al. 1975; ARANCIBIA et al. 1980; LODE et al. 1974). Except for a slight delay in onset, the bioavailability of an oral dose is little affected by food (ESHELMAN and SPYKER 1978). Serum levels approximately double when probenecid is given concomitantly (VITTI et al. 1974; BARBHAIYA et al. 1979). Concomitant administration of oxacillin has no effect on amoxicillin excretion or biotransformation (GRABER et al. 1976).

Amoxicillin is approximately 17%–21% bound to human serum proteins (TAN et al. 1974; BIRD and MARSHALL 1967). Penetration into the CNS is normally poor (CLUMECK et al. 1978) but may be enhanced by meningitis (STRASBAUGH et al. 1978). Serum to tissue concentration ratios are roughly 0.5 in bile and interstitial fluids and about 0.07 in bronchial secretions (TAN et al. 1974; CHELVAN et al. 1979; BERGOGNE-BEREZIN et al. 1978). Insignificant quantities are secreted in human milk (CECCARELLI and CIAMPINI 1979). In patients with pelvic inflammatory disease, peak levels of amoxicillin in peritoneal fluid are similar to those in serum (ONSRUD et al. 1979). Free and total concentrations of amoxicillin in blister fluids are about 70%–80% those in serum (WISE et al. 1980e).

Oral absorption is unreliable during labor and does not improve with the concurrent intramuscular injection of metoclopramide (BUCKINGHAM et al. 1975). Placental transfer appears to be slow, although concentrations in cord blood and amniotic fluid eventually surpass those in maternal serum (BERGOGNE-BEREZIN et al. 1979b). The pharmacokinetics of amoxicillin in infants and children 4 months of age or older are similar to those in adults (GINSBURG et al. 1979; RUDOY et al. 1979). Substantial but variable concentrations are found in bronchial secretions of children (RICHTER 1980).

In the elderly, serum half-lives are prolonged even in the absence of signs and symptoms of renal impairment (BALL et al. 1978b). Urinary recovery of amoxicillin decreases progressively in patients whose creatinine clearances are below 55 ml/min (HUMBERT et al. 1979c). In chronic renal failure, mean serum clearance is about 0.37 ml/min per kilogram between dialyses and 1.16 ml/min per kilogram during hemodialysis (FRANCKE et al. 1979a). Absorption and elimination are not noticeably affected in patients with liver impairment (PARADISI and CIOFFI 1979).

X. Azidocillin

Ampicillin has been identified as a metabolite of azidocillin in the rat, the dog, and man. α-Azidobenzylpenicilloic acid is the major metabolite while α-hydroxybenzylpenicillin is a probable metabolite in rats and dogs (Fig. 9). Following oral and intravenous doses of ^{35}S-azidocillin to dogs and rats, most of the radioactivity in

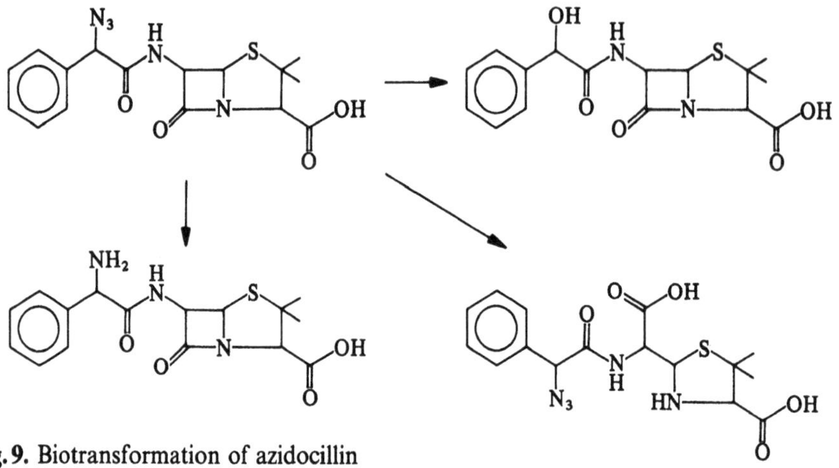

Fig. 9. Biotransformation of azidocillin

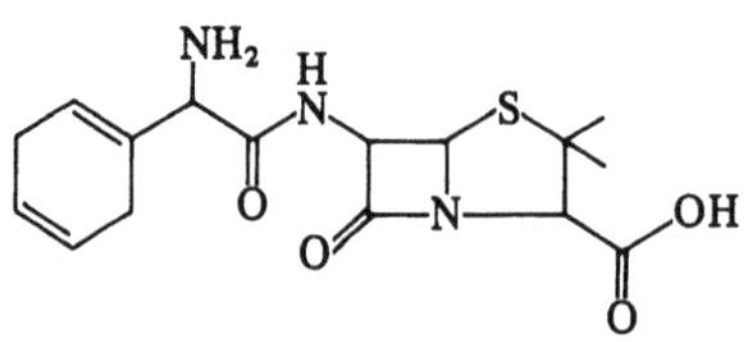

Fig. 10. Structure of epicillin

urine is biologically active while most of that in bile is inactive (ULLMANN and WURST 1979; RAMSAY et al. 1972).

About 5% of the microbiological activity in human urine is attributed to ampicillin. Peak serum activity is similar after an oral dose of the potassium salt and an intramuscular injection. Lower but more sustained levels are achieved after oral doses of dibenzylethylenediamine salt. Urinary recoveries are 85% after an intramuscular dose, 60%–70% following the potassium salt given orally, and somewhat less after the dibenzylethylenediamine salt. Concomitant probenecid administration causes peak serum concentrations to double with little or no effect on urinary recovery (HANSSON et al. 1967).

Azidocillin is about 83%–85% bound to human serum proteins (SJOBERG et al. 1967). Antimicrobial activity is present in human amniotic fluid, fetus, and bronchial secretions (BENGTSSON et al. 1979; WASZ-HOCKERT et al. 1970). In mice, radioactivity is ubiquitously distributed among tissues outside the CNS. Highest concentrations are found in intestinal contents, liver, gall bladder, kidney, urinary bladder, and stomach (RAMSAY et al. 1972).

XI. Epicillin

The chemical structure of epicillin is shown in Fig. 10. Human urine contains an unknown but biologically active metabolite (ULLMANN and WURST 1979). About 27% of an oral dose in man is excreted in the urine as epicillin-like activity (PHILIPSON et al. 1975). Microbiological activity in bile is about 10 times higher than in serum and peaks 1 h after an intravenous dose (BAIER et al. 1980).

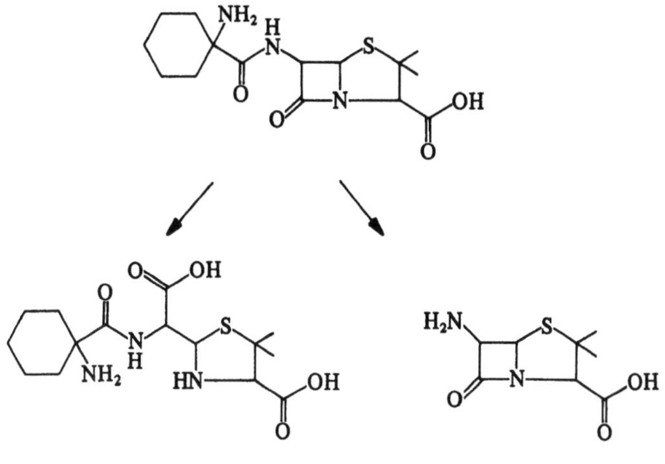

Fig. 11. Biotransformation of cyclacillin

In the rabbit, about 22% of an intravenous dose is eliminated by metabolic inactivation while another 2% is excreted in bile (KIENEL 1976). Serum protein binding is 10%–30%, depending on the concentration (BASCH et al. 1971).

XII. Cyclacillin

The metabolic disposition of cyclacillin is shown in Fig. 11. Following oral administration in man, 50%–70% of the dose is excreted in the urine as unchanged drug, 17% as the penicilloic acid, and about 2% as 1-aminocyclohexanecarboxylic acid (MASHIMO et al. 1970; MIKI et al. 1970; OKUBO et al. 1970; HERTZ 1973). The disposition of 1-aminocyclohexanecarboxylic acid in the rat has been reported by JANSSEN et al. (1976).

The absorption and biotransformation of cyclacillin appears to be independent of dose between 250 and 1,000 mg. The suspension dosages may be slightly less bioavailable than tablets, however (HERTZ 1973). Serum half-life of cyclacillin is normally about 50 min and increases to about 21 h in patients with creatinine clearance of 10 ml/min (UEDA et al. 1970).

Depending on the method of determination, cyclacillin is 18%–23% bound to human serum proteins. Tissue distribution studies in the dog indicated that the drug has the highest affinity for the kidney and the lowest for the spleen. Concentrations in the heart, lung, liver, and muscle are about 5% those in serum at 1 h but much less at later times (ROSENMAN et al. 1967). Biliary clearance in the dog is one-tenth of renal clearance. In the rat, concentrations in the liver and kidney are 2–10 times higher than those in plasma and lungs (MASHIMO et al. 1970; OKUBO et al. 1970).

XIII. Carbenicillin

The two known routes of carbenicillin biotransformation (Fig. 12) are β-lactam cleavage to form the penicilloic acid and α-decarboxylation to form benzylpenicil-

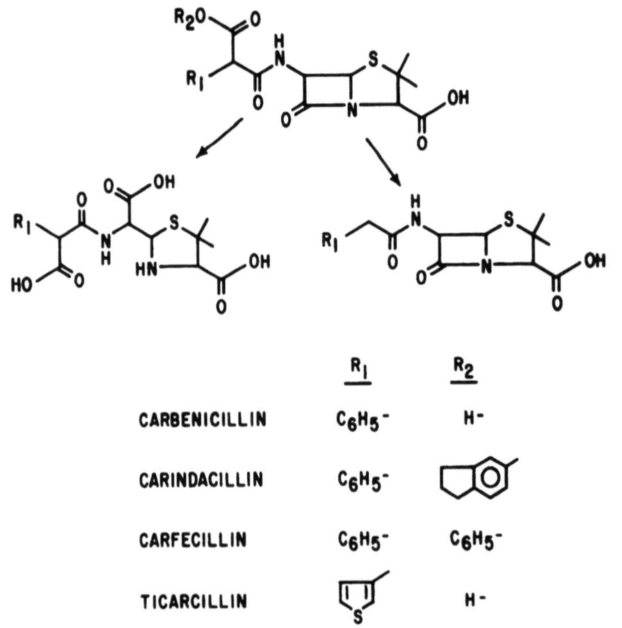

Fig. 12. Biotransformation of ticarcillin, carbenicillin and its prodrugs, carindacillin and carfecillin

lin (Cole et al. 1973; Ullmann and Wurst 1979). Both pathways are minor in that 92% of an intravenous dose is recovered in the urine unchanged. Carbenicillin is administered as a diastereomeric mixture comprising 55% of the D(−)-isomer, the composition of which is unaltered in the urine (Yamaoka et al. 1979). Thus epimerization is not a metabolic event; distribution and elimination are not stereospecific for all practical purposes.

Renal clearance of carbenicillin is essentially the same as glomerular filtration rate (GFR). Since over 90% of an intravenous dose is recovered in the urine unchanged, serum clearance is only slightly above GFR (Libke et al. 1975; Pancoast and Neu 1978). Truncated area estimates or incomplete urine collections are likely causes for the somewhat higher clearances reported by Wirth et al. (1976b) and Meyers et al. (1980). In the presence of probenecid, mean serum concentrations are elevated by about 25% while serum clearance is decreased by a corresponding amount (Libke et al. 1975). Biliary excretion accounts for only 0.1% of the dose (Brogard et al. 1974).

Carbenicillin is about 50% bound to human serum proteins (Rolinson and Sutherland 1967; Libke et al. 1975). Normally, kidney concentrations are several times higher than those in serum; this gradient is greatly diminished in diseased and tumorous kidney tissues (Whelton et al. 1973; Ivan et al. 1972). Relative to plasma, less than 3% are present in rabbit liver and lung. No carbenicillin can be detected in the brain and spleen (Tsuchiya et al. 1972).

Serum clearance rate in the neonate is 2–4 times slower than in the adult and is slowest among those with low birth weight and less than 1 day old (Morehead et al. 1972; Yoshioka et al. 1979a). Elimination is accelerated in children with diabetes mellitus (Mad'acsy et al. 1976).

Liver or kidney dysfunctions have the anticipated effect on carbenicillin. However, clearance in patients with combined hepatorenal failure appears to be disproportionately low. The efficiency of hemodialysis is about 30% compared to that for urea (HOFFMAN et al. 1970). In patients with reduced renal function, there appears to be a fair correlation between creatinine clearance and the cumulative amount of antimicrobial activity excreted in the urine (NAKANO et al. 1977).

Following an intramuscular injection, 80% of the dose is excreted in the urine (ROBINSON 1967). Carbenicillin is poorly transported into and out of the CNS. Therapeutic levels in the CSF can be achieved and maintained for 24 h or more by intraventricular and intrathecal injections (ROBINSON and SUTHERLAND 1967).

Orally, carbenicillin is administered as esters, the improved transport properties of which are necessary for activity. A number of monoesters have been synthesized and characterized (CLAYTON et al. 1975); all of them retain a free carboxyl group on the thiazolidine nucleus and are expected to possess some antibacterial activity per se. In fact, although not identified, a third active substance besides carbenicillin and benzylpenicillin is invariably present in human urine pursuant to the administration of carbenicillin esters (ULLMANN and WURST 1979).

1. Carindacillin

Carindacillin is the 5-indanyl ester of carbenicillin (Fig. 12). About 35% of the administered dose is recovered in the urine as carbenicillin-like activity. Small quantities of benzylpenicillin and unhydrolyzed carindacillin are present in serum (BUTLER 1971; FABRE et al. 1972; ENGLISH et al. 1972; MODR et al. 1977). On the other hand, the other product of hydrolysis, 5-indanol, is quantitatively excreted in the urine, mostly as its sulfate or glucuronide conjugates (HOBBS 1972; KNIRSCH et al. 1972). Thus, lumenal hydrolysis appears to be a major competing pathway to the transport of carindacillin across the gastrointestinal wall; consequently, it is incompletely bioavailable as carbenicillin. By the same token, the gastrointestinal absorption of 5-indanol is efficient and complete.

2. Carfecillin

Carfecillin is the phenyl ester of carbenicillin (Fig. 12). In all respects, its pharmacokinetic characteristics are practically indistinguishable from those of carindacillin in man (CLAYTON et al. 1975; MODR et al. 1977; WILKINSON et al. 1975).

XIV. Ticarcillin

Like carbenicillin, ticarcillin is given as a mixture of diastereoisomers. An active metabolite has been isolated in human urine and tentatively identified as the thiophene analog of benzylpenicillin (ULLMANN and WURST 1979). Small quantities of the α-decarboxylated compound are also present in rat and dog urine (ACRED et al. 1970). The penicilloic acid accounts for 14.6% of an intramuscular dose excreted in human urine (COLE et al. 1973). Thus, the biotransformation of ticarcillin appears to be qualitatively similar to carbenicillin (Fig. 12).

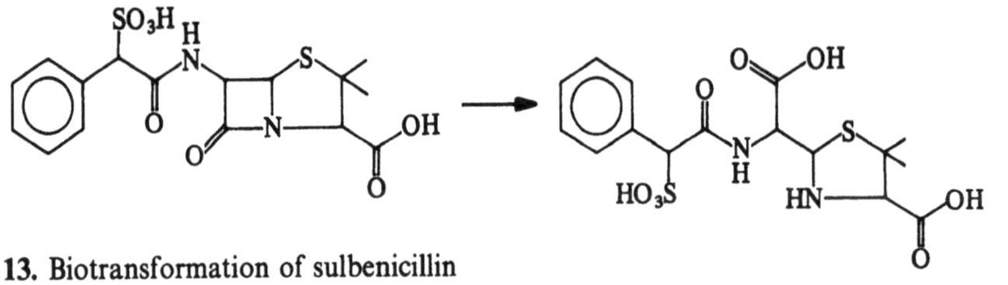

Fig. 13. Biotransformation of sulbenicillin

About 90% of an intravenous dose is recovered in the urine as ticarcillin-like activity (LIBKE et al. 1975; SUTHERLAND and WISE 1970; RODRIQUEZ et al. 1973). Apparent serum clearance is about 145 ml/min and approaches GFR in the presence of probenecid. On the basis of urinary recovery, bioavailability of an intramuscular injection is nearly quantitative. Peak serum concentrations approximately double in the presence of probenecid. It would appear, therefore, that ticarcillin is actively secreted and reabsorbed by the renal tubules. In contrast, tricarcillin is poorly absorbed when given by mouth. Less than 3% of on oral dose is excreted in urine (SUTHERLAND and WISE 1970).

Ticarcillin is 45%–65% bound to proteins in human serum (SUTHERLAND et al. 1970a; LIBKE et al. 1975). In patients in chronic renal failure, hemodialysis appears to be an efficient way to remove ticarcillin. On the other hand, the apparent clearance rate by peritoneal dialysis is only about 5 ml/min (WISE et al. 1974). Ticarcillin passes readly into extravascular fluids. Concentration profiles of unbound ticarcillin in thoracic and peripheral lymph of dogs mirror those in serum with a slight delay in onset (ACRED et al. 1970).

XV. Sulbenicillin

Sulbenicillin is a diastereoisomeric mixture containing 77% of the D(−)-isomer (Fig. 13). About 75% of an intravenous dose is excreted in human urine without change in the ratio of the diastereomers (YAMAOKA et al. 1979). There is no evidence of active metabolites in human, dog, rabbit, rat, and mouse urine (TSUCHIYA et al. 1972). From 10% to 20% of the radioactivity excreted in rat urine and bile has been identified as α-sulfobenzylpenicilloic acid (NAKAI et al. 1972).

From 65% to 80% of the intramuscular dose is excreted in the urine. Disappearance rate of antibacterial activity in serum is greatly attenuated in anuric patients and those with creatinine clearance of 2 ml/min (UEDA et al. 1971; ISHIYAMA et al. 1971; MASHIMO et al. 1971).

Binding to human serum proteins has been estimated to be 2% by gel filtration (NAKAI et al. 1972) and 55% by equilibrium dialysis (ISHIYAMA et al. 1971). Little or no sulbenicillin is found in the brain and spleen of rodents, while the highest levels are located in kidney and liver tissues (TSUCHIYA et al. 1972; NAKAI et al. 1972). Concentrations in rat and rabbit bile are 2–10 times those in serum. Little or no sulbenicillin is present in sheep red blood cells (FUKAYA and KITAMOTO 1971; SHIMIZU and KUNI 1971).

XVI. Ureidopenicillins

The chemical structures of this newest family of penicillins are shown in Fig. 14. To date, there has been no systematic study reported on the biotransformation of

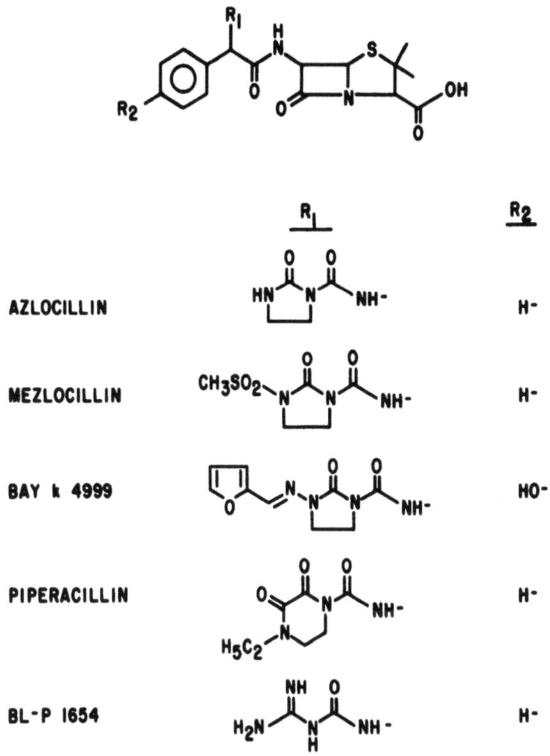

Fig. 14. Structures of ureidopenicillins

these compounds in man, although there does not appear to be active metabolite formation. Therefore, serum and urine antimicrobial activity represents unchanged drug. Limited information on azlocillin, mezlocillin, and piperacillin would suggest that dose-dependent pharmacokinetics may obtain within the therapeutic range.

1. Azlocillin

The penicilloic acid is the major metabolite of azlocillin in human urine (GAU and HORSTER 1979). A polar substance found in human urine is probably not an active metabolite in that it is present in the starting material used (ULLMANN and WURST 1979).

Sixty percent of an intravenous dose is recovered in human urine. Renal clearance is equal to glomerular filtration rate. Following intravenous administration in man, serum concentrations decline biexponentially with a terminal half-life of about 50 min (LODE et al. 1977; WIRTH et al. 1976a; LEROY et al. 1980).

Azlocillin is 25% bound to serum proteins. Although therapeutic concentrations are achieved in bronchial secretions, their relation to corresponding serum levels is not readily discernible (WEINGARTNER et al. 1979; DAIKOS et al. 1979).

In patients with varying degrees of renal insufficiency, FIEGEL and BECKER (1978) found a linear relationship between inulin clearance rate and serum half-life on a log-log scale. In patients with end-stage renal disease, mean serum half-life is about 2 h on dialysis and twice that off dialysis. Over a 4- to 6-h period, 30%–46% of the dose is removed in the dialysate (ALETTA et al. 1980; LEROY et al. 1980). Elimination rate is further attenuated in patients with hepatorenal disease (SCHURIG et al. 1979).

Serum half-life in full-term neonates is about 2.6 h while that in premature infants is 4.7 h. Absorption is rapid following an intramuscular dose (HEIMANN et al. 1979; SITKA et al. 1980). The disposition of azlocillin in healthy children of school age appears similar to that in adults, but renal excretion is greatly accelerated in children with cystic fibrosis (WEINGARTNER et al. 1979; BERGAN and MICHALSEN 1979).

2. Mezlocillin

There is a singular lack of consensus among workers concerning the pharmacokinetics of mezlocillin. After intravenous injections of 1–5 g, BERGAN (1978b) noted that the area under the serum curve increases more rapidly in proportion to dose. At the same time fractional urinary recoveries appear similar; if anything, recovery is lowest during the first 2 h after the 1-g dose. Estimates of apparent serum and renal clearance are considerably higher than those reported by LODE et al. (1977) after a 5-g dose. On the other hand, the corresponding parameters after a 4-g dose (PANCOAST and NEU 1978) are within 10% those of LODE et al. (1977) after a 5-g dose when the difference in urinary recoveries is taken into account. Finally, there is no dose-related trend in apparent serum half-life, including that following a 3-g dose (ISSELL et al. 1978). Within the therapeutic range, dose-dependencies in the pharmacokinetics, if real, are probably unimportant because mezlocillin elimination is so rapid that no unusual accumulation is likely to occur.

There is no evidence of active metabolites in human urine (ULLMANN and WURST 1979). Mezlocillin concentrations in CSF are low except when the meninges are inflamed (MODAI et al. 1979a; LLORENS-TEROL et al. 1979). Concentrations in bile tend to be high compared to serum (ELLIS et al. 1979). About 25% of a 2-g dose is recovered in bile after 8 h. Binding to serum proteins is about 50% (BERGAN 1978b). In patients undergoing hip surgery, bone concentrations tend to be one-fifth to one-tenth those in serum during the first hour (VENT 1979). While significant amounts of mezlocillin are bound to the iris, ciliary body, retina, choroids, sclera, and cornea of the rabbit eye, no mezlocillin can be detected in the lens or the aqueous humor (OISHI et al. 1979).

While probenecid appears to have the expected effect on renal excretion, serum half-life of mezlocillin is little affected (VERBIST et al. 1979). Urinary recoveries of both antibiotics are enhanced when mezlocillin is given simultaneously with oxacillin (ADAM and BAUER 1979).

In patients with varying degrees of renal dysfunction, BERGAN et al. (1979) noted a small increase in apparent half-life from 1.1 to 1.6 h when GFR is below 20 ml/min. KOSMIDIS et al. (1979), on the other hand, reported a linear relationship between serum half-life and serum creatinine. In patients undergoing hemodialysis, serum half-life is about 1.6 h, compared with 5.4 h between dialyses (FRANCKE et al. 1979b).

3. Piperacillin

There are no active metabolites of pipericillin in the urine of man, dogs, monkeys, rats, and mice. The penicilloic acid and a product of piperazine ring cleavage, α-3-[2-(*N*-ethyl-*N*-oxaloamino)ethyl]-ureidobenzylpenicillin, are present in minute amounts in rat urine; neither is present in freshly voided human urine. Whereas piperacillin is excreted predominantly unchanged in rat bile, 94% of the radioactivity in rat feces is the penicilloic acid (SAIKAWA et al. 1977).

Apparent renal clearance of piperacillin decreases continuously with increasing serum concentration (MORRISON and BATRA 1979). Therefore, serum clearance must also change continuously with time. Not surprisingly, areas under the serum concentration curve increase in the ratio of 1:2.6:6.7:12 following intravenous boluses of 1, 2, 4, and 6 g. A similar disproportionate increase obtains following gradated doses given intramuscularly, even though serum levels are 1–2 orders of magnitude lower. There appears to be a slight increase in urinary recovery with dose (TJANDRAMAGA et al. 1978). This trend is less obvious in other studies where different dosage regimens are not compared in the same subjects (BATRA et al. 1979; EVANS et al. 1978, 1979). Pharmacokinetic models to date have failed to recognize these dose-related effects of piperacillin disposition and are therefore neither characteristic nor predictive.

Piperacillin is 21% bound to serum proteins (MORRISON and BATRA 1979). On pretreatment with probenecid, serum concentrations of piperacillin after a 1-g intramuscular injection approximately double, time-averaged renal clearance is about halved, while urinary recovery is unaffected (TJANDRAMAGA et al. 1978). In patients with chronic renal failure, about 50% of the dose is removed in the dialysate during 4 h hemodialysis. However, nonrenal elimination of piperacillin must be extensive since a similar fraction is removed by other means during the same interval (FRANCKE et al. 1979c).

4. Bay k 4999

Resistance of this compound to β-lactamase is between that of ampicillin and carbenicillin (NEU et al. 1979b). Following an intravenous injection in man, serum antibacterial activity declines polyexponentially with a terminal half-life of 1.3 h. Serum clearance is about 275 ml/min while 26% of the dose is recovered in the urine (WISE et al. 1979b). Another 26% of the administered activity is recovered in bile in 24 h (LODE et al. 1980b).

Bay k 4999 is 60% bound to serum proteins. Levels in dermabrasion fluids are similar to those in serum while those in blisters tend to be higher and more sustained after the first hour. Over time, however, mean concentrations of free and total antimicrobial activity in blister fluids are one-half those in serum (WISE et al. 1979b, 1980e).

5. BL-P1654

Following intravenous infusions in man, serum antimicrobial activity declines biexponentially with a terminal half-life of about 2 h. Renal clearance is about 70% of creatinine clearance and urinary excretion accounts for 72%–75% of the dose.

Neither is affected by the concurrent administration of probenecid (CLARKE et al. 1974).

BL-P1654 is 20%–28% bound to human serum proteins and appears to be well absorbed when given by the intramuscular route (PRICE et al. 1970; CLARKE et al. 1974).

C. Cephalosporins

In general, the cephalosporin and cephamycin antibiotics are a family of parenterally administered antimicrobial agents. Notable orally absorbed cephalosporins include cephaloglycine, cephalexin, cephradine, cefadroxil, FR 10612, cefaclor, cefroxadine, and cefatrizine. Urinary excretion is the primary route of elimination for all cephalosporins although biliary excretion and metabolism contribute to the elimination of several. For most, urinary excretion involves both glomerular filtration and renal tubular secretion. As might be expected, kidney dysfunction or the coadministration of probenecid cause dramatic changes in drug elimination.

Cephalosporin antibiotics are remarkably stable in vivo, with only those that are direct descendants of cephalosporanic acid being metabolized extensively. The metabolism of other cephalosporins has generally not been studied with discriminating assay techniques. Those that have been studied in this fashion have shown insignificant metabolism.

Similar pharmacokinetic interpretative cautions, as noted with penicillins, should be exercised with cephalosporins as well.

I. Cephalosporanic Acids

This group of cephalosporin antibiotics is characterized by a 3-acetoxymethyl group which undergoes facile deacetylation both in vitro and in vivo. These antibiotics are also rapidly deacetylated in lysed whole blood (WRIGHT and FROGGE 1980), creating problems when whole blood or tissue samples containing blood must be assayed for unchanged drug. These desacetyl-cephalosporanic acids have been shown to possess antimicrobial activity or are judged to have such by inference. Without an assay procedure whereby both biologically active substances may be distinguished in human and animal biological samples, meaningful pharmacokinetic interpretation of any data collected is nearly impossible. Hence, reference to these antibiotics in plasma or serum will be termed "antimicrobial activity" unless a specific assay procedure was used.

1. Cephalothin

Following parenteral administration, cephalothin is eliminated rapidly from the systemic circulation by way of metabolism and urinary excretion. Bilary excretion is also of some importance (RAM and WATANATITTAN 1974; BROGARD et al. 1973). The major metabolic product is desacetylcephalothin (Fig. 15); hydrolysis is said to occur in the liver or kidneys (LEE et al. 1963). This metabolite has the same antimicrobial spectra, but is much less potent than cephalothin itself (WICK 1966).

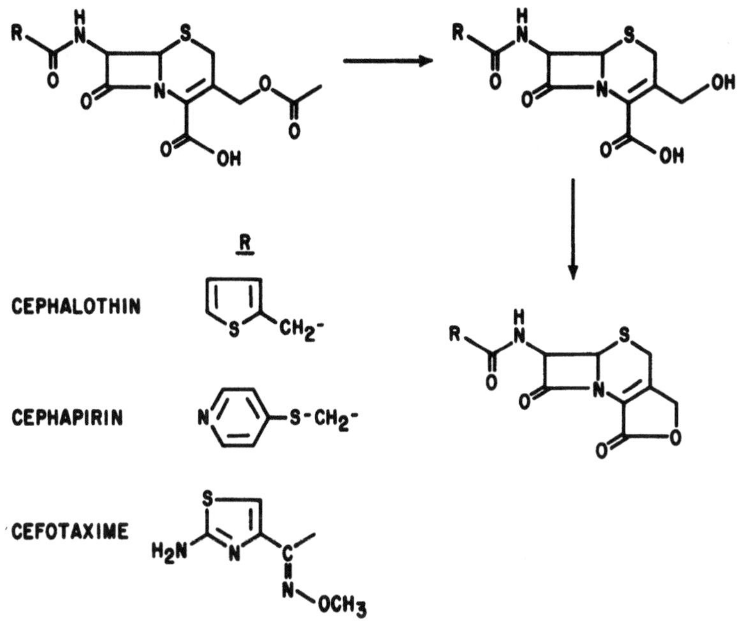

Fig. 15. Biotransformation of cephalothin, cephapirin, and cefotaxime

Several methods are available for the determination of cephalothin and its metabolite in biological fluids (MILLER 1962; HOEHN et al. 1970; COOPER et al. 1973). In healthy volunteers and patients with normal kidney function given cephalothin sodium intravenously, cephalothin serum levels declined with a mean serum half-life of 11.8–13.5 min (COOPER et al. 1973; ROLEWICZ et al. 1977). In subsequent studies by ANDERS et al. (1975) and ROLEWICZ et al. (1977), pediatric subjects received cephalothin sodium intravenously and again a very short mean terminal serum half-life was noted (14.9–18.6 min). Using a nondiscriminating biological assay, the apparent half-life in adult serum was 1.7 times greater (ROLEWICZ et al. 1977). Urine collections through 5 h in this study accounted for a mean of 102% of the administered dose consisting of 35.7% desacetylcephalothin and 66.3% cephalothin. These findings are in general agreement with those of BUHS et al. (1974) and GRIFFITH and BLACK (1971). With more frequent and extensive blood and urine sampling following an intravenous infusion (10 min) of cephalothin sodium, AZIZ et al. (1977) found that cephalothin disappears from serum tri-exponentially with mean serum half-lives of 5, 16, and 102 min respectively. The mean renal clearance of cephalothin is 2.8 ml/min per kilogram, while that for desacetylcephalothin is 9.3 ml/min per kilogram. The mean total plasma clearance of cephalothin is 4.6 ml/min per kilogram. Sixty-one percent of the dose is excreted unchanged in the urine in 24 h. Desacetylcephalothin is recovered in the amount of 34% of the dose.

NILSSON-EHLE and NILSSON-EHLE (1979) administered intravenous doses of cephalothin sodium to uremic patients every 12 or 24 h and to healthy volunteers every 6 or 8 h. Serum levels of cephalothin declined after the first dose in healthy subjects with a mean terminal serum half-life of 28 min. In patients, all of whom had a creatinine clearance of < 10 ml/min, mean serum half-life ranged from 151 to 326 min. Serum concentrations of desacetylcephalothin were variable in volunteers and were undetectable within 6 h. In patients, desacetylcephalothin accumulated in serum, even after the first dose, showing little decline over the first 12–14 h. From infrequent blood samples taken after 2–5 days of drug administration, little, if any, cephalothin accumulation in serum was noted. The same was true for desacetylcephalothin in healthy subjects, but a twofold accumulation of metabolite was noted in some uremic patients. Through 6 h after the first dose in volunteers, a mean of 95% of the dose was recovered in urine; 52% as cephalothin and 43% as desacetylcephalothin. In those patients who were producing urine, desacetylcephalothin represented the major drug-related component, a mean of 5% of the dose through 12 or 14 h. KIRBY et al. (1971) made similar observations in uremic patients using a bioassay with two microorganisms that were felt to be mutually exclusive for cephalothin and desacetylcephalothin. Serum antimicrobial activity is effectively cleared by both hemodialysis (VENUTO and PLAUT 1971) and peritoneal dialysis (PERKINS et al. 1969).

Cephalothin kinetics have also been studied before, during, and after cardiopulmonary bypass surgery (MILLER et al. 1979). Although details of the experiment are somewhat sketchy, it appears that cephalothin pharmacokinetics are different in patients requiring cardiopulmonary bypass surgery. Mean total body clearance is unaltered, but mean renal clearance of cephalothin and estimates of the fraction excreted unchanged in the urine are 50% lower than seen in healthy subjects. During the surgical procedure, both total body and renal clearance are reduced. Postoperatively, estimates of urinary excretion and renal and total body clearance are similar to those reported by AZIZ et al. (1977).

Cephalothin is poorly absorbed following oral administration (GRIFFITH and BLACK 1971). Serum cephalothin levels were detectable in four of ten subjects after a 500-mg dose and only 11 mg was excreted in the urine in 6 h. Studying the situation in rats, SULLIVAN and MCMAHON (1967) found that cephalothin is degraded in the gut. Only 50% of the dosed radioactivity is recovered in urine 40 h after dosing, none of which is unchanged drug.

Intramuscular administration of cephalothin sodium has been studied by numerous investigators (LEE et al. 1963; GRIFFITH and BLACK 1971; DUVAL et al. 1974; GRIFFITH and BLACK 1964; NAUMAN 1967; BRUMFITT et al. 1974). Peak serum levels of antimicrobial activity occur 0.5 h after injection, but dose proportionality is difficult to demonstrate. Recovery in 6-h urine collections accounted for 50%–70% of the dose, with the ratio of cephalothin to desacetylcephalothin being 65:35. Urine collected for 12–24 h after intramuscular doses accounted for 80%–100% of the administered antimicrobial activity. This information indicates that cephalothin is rapidly and reasonably well absorbed following intramuscular administration.

Human serum protein binding of cephalothin is reported to be 71% (SINGHVI et al. 1977), but other literature values vary slightly depending on variations in protein concentration in serum samples and experimental technique (MIYAKE and EBATA 1976; CHISHOLM et al. 1970; MADHAVAN et al. 1973; NISHIDA et al. 1970; WAHLIG et al. 1979). VERONESE et al. (1977) discovered that cephalothin binds to hydrophobic sites on human serum albumin and that its association constant was nearly the same for human, bovine, rabbit, and chicken serum albumins. PITKIN et al. (1980b) found that saturated fatty acids of 10–14 carbon atom chain length markedly inhibit the serum protein binding of cephalothin when the fatty acid to protein molar ratio exceeds 3:1. This effect is shared by organic acids such as probenecid and novobiocin. These findings should be considered when a given disease state might alter the fatty acid content of human serum or when highly protein bound compounds are coadministered with cephalothin. Variations in serum pH between 6.0 and 8.0 have little effect on the serum protein binding of cephalothin (JOHNSON and SABATH 1979).

The tissue and fluid distribution of cephalothin has been studied by a number of investigators. RECORDS (1968) administered intravenous doses of sodium cephalothin to two groups of cataract patients and then sampled venous blood and secondary aqueous humor. Mean serum levels of antimicrobial activity decreased by a factor of 5 within 30 min in both groups while mean activity in secondary aqueous humor remained relatively constant.

MORROW et al. (1968) administered sodium cephalothin intramuscularly to women about to give birth. Serum levels of antimicrobial activity were found in neonates born 15–30 min after the injection. These levels peaked in babies born 46–60 min after injection, but in all cases levels of antimicrobial activity were quite low when compared to maternal serum levels. This indicates rapid, but minimal placental transfer of the antimicrobial activity.

LERNER (1969) found therapeutic levels of antimicrobial activity in CSF after 2–4 g intravenous doses of sodium cephalothin, but only in patients with CSF protein concentration in excess of 50 mg/100 ml. This fact was noted previously by VIANNA and KAYE (1967).

Studies in rabbits with confirmed meningitis would suggest that more than half of the antimicrobial activity detected in CSF may be attributable to desacetylcephalothin (NOLAN and ULMER 1978). The apparent half-life of desacetylcephalothin in rabbit CSF was much greater than cephalothin, and isolated rabbit choroid plexuses demonstrated the ability to metabolize cephalothin to desacetylcephalothin (NOLAN and ULMER 1980).

Low levels of antimicrobial activity were noted in heart muscle samples obtained from children with Fallot's disease 60 min after receiving a 100 mg/kg intravenous dose of sodium cephalothin (ADAM et al. 1976a).

Prostatic tissue levels of antimicrobial activity 30 min after a 2-g i.v. dose of sodium cephalothin were about 25% of serum levels. Only after a 4-g intravenous infusion of drug were levels in brain tissue or CSF detectable in patients with cerebral tumors (ADAM et al. 1976a).

PERKINS and SASLAW (1966) studied a deceased patient who had received 2 g sodium cephalothin intramuscularly every 4 h for 13 days prior to death. Renal cortex levels of antimicrobial activity were 90% of those in blood while levels in myocardium, striated muscle, pleural fluid, gastric wall, and skin were about 30% of blood levels. Antimicrobial activity in cerebral cortex or liver was less than 10% of blood levels. Brain tissue levels of antimicrobial activity after 2-g intravenous doses of sodium cephalothin were more extensively studied by GRIFFITH and BLACK (1971).

Biliary and gall bladder tissue levels of cephalothin related antimicrobial activity following intravenous administration were studied by RAM and WATANATITTAN (1974). Following an 8-g (1 g every 6 h) total dose of sodium cephalothin, levels of antimicrobial activity in gall bladder bile ranged from 3 to 150 times the levels noted in serum, while levels in common duct bile were much lower, but still in excess of serum activity. Patients with indwelling T tubes were given a single 2-g intravenous dose of sodium cephalothin and antimicrobial activity levels were determined serially. Peak levels were noted at 2 h and antimicrobial activity was judged therapeutic for 4–6 h. Gall bladder tissue levels of antimicrobial activity were variable in comparison to serum levels, but generally exceeded them. Similar results were reported by BROGARD et al. (1973).

Levels of antimicrobial activity were measured in skin window chamber interstitial fluid by TAN and SALSTROM (1977) following a 1-g intravenous dose of antibiotic. Levels in interstitial fluid equaled or exceeded serum levels after 2 h. A later study (TAN and SALSTROM 1979) did not confirm this finding. In patients undergoing total hip replacement, the effect of hypotensive anesthesia on cephalothin levels in bone, muscle, and serum was studied by PATEL et al. (1979). Sodium cephalothin was administered as a 20-mg/kg intravenous bolus followed by a 20-mg/kg intravenous infusion (60 min). Mean serum levels of antimicrobial activity were 20%–30% lower under hypotensive anesthesia. Mean bone and muscle levels, however, remained similar to the normotensive situation. Following a 2-g intravenous bolus of cephalothin sodium, peak levels of antimicrobial activity were seen in knee (femoral condyle) and hip (femoral head) within 70 min (SCHURMAN et al. 1980). These levels of activity were only about 5% of serum activity, however. Synovial and wound drainage fluid levels were higher.

Patients undergoing hip arthroplasty received 1 g cephalothin sodium intravenously. Antimicrobial activity in samples of osseous tissue and synovial fluid obtained 1 h after drug administration was 30% and 20%, respectively, of the levels found in serum at that time (FITZGERALD et al. 1978).

PLAUE et al. (1974) administered 50 mg/kg intravenous doses of cephalothin sodium to children and young adults and found that levels in cortical bone remained relatively constant and equaled serum levels of antimicrobial activity after 3.5–4.0 h. Levels in spongiosa bone and cutis were similar to each other. Antimicrobial activity also penetrated subcutis, fascia, and muscle tissue.

Finally, WHELTON et al. (1980) and YAMADA et al. (1980) studied cephalothin levels in the female genital tract in patients undergoing hysterectomy. Levels of antimicrobial activity in endometrium, perimetrium, cervix, fallopian tubes, and ovary were comparable to serum levels. Only levels in myometrium were below serum levels.

The effect of probenecid on cephalothin serum and urine levels of antimicrobial activity has been studied by KLEIN et al. (1964), who administered sodium cephalothin intramuscularly with and without four prior oral doses of probenecid (0.5 g). Peak serum levels of antimicrobial activity were seen within 1 h of injection and those levels were twice as high when probenecid was coadministered. The duration of serum antimicrobial activity was extended by probenecid. Probenecid had little effect on the urine levels of antimicrobial activity. GOODWIN et al. (1974) administered sodium cephalothin intravenously with and without a prior infusion of

1 g probenecid. The apparent serum half-life of antimicrobial activity doubled in the presence of probenecid and there was no effect on 12-h urinary recovery of antimicrobial activity.

2. Cephapirin

Cephapirin is rapidly eliminated by deacetylation and urinary excretion. The desacetyl metabolite (Fig. 15) present in human serum and urine following parenteral drug administration has significant microbiological activity (CABANA et al. 1976). Following intravenous administration, the mean terminal serum half-life of cephapirin is 0.5 h. In 6 h, 48.5% of the dose is excreted unchanged in urine, while 45.3% is excreted as desacetylcephapirin. The mean clearance of cephapirin is 342 ml/min. Biliary clearance of cephapirin or desacetylcephapirin is not an important means of elimination (BODNER and KOENIG 1972).

In a similar study, CABANA et al. (1975) found that 48% of the dose was excreted unchanged in urine; renal clearance was 242 ml/min. Mean cephapirin serum data were fitted to a two-compartment open model, revealing an apparent serum half-life of approximately 0.7 h, a volume of distribution in the central compartment of 6.3 liters, and a serum clearance of 500 ml/min. An unusually high estimate of 1,131 ml/min for the renal clearance of desacetylcephapirin suggests the possibility of renal metabolism of cephapirin. The model, to this effect, describes the mean data adequately. However, intravenous administration of desacetylcephapirin was not pursued to better establish this assumption.

ARVIDSSON et al. (1979a) investigated the possibility of saturable tubular reabsorption of cephapirin using an intravenous infusion of cephapirin in healthy subjects. The 12-h urinary recovery of cephapirin represented 48.6% of the dose, but more importantly it was observed that the renal clearance of cephapirin decreased as plasma drug concentration decreased. There were indications that, at low plasma and urine concentrations, drug was reabsorbed from the kidneys more rapidly than it was secreted. These results do not appear to agree with those of CABANA et al. (1975).

The biotransformation of cephapirin in animals and humans has been studied by CABANA et al. (1976). Studies indicate the presence of cephapirin and desacetylcephapirin in the urine of mice, rats, dogs, and humans, while rat urine also contains trace amounts of desacetylcephapirin lactone.

Cephapirin is apparently not absorbed following oral administration, but is rapidly absorbed following intramuscular administration (LANE et al. 1977; CABANA et al. 1975). Peak levels of plasma antimicrobial activity occur within 1 h of injection, but only CABANA et al. report actual drug levels. The mean percentage dose urinary recovery reported by CABANA et al. (1975) for cephapirin following intramuscular administration is 43.3% in 24 h. Recovery of desacetylcephapirin in 24-h urine collections amounts to 43.4% of the dose. Cephapirin is well absorbed from intramuscular injection sites.

The human serum protein binding of cephapirin is 62% over a concentration range of 2–250 μg/ml using an ultrafiltration technique (ARVIDSSON et al. 1979a; HOTTENDORF et al. 1975; CHISHOLM et al. 1970).

Few studies have been published concerning the distribution of cephapirin and desacetylcephapirin in animal or human tissue and fluids. SCHURMAN et al. (1976)

administered 1- or 2-g intravenous doses of sodium cephapirin to patients about to receive bone prostheses of various kinds. Subchondral bone levels of antimicrobial activity at early collection times (<30 min) averaged about 5%–10% of serum levels, while samples collected after nearly an hour possessed comparable antimicrobial activity (no tourniquet application). Patients treated with tourniquet application tended to have lower bone levels of antimicrobial activity. Synovial fluid contained therapeutic levels of antimicrobial activity for at least 30 min after administration. TAN and SALSTROM (1979) gave a 1-g intravenous infusion of sodium cephapirin and then sampled plasma, urine, and interstitial fluid (TAN et al. 1972) in skin window chambers. The ratio of mean plasma levels of antimicrobial activity to similar interstitial fluid activity approached unity 2 h after drug administration and then declined.

The penetration of cephapirin derived antimicrobial activity into prostatic and seminal vesicle tissues following 1- or 2-g intravenous infusions of sodium cephapirin was studied. After a 1-g dose, mean antimicrobial activity in prostatic tissue nearly equaled that found in plasma; seminal vesicle tissue levels were 50% of plasma. After a 2-g dose, antimicrobial activity in plasma was double that found in prostate and comparable to that in seminal vesicle tissue (RUBI and GALAN 1979).

FRY et al. (1980) were able to obtain gynecologic tissue samples following a 1-gm intravenous infusion of sodium cephapirin. Thirty minutes after the infusion had been completed mean plasma levels of antimicrobial activity were 4 times those seen in fallopian tube tissue and 1.4 times those seen in ovarian tissues or cysts. Sixty minutes following the infusion, antimicrobial activity in fallopian tube tissue, ovarian tissue, uterine wall, vaginal mucosa, and peritoneum was comparable to that observed in plasma.

The effect of probenecid on cephapirin disposition has not been discussed in the literature, but renal clearance estimates suggest that cephapirin is secreted by the renal tubules, and ARVIDSSON et al. (1979a) suggest that the tubular reabsorption of the drug is a saturable process.

MCCLOSKEY et al. (1972) have studied the effects of 1-g intravenous infusions of sodium cephapirin on 16 azotemic patients. Plasma levels of antimicrobial activity were more sustained with time, and urine, when produced, contained bactericidal levels of activity. Hemodialysis was able to remove activity from plasma, but not efficiently.

Some plasma level and urinary excretion data gathered in children have been reported by GORDON et al. (1971). Intramuscular doses of 12.5 mg/kg or 20 mg/kg sodium cephapirin result in rapid appearance of plasma levels of antimicrobial activity. These levels persist through 2 h at the low dose and 3 h at the high dose. Urinary excretion of antimicrobial activity during 4 h after the 20 mg/kg intramuscular dose in one subject represented 53% of the administered activity.

3. Cefotaxime

Deacetylation is again of concern with this antibiotic, and WISE et al. (1980a, d) have shown that desacetylcefotaxime is present in serum following parenteral administration of cefotaxime and that it is at least one-tenth as active as the parent against common *Enterobacteriaceae*, *Staphylococcus aureus*, and *Bacillus fragilis*.

Following intravenous infusions of sodium cefotaxime, LUTHY et al. (1979) observed dose-proportional responses in serum levels of antimicrobial activity and a rapid disappearance of that activity at all doses. Mean urinary excretion of antimicrobial activity within 24 h of infusion amounted to 63% of the dose.

FU et al. (1979) followed serum and urine levels of apparent cefotaxime subsequent to intravenous administration of the antibiotic. They confirmed the presence of both compounds in urine, but quantitated only apparent cefotaxime. The mean terminal half-life of apparent cefotaxime serum levels was 1.13 h. The mean 24-h urinary recovery of apparent cefotaxime accounted for 22%–66% of the dose. NEU et al. (1980) reported similar results. In their study, mean 24-h urinary recovery of apparent cefotaxime ranged from 50% to 59% of the dose. On a multiple intravenous dose regimen of 1.0 g sodium cefotaxime infused every 6 h for 14 days, little accumulation of apparent cefotaxime in serum was seen.

Following an intravenous bolus of the drug, the mean terminal serum half-life of apparent cefotaxime was 1.2 h and mean estimates of apparent volume of distribution, total body clearance, and renal clearance were 10.6 liters, 208 ml/min, and 105 ml/min respectively (WISE et al. 1980b). The mean 24-h urinary excretion of apparent cefotaxime represented 50.5% of the dose.

BAX et al. (1980) studied the pharmacokinetics of cefotaxime following intravenous administration and observed a linear serum level response. The mean terminal serum half-life of cefotaxime is 1.14 h with a mean total body clearance of 273 ml/min. The mean volume of distribution of cefotaxime in the vascular compartment is 10.7 liters. The renal clearance of unchanged drug is 164 ml/min, with 61% of the dose being recovered unchanged in urine. The desacetyl metabolite's recovery in urine accounts for another 24% of the dose. Similar plasma level and urinary excretion data were observed by NAKAYAMA et al. (1980b).

There is evidence to suggest that cefotaxime and/or desacetylcefotaxime are also excreted via the bile (WITTMAN et al. 1980).

It seems evident that all non-chemically-specific assay techniques yield results that underestimate cefotaxime concentration, especially in urine.

A complete study of the biotransformation of cefotaxime in animals or man has not been published. As noted earlier, the presence of desacetylcefotaxime in serum and urine has been confirmed in man after intravenous or intramuscular administration of cefotaxime (Fig. 15).

WISE et al. (1980a, d) have estimated that metabolite levels in serum are 10%–20% of cefotaxime concentrations 15 min after an intravenous injection of the antibiotic. By 4 h after administration desacetylcefotaxime serum levels exceed those of cefotaxime.

There are no studies published concerning cefotaxime administration by other than parenteral routes. Single and multiple intramuscular administration of sodium cefotaxime have been studied in healthy volunteers (FU et al. 1979, NEU et al. 1980). Single intramuscular injections produced mean serum levels of apparent cefotaxime which were dose proportional and which peaked at 30 min. Mean 24-h urinary recovery of apparent cefotaxime represented 33%–39% of the dose. Multiple intramuscular injections of sodium cefotaxime (0.5 g given every 8 h for 10 days) produced no accumulation of cefotaxime in serum. Mean peak serum concentrations of apparent cefotaxime occurred 30 min after the first and last dose.

The data suggested that the excretion of cefotaxime was changing with time in this study since mean 6-h urinary recovery of apparent cefotaxime was 315 mg and 195 mg after the first and last dose, respectively. The authors considered this difference insignificant. BAX et al. (1980) found no such changes following intravenous and intramuscular administration of sodium cefotaxime. These investigators also suggest that concomitant administration of sodium cefotaxime and lidocaine causes a slight increase in the renal clearance of the antibiotic. These data indicate that cefotaxime is well absorbed following intramuscular administration.

The serum protein binding of cefotaxime is reported to be in the range of 27%–60% (LUTHY et al. 1979; NEU et al. 1979a; WISE et al. 1980b; KEMMERICH et al. 1980).

The human tissue and fluid distribution of cefotaxime or cefotaxime-derived antimicrobial activity has not been extensively studied. After a 2-g bolus intravenous injection of sodium cefotaxime (WITTMAN et al. 1980), antimicrobial activity in spongiosa or cortical bone was 5%–10% of that detected in serum for 2 h after drug administration. Levels of antimicrobial activity in peritoneal exudates exceeded serum levels by 1.5 h and remained at least 100% higher as long as activity was detectable. The levels of antimicrobial activity in T tube bile were comparable to serum levels after 1.5 h. The concentration of cefotaxime and desacetylcefotaxime in common duct bile, gall bladder bile, and serum have been reported by MCKENDRICK et al. (1980).

WISE et al. (1980b) observed mean concentrations of cefotaxime in superficial blister fluid that were less than 10 μg/ml at all time points following a 1-g intravenous bolus of sodium cefotaxime. Cefotaxime disappeared from this tissue fluid at a rate similar to its decay in serum.

Relatively high levels of antimicrobial activity are found in CSF following a 2-g intravenous dose of sodium cefotaxime given to healthy adults (BELOHRADSKY et al. 1980). Results in patients were similar (SHAH et al. 1979). MCKENDRICK et al. (1980) could not confirm these results, however.

GRASSI et al. (1980) studied patients with an upper respiratory infection who had received a 2-g intravenous bolus or 1-g intramuscular injections (every 8 h) of sodium cefotaxime. Levels of antimicrobial activity in sputum or bronchial secretions increased with time after either regimen but the ratio to serum activity never exceeded 50%. Bronchial and pulmonary tissue antimicrobial activities 1 h after the intravenous bolus were considered therapeutic.

In a study by BAX et al. (1980), the investigators studied intravenous administration of sodium cefotaxime with and without concomitant administration of probenecid. Probenecid creates serum concentrations of cefotaxime and desacetylcefotaxime that are higher and more sustained than those following administration of the antibiotic alone. The mean serum half-life of cefotaxime increases by 50% and mean total body clearance decreases by 30% under the influence of probenecid. Mean renal clearance decreases by 25%. This confirms assertions by earlier investigators (LUTHY et al. 1979) that renal tubular secretion of cefotaxime plays an important role in the renal elimination of the drug.

WRIGHT and WISE (1980) followed cefotaxime elimination in patients with liver and renal dysfunction. The mean terminal serum half-life of cefotaxime in healthy volunteers following intravenous administration is 0.82 h. Eight-hour urine collections contained cefotaxime accounting for 68% of the dose. For patients with creatinine clearance between 5 and 30 ml/min, the serum half-life of drug increases to 1.87 h and 8-h urinary recovery of cefotaxime is 21% of the dose. The serum half-life increases to 4.2 h when creatinine clearance drops to between 0 and 5 ml/min. Twenty-four-hour urinary recovery of unchanged drug is 14.7% of the dose. The desacetyl metabolite accumulates rapidly in these patients and hemodialysis, but not peritoneal dialysis, is effective in clearing cefotaxime from serum. Hepatic necrosis markedly reduces cefotaxime metabolite formation.

BELOHRADSKY et al. (1980) administered sodium cefotaxime intravenously (50 mg/kg bolus) to 13 children with meningitis. In general, CSF levels of antimicrobial activity exceeded serum levels considerably 2–4 h after injection.

IWAI et al. (1980) gave children 15 mg/kg intravenous injections of sodium cefotaxime and were able to detect serum levels of antimicrobial activity for 4 h. In 6 h, 51.8% of the administered antimicrobial activity was recovered in urine. In a patient with suppurative meningoencephalitis, a 51.9 mg/kg intravenous injection of antibiotic produced measurable levels of antimicrobial activity in CSF for 4 h.

4. Cephaloglycine

Cephaloglycine is eliminated rapidly from serum by deacetylation and urinary excretion (WICK and BONIECE 1965). The same investigators also found that degradation is a concern in vitro when the extreme lability of the drug in broth solutions was noted. SULLIVAN et al. (1969 a) administered radio-labeled cephaloglycine and its biologically inactive L-isomer to rats, both orally and intraperitoneally. After oral administration of D-cephaloglycine, 20% of the radioactivity was recovered in urine within 24 h. Fecal samples collected over 24 h accounted for 70% of the radioactivity. Two percent of the dose was excreted as desacetylcephaloglycine, 8.5% as 2-phenylglycine, 5.0% as benzoylformic acid, and 3.0% as an unidentified polar metabolite. Larger oral doses (200 mg/kg) increased the amounts of desacetylcephaloglycine found in urine, revealed the presence of the lactone of desacetylcephaloglycine, and allowed detection of unchanged drug (Fig. 16). After intraperitoneal injection, 79% of the radioactivity was recovered in urine in 24 h, with 13.5% being cephaloglycine, 28.6% being desacetylcephaloglycine, 11.3% being D-s-phenylglycine, 7.8% being benzoylformic acid, 6.0% being mandelic acid, and 3.8% being unknown polar metabolite. Eight percent of the dose was excreted in the bile. Intraperitoneal or oral administration of L-cephaloglycine led to its complete metabolism, but no L-desacetylcephaloglycine or its lactone was found.

HOEHN and PUGH (1968) detected and quantified cephaloglycine and its metabolites in serum and urine. Desacetylcephaloglycine was confirmed in human urine by SHIMIZU and NISHIMURA (1970), who identified it after oral administration and demonstrated the differing activities of cephaloglycine and desacetylcephaloglycine against commonly used test organisms. They found that almost all antimicrobial activity in urine after an oral dose is attributable to the desacetylmetabolite.

The antibacterial activity of desacetylcephaloglycine is equal to cephaloglycine against gram-positive organisms, but less active against gram-negative bacilli (WICK et al. 1971). Urinary antimicrobial activity is composed of less than 10% cephaloglycine, and both cephaloglycine and desacetylcephaloglycine degrade to

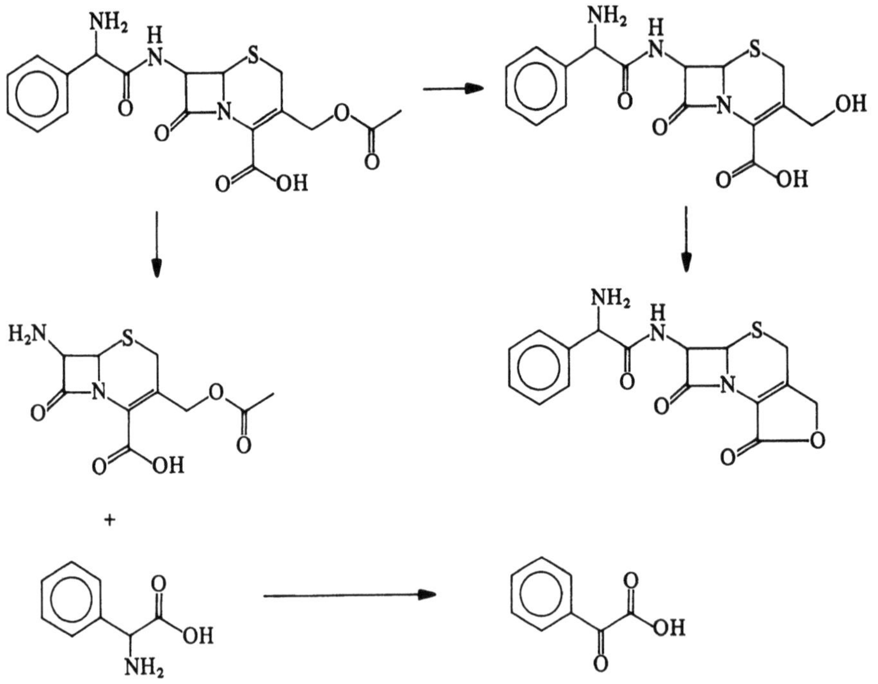

Fig. 16. Biotransformation of cephaloglycine

inactive species rather rapidly in vitro in human serum at 37 °C. The parent drug degrades twice as fast as the desacetylmetabolite.

Intravenous administration of cephaloglycine has not been reported and, therefore, its disposition has not been well assessed. GRIFFITH and BLACK (1971) administered cephaloglycine orally as capsules or suspension at dose levels of 250 and 500 mg. Peak levels of antimicrobial activity in serum were noted at 1 h with the suspension and at 2 h with capsules. Serum levels of antimicrobial activity were much higher after capsule administration at the 500-mg dose. At either dose level, 22%–24% of the dose appears in the urine within 6–8 h. Cephaloglycine represents 10% of the urinary antimicrobial activity while desacetylcephaloglycine represents 90%. Food has no affect on the absorption or excretion of cephaloglycine. Three individuals also received 250 mg cephaloglycine intramuscularly. Peak serum levels of antimicrobial activity were observed in 30 min and 100% of the dose was recovered in 8-h urine collections. This suggests that approximately 25% of an oral dose of cephaloglycine is absorbed.

HAGINAKA et al. (1979) investigated the degradation of cephaloglycine in acidic media. Kinetic rate constant estimates show that the deacetylation of cephaloglycine is the rate-determining step in the formation of the lactone. In a subsequent study HAGINAKA et al. (1980) administered 250-mg capsules of cephaloglycine to four volunteers and found that within 12 h of oral administration 0.5% of the dose is excreted is urine as cephaloglycine, 17.1% as desacetylcephaloglycine, 0.4% as the lactone, and 0.9% as benzoylformic acid, a product of the hydrolysis of the amide linkage in the substituent at the 7-position of the cephem ring.

BINDERUP et al. (1971) reported the enhanced oral absorption of two esters of cephaloglycine, the acetoxymethyl and the pivaloyloxymethyl ester. Neither advanced into pharmaceutical development with the advent and use of cephalexin as an orally absorbed antibiotic.

The human serum protein binding of cephaloglycine has not been accurately determined, but information reported by WICK (1967) would suggest that it is approximately 24% bound.

The tissue and fluid distribution of cephaloglycine in humans has not been reported.

Information concerning the distribution of cephaloglycine in rats is presented by BINDERUP et al. (1971).

Prior probenecid administration slightly increases the magnitude and duration of serum antimicrobial activity following 500-mg oral doses of cephaloglycine (APPLESTEIN et al. 1968). The rate of excretion of urinary antimicrobial activity decreases, however.

The pharmacokinetics of cephaloglycine in patients with urinary dysfunction have not been studied using discriminating assay methods. Suffice it to say, from what is known, the species of concern is desacetylcephaloglycine and it is expected to accumulate in serum as renal function decreases. Neither peritoneal dialysis nor hemodialysis appears to clear cephaloglycine-derived antimicrobial activity from serum (JOHNSON et al. 1968; STEIN et al. 1974).

Finally, studies of the disposition of cephaloglycine in children are scarce, although some information may be obtained from MATSEN (1971).

5. Cephacetrile

Following intravenous administration of ^{14}C-cephacetrile sodium to two male volunteers, 98% of the radioactivity was recovered via the urine within 24 h. An average of 76% of the ^{14}C-dose was excreted as intact drug with approximately 21% of the recovery being a hydrolysis product, desacetylcephracetrile (Fig. 17). An insignificant amount of cyanoacetic acid was found (DORHOFER and FAIGLE 1976).

By inference from other cephalosporins of this type, it is safe to assume that desacetylcephacetrile is present in serum after administration of cephacetrile and that its intrinsic antimicrobial activity is great enough to interfere with most bioassay techniques.

Other investigators (DVORACEK et al. 1974; WESTENFELDER et al. 1974; BROGARD et al. 1976a; NISSENSON et al. 1972; SPRING et al. 1974) have shown nearly quantitative urinary recovery of antimicrobial activity following intravenous administration of cephacetrile sodium with 80% of the total being recovered within 2 h. Antimicrobial activity in serum declines with an apparent terminal half-life of approximately 1 h. Following intramuscular injection of cephacetrile sodium, peak serum concentrations of antimicrobial activity are seen within 1–2 h and the 24-h urinary excretion of drug and metabolite(s) nearly equaled that observed after intravenous drug administration (DUVAL et al. 1974; DVORACEK et al. 1974). The rate of drug absorption or metabolism after intramuscular administration appears to be site dependent (WISE and REEVES 1975).

Decreasing renal fuction causes the expected rise in serum antimicrobial activity, while activity in urine is decreased. Also, the fact that antimicrobial activity is

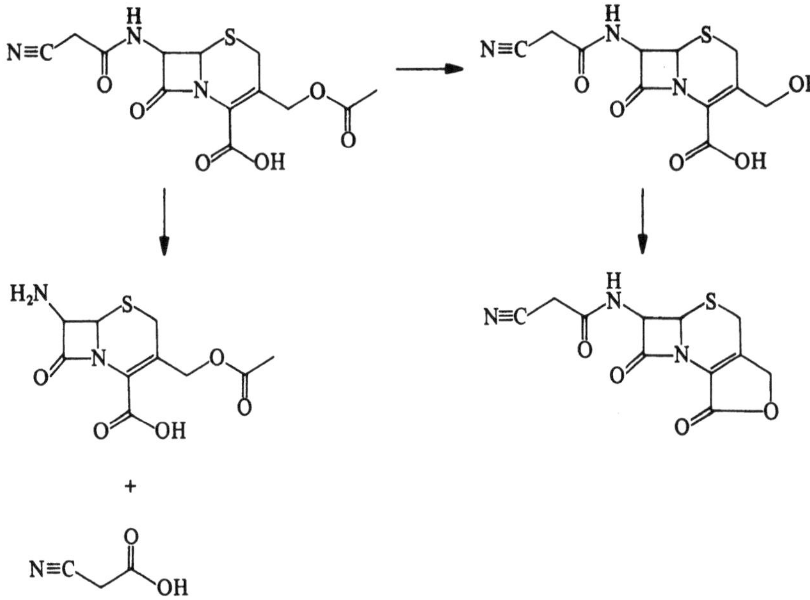

Fig. 17. Biotransformation of cephacetrile

cleared from serum by renal tubular as well as by glomerular filtration, was established by prior or simultaneous administration of oral or intravenous probenecid (Westenfelder et al. 1974). Brogard et al. (1976a), Zech et al. (1974), Nissenson et al. (1972), Reutter and Maurice (1974), Spring et al. (1974), and Malandain et al. (1973) have administered sodium cephacetrile intravenously to patients with varying degrees of renal dysfunction and found that the apparent terminal serum half-life of antimicrobial activity increased in a fashion that correlated well with decreasing creatinine clearance. Dosage adjustments were offered based on the individual's creatinine clearance. For those patients who require hemodialysis, antimicrobial activity is cleared from blood effectively by conventional dialysis units (Zech et al. 1974; Nissenson et al. 1972; Malandain et al. 1973).

Cephacetrile is poorly absorbed after oral administration to rabbits (Luscombe et al. 1974) and no studies of human oral absorption have been reported. In vitro estimates place the protein binding of the drug at 20%–30% (Luscombe et al. 1974; Naber et al. 1976; Naber et al. 1976; Meyer-Brunot et al. 1976).

Cephacetrile-related antimicrobial activity distributes widely into body tissues and fluid following intravenous administration. Kiss et al. (1977) gave a 3-g intravenous dose of the drug to patients 60–120 min before a scheduled operation and repeated the dose 10 min prior to surgery. At the time of surgery, antimicrobial activity in skin, subcutis, and skeletal muscle represented 9%, 5%, and 4% respectively of that measured in serum. Thirty to 60 min after the second dose, antimicrobial activity in normal, inflamed, and tumorous pulmonary tissue was 10%–20% of serum levels. During a similar period, levels in pericardial fluid were 15%–25% of those in serum. Antimicrobial activity in resected atrial auricle was 10%–20% of that found in serum. Aortic valve and mitral valve levels were comparable to serum levels, while papillary muscle levels only reached 10% of serum levels. Antimicrobial activity in stomach wall and greater omentum was 10%–30% of that in serum. Very low levels were found in the spleen and in cholecystic bile when the cystic duct was closed. An open cystic duct evidently led to the 4%–7% levels found in cholecystic bile. Levels in liver were low while activity in choledochus bile and gall bladder wall reached 13%–20% and 20%–33%, respectively, of that in serum. Similar results in myocardial tissue have been reported by ADAM et al. (1976b).

During a constant 500 mg/h infusion (24 h) of cephracetrile sodium to pregnant women, HIRSCH et al. (1974) found that in 3–5 h cord serum and amniotic fluid antimicrobial activity levels are high enough to inhibit gram-positive and the more sensitive gram-negative organisms. Hirsch also found that a 1-g intramuscular injection of cephacetrile sodium given every 2 h for 24 h, led to higher levels in both fluids (see also DUVAL et al. 1974; WIDHOLM and RENKONEN 1973).

FRIEDRICH et al. (1979) reported that 2- to 4-g doses of cephracetrile sodium given every 6 h led to no detectable antimicrobial activity in CSF even after 5 days of therapy, suggesting that penetration may result only when there is inflammation or other impairement of the blood–cerebrospinal fluid barrier as observed by DUVAL et al. (1974). This may have been alluded to in a study by DETTLI et al. (1976), who reported that 3 g cephacetrile injected intravenously every 6 h to patients with bacterial meningitis led to significant CSF levels of antimicrobial activity.

WINDORFER and GASTEIGER (1977) found that the disappearance of antimicrobial activity from the serum of premature and full-term babies was 3–5 times slower than from adult serum.

Finally, STUFLESSER et al. (1978) reported on the ability of cephacetrile-related antimicrobial activity to enter bone tissue. The drug was administered intravenously, and at steady-state, levels of activity in blood-free spongiosa averaged 20% of the levels in serum. Levels in this tissue then declined more slowly than in serum following termination of the infusion. HIERHOLZER et al. (1974) found that a short 2-g intravenous infusion of cephacetrile sodium led to levels of antimicrobial activity in aseptic and chronically inflammed bone tissue capable of inhibiting all sensitive gram-positive organisms and many clinically important gram-negative organisms.

The concomitant intravenous administration of cephacetrile sodium and probenecid decreases the mean urinary recovery of antimicrobial activity, and increases the mean apparent serum half-life of the same, in rabbits (LUSCOMBE et al. 1974). This suggests the presence of renal tubular secretion of the drug in this animal.

DUVAL et al. (1974) administered 50-mg intramuscular doses of sodium cephacetrile to premature infants. Peak serum levels of antimicrobial activity were seen in 30–60 min, and 40%–70% of the administered activity was recovered in 12-h urine collections.

II. Desacetoxycephalosporanic Acids

1. Cephalexin

The elimination of cephalexin (Fig. 18) proceeds rapidly by urinary excretion. The terminal serum half-life is around 45 min (GREEN et al. 1976). There have been a

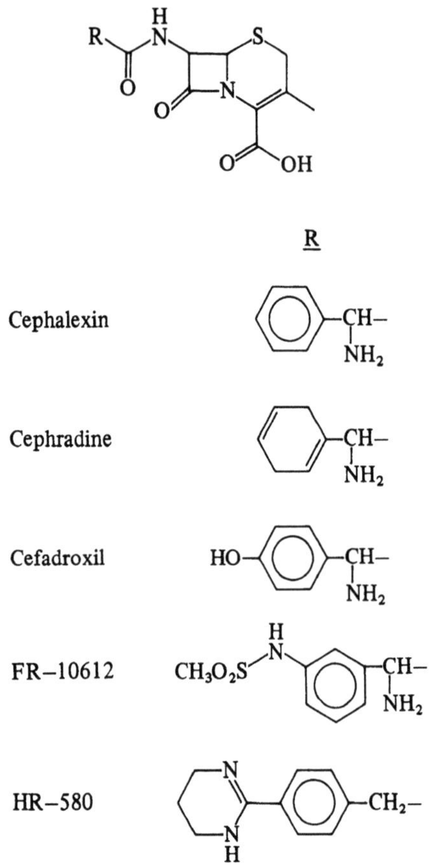

Fig. 18. Structures of desacetoxycephalosporanic acid derivatives

number of studies conducted in which sodium cephalexin was administered by intravenous infusion or injection (DEMAINE and KIRBY 1970; GOWER et al. 1973; REGAMEY et al. 1974; GREENE et al. 1976; KIRBY et al. 1971; DAVIES and HOLT 1972).

Most who estimate it report a mean serum clearance for cephalexin of 250–290 ml/min and in studies where quantitative urine collections were carried out the renal clearance of cephalexin nearly equaled that value. Hence, nearly 100% of the intravenous dose cephalexin is recovered in 24-h urine collections. GREENE et al. (1976) have shown that a two-compartmental analysis of cephalexin serum concentration data wherein elimination occurs only from the central compartment provides parameter estimates which adequately describe the time course of cephalexin in the body. Using this model, the mean volume of distribution of cephalexin in the vascular compartment is 10.9 liters and the mean elimination rate constant is $1.62\ h^{-1}$.

There is evidence that cephalexin is excreted via the bile (IRMER et al. 1971; SALES et al. 1972). However, it would appear that the drug may be reabsorbed from the gut since drug appears quantitatively in the urine after an intravenous dose.

The biotransformation of cephalexin has been studied in rats and mice (SULLIVAN et al. 1969b). Following oral doses of a solution of ^{14}C-cephalexin in both species, 84%–89% of the label was recovered in 24-h urine collections with the remainder appearing in feces. The investigators attributed the fecal recovery to biliary excretion of cephalexin. Only unchanged cephalexin was found in urine specimens. No metabolites of cephalexin have been identified following any route of drug administration in man.

The absorption of cephalexin following intramuscular or oral administration is quite good. Following a single intramuscular injection of cephalexin as the sodium or lysine salt, peak concentrations of cephalexin in serum occur in 30–60 min (REGAMEY et al. 1974; GOWER et al. 1973; BARRIOS et al. 1975). The drug was recovered quantitatively in the urine within 24 h with 40% and 80% of dose appearing within 2 and 6 h respectively (REGAMEY et al. 1974; GOWER et al. 1973; BARRIOS et al. 1975). Serum levels appear to be dose proportional. BARRIOS et al. (1975) have suggested that sodium cephalexin is not well absorbed after intramuscular injection, but it appears that intramuscularly administered sodium cephalexin is rate limited in its absorption when compared to oral doses. Urinary recovery, however, is independent of route of administration or dose. Solubility at the site of injection could be creating a depot-like effect, as suggested by GOWER et al. (1973).

As suggested earlier, cephalexin is well absorbed following a wide range (0.125–2.0 g) of oral doses administered as capsule, tablet, solution, or suspension (THORNHILL et al. 1969; GOWER and DASH 1969; BERGAN et al. 1970; GRIFFITH and BLACK 1971; O'CALLAGHAN et al. 1971; LODE et al. 1979; BARRIOS et al. 1975; ACTOR et al. 1976a; PFEFFER et al. 1977; HARTSTEIN et al. 1977; HENNESS et al. 1978; FINKELSTEIN et al. 1978; CHOW et al. 1979; BUSTRACK et al. 1980; SIMON 1980a; LECAILLON et al. 1980; LODE et al. 1980c). Peak serum concentrations of cephalexin occur within 1–2 h, dependent upon the formulation. Nearly 100% of the oral dose may be recovered in urine within 6–12 h of drug administration. Serum levels are proportional to dose, and administering the drug with food has only a slight effect on the rate and extent of drug absorption. Multiple oral dose administration (0.75, 1.0, or 2.0 g every 6 h or 1.0 g every 4 h) resulted in no drug accumulation in serum (GOWER and DASH 1969; BERGAN et al. 1970; LODE et al. 1979; GRIFFITH and BLACK 1971; CHOW et al. 1979; LECAILLON et al. 1980; HENNESS et al. 1978; FINKELSTEIN et al. 1978). However, some accumulation may occur on a regimen of 1.5 g every 6 h (JOLLY et al. 1977). The absorption of cephalexin after oral administration has been studied in several disease states and in elderly subjects (DEAN et al. 1979; DAVIES and HOLT 1975). No problems were noted in patients with congestive cardiac failure, pneumococcal pneumonia, severe hypertension, obstructive jaundice, gastric achlorhydria, or partial gastrectomy or in the elderly. Elderly subjects do not eliminate cephalexin as rapidly as younger, healthy volunteers.

The human serum protein binding of cephalexin is approximately 10%–17% (KIRBY and REGAMEY 1973; NISHIDA et al. 1970; BUCK and PRICE 1977; SINGHVI et al. 1977) over the range of therapeutic serum concentrations. VERONESE et al. (1977) suggested that cephalexin binds (10%) to hydrophobic sites on serum albumins. These investigators found little difference in the association constant of cephalexin to bovine, rabbit, chicken, and human serum albumins.

ORSOLINI (1970) studied the tissue distribution of cephalexin after 500-mg or 1,000-mg oral doses in 45 patients. Over a period of 4 h after drug administration, cephalexin concentrations in stomach, appendix, gall bladder, and omentum tissue ranged from 5%–50% of serum levels. Vascular and tumorous tissue cephalexin levels were relatively constant at 50% and 33% of serum levels respectively. BOYLE et al. (1970) gave 1.0- to 3.0-g oral doses of cephalexin to cataract patients 1–15 h before surgery. In general, cephalexin concentration in aqueous humor was not detectable earlier than 2 h or later than 12 h after drug administration. This was true at all dose levels except for the 3-g dose, where aqueous humor levels were still measurable 13–14 h after administration. SIMON (1980a) administered 1-g oral doses and found drug levels in artificial skin blister fluid to be comparable to serum levels 2 h after dosing.

The concentration of cephalexin in the bile of patients with some form of biliary tract disease was investigated by SALES et al. (1972). After a single oral dose of cephalexin (0.5 g), peak drug levels occurred in bile within 2–3 h, but levels were generally less than 10 μg/ml. After multiple oral doses (0.5 g every 6 h for 5 days), biliary levels of cephalexin were in excess of 40 μg/ml in patients with functioning gallbladders, but less than 10 μg/ml in those with nonfunctioning gallbladders. IRMER et al. (1971) confirmed these biliary results, but also found measurable cephalexin levels in bone marrow and peritoneal exudate after single and multiple 1-g oral doses of the antibiotic. DUVAL et al. (1972) has found cephalexin easily passes the placental barrier. VALDIVIESO et al. (1977) administered 500-mg oral doses to pregnant women 2 h before caesarian section. Drug levels in fetal serum were 33% of maternal serum levels. Drug concentration in fetal urine, placenta, amniotic fluid, umbilical cord, and fallopian tube was 8%–25% of the concentration in maternal serum. SYMES et al. (1974) found cephalexin levels in semen and prostatic tissue to be low after 0.5-g or 1.0-g oral doses. KOERNER and JAESCHKE (1974) found that cephalexin must be dosed at 3 g per day for at least 3 days before significant drug levels could be found in epididymis, fat tissue, and muscle tissue. Sinus mucosa and secretion contained therapeutic levels of cephalexin after 15 mg/kg oral doses (KOHONEN et al. 1975). HALPRIN and MCMAHON (1973) studied the appearance of cephalexin in sputum following multiple oral doses of the drug in patients with acute respiratory infections. Also, following a single oral dose of cephalexin (1 g), the drug's presence in skin abrasion exudates remained fairly constant at a level that was 70% of the serum concentration for at least 3 h after dosing (GILLETT and WISE 1978). Penetration of cephalexin into CSF following single (DAVIES et al. 1970) or multiple (BERGAN et al. 1970) oral doses in subjects not exhibiting meningeal irritation is minimal.

Oral doses of cephalexin accompanied and/or preceded by oral doses of probenecid led to serum concentrations of cephalexin higher and more sustained than when cephalexin was given alone. Six-hour urinary excretion of cephalexin was also lower. The serum half-life of cephalexin doubled and serum concentrations of cephalexin were up to 134% higher (THORNHILL et al. 1969; GOWER and DASH 1969). REGAMEY et al. (1974) gave 1 g probenecid 1 h before a 20-min intravenous infusion of sodium cephalexin (0.5 g). The terminal serum half-life of cephalexin doubled. The mean renal clearance dropped by 50% as compared to intravenous administration of the antibiotic alone. This information suggests that the drug is eliminated by renal tubular secretion, but ARVIDSSON et al. (1979b) feel that it is not reabsorbed via kidney tubules.

The effect of decreasing renal function on serum and urine cephalexin concentrations after oral cephalexin has been reported (BAILEY et al. 1970; BROGARD et al. 1975a; SPYKER et al. 1978). As creatinine clearance fell below 30 ml/min, the serum half-life of cephalexin increased rapidly and peak serum levels were delayed for several hours. In patients whose creatinine clearance was below 20 ml/min, less than 60% of the cephalexin dose could be recovered in urine in 48 h. Hemodialysis was effective in clearing cephalexin from the blood.

Sodium cephalexin was given intravenously (0.5 g) to three anuric patients during and between dialysis sessions (DEMAINE and KIRBY 1970). The apparent serum half-life of cephalexin in these patients was 18 h while not being dialyzed and approximately 3.6 h during hemodialysis.

Oral doses of cephalexin (15–50 mg/kg) were given to newborn infants for 3 days after birth (BOOTHMAN et al. 1973). During the second or third day, male infants excreted a mean of 30%–39% of the daily cephalexin dose in their urine.

In older infants and children given a cephalexin oral dose of 15 mg/kg (McCRACKEN et al. 1978a), peak serum levels of antibiotic were seen in 0.5 h. Lower serum concentrations were observed when cephalexin was taken with food. Mean saliva and tear drug concentrations were less than 1 μg/ml. These results appear to have been coinfirmed by TETZLAFF et al. (1978) although unreliable serum sampling techniques were used.

2. Cephradine

Cephradine (Fig. 18) is eliminated primarily by the kidneys with a terminal serum half-life of less than 50 min (HOFFLER and KOEPPE 1975; SIMON et al. 1973). SIMON et al. (1973) have given the drug by bolus intravenous injection and by infusion at a dose of 1 g. The volume of distribution for cephradine in the vascular compartment is 9.6 liters and total body clearance is 412.8 ml/min. The urinary recovery of cephradine through 9 h represented 70% of the dose. Following an intravenous infusion of sodium cephradine (0.166 g/h for 4 h), total body clearance was estimated to be 577 ml/min while renal clearance was 378 ml/min. Data suggest that cephradine is also cleared metabolically or via biliary secretion (MAROSKE et al. 1976; BERGOGNE et al. 1976).

Studies of the biotransformation of cephradine have been carried out in mice and dogs (WELIKY et al. 1974). After subcutaneous injections into rats and oral administration to dogs, only cephradine was recovered in urine. In mice, 6-h urinary excretion of cephradine accounted for 84% of the dose and in dogs the entire dose could be accounted for in urine and feces after 24 h with 70% of the dose appearing in urine. No metabolites of cephradine have been found in humans (NEISS 1973; ZAKI et al. 1974).

Cephradine is rapidly and well absorbed following oral and intramuscular administration (RATTIE et al. 1976; WELIKY and LEITZ 1976; FINKELSTEIN et al. 1978; HARVENGT et al. 1973; ZAKI et al. 1974; MISCHLER et al. 1974b; CHOW et al. 1979). Peak serum levels of cephradine occur within 1 h for capsule, solution, or suspension formulations. There is no accumulation of drug in serum, at least up to oral doses of 2 g every 6 h, and renal clearance ranges from 239 to 308 ml/min. Urinary recovery of cephradine in 24-h urine collections after oral administration is nearly total. Serum levels of cephradine are proportional to dose. Administration with food decreases the rate but not the extent of absorption.

After intramuscular injection of cephradine, peak serum concentrations of antibiotic occur within 30–60 min. Serum levels are proportional to dose, but it appears that cephradine may be slightly less bioavailable by this route of administration. Peak serum concentrations are less than after equivalent oral doses and total urinary recovery of drug averages 80%–85% of the dose. VUKOVICH et al. (1975b) found that using a 2% procaine hydrochloride solution as diluent for an intramuscular injection of cephradine has no effect on its bioavailability. Intramuscular cephradine is less bioavailable in women than in men; the degree of difference was dependent upon the muscle mass chosen for injection (VUKOVICH et al. 1975a).

The serum protein binding of cephradine ranges from 6% to 14% (NEISS 1973; WELIKY and LEITZ 1976; SINGHVI et al. 1978). There have been suggestions that the serum protein binding of cephradine varies with the concentration of drug in serum, but GADEBUSCH et al. (1972) found no difference in MIC of cephradine against *Staphylococcus aureus* and *Escherichia coli* when determined in buffer or human serum. JOHNSON and SABATH (1979) report that pH has little effect on the serum protein binding of cephradine.

ADAM et al. (1976a) found that drug levels ranged from 10% to 60% of serum levels in heart muscle, prostatic tissue, and brain tissue after intravenous administration of cephradine to children with Fallot's disease, patients with prostatic adenoma, and patients with cerebral tumors respectively. Drug levels in CSF were very low after administration to patients with no meningitis. The presence of cephradine in CSF was not predictable in children with purulent meningitis after 75 mg/kg cephradine intravenously (BERGOGNE et al. 1976).

MAROSKE et al. (1976) administered 2 g cephradine intravenously to surgical patients and monitored drug concentration in liver tissue and bile. Thirty minutes after dosing, the ratio of drug concentration in liver tissue to that in serum ranged from 0.36 to 0.83. T-tube bile from cholecystectomized patients contained mean cephradine concentrations of 86.4 µg/ml 75 min after 2 g antibiotic given intravenously. Similar observations were made by BERGOGNE et al. (1976).

PARSONS et al. (1976a) administered cephradine intravenously and intramuscularly to patients about to undergo total hip replacement. Cephradine penetrated cancellous bone, cortical bone, and mixed cancellous and cortical bone, as well as hip capsule. Bone levels were dependent upon the dose size and the route of administration. Therapeutic drug levels were more easily attained in drain fluid.

BERGOGNE et al. (1976) showed that cephradine crossed the placental barrier easily. Drug concentrations in cord blood and amniotic fluid could be brought to therapeutic levels after intravenous or oral drug administration. CRAFT and FORSTER (1978) administered 2 g cephradine intravenously to women about to undergo therapeutic abortion and obtained placental and fetal tissue samples. On average, tissue levels of cephradine were less than 10% of maternal serum levels. Women undergoing caesarian section (late pregnancy) were also studied. Ten to thirty minutes after drug administration, cephradine concentration in myometrium, cord blood, and placental tissue was 25% of maternal serum levels. Cord tissue drug concentration was 10% of maternal serum levels. Milk samples collected over a period of 6 h after the last dose from lactating women who had received 0.5 g cephradine every 6 h for 2 days contained unchanging concentrations of cephradine that averaged 0.6 μg/ml (MISCHLER et al. 1974a).

Thirty minutes following a 2-g intravenous infusion of cephradine, concentrations of drug in lung tissue were at least 40% of serum levels (MOATTI et al. 1978). As time progressed, drug concentration in the two media grew more similar.

In patients about to undergo peripheral vascular reconstruction or amputation, 1 g cephradine was given intramuscularly 1 h preoperatively and then intravenously with anesthetic induction. Cephradine concentration in subcutaneous fat and voluntary muscle tissue averaged 10% and 20% of serum levels respectively (MATHARU et al. 1978). In similar patients, RYLANDER et al. (1979) found that the presence of peripheral vascular disease did not keep cephradine concentrations in wound secretions (ulcerative foot lesions) from matching serum levels after a 1-g intravenous bolus.

High levels of cephradine in normal renal tissue (>100 μg/g) were found after a 2-g intravenous bolus of the antibiotic (ADAM and TUNN 1979). Drug concentration in chronically inflamed kidney tissue was 3–5 times less.

Cephradine concentration in heart valves remained above 8 μg/g for 2 h following a 1-g i.v. infusion (5 min) of the antibiotic (DASCHNER et al. 1979b). Subcutaneous fat and muscle levels were somewhat less.

SIMON et al. (1973) measured cephradine concentration in artificially produced skin blister fluid following an intravenous infusion (0.5 g) of drug. Blister fluid levels at the end of the infusion were 71% of serum concentrations.

In a study where oral and intramuscular doses of cephradine were administered, with and without oral probenecid, MISCHLER et al. (1974b) observed the expected elevated and prolonged serum concentration profile. During concomitant administration of probenecid and cephradine, the apparent serum half-life of cephradine approximately doubled. Probenecid had no effect on the 24-h urinary recovery of unchanged antibiotic.

SOLOMON et al. (1975) administered single and multiple oral doses of cephradine to patients in renal failure. Creatinine clearance ranged from 31 to 0 ml/min. As renal function decreased, peak serum concentrations increased, as did the time to peak. Serum concentrations became more sustained with time and drug accumulation in serum became more and more apparent upon multiple dosing. In patients requiring dialysis, serum drug concentrations remained above 4 μg/ml for 36 h after a single oral 250-mg dose between dialysis sessions. After a similar dose, serum cephradine concentrations were between 5 and 10 μg/ml at the end of a 9-h dialysis session.

HOFFLER and KOEPPE (1975) administered 1 g cephradine by intravenous injection to a group of patients with a wide range of kidney function. The terminal serum half-life of cephradine ranged from 41 min in patients with normal renal function to 348 min in patients requiring hemodialysis. These investigators found that their estimates of cephradine half-life in these patients correlated well with the individual's creatinine clearance in a log-log fashion.

The oral absorption of cephradine in children has been studied by ZAKI et al. (1974) and GINSBURG and MCCRACKEN (1979). Oral suspension formulations were rapidly absorbed with peak serum concentrations occurring in 30 min. Serum levels were proportional to dose. Administration of cephradine with milk decreased the peak serum concentration of drug but appears only to slow the rate of drug absorption. Drug was detectable in the saliva of some subjects 2–6 h after drug administration.

3. Cefadroxil

Cefadroxil (Fig. 18) is a semisynthetic cephalosporin which is eliminated from the systemic circulation by urinary excretion. Biliary levels of cefadroxil have been reported (Palmu et al. 1980), but, since the drug is well absorbed orally, this may not be an effective route of elimination.

There have been no reports of intravenous administration of the drug. Studies of its biotransformation in animals or man are limited to a study in mice (Buck and Price 1977) where no biologically active metabolites were found. One study in rats (Esumi et al. 1979 b) where radioactive cefadroxil was given orally, reports finding no radioactivity in expired air within 24 h. No metabolites were found in urine.

As mentioned, the drug is absorbed after oral administration. Peak serum levels of cefadroxil occurred 1.5–2 h after oral doses ranging from 300–1,000 mg and at 3 h after a 1,500-mg dose. Serum levels were not proportional to dose. Thirty-eight percent to 58% of the dose was excreted unchanged in urine in 3 h and 85%–93% was recovered in 24 h. Regimens of 500–1,000 mg every 6 h did not lead to drug accumulation in serum, whereas 1,500 mg every 6 h led to a small amount of accumulation. The apparent serum half-life of cefadroxil appears to be approximately 1–1.5 h. Administration with food does not affect the plasma levels or urinary recovery of cefadroxil (Hartstein et al. 1977; Pfeffer et al. 1977; Jolly et al. 1977; Henness et al. 1978; Lode et al. 1980c; Simon 1980a; Prenna and Ripa 1980).

Buck and Price (1977) determined the serum protein binding of cefadroxil to be 20% by ultrafiltration over a drug concentration range of 10–25 μg/ml.

The distribution of cefadroxil in human tissues has not been extensively studied. Levels of cefadroxil in artificial skin blister fluid are comparable to serum levels 3 h after a single 1-g oral dose (Simon 1980 a). One gram of cefadroxil given every 12 h the day before surgery led to T-tube bile levels that were 10%–20% of serum levels at surgery. Levels in gallbladder bile and common duct bile were much higher. Gallbladder and liver tissue levels were 75%–90% of serum levels (Palmu et al. 1980).

Valdivieso et al. (1977) gave a single 500-mg oral dose to pregnant women 2 h before they were to undergo caesarian section. Drug levels in fetal serum, fetal urine, and placenta were comparable and about 15% of maternal serum levels. Levels in amniotic fluid, umbilical cord, and fallopian tube were 50% lower.

Distribution in rats has been reported by Esumi et al. (1979 a, b). After oral administration of ^{14}C-cefadroxil, highest levels of radioactivity were found in kidney, liver, and bladder tissue and in the small intestinal contents.

Cefadroxil has been administered to patients with renal insufficiency. Cutler et al. (1979) gave 1-g oral doses to patients whose creatinine clearance ranged from 113–0 ml/min. Peak serum concentrations were higher and appeared later as kidney function decreased. Urinary recovery, from patients producing urine, over a 48-h period ranged from 100%–11%, decreasing as renal insufficiency increased.

In a similar study, HUMBERT et al. (1979 b) administered 1-g oral doses. In normal subjects, 93% of the dose was recovered in 24-h urine collections. Results in uremic patients were similar to the previous study. Cefadroxil is effectively cleared from blood by hemodialysis.

Cefadroxil has been studied in children who received 10–15 mg/kg doses as an oral suspension. Peak serum concentrations of drug were seen in 1 h; drug was detected in saliva, and administering the drug with milk appeared to have no effect on its absorption (GINSBURG et al. 1978).

4. FR-10612

FR-10612 is a new, broad-spectrum, orally absorbed cephalosporin derivative which is similar to cephalexin (Fig. 18). The drug is eliminated primarily by urinary excretion. Nearly 90% of an oral dose is recovered in 24-h urine collections. The apparent serum half-life of the drug is 2–4 h.

After oral doses of FR-10612 to rats, dogs and monkeys, 60%, 50%, and 18% of the dose respectively was excreted in 24-h urine collections. After oral doses of FR-10612 to bile-duct cannulated rats, 68% of the dose was recovered in 24-h bile collections. Secretion of drug into bile appears to be a major route of FR-10612 elimination in the rat. Some drug may be reabsorbed from the gut following bile dumping.

Tissue distribution patterns were similar in rats and mice. Highest drug concentrations were found in kidneys, liver, and serum, with significantly lower levels being found in lungs, heart, and spleen. Drug concentrations in kidneys and liver exceed serum levels in both animals through 6 h after drug administration. Drug concentrations in peripheral granuloma pouch exudates following oral drug administration to rats increased gradually with time and matched levels in serum by 8 h. No biologically active metabolites were found in the urine of any species studied (NISHIDA et al. 1976 b).

Healthy volunteers received 250-mg and 500-mg oral doses of FR-10612 while fasting. Peak serum concentrations were reached in 2–3 h and were not dose proportional. Urinary recovery of FR-10612 in urine for 24 h after the oral dose accounted for 89% of that dose. No biologically active metabolites were found in urine.

The serum protein binding of FR-10612 was determined by ultrafiltration. The percent bound in human, dog, rabbit, and rat serum is 13%, 17%, 15%, and 29% respectively (NISHIDA et al. 1976 b).

5. HR-580

DELL and INGS (1978) conducted a study in three healthy volunteers, who received 500-mg intravenous doses of HR-580 (Fig. 18). The mean terminal serum half-life of HR-580 is 2.2 h. The mean total body clearance of the drug is 133 ml/min and renal clearance is 128 ml/min. On average, 88% of the dose was recovered in 6-h urine collections. The volume of distribution of HR-580 in the vascular compartment ranged from 8.3 to 20 liters. There were differences between the results of microbiological and liquid chromatographic assays.

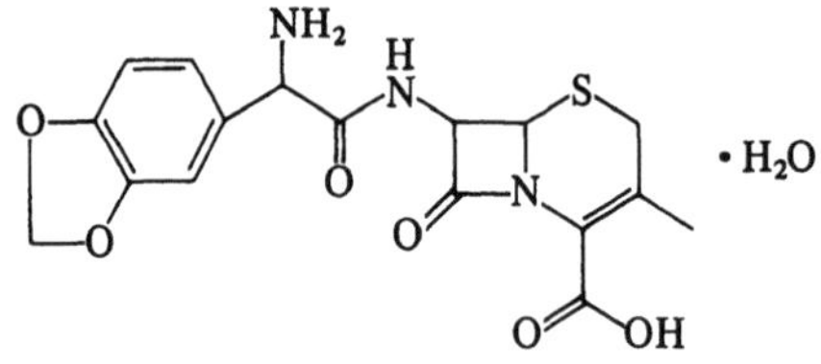

Fig. 19. Structure of RMI 19,592

6. RMI 19,592

RMI 19,592 (Fig. 19) is an investigational oral cephalosporin antibiotic which is in very early stages of human testing (BUSTRACK et al. 1980). Following oral doses ranging from 250–1,000 mg, plasma levels of RMI 19,592 peaked within 1 h of dosing. Eighty percent to 90% of the dose was recovered in 24-h urine collections. The apparent plasma half-life of RMI 19,592 is between 1 and 1.5 h. Renal clearance ranges between 195 and 225 ml/min. Elimination is thought to proceed via glomerular filtration and renal tubular secretion.

III. 3-(5-Methyl-1,3,4-thiadiazol-2-ylthiomethyl)ceph-3-em-4-oic Acids

1. Cefazolin

The elimination of cefazolin (Fig. 20) proceeds chiefly by glomerular filtration and renal tubular secretion. There is a minor elimination pathway which involves biliary excretion (THYS et al. 1976). The terminal serum half-life of cefazolin ranges from 1.25–2 h (SIMON et al. 1973; BERGAN 1977; RATTIE and RAVIN 1975; LODE et al. 1975; BASSARIS et al. 1976; LEOPOLD et al. 1977; PABST et al. 1979; HITZENBERGER and JASCHEK 1980; NIGHTINGALE et al. 1975a). BRISSON et al. (1980) feel that cefazolin serum levels decline triexponentially with time following intravenous administration and they report a terminal serum half-life for cefazolin of 2.6 h. The total body clearance is usually estimated to be in the range of 60–100 ml/min and estimates of renal clearance closely approximate this value (SIMON et al. 1973; KIRBY and REGAMEY 1973; RATTIE and RAVIN 1975; LODE et al. 1975; NIGHTINGALE et al. 1975a; LEOPOLD et al. 1977; PABST et al. 1979; HITZENBERGER and JASCHEK 1980; BRISSON et al. 1980). The urinary recovery of cefazolin ranges from 76%–92% of the dose in 6–12 h (ADAM and PATZOLD 1977; SIMON et al. 1973; RATTIE and RAVIN 1975; THYS et al. 1976; BRISSON et al. 1980) to nearly 100% in 24 h (KIRBY and REGAMEY 1973; HITZENBERGER and JASCHEK 1980; NIGHTINGALE et al. 1975a). The volume of distribution of cefazolin in the vascular compartment is 3–6 liters (LODE et al. 1975; NIGHTINGALE et al. 1975a; RATTIE and RAVIN 1975; BASSARIS et al. 1976; BERGAN 1977; LEOPOLD et al. 1977; PABST et al. 1979; BRISSON et al. 1980).

Serum antibiotic concentrations appear to be proportional to dose after intravenous administration (BERGAN 1977). SIMON et al. (1973) found a mean steady-state serum concentration of 25 μg/ml following a 4-h, 0.166-g/h sodium cefazolin infusion.

MILLER et al. (1980) studied the effect of cardiopulmonary bypass surgery on the pharmacokinetics of cefazolin. Before surgery renal clearance was similar to

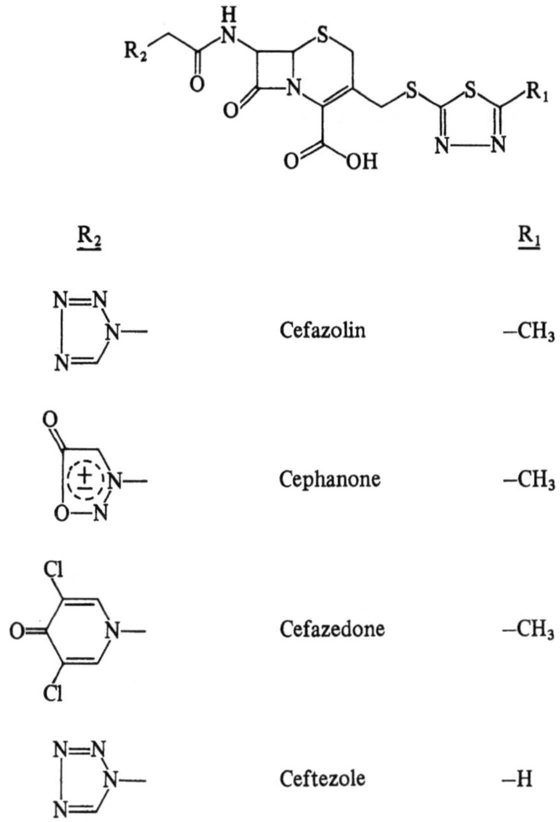

Fig. 20. Structure of 3-(5-methyl-1,3,4-thiadiazol-2-ylthiomethyl)-ceph-3-em-4-oic acid derivatives

total body clearance and the terminal serum half-life was 2.5 h. These parameters changed dramatically during the surgical procedure and had not returned to presurgical estimates on the day after surgery.

SIMON et al. (1976b) report the disposition of cefazolin to be different in geriatric subjects as compared to younger adults. In the absence of renal disease, the mean terminal serum half-life doubled and mean renal clearance was 50% of the values estimated in young volunteers.

At most, the biotransformation of cefazolin represents an insignificant elimination pathway in humans. No metabolites possessing antimicrobial activity have been found in human urine (NISHIDA et al. 1969, 1970). Small amounts of metabolites may have been identified in rats (LEROY et al. 1974), but this is contrary to the findings of ISHIYAMA et al. (1971).

Cefazolin is apparently not absorbed after oral administration. Following intramuscular administration, peak serum concentrations are observed in 30–90 min and 75%–95% of the dose is recoverable in 24-h urine collections (NISHIDA et al. 1969, 1970; ISHIYAMA et al. 1970; DESCHEPPER et al. 1973; CRAIG et al. 1973; KIRBY and REGAMEY 1973; REIN et al. 1973; CAHN et al. 1974; LEROY et al. 1974; RATTIE and RAVIN 1975; ACTOR et al. 1976a; PARADELIS et al. 1977; PABST et al. 1979). Serum levels of cefazolin are proportional to intramuscular doses (NISHIDA et al.

1969, 1970; CAHN et al. 1974). Similar serum level information was obtained from bedridden patients with normal renal function (MADHAVAN et al. 1973; BERGAN et al. 1978 b).

Cefazolin is extensively bound to human serum proteins, with values of 70%–90% being reported over a drug concentration range of 10–500 µg/ml (PARADELIS et al. 1977, KIRBY and REGAMEY 1973; WAHLIG et al. 1979; MADHAVAN et al. 1973; MIYAKE and EBATA 1976; HOTTENDORF et al. 1975; CRAIG et al. 1973; NISHIDA et al. 1969). PITKIN et al. (1980 b) showed that saturated fatty acids of 10–14 carbon atoms could greatly inhibit the serum protein binding of cefazolin. The effect was concentration dependent. However, slight changes in serum pH had little effect on cefazolin binding (JOHNSON and SABATH 1979). Cefazolin is 73% bound to serum protein in uremic patients immediately before hemodialysis. This value dropped to a mean of 22% in the same patients after dialysis (GREENE et al. 1977).

As mentioned earlier, a small amount of cefazolin is eliminated by biliary excretion. In patients with chronic cholecystitis and cholelithiasis without obstruction, MADHAVAN et al. (1975 b) found drug concentration in gall bladder bile to be low and rather variable 1 h after an intramuscular dose. One hour after an intravenous dose, gallbladder bile levels of drug were up to 8 times the levels observed in serum at corresponding time points. Mean gallbladder tissue concentrations of cephazolin were 58.2 µg/g, 90–120 min after intravenous injection. The intramuscular dose of cefazolin led to drug concentrations in common duct bile that ranged from equivalent to twice those concentrations found in serum from 1–2.5 h after dosing. In a single patient, the T-tube bile drainage collected for 6 h after an intramuscular injection of sodium cefazolin contained 0.19% of the dose. Similar results had previously been reported by RATZAN et al. (1974). BROGARD et al. (1975 b) studied the biliary excretion of cefazolin in normal subjects and in patients after intravenous doses of the antibiotic. Cefazolin concentration in the duodenal-tube fluid ranged from 60% down to 40% of serum levels over a 4-h period. In 4 h, 0.15% of the dose was recovered in this fluid. In cholecystectomized patients with external biliary drainage, an intravenous dose of cefazolin produced biliary drug concentrations that were approximately 20% of serum levels at 1 h after administration and declined progressively to zero by 9–10 h. Similar results were later reported by THYS et al. (1976). Data gathered during surgery 1 h after an intravenous dose of cefazolin (BROGARD et al. 1975 b) revealed comparable drug concentrations in serum and common duct bile, while levels in gallbladder bile were only 15% of those in serum. In a larger patient study, RAM and WATANATITTAN (1976) administered 500-mg intramuscular doses of sodium cefazolin every 6 h. In samples obtained 90–120 min after the last dose, drug levels in gallbladder bile were much higher than serum levels in the absence of obstructive jaundice or obstructed cystic duct, while gallbladder tissue drug concentrations were twice as high as serum. Obstructed cystic duct greatly reduced biliary excretion of cefazolin, but did not affect gallbladder tissue levels. Obstructive jaundice nearly precluded the presence of cefazolin in gallbladder bile. A similar study was reported by MCLEISH et al. (1977).

COLE and PUNG (1977) report that the pleural fluid penetration of cefazolin appears to be better after intramuscular administration than following intravenous doses, but therapeutic concentrations of drug were present after either route. LITVAK et al. (1976) reported on the penetration of cefazolin into prostatic tissue. Following 1-g i.v. doses of sodium cefazolin given to patients scheduled for total joint replacement, SCHURMAN et al. (1978) found mean drug concentrations in synovial fluid to be in excess of 20 μg/ml for at least 45 min after administration, but bone levels rarely exceeded 10 μg/g. After infusing sodium cefazolin at 0.166 g/h for 4 h SIMON et al. (1973) noted that drug levels in artificially produced skin blister fluid were 34% of serum levels. Lower cefazolin interstitual fluid penetration was reported by TAN and SALSTROM (1977). Cefazolin concentration in psoas muscle was between 10 and 20 μg/g for 3 h following a 25-min 2-g i.v. infusion of drug (SINAGOWITZ et al. 1976a, b). Also, after a 50-mg subconjunctival injection of sodium cefazolin, drug concentrations in aqueous humor quickly reached minimum inhibitory levels (SAUNDERS and MCPHERSON 1980). KESTER et al. (1979) report good penetration of cefazolin into subcutaneous fat and skeletal muscle of atherosclerotically diseased lower limbs. After intravenous administration of cefazolin, RYLANDER et al. (1979) reported the presence of drug in wound secretions of patients with foot ulcers.

Penetration of cefazolin into the breast milk of lactating women is minimal (YOSHIOKA et al. 1979b). However, drug concentrations in perimetrial, myometrial, and endometrial tissue after a 2-g intravenous bolus of the antibiotic were well above levels needed for therapeutic effectiveness (YAMADA et al. 1980).

BERNARD et al. (1977b) studied the maternal-fetal transfer of cefazolin following administration of 14 mg/kg intramuscular doses of the drug to women scheduled for elective therapeutic abortion and sterilization by hysterectomy. Drug concentration in placenta and amniotic fluid was low at all sampling times. Cord serum levels appear to peak much later than maternal serum drug concentrations and persist up to 10 h after injection. Drug was detected in fetal urine for up to 20 h after the dose, but no antimicrobial activity at any time could be demonstrated in fetal CSF, fetal lung, fetal liver, or fetal kidney. DEKEL et al. (1980) reports that cefazolin crosses the placenta more easily during the second and third trimesters of pregnancy than during the first. Similar studies have been conducted by VON KOBYLETZKI et al. (1974).

ISHIYAMA et al. (1970), BASSARIS et al. (1976), and THYS et al. (1976) report that cefazolin does not penetrate the CSF of subjects with noninflamed meninges after single or multiple intravenous doses. However, in the presence of the compromising physiological conditions, wherein cefazolin has accumulated in serum to levels as high as 1,000 μg/ml, the penetration of drug into CSF has been noted and so-called antibiotic-induced seizures have occurred (BECHTEL et al. 1980; GARDNER et al. 1978).

The concomitant administration of probenecid and cefazolin produced a significant increase and prolongation in serum levels compared to antibiotic given alone (KIRBY and REGAMEY 1973). This effect of probenecid on cefazolin serum levels may also aid the penetration of the drug into CSF (BAKER et al. 1975). REIN et al. (1973) gave four oral doses of probenecid (500 mg) at 6-h intervals while giving 500 mg sodium cefazolin intramuscularly 1 h after the initial probenecid dose. Peak serum concentrations of cefazolin were slightly elevated in the presence of probenecid and the apparent serum half-life of cefazolin was approximately 30% longer.

MADHAVAN et al. (1973) reported serum cefazolin concentrations from five azotemic patients after a single 500-mg intramuscular injection. Drug levels were elevated over those observed in healthy subjects, with detectable levels persisting for at least 24 h after dosing when creatinine clearance dropped below 12 ml/min. LEVISON et al. (1973) and REIN et al. (1973) administered a single 500-mg intramuscular dose of sodium cefazolin to patients with normal or abnormal renal function. Peak serum concentrations tended to increase slightly and serum drug levels persisted longer as kidney function decreased, especially as creatinine clearance dropped below 20 ml/min (CRAIG et al. 1973; CZERWINSKI et al. 1974). Recovery of drug in urine decreased as renal impairment increased. Hemodialysis was effective in slowly removing cefazolin from blood, but peritoneal dialysis was not particularly successful. Similar findings were reported by CRAIG et al. (1973), CZERWINSKI et al. (1974), LEROY et al. (1974), MADHAVAN et al. (1975a), HUMBERT et al. (1975), and BERGAN et al. (1977). BRODWALL et al. (1977) found no change in the serum protein binding of cefazolin in patients as inulin clearance dropped from 148 ml/min down to 10 ml/min, but CRAIG et al. (1973) reported the binding to be more variable as kidney function decreased. The renal clearance of cefazolin correlated well with inulin clearance in a log-log fashion. CZERWINSKI et al. (1974) found reasonable linear correlations between serum half-life and serum creatinine concentrations and between cefazolin renal clearance and creatinine clearance. Similar correlations were observed by BROGARD et al. (1977b).

KAYE et al. (1978) added cefazolin to the dialysis fluid (50 mg/ml or 150 mg/ml) of patients undergoing peritoneal dialysis. Drug was absorbed into the systemic circulation and therapeutic levels were attained. When drug was no longer added to the dialysis fluid, cefazolin was slowly cleared from the body. Several patients similarly received intraperitoneal injections (1 g) of cefazolin. Peak serum levels were attained in 2 h and 22 h later had dropped by 65% without dialysis.

BEGUE et al. (1977) administered cefazolin intramuscularly every 12 h to children ranging in age from less than 30 months to 14 years. Dose size was 10 mg/kg per dose or 20 mg/kg per dose. Mean peak serum levels were seen 30 min after injection. No accumulation of cefazolin in serum was observed after 8 days of therapy. HINER et al. (1980) administered sodium cefazolin (7 mg/kg) intravenously to children with varying degrees of renal insufficiency. Generally the apparent serum half-life of cefazolin increased as creatinine clearance declined. Hemodialysis slowly cleared cefazolin from the blood of children who required such treatment.

2. Cephanone

Cephanone (Fig. 20) is a semisynthetic cephalosporin derivative which has been withdrawn from clinical trials (NIGHTINGALE et al. 1975b). The drug is eliminated from blood by urinary excretion. Following intravenous administration, the terminal serum half-life for cephanone is 2 h (MEYERS et al. 1972). Serum levels appear to be proportional to dose after 0.5 g and 1.0 g intravenous doses. KIRBY and REGAMEY (1973) and REGAMEY and KIRBY (1973) find the total body clearance of cephanone to be 56 ml/min per 1.73 m^2 while renal clearance is 47 ml/min per 1.73 m^2. The terminal serum half-life of cephanone in this study was 2.5 h. Investigators cited have reported near-total recovery of cephanone in urine within 24 h of intravenous dosing. Half of the dose is recovered in 4 h, 80% in 8 h, and 92% in 24 h.

The biotransformation of cephanone in animals or man has not been reported.

Intramuscular administration of cephanone by MEYERS et al. (1972) resulted in peak serum concentrations of drug in 60 min. These investigators could only account for 60% of the dose in 24-h urine collections. REGAMEY and KIRBY (1973) and KIRBY and REGAMEY (1973) report peak serum concentrations of cephanone occurring between 0.75 and 1.5 h after intramuscular injection. The 24-h urinary recovery of cephanone after intramuscular injection represents 92% of the dose.

The human serum protein binding of cephanone is 88% at a serum drug concentration of 30 µg/ml (KIRBY and REGAMEY 1973) and may be concentration dependent (WICK and PRESTON 1972).

3. Cefazedone

Cefazedone (Fig. 20) is eliminated principally by urinary excretion and insignificantly by biliary excretion (KRATOCHVIL et al. 1979). The terminal serum half life of cefazedone is 1.6 h (LEOPOLD et al. 1977; PABST et al. 1979; HITZENBERGER and JASCHEK 1980). Plasma levels are proportional to dose. The total body clearance of cefazedone is approximately 90 ml/min. The 24-h urinary recovery of unchanged drug represents 80% of the dose and the renal clearance is therefore approximately 70–75 ml/min. The vascular compartment volume of distribution of the antibiotic is 6 liters. In another intravenous study, the 24-h urinary recovery of cefazedone was 87.5% of the dose. Total body clearance was slightly less than 80 ml/min and renal clearance was approximately 70 ml/min (UNGETHUM et al. 1979).

The presence of cefazedone metabolites has not been demonstrated in human serum or urine. In a study carried out in rats, dogs, and monkeys (SAILER et al. 1979), metabolites or decomposition products of cefazedone were observed in rat serum and late urine specimens (8–24 h) in all species. These chemical species were not identified.

Cefazedone is a semisynthetic cephalosporin intended for parenteral administration. Following intramuscular injection, peak serum concentrations of drug are seen in 1–2 h with 60% of the dose being recovered in 24-h urine collections. Twenty-four hours of urine collection may not have afforded time for complete recovery of cefazedone. Using a lidocaine hydrochloride solution as diluent for intramuscular injection did not appear to effect absorption (LEOPOLD et al. 1977). Comparison of serum level information and urinary excretion data after intravenous and intramuscular administration would indicate that cefazedone is well absorbed from intramuscular injection sites.

The human serum protein binding of cefazedone using an ultrafiltration technique is 93%–96% at cefazedone serum concentrations of 10–40 µg/ml (WAHLIG et al. 1979).

The distribution of cefazedone in body tissues and fluids has been studied in rats and to a limited extent in humans. One hour after intravenous and intramuscular injection of radiolabeled cefazedone to rats (SAILER et al. 1979), radioactivity was most prevalent in small intestine, urinary bladder, kidney, lung, liver, and bone marrow. Only bladder and small intestinal levels exceeded plasma levels. About one-half of the small intestinal radioactivity was found in the contents thereof. The biliary excretion of the drug in rats represented 37% of the dose in 24 h.

In human patients undergoing hip joint surgery, cefazedone levels in wound secretions, bone, and hip capsule were antimicrobially significant for 10 h after intravenous (1-g) drug administration. VON KOBYLETZKI et al. (1979) followed cefazedone levels in endometrium, myometrium, fallopian tubes, and ovaries after single- and multiple-dose intravenous regimens in gynecological patients. Sixty to 75 min after the last dose of cefazedone, tissue levels averaged 50%–75% of serum concentrations. In patients studied in early pregnancy, similar intravenous doses led to drug levels in decidua that were 33% of serum levels. Much lower levels were noted in placenta and embryo. Patients studied during late pregnancy exhibited comparable cefazedone levels in maternal serum, cord blood, placenta, and amniotic fluid. Significant drug levels were found in the urine of newborn infants, but very little penetration of drug into human breast milk was noted. Bile concentrations in patients 1 h after a 1-g intravenous injection of cefazedone were, in general, well in excess of serum levels (KRATOCHVIL et al. 1979).

ADAM et al. (1979c) administered intravenous doses of cefazedone to surgical patients and monitored drug presence in cardiac muscle, prostatic and skin tissue, and bile. Thirty to eighty minutes after a 100-mg/kg intravenous injection of antibiotic, drug concentrations in cardiac muscle were 10%–50% of serum levels. A 2-g intravenous bolus of cefazedone resulted in prostatic tissue levels that were 25% of serum concentrations. Intravenous doses to patients with biliary T tubes led to bile concentrations between 71 and 210 μg/ml. Two hours after drug administration, bile levels were 4 times greater than serum concentrations. Skin drug levels were high 3 h after a 2-g intravenous injection of cefazedone.

In one study where intravenous cefazedone was administered with and without oral probenecid (UNGETHUM et al. 1979), serum antibiotic concentrations were elevated and sustained in the presence of probenecid. The terminal serum half-life of cefazedone more than doubled and urinary excretion of unchanged drug was not complete within 24 h of administration.

4. Ceftezole

Ceftezole (Fig. 20) is a cephalosporin derivative that is eliminated from the systemic circulation primarily by urinary excretion, but the drug is eliminated in the bile of rats and and dogs (NISHIDA et al. 1976a; HARADA et al. 1976). After intravenous doses, more than 80% of the dose is recovered in 6-h urine collections (OHKAWA and KURODA 1980). The terminal serum half-life appears to be less than 60 min and apparent renal clearance is 217 ml/min.

After intravenous or intramuscular administration, rats excrete 70%–80% of the dose in 24-h urine collections. Urinary excretion accounts for 75%–85% of the dose in dogs, and rabbits excrete over 90% in this manner (NISHIDA et al. 1976a; ISHIYAMA et al. 1976; HARADA et al. 1976).

Twenty-four-hour urinary recovery in monkeys was 73% after intramuscular injection. In 24 h, approximately 4%–5% of an intravenous or intramuscular dose in rats is excreted in bile, and dogs excrete 1.4% in the same manner. Following intravenous or intramuscular doses in rats, drug levels were highest in kidney followed by liver, lung, heart, and spleen. In rabbits an intravenous dose again showed up most prominently in kidney tissue followed by heart, lung, liver, and spleen tissue. Drug concentration in rat lymph peaked in 30–60 min and was still measurable 5–8 h after intramuscular doses. It was shown that intravenous drug administration led to higher drug concentration in rat inflammatory pouch exudates than did intramuscular injection. After intravenous dosing, ceftezole penetrated rabbit CSF better when meningitis was present. Twice-daily intramuscular administration of ceftezole (20 mg/kg) led to no serum accumulation or change in urinary excretion in rabbits. No microbiologically active metabolites were found in rat, dog, or monkey urine. OISHI et al. (1976) determined that ceftezole penetrated the aqueous humor of rabbits after intravenous or intramuscular injection.

Following intramuscular injection in human volunteers, serum ceftezole concentration peaked in 15–30 min. In 24 h, 87%–93% of intramuscular doses was recovered as unchanged drug in urine. No microbiologically active metabolites were found in human urine (ISHIYAMA et al. 1976; NISHIDA et al. 1976a; HARADA et al. 1976).

The serum protein binding of ceftezole has been determined to be 86%, 19%, 97%, 90%, and 27% respectively in human, dog, rabbit, rat and mouse sera (NISHIDA et al. 1976a).

Ceftezole penetrates into sputum following intravenous administration (KIKUCHI et al. 1980).

OHKAWA and KURODA (1980) administered ceftezole intravenously to patients with varying degrees of renal function. Serum levels increased as renal function decreased and the apparent terminal serum half-life became longer. Mean 6-h urinary excretion of drug decreased as creatinine clearance decreased.

IV. 3-(1-Pyridylmethyl)-ceph-3-em-4-oic Acids

1. Cephaloridine

Elimination of cephaloridine (Fig. 21) from the body proceeds by glomerular filtration, a small amount of renal tubular secretion, and biliary excretion. Following intravenous administration, the terminal serum half-life of cephaloridine is 72–108 min. Serum drug levels are proportional to dose. On average the total body clearance of drug is 170–280 ml/min and renal clearance is 125–200 ml/min. Twenty-four-hour urine collections contain over 80% of the dose as unchanged antibiotic (KISLAK et al. 1966; PRYOR et al. 1967; ARVIDSSON et al. 1979a; DEMAINE and KIRBY 1970; KIRBY and REGAMEY 1973; GRIFFITH and BLACK 1971). Alteration of urine pH between 4.5 and 7.6 seemed to have little effect on the renal clearance of cephaloridine (ASSCHER et al. 1970). The terminal serum half-life of this antibiotic appears longer when administered to patients under general anesthesia (MATHEWS 1975). It was suggested by ARVIDSSON et al. (1979a) that the renal tubular reabsorption of cephaloridine is saturable (i.e., an active or carrier-mediated process) causing the renal clearance of drug to increase as serum drug levels increase. Elimination of cephaloridine via biliary excretion is of minor importance. An intramuscular regimen of 1 g every 6 h created biliary levels of drug that were

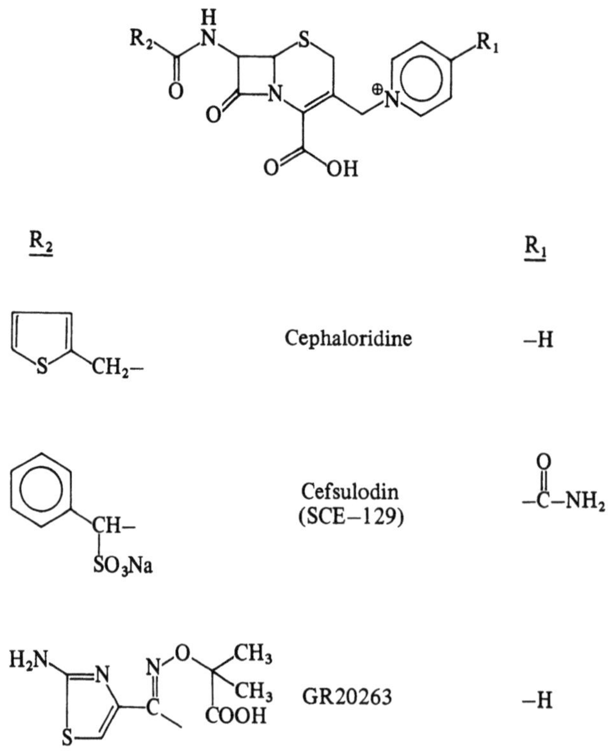

Fig. 21. Structure of 3-(1-pyridylmethyl)-ceph-3-em-4-oic acid derivatives

commonly 50% of serum concentrations. However, after two doses of 0.5 g given at an interval of 6 h less than 2 mg of drug was recovered in 12-h bile collections (APICELLA et al. 1966; ACOCELLA et al. 1968).

The biotransformation of cephaloridine in the rat has been studied by SULLIVAN and MCMAHON (1967). After oral dosing of radiolabelled compound, 50% of the radioactivity was recovered in 40-h urine collections. Only 5% of the dose was found in urine as unchanged drug. Thirty percent of urinary radioactivity was characterized as thienylacetylglycine and 17% was found to be thienylacetamidoethanol. In rat urine collected 2 h after subcutaneous injection, cephaloridine was the only biologically active component found (WICK and PRESTON 1972).

Following intramuscular administration of cephaloridine to humans, no biologically active compounds other than cephaloridine itself were found in 24-h urine collections (MUGGLETON et al. 1964).

Cephaloridine is not well absorbed following oral administration to humans. Only 1%–4% of an oral dose is recovered unchanged in urine (MUGGLETON et al. 1964; GRIFFITH and BLACK 1971). Following intramuscular administration, peak serum concentrations of cephaloridine occur in 30–60 min. As much as 65%–85% of an intramuscular dose may be recovered as unchanged drug in 24-h urine collections. Serum concentrations are proportional to dose and the renal clearance of drug is 165 ml/min (MUGGLETON et al. 1964; CURRIE 1967; KISLAK et al. 1966; GRIFFITH and BLACK 1971; PARADELIS et al. 1977; NISHIDA et al. 1970; DESCHEPPER et al. 1973; CAHN et al. 1974). Slight accumulation of drug in serum was noted on a cephaloridine regimen of 1 g intramuscularly every 6 h (APICELLA et al. 1966).

Most investigators find the human serum protein binding of cephaloridine to be in the 10%–30% range (CURRIE 1967; KIND et al. 1968; WICK and PRESTON 1972; KIRBY and REGAMEY 1973; NISHIDA et al. 1970; SINGHVI et al. 1978; PARADELIS et al. 1977; ARVIDSSON et al. 1979a). MIYAKE and EBATA (1976) measured the human serum protein binding of cephaloridine over a concentration range of 20–100 μg/ml. At low drug concentration 60% binding was reported and at high concentration the binding was 10%. Different results were observed using purified human serum albumin. These results disagree in general with those of other investigators. VERONESE et al. (1977) found that the protein binding of cephaloridine is 20% and that the association constant is similar for bovine, rabbit, and chicken serum albumins at hydrophobic sites.

Following intramuscular and subcutaneous injection to rats, cephaloridine levels were highest in kidney tissue. Much lower levels were found in liver, lung, heart, and spleen. A similar pattern was noted in rabbits after intravenous, intramuscular, or subcutaneous administration. Biliary excretion in these two species and in dogs is minimal (NISHIDA et al. 1970).

In human studies (MURDOCH et al. 1964) cephaloridine levels in pleural effusions were in excess of 30 μg/ml following daily 2-g doses. Low drug levels were noted in CSF 1–2 h after a single 500-mg intramuscular injection. LERNER (1971) finds no cephaloridine penetration into the CSF of patients without meningitis after single or multiple 1-g doses. Patients with acute bacterial meningitis showed CSF levels of cephaloridine that ranged from 0.4–5.6 μg/ml, 1.5–4 h after intravenous or intramuscular drug administration. Similar levels were described in azotemic patients with no bacterial meningitis (KABINS and COHEN 1965). Tissue levels of cephaloridine from a deceased patient who had received 1 g of drug every 4 h for 36 h prior to death were studied (APICELLA et al. 1966). Drug levels in liver were 60% of serum concentration while spleen levels were 40%. Stomach and lung levels were just over 20% of those in serum and brain tissue levels were at 5%. These investigators also found biliary levels of antibiotic that are 50% of those in serum in patients on a regimen of 1 g every 6 h. ACOCELLA et al. (1968) reported similar findings.

Cephaloridine penetration into aqueous humor, secondary aqueous humor, and subretinal fluid is excellent after intravenous, intramuscular, or subconjunctival injection (RILEY et al. 1968; RECORDS 1969; MOLL et al. 1971).

GRIFFITH and BLACK (1971) were able to detect cephaloridine in brain tissue 2–4 h after a single 2-g intravenous dose.

In women experiencing induced childbirth, up to three 1 g intramuscular doses of cephaloridine were given every 12 h during labor (STEWART et al. 1973). Peak levels in amniotic fluid were reached in 3 h and nearly equaled maternal serum levels. Cord serum levels peaked in 1 h and were 20% or more of maternal serum concentration. Drug was present in fetal urine. Relatively high fetal serum levels were noted after a 1-g dose (BARR and GRAHAM 1967). Similar studies have been reported by PRAKESH et al. (1970).

Fifteen to fifty minutes after a 1-g intravenous injection of cephaloridine to patients undergoing hip joint replacement (HUGHES et al. 1975), drug levels in synovial fluid closely approximated serum levels, while levels in synovial capsule and bone were generally 50% or less of serum concentration.

In general, co-administration of oral probenecid and intravenous or intramuscular cephaloridine caused a slight elevation of serum levels (20%) of antibiotic, but did not alter the urinary excretion rate to any extent. Total urinary recovery was not affected. Hence the apparent renal clearance of drug decreased 25%. It therefore appears that renal tubular secretion plays a minor role in the urinary excretion of cephaloridine (KISLAK et al. 1966; TUANO et al. 1966b; FOLEY et al. 1967).

As with other cephalosporins, the urinary excretion of cephaloridine is decreased as renal function worsens in the uremic patient (KABINS and COHEN 1965; APICELLA et al. 1966; FOLEY et al. 1967; RUEDY 1967; PRYOR et al. 1967; CURTIS and MARSHALL 1970; DEMAINE and KIRBY 1970; BROGARD et al. 1976b). The degree of renal dysfunction did not seem to affect consistently peak serum concentrations of drug after 0.5-g i.m. injection until 4.0-g doses were used. Upon multiple dosing, drug accumulation in serum of azotemic patients was observed on regimens such as 1 g every 48 h. One gram every 4 h in patients with normal renal function caused antibiotic to accumulate in serum. The apparent terminal serum half-life of cephaloridine ranged from 1.5 h in patients with normal renal function to 20–24 h in patients with creatinine clearance less than 2 ml/min. Half-life appeared to be log-linearly related to creatinine clearance. Urinary recovery of unchanged drug during 8 h after intravenous or intramuscular injection ranged from nearly 90% for patients with normal kidneys to less than 8% when creatinine clearance was less than 10 ml/min. Hemodialysis seems to be more efficient than peritoneal dialysis in clearing cephaloridine from blood. In eight patients with creatinine clearance between 2.6 and 88 ml/min who received cephaloridine intravenously, the renal clearance of antibiotic closely approximated their creatinine clearance. The volume of distribution of drug in the vascular compartment of one patient with no renal function who also received cephaloridine intravenously was 16–20 liters. The terminal serum half-life of cephaloridine in this patient, who had been maintained on chronic intermittent hemodialysis for nearly 2 years, decreased by 50% over that time period (PRYOR et al. 1967). A similar phenomenon is reported by CURTIS and MARSHALL (1970).

2. Cefsulodin (CGP 7174/E, SCE-129)

Cefsulodin (Fig. 21) is a semisynthetic parenteral cephalosporin with antipseudomonal activity (AHRENS et al. 1979). It is eliminated from the systemic circulation via urinary excretion and possibly biliary excretion (TANAYAMA et al. 1978). Following intravenous infusion of sodium cefsulodin, AHRENS et al. (1979) and BAKER et al. (1980) estimate its terminal serum half-life to be approximately 90 min. Renal clearance is 77 ml/min and the volume of distribution of the drug in the vascular compartment appears to be 7–9 liters. In 24 h, 78% of the dose is recovered unchanged in urine.

Thorough metabolism studies have not been completed, but no biologically active metabolites have been found in rats or dogs (TANAYAMA et al. 1978).

AHRENS et al. (1979) have also administered intramuscular doses to healthy subjects and have observed rapid absorption. Peak plasma levels are reached in

30 min and appear to be proportional to dose. Twenty-four-hour urine collections contained 74% of the dose, with most drug appearing in 8 h. Hence, drug absorption following intramuscular doses appears to be quantitative.

The human serum protein binding of cefsulodin is 30% (WISE et al. 1980e). TANAYAMA et al. (1978) found that cefsulodin does not appreciably penetrate rat and dog erythrocytes. After a radioactive intramuscular dose of cefsulodin to rats, levels of radioactivity were highest in the kidney, followed by plasma, adrenals, lung, heart, thymus, gastrointestinal wall, and liver. Levels were lowest in brain tissue. Radioactivity remained significant in kidney tissue 24 h after the dose. The drug was not shown to cross the rat placenta. In bile-cannulated rats, 4% of an intramuscular dose was excreted via the bile within 24 h of drug administration. Concentrations of cefsulodin in rat milk after intramuscular administration were comparable to those seen in plasma.

In limited human tissue distribution studies, WITTKE and ADAM (1980) gave intravenous bolus doses of cefsulodin preoperatively to surgical patients. They found drug levels in skin, fat, fascia, muscle, peritoneal secretions, and wound exudates to be well above minimum inhibitory concentrations for as long as 6 h. Sputum levels of cefsulodin after intramuscular injection or intravenous infusions are low (NAKATOMI et al. 1980). Drug rapidly penetrates artificial skin blister fluid (BAKER et al. 1980).

3. GR20263

The structure of GR20263 is shown in Fig. 21. The drug is eliminated by urinary excretion. Other routes of elimination have not been studied. Serum drug levels following intravenous doses are not proportional to dose. Apparent renal clearance increases with dose, as does the apparent serum half-life. Serum levels following a 500 mg intravenous dose were above 8 μg/ml for 2.6 h. Only 50%–78% of the intravenous dose was recovered in urine, but investigators state that the usual 12-h recovery is about 90%. No microbiologically active metabolites were found in urine (O'CALLAGHAN et al. 1980).

The drug appears to be well absorbed after intramuscular administration, but again serum levels are not proportional to dose (O'CALLAGHAN et al. 1980; ACRED et al. 1980). In this instance apparent renal clearance tended to decrease as dose increased. Urinary recovery ranged from 48%–88% of the dose.

The serum protein binding of GR20263 at a serum concentration of 25 μg/ml was 13%, 19%, 11%, 20%, 8%, and 17% for mice, rats, rabbits, dogs, monkeys, and humans respectively (O'CALLAGHAN et al. 1980).

Concomitant administration of oral probenecid and intravenous GR20263 had little apparent effect on drug elimination. Serum concentrations were slightly elevated, but the urinary excretion rate was not affected (O'CALLAGHAN et al. 1980).

V. 3-{[(1-Methyl-1H-tetrazol-5-yl)thio]methyl}-ceph-3-em-4-oic Acids

1. Cefamandole Nafate

Cefamandole nafate (Fig. 22) is the *O*-formyl ester of the more potent antimicrobial species cefamandole. The drug formulation contains 68 mg sodium carbonate

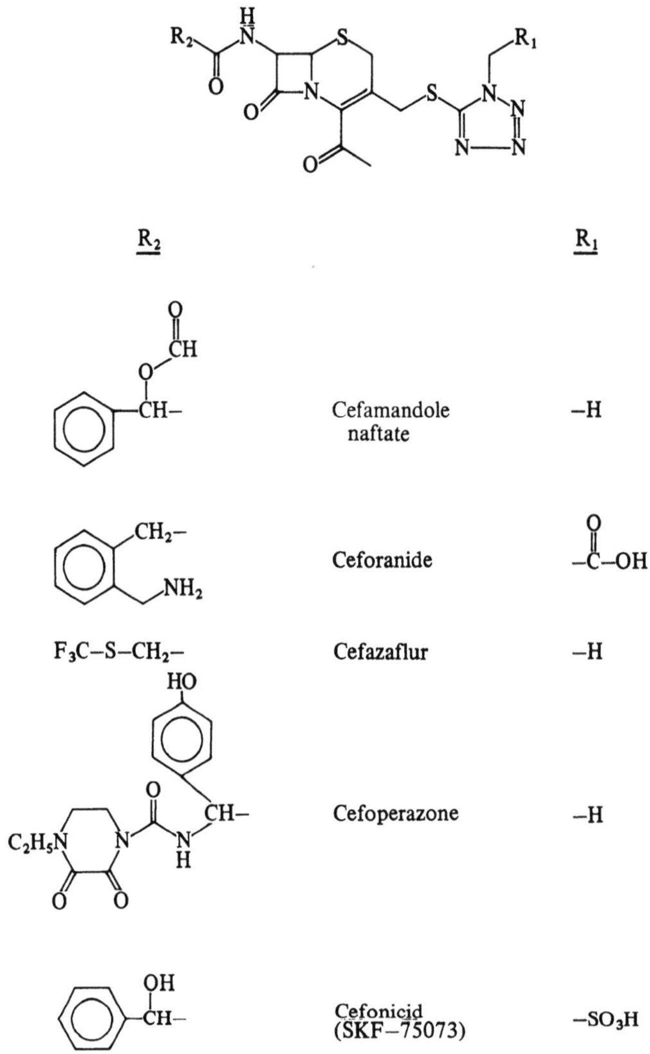

Fig. 22. Structure of 3-{[(1-methyl-1*H*-tetrazol-5-yl)thio]methyl}-ceph-3-em-4-oic acid derivatives

for each 1.11 g cefamandole nafate to facilitate the hydrolysis of the ester to cefamandole upon addition of diluent. This hydrolysis is both pH and temperature sensitive as well as self-quenching (INDELICATO et al. 1976). Hence, upon dilution, only 30% of the ester is hydrolyzed in 30 min (25 °C), at which time the reaction has essentially stopped. Upon intravenous injection, the in vivo hydrolysis of cefamandole nafate is rapid (WOLD et al. 1978). After intravenous administration of partially hydrolyzed nafate, these investigators followed the degradation of the nafate ester in plasma and detected unchanged cefamandoel nafate in the urine of normal subjects. NIELSEN et al. (1979) demonstrated the presence of cefamandole nafate and cefamandole in the plasma of both normal subjects and uremic patients under similar conditions. Although most investigators contend that the two compounds are indistinguishable with regard to antimicrobial potency, TURNER et al. (1977)

have shown a 5- to 10-fold higher potency of cefamandole for certain organisms. Similar results were reported by WINELY et al. (1979).

Since cefamandole is the intended therapeutic agent and the predominant species in vivo, the discussion of its human pharmacokinetics will be limited to results published by investigators who have used a discriminating assay or taken the precaution of administering only cefamandole. Publications by other authors will be mentioned for completeness. The term "antimicrobial activity" will be used to describe the mixed presence of the two species in biological fluids and tissues.

The elimination of cefamandole from the systemic circulation proceeds rapidly by glomerular filtration and renal tubular secretion. Biliary clearance plays a minor role in the elimination process (BROGARD et al. 1977a). Following intravenous doses to healthy volunteers (AZIZ et al. 1978), the terminal serum half-life averages 74 min with serum concentrations still detectable at 6 h. The total body clearance of drug is 196.7 ml/min and renal clearance is 189.7 ml/min. Hence, 96% of the dose can be recovered unchanged in complete urine collections. The volume of distribution of cefamandole in the vascular compartment is 4.3 liters. There appears to be a linear serum level response to increases in dose. POLK et al. (1978) concluded that the elimination of cefamandole is reduced in patients undergoing cardiopulmonary bypass surgery after administration of the drug intravenously at the time of anesthesia induction. Other investigators have followed the time course of antimicrobial activity in serum following intravenous doses of mixtures of cefamandole and cefamandole nafate (GRIFFITH et al. 1976; BROGARD et al. 1977a; BARZA et al. 1976; FONG et al. 1976; LEROY et al. 1977; NEU 1978; RIZZO et al. 1979; MEYERS et al. 1976; GROSE et al. 1976). No accumulation of antimicrobial activity in serum was seen on intravenous regimens as high as 2 g every 6 h (GROSE et al. 1976).

The biotransformation of cefamandole in man has not been studied. It may be inferred from studies by SULLIVAN et al. (1977) in rats and dogs that cefamandole, once formed by hydrolysis of its nafate precursor, does not undergo further metabolism in man.

Cefamandole nafate is intended for parenteral administration and no studies have been published detailing its lack of oral absorption. Following intramuscular administration, it is well absorbed. Peak serum levels of antimicrobial activity appear in 30–60 min and are proportional to dose. At least 80%–90% of the dose is recovered in 24-h urine collections (MEYERS et al. 1976; GROSE et al. 1976; SHEMONSKY et al. 1975; GRIFFITH et al. 1976; NEU 1978; FONG et al. 1976; LEROY et al. 1977; FOSTER et al. 1980). Intramuscular doses of 1 g every 4 h did not cause accumulation of antimicrobial activity in serum (SHEMONSKY et al. 1975). Using a 1% lidocaine solution as a diluent for intramuscular injection of cefamandole nafate has no effect on the bioavailability of the drug (FOSTER et al. 1980).

The human serum protein binding of cefamandole is 70%–80% over a concentration range of 5–40 µg/ml (FONG et al. 1976; NEU 1978; GRIFFITH et al. 1976). Other investigators report the value as 67%–70% over a concentration range of 20–40 µg/ml (NEU 1978; BARZA et al. 1976).

In dogs, 20 mg/kg intravenous doses of cefamandole nafate produced interstitial fluid, bile, and renal interstitial fluid levels of antimicrobial activity that exceeded serum levels at 2 h and then declined in a manner similar to serum level decay (WATERMAN et al. 1976). Tissue distribution studies in rats after intravenous administration of ^{14}C-cefamandole nafate showed highest amounts of radioactivity in the kidney, followed by fat, liver, sciatic nerve, and lung. Low levels were found in eye lens, brain, and spleen. Similar studies in dogs led to high levels of radioactivity in bile, kidney, and liver (SULLIVAN et al. 1977).

In human studies, STEINBERG et al. (1977) demonstrated the presence of minimal antimicrobial activity in CSF following a 33 mg/kg i.v. dose of cefamandole nafate to patients with proven bacterial meningitis. KORZENIOWSKI et al. (1978) found that CSF levels of antimicrobial activity increased in proportion to increasing serum levels as well as increasing protein levels in CSF. Co-administration of probenecid may facilitate the process, but penetration does not appear to be facile (BAKER et al. 1975).

In three cholecystectomized patients with T-tube drainage, high levels of antimicrobial activity were observed in bile following a 1-g i.v. bolus of drug (BROGARD et al. 1977a). Little drug was recovered in bile, however. Slightly better recovery was reported by RATZAN et al. (1978) after a similar study. Levels were also high in gallbladder tissue (QUINN et al. 1978).

AXELROD and KOCHMAN (1978) could not detect antimicrobial activity in the aqueous humor of cataract patients up to 4 h after a 1-g intramuscular injection of cefamandole nafate. Very low levels were detected after an intravenous injection of 1 g, but levels were higher after a 2-g intravenous dose. Aqueous humor levels were no different in patients with some degree of renal insufficiency.

MADHAVAN et al. (1979) report very little antimicrobial activity in saliva after 2-g intramuscular injections of cefamandole nafate with or without concomitant probenecid administration.

BULLEN et al. (1979) have administered intravenous or intravenous–intramuscular combination doses to patients with ischemic lower limbs and found therapeutic levels of antimicrobial activity in muscle and subcutaneous fat. Levels decreased the farther down the limb that samples were taken.

Heart valve and atrial appendage levels of antimicrobial activity following a 20 mg/kg i.m. injection of cefamandole nafate were comparable to or slightly lower than plasma levels (ARCHER et al. 1978). Following a 2-g i.v. bolus of cefamandole nafate, peak levels of antimicrobial activity in pulmonary tissue were seen within 1 h and levels averaged 40%–50% of serum levels. Antimicrobial activity in subcutaneous fat was much lower (DASCHNER et al. 1979a).

Levels of antimicrobial activity in cancellous bone were well in excess of therapeutic levels after a 2-g bolus injection followed by a 2-g infusion of cefamandole nafate in patients undergoing hip arthroplasty (QUINN et al. 1978).

Antimicrobial activity penetrates knee (femoral condyle) and hip (femoral head) bone rapidly following a 2-g i.v. bolus injection. Peak levels were attained in 30 min and levels remained at about 10% of serum values through time (SCHURMAN et al. 1980). Synovial and wound drainage fluid levels were higher.

TAN and SALSTROM (1977) report penetration of cefamandole-nafate-derived antimicrobial activity into human interstitial fluid following a 1-g intravenous dose.

Levels of antimicrobial activity were observed in corticalis, spongiosa, cutis, subcutis, fascia, and muscle after three different intravenous regimens of cefamandole nafate (PLAUE et al. 1978). After a 2-g intravenous dose of cefamandole nafate, levels of antimicrobial activity in prostatic tissue were about 30% of serum levels (ADAM et al. 1979 b).

As might be expected for a drug cleared from the body in the way that cefamandole is, the concomitant administration of probenecid and cefamandole nafate elevated serum levels of antimicrobial activity and decreased apparent total body clearance by 70% (GREENE et al. 1977). Similar observations were made by NEU (1978) and MELLIN et al. (1977). There was no effect on the amount of antimicrobial activity eventually excreted in urine.

There have been a number of studies involving the intravenous or intramuscular administration of cefamandole nafate to patients with varying degrees of renal dysfunction (HOFFLER et al. 1978; APPEL et al. 1976; AHERN et al. 1976; MELLIN et al. 1977; MEYERS and HIRSCHMAN 1977; LEROY et al. 1977; CAMPILLO et al. 1979; BROGARD et al. 1979 a; RIZZO et al. 1979; CZERWINSKI and PEDERSON 1979). In general, serum levels of antimicrobial activity were elevated and the apparent serum half-life increased as kidney function decreased. Urinary recovery of drug also decreased as the degree of renal impairment advanced. Hemodialysis removes cefamandole nafate-related antimicrobial activity slowly from serum and peritoneal dialysis is even less efficient.

In a study by GAMBERTOGLIO et al. (1979), the terminal serum half-life of cefamandole in patients requiring hemodialysis was in excess of 9 h. During dialysis, half-life decreased by 60%–70% to around 4 h. Total body clearance in these patients was 7.7 ml/min. The mean clearance of cefamandole by hemodialysis was 23 ml/min and recovery of drug in dialysate during a 5-h session averaged 35% of the dose.

Finally, in a study by NIELSEN et al. (1979), the disappearance of cefamandole nafate and cefamandole were followed in both normal subjects and dialysis patients while off dialysis. In healthy subjects the half-life of cefamandole nafate in plasma is about 8–12 min while that for dialysis patients is 13–25 min. The mean terminal plasma half-life of cefamandole in both groups was much longer, being greatly extended in dialysis patients.

Cefamandole nafate has been administered both intravenously and intramuscularly to infants and children and their plasma or serum level response and urinary excretion has been observed (CHANG et al. 1978; RODRIQUEZ et al. 1978; WALKER and GAHOL 1978; AGBAYANI et al. 1979). The time course of plasma or serum and urine levels of antimicrobial activity appears similar to that in adults except in children less than 1 year of age, where elimination is slower. Penetration of antimicrobial activity into CSF was better in the presence of meningitis.

2. Ceforanide

Ceforanide (see Fig. 22) is eliminated via the kidneys by glomerular filtration and renal tubular secretion (PFEFFER et al. 1980). Following intravenous infusions of the lysine salt of ceforanide, the 12-h urinary recovery is 85%–91% of the dose. The mean apparent terminal serum half-life for ceforanide was 3 h. Serum levels of ceforanide are proportional to dose. No accumulation of drug in serum was noted on multiple doses of 1.13 g or 2.26 g given every 12 h. SMYTH et al. (1979)

gave single 2-g, 3-g, and 4-g intravenous doses (30 min infusion) and found that at the higher doses the area under the serum concentration-time curve did not increase in proportion to dose. The 24-h urinary recovery of ceforanide was approximately 90% of the dose at all dose levels. The suggested nonlinearity was attributed to a decrease in the percentage of drug bound at serum ceforanide concentration in excess of 200 μg/ml. The data are not entirely supportive of this, however. The apparent terminal serum half-life for ceforanide did not change across the dose range. Mean renal clearance ranged from 44–49 ml/min and did not change upon multiple intravenous doses of 4.0 g (30 min infusion) given every 12 h for 19 doses. The nonlinear increases in total area under the curve may be attributed to the fact that the area was estimated from pharmacokinetic parameters and not by model independent methods. One estimate of the volume of distribution of ceforanide in the vascular compartment was around 8 liters, but this was obtained from mean serum profiles (PFEFFER et al. 1980). LEE et al. (1980) estimated the total body volume of distribution ($V\beta$) to be 0.2 liters/kg.

All investigators mentioned who have studied ceforanide pharmacokinetics have asserted that the antibiotic undergoes no metabolism in humans. The only finding they cite is that they have detected no biologically active metabolites in the urine of their subjects using bioautographical techniques.

The plasma protein binding of ceforanide is approximately 80% over a concentration range of 25–200 μg/ml (LEE et al. 1980; PFEFFER et al. 1980). However, the protein binding dropped to 65% at 400 μg/ml (SMYTH et al. 1979). Seldom are such plasma concentrations attained in therapeutic regimens.

Ceforanide is intended for parenteral administration although no studies proclaiming its lack of oral efficacy have been published. PFEIFFER et al. (1980) studied single and multiple (every 12 h) intramuscular doses at 0.57-g and 1.13-g dose levels. Peak concentrations of ceforanide in plasma were noted in 1 h and plasma levels were dose proportional. Renal clearance of drug and percent dose urinary recovery were the same as results obtained after intravenous administration of the antibiotic. Similar serum level observations were made by BURCH et al. (1979).

HESS et al. (1980) administered sodium ceforanide by intravenous infusion to two groups of patients with end-stage renal disease. The mean terminal serum half-life of ceforanide between dialysis sessions was 19.1 h, while in patients on dialysis it was 5 h.

3. Cefazaflur

Elimination of cefazaflur (Fig. 22) is rapid via urinary excretion. Following an intravenous bolus dose of drug, the terminal serum half-life appears to be approximately 30 min and 70% of the dose is recovered in urine within 6 h of administration (ACTOR et al. 1976b). After intramuscular administration, peak serum levels of drug occur in 30 min and 76% of the dose is recovered in urine in 6 h. After 24 h, 93% of the cefazaflur dose is recovered in urine (HARVENGT et al. 1977). The antibiotic appears to be rapidly and well absorbed after intramuscular administration. Although it is apparently not absorbed orally, no documentation of this is found in the literature.

The antibiotic was 2-fold less active in vitro against many common organisms in studies run in 50% human serum protein as compared to broth. The human serum protein binding is reportedly the same as cephalothin (ACTOR et al. 1977).

4. Cefoperazone

Cefoperazone is a semisynthetic piperazine cephalosporin (see Fig. 22) which deviates from other cephalosporins in that its major route of systemic elimination is not via urinary excretion. Biliary excretion may play a major role in the total body clearance of cefoperazone (BALANT et al. 1980).

Following intravenous administration, the terminal serum level half-life of cefoperazone is 1.6–2 h. The total body clearance of drug is 80–100 ml/min and the renal clearance is 20–30 ml/min. Only 25% of the dose is recovered unchanged in urine in 24-h collections. The volume of distribution of drug in the vascular compartment appears to be 7–11 liters (LODE et al. 1980a; BALANT et al. 1980; ALLAZ et al. 1979; CRAIG 1980; WATANABE et al. 1980; SHIMIZU 1980). Slight accumulation of drug is seen on a regimen of 2 g administered intravenously every 12 h (BALANT et al. 1980). The biliary excretion of cefoperazone has been reported in animals and man, but has not been quantitated to estimate its contribution to total body clearance (WATANABE et al. 1980; SHIMIZU 1980; AOKI et al. 1980). There was a suggestion of dose-dependent kinetics with cefoperazone (CRAIG 1980), but further study is necessary.

No biologically active metabolites have been observed in man (SHIMIZU 1980). However, SAIKAWA et al. (1980) found two minor metabolites, 7-[D(−)-α-3-[2-(*N*-ethyl-*N*-oxaloamino)ethyl]ureido-α-(4-hydroxyphenyl)acetamido]-3-[(1-methyl-1*H*-tetrazol-5-yl)thiomethyl]-3-cephem-4-carboxylic acid and 5-mercapto-1-methyl-1*H*-tetrazole, in urine.

The drug is apparently not absorbed after oral administration. Peak serum concentrations of cefoperazone are observed within 60 min after intramuscular administration. No accumulation is seen on regimens administered at 12-h intervals. In 6 h, 14%–18% of the dose had been excreted in urine (SHIMIZU 1980).

Over a concentration range of 10–250 μg/ml cefoperazone is 89%–94% bound. At 5,000 μg/ml the bound fraction dropped to 0.43 (ALLAZ et al. 1979; CRAIG 1980; WATANABE et al. 1980).

The distribution of cefoperazone in biological tissues and fluids has not been widely studied. In rabbits (WATANABE et al. 1980), 20% of a 20 mg/kg intravenous dose was excreted in 4 h. In rats, 1 h after a 100 mg/kg intraperitoneal dose of radiolabeled cefoperazone, radioactivity concentrated in stomach, liver, renal cortex, and renal medulla (FABRE et al. 1980). In humans, AOKI et al. (1980) administered 2 g cefoperazone by intravenous infusion (2 h), finding maximum biliary concentrations 5 h after the infusion. At a similar dose, the concentration of cefoperazone in bile 6 h after the infusion was nearly 1 mg/ml (SHIMIZU 1980). In patients with respiratory diseases, 0.5- to 3-g intravenous infusions of cefoperazone resulted in sputum concentrations ranging from 0.1–6 μg/ml. After 3 days on a regimen of 1 g cefoperazone intravenously every 12 h, antibiotic concentration in peritoneal exudates was 64 μg/ml. In tissue and fluid samples taken 1 h after 1- to 2-g intravenous doses of cefoperazone, the transplacental transfer of drug was demonstrated. Levels in cord blood and amniotic fluid were quite significant, while concentrations in endometrium, myometrium, and serous membrane ranged from 30%–90% of serum levels. MATSUDA et al. (1980) found similar ratios after intramuscular injection of drug. SHIMIZU (1980) found levels of cefoperazone in tonsils and maxillary sinus mucosa to be above 6 µg/ml 90 min after intramuscular doses. A 2-g intravenous infusion produced 3 µg/ml concentrations in otorrheal fluid in patients with otitis media.

A single oral dose of probenecid (0.5 g) given 30 min before a 1-g intravenous infusion of cefoperazone had only a slight effect on the serum levels and urinary excretion of antibiotic, implying that renal tubular secretion of cefoperazone is not significant (SHIMIZU 1980).

The disposition of cefoperazone after 2-g intravenous infusions has been studied in patients with creatinine clearance ranging from 17–9 ml/min (BALANT et al. 1980). The terminal serum half-life of cefoperazone ranged from 2.9–1.3 h in these patients. In one patient with normal kidney function, but who had biliary obstruction because of hepatoma, the half-life of drug in serum was 14 h and the serum concentration at 24 h was above 30 µg/ml. Again in the patients with renal dysfunction, 12-h urinary recovery of cefoperazone ranged from 8.4%–1.5% of the dose. The patient with biliary obstruction excreted over 30% of the dose in 20-h urine collections.

5. Cefonicid (SKF-75073)

Cefonicid is a new parenteral cephalosporin that is structurally similar to cefamandole (Fig. 22). After intravenous administration to humans the mean terminal serum half-life is 212 min and 98% of the dose is recovered in 24-h urine collections (PITKIN et al. 1980a). Biliary excretion of cefonicid is of importance in rats (INTOCCIA et al. 1978), but appears to be absent in humans.

It would appear from animal studies that cefonicid is not metabolized (INTOCCIA et al. 1978). Studies in humans have not been reported.

The human serum protein binding of cefonicid is 98% (ACTOR et al. 1978). PITKIN et al. (1980b) have shown that saturated fatty acids of 10–14-carbon chain length can greatly affect the serum protein binding. At a molar ratio of 10:1 (fatty acid:serum protein), a 12-carbon fatty acid will cause cefonicid serum protein binding to drop nearly to zero.

As mentioned earlier, cefonicid is a parenteral cephalosporin. After intramuscular administration to healthy volunteers, it is well absorbed, with maximum serum levels appearing in 1–2 h. Twenty-four-hour urinary recovery of drug is total (PITKIN et al. 1980a).

Tissue distribution studies in rats have been reported by INTOCCIA et al. (1978). Thirty minutes after a 20 mg/kg intravenous dose of ^{14}C-cefonicid, tissue levels of radioactivity were highest in the kidney, followed by the gastrointestinal tract, lung, liver, heart, and adrenals. By 2 h, the gastrointestinal tract exhibited the highest levels of radioactivity, with the kidney close behind. At all time points, levels were low in brain and red blood cells. These investigators also studied the penetration of ^{14}C-cefonicid into inflammatory pouch exudates in rats following intramuscular injection. At 2 h after administration radioactivity in exudates was about 40% of serum levels, but by 6 h exudate levels exceeded serum levels. Bioassay results were similar. Cefonicid is 97% bound to rat serum proteins.

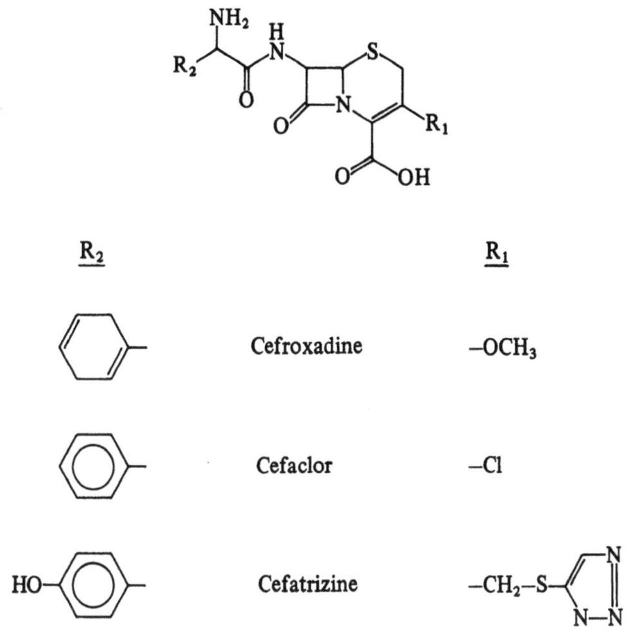

Fig. 23. Structure of 3-desacetoxymethylcephalosporanic acid derivatives

VI. Derivatives of 3-Desacetoxymethylcephalosporanic Acid

1. Cefroxadine

Cefroxadine (Fig. 23) is a new cephalosporin derivative which is absorbed after oral ingestion. The drug is rapidly eliminated from the systemic circulation by both glomerular filtration and renal tubular secretion.

After intravenous bolus administration of sodium cefroxadine to healthy volunteers (HIRTZ et al. 1980), the terminal plasma half-life of the antibiotic is 44 min. The total body clearance of cefroxadine is approximately 340 ml/min and renal clearance is nearly 250 ml/min. Nearly 90% of the dose was recovered unchanged in total urine collections. Similar observations were reported by WIRZ et al. (1978).

No reports of metabolism of cefroxadine have been published following drug administration to animals or humans. NAKAYAMA et al. (1980a), however, report that bioassay and high-performance liquid chromatographic assay techniques yield reasonably comparable estimates of serum and urine drug levels.

As mentioned earlier, cefroxadine is well absorbed following oral administration. Oral doses of solution or tablets ranging from 125–1,500 mg given to healthy volunteers, produced peak plasma levels of drug in 30–90 min. Plasma levels are proportional to dose and 88%–96% of the dose is recovered unchanged in urine in 12 h. Renal clearance ranged from 240–340 ml/min in the different groups studied (WIRZ et al. 1979; LODE et al. 1979; LECAILLON et al. 1980; BERGAN 1980). Ingesting an oral dose of cefroxadine with food delays the time of peak plasma levels of drug and reduces absorption by 5%–10% (LECAILLON et al. 1980). Multiple doses (500 mg given every 6 h while awake for 4.5 days) of cefroxadine were administered to healthy volunteers (HOLT et al. 1978). No accumulation of drug in serum was noted and total urinary recovery during the study contained over 90% of the total dose.

Over a concentration range of 4–33 μg/ml, the human serum protein binding of cefroxadine (equilibrium dialysis) is 8.5% (WIRZ et al. 1978).

ARMBRUSTER et al. (1980) report that, after 500-mg and 1,000-mg oral doses of cefroxadine, drug concentrations in wound secretions exceeded plasma levels at 4–6 h after drug administration. Similarly, after a 1-g oral dose, GILLETT and WISE (1978) report interstitial fluid levels of cefroxadine that are 60%–80% of serum levels for 3 h after drug administrations.

2. Cefaclor

Cefaclor (see Fig. 23) is an orally effective semisynthetic cephalosporin. Elimination from the systemic circulation proceeds via urinary and biliary excretion. The disposition of cefaclor following intravenous administration has not been studied in man. It is noted, however, that special handling of biological samples containing cefaclor is required because of the extreme instability of cefaclor at alkaline pH and temperatures above 4 °C (FOGLESONG et al. 1978).

Following oral administration of doses ranging from 100–1,000 mg, peak serum concentrations of cefaclor were observed in 45–60 min. The apparent terminal serum half-life of cefaclor is between 0.5 and 1 h. Within 6 h of dose ingestion, 50%–70% of the dose was recovered in urine. Very little drug was recovered in urine thereafter. Plasma levels are proportional to dose (KORZENIOWSKI et al. 1977; GLYNNE et al. 1978; BLOCH et al. 1977; LEVISON et al. 1979; SANTORO et al. 1978; SPYKER et al. 1978; HODGES et al. 1978; MEYERS et al. 1978; WELLING et al. 1979; LODE et al. 1979; FILLASTRE et al. 1980; LODE et al. 1980c; SIMON and GATZEMEIER 1979). No accumulation of drug in serum was noted on multiple-dose regimes of 250–1,000 mg given every 6 h (KORZENIOWSKI et al. 1977; HODGES et al. 1978; MEYERS et al. 1978). Concomitant ingestion of food only slows absorption (GLYNNE et al. 1978).

No biologically active metabolites of cefaclor were found in human urine (GLYNNE et al. 1978). Disposition studies in animals (SULLIVAN et al. 1976) have shown that 38% of an oral dose in rats is eliminated via biliary excretion. However, most of this material was an unknown polar metabolite. In urine, 70% of recovered radioactivity was unchanged cefaclor. Similar results were found in mice. In dogs, after intravenous injection, 79% and 3.5% of the total administered radiocarbon appeared within 6 h in urine and bile respectively. However, only approximately 60% of the radioactivity in urine was unchanged drug. After oral administration less than 40% of radioactivity excreted in urine was unchanged cefaclor. Levels of radioactivity and antimicrobial activity in blood differed significantly after oral and intravenous administration of ^{14}C-cefaclor in dogs.

The human serum protein binding of cefaclor at concentrations of 10–50 μg/ml is 50% (TALLY et al. 1979).

The tissue distribution of cefaclor in mice, rats, and dogs has been studied by SULLIVAN et al. (1976). After oral administration of ^{14}C-cefaclor to mice and rats, highest levels of radioactivity were found in kidney, liver, heart, spleen, and lung tissue. Low levels were found in brain tissue. Similarly, in dogs 90 min after dose administration, only bile, urine, blood, and synovial fluid contain unchanged cefaclor. As in rats and mice levels of radioactivity were highest in kidney and liver.

In adult patients, multiple oral doses of cefaclor produced sputum levels of drug that were usually less than 0.5 μg/ml regardless of sampling time (SIMON and GATZEMEIER 1979). AXELROD and KOCHMAN (1980) have shown that low, but therapeutic, levels of cefaclor may be achieved in aqueous humor following single 0.5- or 1.0-g oral doses.

It has also been shown that cefaclor penetrates into spongy bone, muscle, fascia, cutis, and subcutis following 1-g oral doses (PLAUE et al. 1979a). A 1-g oral dose of probenecid taken 0.5 h before a 500-mg oral dose of cefaclor only slightly elevated and sustained plasma levels of cefaclor. The excretion rate of drug in urine was slowed (LEVISON et al. 1979; SANTORO et al. 1978).

In patients with varying degrees of renal dysfunction, the apparent terminal plasma half-life of cefaclor increased as creatinine clearance decreased. The amount of drug appearing in urine decreased accordingly. In patients with creatinine clearance less than 5 ml/min, no drug was detectable in plasma 24 h after a 1-g oral dose. Hemodialysis is effective in clearing cefaclor from blood. Doses of 500 mg given every 6 h to these patients did not cause drug accumulation in plasma (BLOCH et al. 1977; BERMAN et al. 1978; SANTORO et al. 1978; FILLASTRE et al. 1980; SPYKER et al. 1978).

Serum, urine, saliva, and tear levels of cefaclor following multiple oral doses in fasting and fed infants and children have been studied by MCCRACKEN et al. (1978b).

3. Cefatrizine

Cefatrizine (see Fig. 23) is a new orally effective semisynthetic cephalosporin. The drug is eliminated chiefly by urinary excretion. Metabolism and biliary excretion do contribute to the process (GAVER and DEEB 1980). Pharmacokinetic studies following intravenous administration of the drug have not been published.

The drug is absorbed following oral and intramuscular administration. Following oral doses (MATSUZAKI et al. 1976a, b; ACTOR et al. 1976a), peak plasma concentrations occurred in 1.5–3 h and were proportional to dose. Thirty-five percent of the dose was recovered unchanged in 12-h urine collections and 77%–82% was recovered in 24 h. The apparent terminal serum half-life of cefatrizine is between 1 and 2 h. No differences were noted after multiple doses of 500 mg given every 6 h (DELBUSTO et al. 1976; KOSMIDIS et al. 1978). After intramuscular injection, peak serum concentrations were observed in 30–60 min. In 12-h urine collections, 45% of the dose was recovered unchanged. Drug availability following intramuscular or oral doses would appear to be comparable.

Analysis of 24-h urine collections by MATSUZAKI et al. (1976b) revealed only small amounts (< 1%) of p-hydroxyphenylglycine and an unidentified polar metabolite in addition to over 80% of the dose as unchanged cefatrizine. Other metabolites were isolated in the urine of rats, rabbits, dogs, and monkeys, but the sum of their presence in urine never exceeded 1.5% of the antibiotic dose. However, in metabolism studies conducted in humans (GAVER and DEEB 1980), oral solutions of ^{14}C-cefatrizine were administered at 490-mg and 1,100-mg dose levels. Significant plasma levels of metabolite (not microbiologically active) were observed by 4 h. The radioactivity associated with metabolite disappeared from plasma more slowly than cefatrizine and constituted most of plasma radioactivity after 8 h. Seventy-two-hour urine collections accounted for 50%–60% of administered radioactivity. Approximately 30% of the radioactivity was recovered in feces. Eighty percent of urine radioactivity was cefatrizine; the other 20% was composed of three microbiologically inactive metabolites. Little cefatrizine was found in feces. It was suggested that biliary excretion of cefatrizine or its metabolites is an operative route of antibiotic elimination in man.

Over a concentration range of 2–50 µg/ml, LEITNER et al. (1975) report the human serum protein (95%) binding of cefatrizine to be 58%.

BERNARD et al. (1977a) administered single 1-g oral doses of cefatrizine to women during early pregnancy within 46 h of elective therapeutic abortion. Placental levels of cefatrizine were present as early as 2 h after drug administration but were nonexistent by 17 h. Similar presence was detected in fetal serum. Low levels of cefatrizine activity were also noted in fetal kidney and urine, fetal lung, fetal bile, and amniotic fluid. Drug levels were not measurable in fetal brain, CSF, or liver. Drug was not detectable in any of these fluids or tissue when abortion was induced by intra-amniotic injection of prostaglandin $F_2\alpha$.

VII. Cefuroxime

Cefuroxime (Fig. 24) is a semisynthetic cephalosporin which is almost totally eliminated from the systemic circulation by urinary excretion. Biliary excretion is of minor importance.

Following intravenous injection, the terminal serum half-life of cefuroxime is approximately 1–1.5 h. The 24-h urinary excretion accounts for nearly 95% of the dose. The total body clearance is 140–180 ml/min and renal clearance is 140–160 ml/min. Renal tubular secretion undoubtedly plays a role in cefuroxime elimination. The volume of distribution of cefuroxime in the vascular compartment is 5–9 liters. Serum levels appear to be proportional to dose over a range of 250–3,000 mg, although FOORD (1976) suggested otherwise (GOWER and DASH 1977; FOORD 1976; GOODWIN et al. 1977; NAKAGAWA 1977; O'CALLAGHAN and HARDING 1977; DAIKOS et al. 1977a, b; NORRBY et al. 1977b; ORSOLINI et al. 1979; SIMON and MALERCZYK 1977; BROGARD et al. 1979b; SIMON 1980b; BROGDEN et al. 1979; HARDING 1980).

After intravenous administration in elderly patients, the terminal plasma half-life is related to the individual's creatinine clearance. Although kidney function appears normal in these patients, advancing age has its affect on renal clearance and therefore on cefuroxime elimination (DOUGLAS et al. 1980; ROBERTSON 1980).

As shown by FOORD (1976), using a high-performance liquid chromatographic assay, all of the material excreted in urine after an intramuscular or intravenous dose of sodium cefuroxime is unchanged drug.

Cefuroxime is not absorbed after oral administration (FOORD 1976). Less than 1% of an oral dose is recovered in urine.

The drug is well absorbed after intramuscular injection. In early studies, the form of the drug supplied allowed solutions to be formed upon addition of diluent.

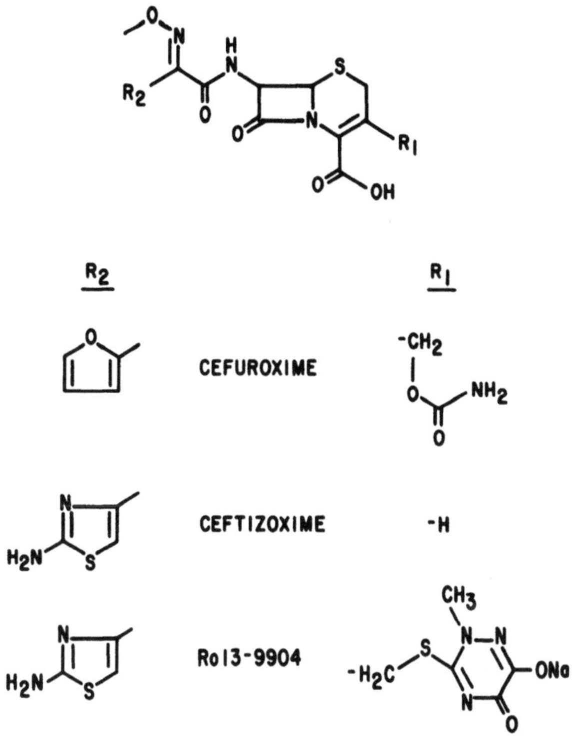

Fig. 24. Structure of cefuroxime, ceftizoxime, and Ro 13-9904

Later intramuscular formulations formed suspensions upon dilution and the only effect noted was slightly decreased absorption (O'CALLAGHAN and HARDING 1977). Serum concentrations, after intramuscular doses ranging from 0.25–1.0 g, tend to peak at later times as the dose increases. Total absorption is independent of dose and at least 95% of the dose is recovered in 24-h urine collections. FOORD (1976) felt that renal clearance increased as dose increased, but too little information is presented to verify the suggestion. In any event, serum levels after intramuscular injection are not strictly proportional to dose (NAKAGAWA 1977; O'CALLAGHAN and HARDING 1977; DAIKOS et al. 1977a, b; NORRBY et al. 1977b; HARDING et al. 1979). Multiple intramuscular injections of 0.75 g given every 8 h did not cause drug to accumulate in serum (NAKAGAWA 1977). HARDING et al. (1979) did show some site dependence in the rate of cefuroxime absorption following intramuscular injection in female subjects. There was also exercise dependence in the rate of absorption in males.

The human serum protein binding of cefuroxime ranges from 33%–41% (FOORD 1976; O'CALLAGHAN et al. 1976; GOTO 1977; WISE et al. 1980e).

The human tissue and fluid distribution of cefuroxime has been evaluated by a number of investigators. Following a 1-g intravenous injection, interstitial fluid levels of cefuroxime closely approximated serum concentrations (GILLETT and WISE 1978). Similar findings were reported by SIMON and MALERCZYK (1977) and SIMON (1980b).

After single or multiple intravenous or intramuscular administration, cefuroxime concentrations in surgically sampled or T-tube bile and in liver tissue were comparable to serum levels. Common duct bile and gallbladder tissue levels were 30%–50% lower. In patients with nonfunctioning gallbladders, gallbladder bile concentrations of cefuroxime were quite low. Muscle and skin antibiotic concentrations were even lower, but still of therapeutic value (DAIKOS et al. 1977a; GEDDES et al. 1978; NAKAGAWA 1977; SALES and RIMMER 1977; SEVERN and POWIS 1979). DAIKOS et al. (1977a) and GEDDES et al. (1978) reported finding low levels of cefuroxime in sputum after multiple intramuscular doses. BERGOGNE-BEREZIN et al. (1979c) reported that cefuroxime levels in bronchial secretions never exceeded 20% of serum levels.

After 3 days of 750- or 1,500-mg intramuscular injections of cefuroxime every 8 h, bone levels of antibiotic exceeded 3 and 10 μg/gm respectively. After three intravenous doses of 750 mg given at 8-h intervals, levels of cefuroxime in hip bone were low (DORNBUSCH et al. 1980). After a single 750-mg intramuscular dose of cefuroxime, knee synovial fluid levels of drug were comparable to serum levels (LEV-EL et al. 1980). One gram of cefuroxime given intravenously at the time of anesthetic induction produced femoral head and lower femur levels of 12–15 μg/g. Capsule levels were 18–22 μg/gm in knee and hip joint respectively (HARDING 1980).

Cefuroxime was able to penetrate into peritoneal dialysate, and 4 h after a 1,500-mg intramuscular injection, cefuroxime levels in pleural fluid were 60% of serum levels (DAIKOS et al. 1977a).

After 1- to 1.5-gm intravenous injections or 1-g intramuscular injections of sodium cefuroxime, drug levels in aqueous humor reflected the route of administration. Aqueous humor levels of cefuroxime rose slowly after 1-g intramuscular doses, while after 1- to 1.5-g intravenous doses, levels remained rather constant for up to 3 h after administration. Levels rarely exceeded 3 μg/ml (RICHARDS et al. 1979).

Single 1.5-g intravenous doses of cefuroxime produced prostatic tissue levels that were 20% of serum levels (ADAM et al. 1979a). Cefuroxime levels in renal tissue often exceeded serum levels, while testicular levels ranged from 10%–30% of serum levels. Fat levels were quite low.

After various intramuscular and intravenous doses of sodium cefuroxime, penetration into CSF was poor to nonexistent in patients with no meningeal inflammation (DAIKOS et al. 1977a; HARDING 1980; FRIEDRICH et al. 1980; MULLER et al. 1980). In patients with varying degrees of meningeal inflammation, intravenous doses of 1–2 g given every 8 h for up to 2 weeks achieved peak levels of 3–7.5 μg/ml in CSF (FRIEDRICH et al. 1980). Severe inflammation allowed levels to approach serum levels (NORRBY et al. 1977a). CSF levels of cefuroxime 30, 90, and 180 min after a 1-g intravenous dose ranged from less than 0.6% to 73% of serum levels (MODAI et al. 1979b). Similar results were reported by MULLER et al. (1980).

After a 1.5-g intravenous bolus, cefuroxime levels in uterine and ovarian tissue were 38%–49% of serum levels 46 min after the injection (VERBIST and VANDERHEYDEN 1980). After a regimen of multiple 1.5-g intramuscular doses, the uterine level of cefuroxime was 48% of serum levels 48 min after the last dose, while ovarian tisue levels were 56% of serum levels 70 min after the last dose. Women in labor or about to undergo caesarian section received 750 mg cefuroxime intramuscularly. Levels in amniotic fluid ranged from 2–19 μg/ml. Cord blood levels were 5–6 μg/ml and placental cord and membrane tissue levels were 2–4 μg/g (HARDING 1980).

Oral probenecid (0.5 g) doses given 2 h before and 1 h after intramuscular injections of cefuroxime (0.5 g), decreased the renal clearance of drug by 40% (FOORD 1976). The urinary excretion rate of cefuroxime was slowed, but the 24-h urinary recovery of drug did not change.

The apparent terminal serum-half life of cefuroxime increased rapidly in uremic patients when creatinine clearance dropped below 25 ml/min. Serum levels persisted for 24 h in these seriously uremic subjects and urinary recovery of drug fell to 5.4% of the dose (KOSMIDIS et al. 1977). In anuric patients the apparent half-life increased to 16–22 h, but hemodialysis shortened this to approximately 3.5 h. Peritoneal dialysis was not nearly as effective (GOWER et al. 1977; KOSMIDIS et al. 1977). Dosage recommendations were proposed by BROGARD et al. (1979 b).

The time course of cefuroxime in serum of infants and children after intravenous administration has been investigated by NISHIMURA et al. (1979 a), and SORIN et al. (1977). CSF penetration of cefuroxime in children has been shown to follow patterns noted earlier for adults (CORBEEL et al. 1979; KUZEMKO and WALKER 1979; RENLUND and PETTAY 1977; HARDING 1980).

VIII. Ceftizoxime

Ceftizoxime (Fig. 24) is a new parenteral, semisynthetic cephalosporin which is eliminated by urinary excretion and to a limited extent by biliary excretion. In human pharmacokinetic studies (NAKASHIMA 1980), intravenous doses of sodium ceftizoxime produced serum level profiles which declined with a terminal half-life of 1.35 h. In 24-h urine collections, 89% of the dose was excreted unchanged. Multiple intravenous doses of 1,000 mg given twice daily for 5 days caused no accumulation of ceftizoxime in serum. After intramuscular injections, peak serum concentrations of ceftizoxime occurred in 30 min and 90% of the dose was excreted in urine in 24 h.

No biologically active metabolites have been identified in animal urine (MURAKAWA et al. 1980), and no studies in humans have been published.

As determined in 90% human serum, the protein binding of ceftizoxime (30 μg/ml) is 31% (MURAKAWA et al. 1980).

Tissue and fluid distribution studies have been conducted in animals (MURAKAWA et al. 1980). Fifteen to 30 min after a single 20-mg/kg intramuscular dose in rats, tissue levels of ceftizoxime were highest in kidney, liver, lung, and heart. The 24-h biliary excretion of ceftizoxime in rats after a 20-mg/kg intraperitoneal injection was 3.7% of the dose. The biliary excretion of drug was even lower (0.59%) in dogs after a 20-mg/kg intravenous dose. As mentioned, no biologically active metabolites have been observed in mouse, rat, dog, or monkey urine. However, a zone of inhibition with an R_f value different from ceftizoxime was observed in rat bile. This metabolite has not been identified.

IX. Ro 13-9904

Ro 13-9904 is a new semisynthetic cephalosporin (see Fig. 24). Elimination from systemic circulation proceeds slowly. Following an intravenous bolus of sodium

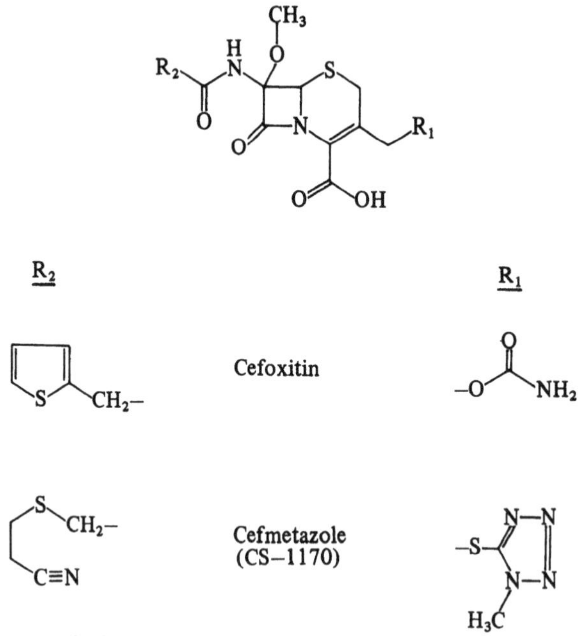

Fig. 25. Structure of cefoxitin and cefmetazole

Ro 13-9904, the terminal serum half-life of the drug averaged 8.8 h (SEDDON et al. 1980). The total body clearance of Ro 13-9904 is 14 ml/min and renal clearance is 8.6 ml/min. Urinary recovery of unchanged drug in total urine collections represented 60% of the dose. The volume of distribution of Ro 13-9904 in the vascular compartment is 4.3 liters. It is felt that biliary excretion of Ro 13-9904 is extensive and metabolism, if it exists, is minimal. The drug is 95% bound to human serum proteins.

The antibiotic does penetrate into the fluid of artificial skin blisters, in which Ro 13-9904 concentration exceeds serum levels by 6.5 h and then declines in a fashion similar to the levels in serum.

X. Cephamycins

The cephamycins are a family of β-lactam antibiotics characterized by a 7-α-methoxy group on the cephem nucleus. The presence of this functionality confers upon the molecule a greater degree of β-lactamase resistance when compared to cephalosporins of similar structure.

1. Cefoxitin

Cefoxitin (Fig. 25) is a semisynthetic cephamycin antibiotic which is effective after intravenous and intramuscular administration. The drug is eliminated from the systemic circulation chiefly by glomerular filtration and renal tubular secretion. Excretion in the bile and metabolism play minor roles in this elimination process (LOGAN et al. 1979; GEDDES et al. 1977; GOODWIN et al. 1974; SONNEVILLE et al. 1976). Following intravenous administration drug disappears rapidly from serum, with a terminal serum half-life of 30–50 min. The total body clearance of cefoxitin ranges between 250 and 350 ml/min, while renal clearance is 200–300 ml/min. Total urine collections contain at least 90% of the dose as unchanged drug. Less than 5% of the dose is eliminated by metabolism and biliary clearance (BUHS et al. 1974; GEDDES et al. 1977; LOGAN et al. 1979). Serum levels are proportional to dose over a dose range of 0.25–3 g. Multiple doses in this range given every 4 h do not cause accumulation of cefoxitin in healthy volunteers. The volume of distribution experienced by cefoxitin in the vascular compartment is approximately 8 liters (SIMON et al. 1978 b; SONNEVILLE et al. 1976; PAZIN et al. 1979; SCHROGIE et al. 1978, 1979; GOODWIN et al. 1974; BRUMFITT et al. 1974; BRISSON et al. 1980; WISE et al. 1979 a; VLASSES et al. 1980). Longer apparent serum half-lives were reported by CHRISTOPHIDIS et al. (1978) in older patients with osteoarthritis.

The biotransformation of cefoxitin is limited. GOODWIN et al. (1974) and SONNEVILLE et al. (1976) detected from 1%–6% of the cefoxitin dose in urine as the descarbamoyl metabolite. This metabolite could not be found in the urine of all subjects. Co-administration of probenecid created the opportunity for more metabolite to be formed (BUHS et al. 1974; GOODWIN et al. 1974).

Cefoxitin is not well absorbed after oral administration. However, after intramuscular administration of cefoxitin, drug is rapidly and completely absorbed. Peak serum levels of cefoxitin are attained in 30 min or less. Serum levels are proportional to dose, and 85%–95% of the intramuscular dose is recovered in urine within 12 h of administration. The renal clearance of cefoxitin after intravenous and intramuscular administration is similar. Use of a 0.5% or 1% lidocaine solution as diluent for the intramuscular dosage has no effect on the absorption or disposition of cefoxitin (SONNEVILLE et al. 1977; BRUMFITT et al. 1974; WISE et al. 1979 a, 1980 e).

The human serum protein binding of cefoxitin at serum concentrations of 10–100 µg/ml is 73% (SCHROGIE et al. 1978; WISE et al. 1980 e).

The tissue and body fluid distribution of cefoxitin has been studied in animals and man. After intramuscular administration of radiolabeled cefoxitin to rats (NAKAYAMA et al. 1978), highest levels of radioactivity were found in kidney, liver, and lung. Low amounts of radioactivity were observed in brain tissue and spleen. Similar distribution was seen after subcutaneous administration to mice (MILLER et al. 1974).

Following intravenous bolus doses of cefoxitin, T-tube bile levels of drug greatly exceeded serum levels for at least 4 h. In general, levels in common duct bile were higher in patients with functioning gallbladders. Gallbladder bile levels were more variable (GEDDES et al. 1977, 1978; LOGON et al. 1979).

Following intravenous administration, cefoxitin levels in skin abrasion fluid (GILLETT and WISE 1978) were very similar to serum levels 1 h after dosing and exceeded serum levels thereafter. Similar observations were made in artificial skin blister fluid after intramuscular administration (WISE et al. 1979 a). Cefoxitin was 60% bound to the protein in this fluid. Four hours after the start of a 0.166 g/h intravenous infusion of cefoxitin, drug levels in interstitial fluid were 77% of serum concentrations (SIMON et al. 1978 b).

After a 2-g intravenous infusion of cefoxitin, drug levels in ascites peaked at 2 h and were still detectable 8 h after the infusion. No serum accumulation of drug was noted in a similar group of patients who had received 2-g infusions of cefoxitin every 8 h for 10 days. Similar trends were observed in the ascitic fluid (BOURREILLE et al. 1979). Two to three hours after a 2-g intravenous infusion of cefoxitin, drug concentration in bronchial secretions was 25% of serum levels. Levels in bronchial secretions were slightly higher after multiple doses (BERGOGNE-BEREZIN et al. 1979a, c). PLAUE et al. (1979b) found that therapeutic levels of cefoxitin were easily attained in cortical bone, spongy bone, muscle, fascia, cutis, and subcutis.

Penetration of cefoxitin into CSF was minimal after single 2-g intravenous infusions with or without concurrent probenecid administration. Only those patients with chronic meningitis consistently had cefoxitin in their CSF. Better penetration in patients without inflamed meninges was noted after multiple intravenous doses of cefoxitin, but when probenecid was given with each dose of cefoxitin, all patients had drug in their CSF (HINTHORN et al. 1978). Similar results are reported by HUMBERT et al. (1980), GALVAO et al. (1980), and GEDDES et al. (1977).

After a 1-g intramuscular injection of cefoxitin to women about to undergo caesarian section, drug levels in cord blood and amniotic fluid were relatively low (BERGOGNE-BEREZIN et al. 1979a). Levels of cefoxitin in these two fluids rose more rapidly following a intravenous infusion of cefoxitin (2 g) and exceeded serum drug levels by 1.5 h. GEDDES et al. (1977) report that 2 h after a 1-g intravenous dose of cefoxitin, drug levels in breast milk of one lactating woman reached 5.6 μg/ml.

The oral or intravenous administration of probenecid concurrent with intramuscular or intravenous injections of cefoxitin has a pronounced effect on the time course of the antibiotic in serum. GOODWIN et al. (1974) noted that prior intravenous infusion (30 min) of probenecid, caused the terminal serum half-life of cefoxitin to double while renal clearance of the antibiotic dropped below 100 ml/min. Urinary recovery of cefoxitin through 12 h after intravenous administration also decreased slightly. HEKSTER et al. (1980) noted similar occurrences. In a study by VLASSES et al. (1980) it was shown that administering probenecid orally 60 min before an intravenous bolus dose of cefoxitin was given allowed the full effect of probenecid to be exerted. Renal clearance of cefoxitin was below 100 ml/min. Concurrent administration of the two drugs caused the renal clearance of cefoxitin to decrease with time as probenecid was being absorbed. Total urinary recovery of cefoxitin was not affected by probenecid administration. A 2-g oral dose of probenecid had a greater effect on the disposition of cefoxitin (2 g intramuscularly) than did a 1-g oral dose. These studies suggest that much of the renal elimination of cefoxitin occurs by renal tubular secretion, and studies by ARVIDSSON et al. (1979b) further suggest that little if any tubular reabsorption of cefoxitin occurs.

As might be expected, the elimination of cefoxitin from the systemic circulation changes drastically as kidney function decreases. Following intravenous doses of the antibiotic to patients with varying degrees of renal insufficiency, the terminal serum half-life of cefoxitin ranged from 0.8 h in normal patients, to 6 h in patients with creatinine clearance of 10–30 ml/min, to over 20 h in patients requiring hemodialysis (FILLASTRE et al. 1978; HUMBERT et al. 1979a; PAZIN et al. 1979; GARCIA et al. 1979a). It also appeared that the volume of distribution of cefoxitin in the vascular compartment was increasing. Urinary excretion of the drug decreased as renal function decreased. Hemodialysis is effective in clearing cefoxitin from blood.

The plasma protein binding of cefoxitin is 40% during hemodialysis and less than normal in all degrees of renal impairment (GARCIA et al. 1979a, b).

In rabbits with increasing degrees of renal impairment, the biliary excretion of the drug also increases (GARCIA et al. 1980).

As in adults, urinary recovery of cefoxitin is about 90% of the dose in infants and children. However, the apparent serum half-life is shorter in children 2–11 years of age than in adults and approaches 3 h in premature infants and neonates (WARREN et al. 1979; ROOS et al. 1979; MARGET et al. 1979; WILKINSON et al. 1979; FELDMAN et al. 1980; OLEGARD et al. 1979). BUCHANAN et al. (1980) noted no large differences in the disposition of cefoxitin in children during kwashiorkor and after the disease was cured.

2. Cefmetazole (CS-1170)

Cefmetazole (Fig. 25) is a semisynthetic cephamycin derivative which is eliminated by urinary excretion and, to a very minor degree, by biliary excretion (MASHIMO et al. 1978; SHIBATA et al. 1978).

Following intravenous administration to healthy volunteers, the terminal serum half-life of cefmetazole is 0.5–1 h. The renal clearance of cefmetazole is 80–100 ml/min and 70%–95% of intravenous doses is recoverable in 6- to 8-h urine collections. Hence, one would expect that total body clearance would only slightly exceed renal clearance. Serum levels are proportional to dose. A multiple intravenous dose regimen of 2 g given every 8 h led to a small amount of cefmetazole accumulation in plasma (KISHI et al. 1978; MIYAMOTO et al. 1978; FUJIMOTO et al. 1978; HINENO et al. 1978; SAKAI et al. 1978; OHKAWA et al. 1978, 1980; YAMASAKU and SUZUKI 1978; UEDA et al. 1978; SAITO et al. 1978; TAKAMOTO et al. 1978).

No microbiologically active metabolites of cefmetazole have been found in human urine (ISHIYAMA et al. 1978; KAWADA 1980).

Cefmetazole is apparently not absorbed after oral administration. The drug is well absorbed, however, after intramuscular administration. Peak serum concentrations of cefmetazole occur within 30 min of injection and 55%–90% of the dose can be recovered in 6- to 8-h urine collections. A total of 96% of the dose is recovered in 24-h urine collections. Administration of 0.5 g at 8-h intervals led to little accumulation of cefmetazole in serum. Serum levels are proportional to dose (ISHIYAMA et al. 1978; SAITO et al. 1978; MASHIMO et al. 1978; FUJIMOTO et al. 1978; MIYAMOTO et al. 1978; KAWADA 1980).

At a concentration of 30 μg/ml, the human serum protein (90%) binding of cefmetazole is 66% (MURAKAWA et al. 1980).

The body tissue and fluid distribution of cefmetazole has been studied in animals and man. In the rat, 79% of a 20 mg/kg intraperitoneal dose of cefmetazole was recovered in 24-h bile collections. Intramuscular injection of radiolabeled antibiotic produced tissue levels of radioactivity that were highest in kidney, followed by liver, lung, and heart (NAKAYAMA et al. 1978; MURAKAWA et al. 1980). Similar findings were reported by other investigators (OKAMATO et al. 1978; ISHIYAMA et al. 1978). Injection of the dose subcutaneously changed the distribution pattern somewhat (YAMAMOTO et al. 1978a). Low levels of radioactivity were detected in brain and spleen tissue (ISHIYAMA et al. 1978; NAKAYAMA et al. 1978).

In humans, a wide range of biliary cefmetazole concentrations have been reported depending upon disease state, and bile type. After 1- to 2-g intravenous infusions of cefmetazole, biliary levels of antibiotic ranged from 20 μg/ml to 250 μg/ml over a time frame of 2–6 h (KAWADA 1980; ISHII et al. 1978; NAKATOMI et al. 1978; YAMAMOTO et al. 1978b; SAKATSUGE et al. 1978). In patients with T-tubes, as much as 2% of a 500-mg intramuscular dose of cefmetazole was recovered in 6-h bile collections (SHIBATA et al. 1978). When hepatic function was greatly decreased, biliary levels of drug were low (NISHIKATA 1978). Cefmetazole levels in pancreatic juice were low after a 2-g intravenous bolus of the antibiotic (SAKATSUGE et al. 1978). Similar cefmetazole levels were detected in sputum after 1-g intravenous doses (NAKATOMI et al. 1978; KAWADA 1980). Drug levels in urogenital tissues have been measured after 1- or 2-g intravenous doses of cefmetazole. Kidney tissue levels were much higher than corresponding serum concentrations of drug while prostate levels were only 20% of serum values (TAKAMOTO et al. 1978). Drug levels of therapeutic value have also been reported in testicular and prepucular tissue and in hydrocele fluid (KAWAMURA et al. 1978).

In gynecological studies, 1-g intravenous doses of cefmetazole produced drug levels in uterine wall, fallopian tube, and ovarian tissue that were respectively 40%, 11%, and 8% of serum levels 100 min after injection (MATSUDA et al. 1978; KAWADA 1979). Drug was also detectable in oviduct, endometrium, myometrium, serosa, and cervix (HIRABAYASHI et al. 1978).

Forty-five minutes after 1-g injections of cefmetazole, umbilical cord blood levels of antibiotic were 30% of serum levels (MATSUDA et al. 1978). Cord blood levels did not decline as rapidly as maternal blood levels. Amniotic fluid levels were low. Similar observations were made by TAKASE et al. (1978) and MOTOMURA et al. (1978), but the former group report amniotic fluid levels of 4 μg/ml 2.5 h after the intravenous injection. More facile placental transfer of cefmetazole was observed by CHO et al. (1979b).

After 1-g intravenous doses in patients with renal dysfunction, serum levels of cefmetazole were elevated compared to those in healthy subjects. As creatinine clearance dropped below 25 ml/min, the 6-h urinary recovery of drug fell sharply and the apparent serum half-life of the drug increased dramatically (OHKAWA et al. 1980; SAKAI et al. 1978; YAMASAKU and SUZUKI 1978; UEDA et al. 1978; SAITO et al. 1978).

CHO et al. (1979a) and NISHIMURA et al. (1979b) administered intravenous doses of cefmetazole to children from 1–9 years of age and followed plasma levels and urinary excretion of the antibiotic. Elimination of the drug seems to reflect the age of the patient and the ease of urine collection. Apparent serum half-lives are similar to adult values, but recovery of drug in the urine was variable. Drug is also eliminated to a minor extent in feces (MINAMITANI et al. 1980).

D. Other β-Lactam Antibiotics

I. Moxalactam (LY 127935)

Moxalactam (Fig. 26) is a semisynthetic oxa-β-lactam having a dihydro-oxazine ring in place of the dihydrothiazine ring that is common to cephamycins and ce-

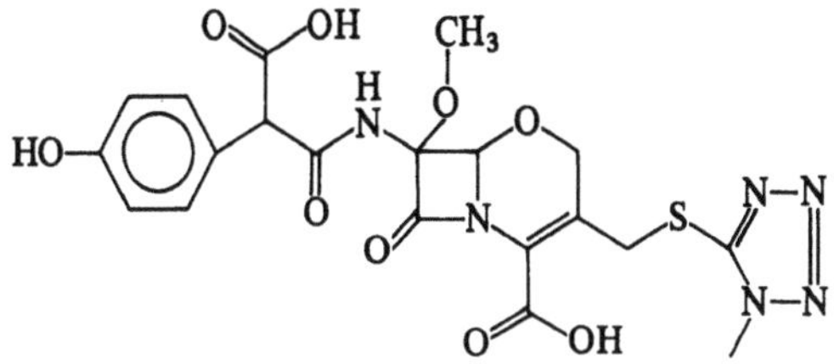

Fig. 26. Structure of moxalactam

phalosporins. The drug is eliminated via urinary excretion and, to a minor extent, biliary excretion (ISRAEL et al. 1980).

Following intravenous administration of moxalactam, serum concentrations decline with a terminal half-life of 1.5–2.5 h. The total body clearance of moxalactam is approximately 55–75 ml/min and renal clearance is 50–55 ml/min. Approximately 70%–90% of the dose is recovered in 24-h urine collections. The volume of distribution for moxalactam in the vascular compartment is approximately 6 liters (WISE et al. 1980b, c; PARSONS et al. 1980; MATSUMOTO et al. 1980; KURIHARA et al. 1980; SHIMADA et al. 1980). Serum levels are proportional to dose (ISRAEL et al. 1980) and regimens up to 1 g given every 12 h cause no accumulation of moxalactam in serum (KURIHARA et al. 1980).

No metabolites of moxalactam have been identified in plasma or urine (KURIHARA et al. 1980).

Moxalactam is a parenteral antibiotic. After intramuscular administration peak levels of drug in serum occur in 30–60 min and are proportional to dose (PARSONS et al. 1980; ISRAEL et al. 1980; KURIHARA et al. 1980). Recovery of unchanged drug in urine is comparable to that seen after intravenous drug administration.

Moxalactam is reportedly 50%–55% bound to human serum proteins (PARSONS et al. 1980; WISE et al. 1980c).

Drug concentrations in artificial skin blisters exceed serum levels by 2 h after a 1-g intravenous injection of moxalactam (WISE et al. 1980b). After a 2-g intravenous dose, sputum levels of moxalactam never exceeded 2.3% of serum levels (MATSUMOTO et al. 1980). Moxalactam reportedly penetrates into CSF rather easily in patients with or without meningitis after single or multiple doses (LANDESMAN et al. 1980; MATSUMOTO et al. 1980).

Oral doses of probenecid (0.5 g) given 30 min before a 1 g intravenous infusion of moxalactam had little effect on the antibiotic's disposition. Apparent serum half-life increased by 10% and the urinary excretion of drug during an 8-h period immediately following the dose decreased by 14% (SHIMADA et al. 1980).

In uremic patients with a creatinine clearance of 10 ml/min, the apparent serum half-life of moxalactam increased to 5 h. Hemodialysis and peritoneal dialysis were not very efficient at clearing moxalactam from blood (SHIMADA et al. 1980).

II. Clavulanic Acid

Clavulanic acid (Fig. 27) is a broad-spectrum β-lactam derivative that has weak antibacterial activity but which is a potent irreversible inhibitor of β-lactamases (BROWN et al. 1976; BALL et al. 1980). Assuming that its most probable use will

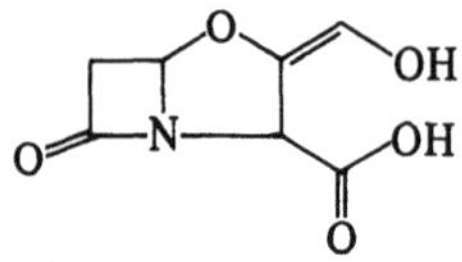

Fig. 27. Structure of clavulanic acid

be in combination with other β-lactam antibiotics to fend off β-lactamases which cause resistance of bacteria to more potent antibiotics, relevant information is presented for completeness.

The only published information concerning the disposition of clavulanic acid deals with oral administration of the drug (BALL et al. 1980; MUNCH et al. 1980). After oral doses of 125 or 250 mg, 35%–45% of the dose was recovered in 6-h urine collections. Only 2%–3% of the dose was recovered in the 4- to 6-h urine collection interval. Lack of fecal studies or information gathered after intravenous administration of the drug preclude estimates of absorption or metabolism. Serum levels are proportional to dose, peak 1 h after administration, and decline with an apparent serum half-life of 1 h. MUNCH et al. (1980) also report wide variation in urinary recovery after 250-mg oral doses in 20 volunteers. These investigators noted little CSF penetration of clavulanic acid in healthy volunteers, but levels in neurosurgical patients were comparable to serum levels at 6 h. They also found that the drug degrades at the rate of 10% per hour in serum at 37 °C. Elimination is delayed as renal function decreases (HOFFLER and DALHOFF 1980).

III. Mecillinam

Mecillinam is a derivative of penicillanic acid in which the 6β-acylamido side-chain of the penicillins is replaced by substituted amidino group (Fig. 28). Mecillinam per se is poorly absorbed when given by mouth and is administered orally as the pi-

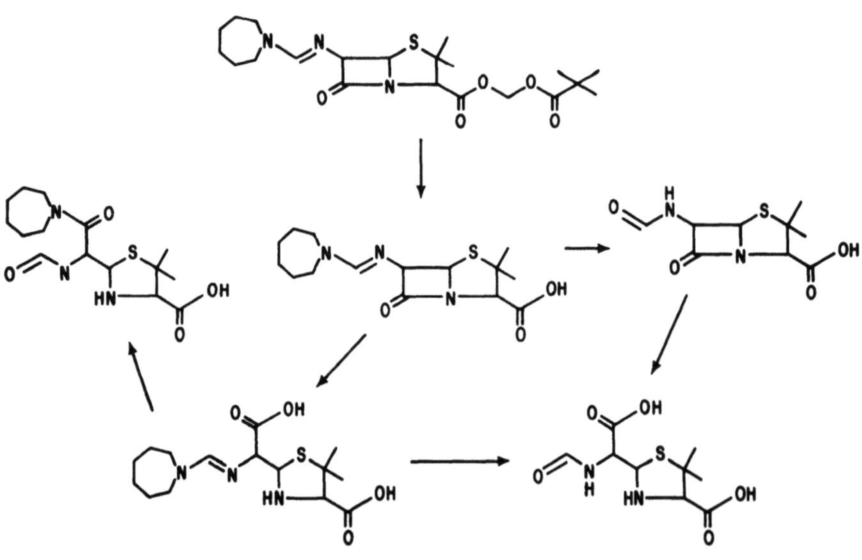

Fig. 28. Biotransformation of mecillinam (*center*) and its prodrug, pivmecillinam

valoyloxymethyl ester, pivmecillinam (LUND et al. 1976b). About 6% of an oral dose is excreted in the human urine as the penicilloic acid, another 2%–6% as the formamide of 6-aminopenicillanic acid and penicic acid (ROHOLT 1977; HATTORI et al. 1977; STROJNY and DESILVA 1980).

Following an intravenous dose in man, serum concentrations of mecillinam decline with a terminal half-life of about 50 min. Serum and renal clearances are respectively 3.52 and 2.50 ml/min per kilogram (GAMBERTOGLIO et al. 1980). Absorption is rapid and essentially complete following intramuscular injection (ROHOLT et al. 1975; WILLIAMS et al. 1976; ROHOLT 1977).

Pivmecillinam is a prodrug which relies on hydrolysis to mecillinam for activity. The bioavailability of orally administered pivmecillinam has been estimated to be 66%–80% as mecillinam. Absorption does not appear to be affected by the form of dosage, the concurrent ingestion of food, or coeliac disease (ROHOLT et al. 1975; MITCHARD et al. 1977; ANDERSON and ADAMS 1979; PARSONS et al. 1976b; ROHOLT 1977).

On the other hand, serum levels of mecillinam can be influenced by age, physical activity, and probenecid. BALL et al. (1978a) reported a mean serum half-life of 4 h in elderly patients with normal renal function. Peak serum levels are significantly lower in supine, resting subjects than in moderately active ones (ANDREWS et al. 1976). Mean serum levels of mecillinam double following co-administration of probenecid (ROHOLT et al. 1975; ANDREWS et al. 1976).

In patients with end-stage renal disease, serum clearance rate is about 67 ml/min, which is essentially identical to nonrenal clearance of mecillinam in normal subjects. Serum clearance is approximately double during hemodialysis (BAILEY et al. 1980).

About the same percentage of radioactivity is recovered in urine and feces following ^{14}C-pivmecillinam administration to the dog. Besides urine and bile, the highest concentrations are located in the liver and the kidneys; the lowest are in the brain. Significant levels are found in the fetus of pregnant rabbits, while insignificant quantities are secreted in the milk of lactating cows (ROHOLT 1977).

Acknowledgements. The authors are grateful to Miss Florence Berg, Miss Tse-Wei Chu, and Mrs. Gale Hobart for their assistance with the literature search, and to Mrs. Gail Landes for the typing and the overall coordination of this project.

References

Abraham EP, Chain E (1940) An enzyme from bacteria able to destroy penicillin. Nature 146:837

Acocella G, Maltussi R, Nicolis FB, Pallanza R, Tenconi LT (1968) Biliary elimination of antibiotics. Gut 9:536–545

Acred P, Hunter PA, Mizen L, Rolinson GN (1971) α-Carboxy-3-thienylmethylpenicillin (BRL 2288), a new semisynthetic penicillin: in vivo evaluation. In: Hobby GL (ed) Antimicrobial agents and chemotherapy – 1970. American Society for Microbiology, Bethesda, pp 396–401

Acred P, Ryan DM, Harding SM, Muggleton PW (1980) In vivo properties of GR 20263. In: Nelson JD, Grassi C (eds) Current chemotherapy of infectious diseases: proceedings of the 11th international congress of chemotherapy 1979. American Society for Microbiology, Washington DC, pp 271–273

Actor P, Pitkin DH, Lucyszyn G, Weisbach JA, Bran JL (1976a) Cefatrizine (SK&F 60771), a new oral cephalosporin: serum levels and urinary recovery in humans after oral or intramuscular administration – comparative study with cephalexin and cefazolin. Antimicrob Agents Chemother 9:800–803
Actor P, Pitkin DH, Lucyszyn G, Weisbach JA (1976b) A new parenteral cephalosporin. SK&F 59962: serum levels and urinary recovery in man. In: Williams JD, Geddes AM (eds) Chemotherapy, vol 5. Plenum, New York, pp 253–257
Actor P, Guarini JR, Uri J, Bartus HF, Zajac I, Wersbach JA (1977) In vitro studies with cefazaflur and other parenteral cephalosporins. J Antibiot 30:730–735
Actor P, Uri JV, Zajac I, Guarini JR, Phillips L, Pitkin DH, Berges DA, Dunn GL, Hoover JRE, Weisbach JA (1978) SK&F 75073, new parenteral broad-spectrum cephalosporin with high and prolonged serum levels. Antimicrob Agents Chemother 13:784–790
Adam D, Bauer W (1979) Pharmakokinetische Untersuchungen mit der Kombination Mezlocillin – Oxacillin. Arzneimittelforsch 29 II:1971–1972
Adam D, Patzold J (1977) Serumkonzentrationen und Kinetik nach Kurzinfusion von vier Gramm Cefazolin. Infection 5:228–231
Adam D, Tunn U (1979) Konzentrationen von Cefradin im Nierengewebe. Muench Med Wochenschr 121:1367–1369
Adam D, Hofstetter AG, Jacoby W, Reichardt B (1976a) Studies on the diffusion of cephradine and cephalothin into human tissue. Infection 4:105–107
Adam D, Patzold J, Reichardt B (1976b) Konzentration von Cephacetril im Herzmuskelgewebe, Infection 4:S215–S216
Adam D, Schalkhauser K, Boettger F (1979a) Zur Diffusion von Cefuroxim in das Prostata- und andere Gewebe des Urogenitalbereichs. Med Klin 74:1867–1870
Adam F, Hofstetter AG, Eisenberger F (1979b) Zur Diffusion von cefamandol in das Prostatagewebe. Med Klin 74:235–238
Adam D, Hofstetter AG, Reichart B, Schneider CH, Wolff H, Koch E (1979c) Zur Diffusion von Cefazedon in das Herzmuskel-, Prostata- und Hautgewebe sowie in die Gallenflüssigkeit. Arzneim Forsch 29:1901–1906
Agbayani MM, Khan AJ, Kemawikasit P, Rosenfeld W, Salazar D, Kumar K, Glass L, Evans HE (1979) Pharmacokinetics and safety of cefamandole in newborn infants. Antimicrob Agents Chemother 15:674–676
Agersborg HPK, Batchelor A, Cambridge GW, Rule AW (1966) The pharmacology of penamecillin. Br J Pharmacol 26:649–655
Ahern MJ, Finkelstein FO, Andriole VT (1976) Pharmacokinetics of cefamandole in patients undergoing hemodialysis and peritoneal dialysis. Antimicrob Agents Chemother 10:457–461
Ahrens T, Vischer W, Imhof P, Fullhaas J, Zak O, Kradolfer F (1979) Human pharmacology of CGP 7174/E (SCE-129) and initial results of clinical trials in Europe. Drugs Exp Clin Res 5:61–70
Aletta JM, Francke EF, Neu HC (1980) Intravenous azlocillin kinetics in patients on long-term hemodialysis. Clin Pharmacol Ther 27:563–566
Alicino JF (1946) Iodometric method for the assay of penicillin preparations. Ind Eng Chem [Anal Ed] 18:619–620
Allaz A-F, Dayer P, Fabre J, Rudhardt M, Balant L (1979) Pharmacocinetique d'une nouvelle cephalosporine, la cefoperazone. Schweiz Med Wochenschr 109:1999–2005
Anders MW, Cooper MJ, Rolewicz TF, Mirkin BL (1975) Application of highpressure liquid chromatography in pediatric pharmacology: pharmacokinetics of cephalothin in man. In: Morselli PL, Garanttini S, Sereni F (eds) Basic and therapeutic aspects of perinatal pharmacology. Raven, New York, pp 405–409
Anderson JD, Adams MA (1979) Urinary excretion of mecillinam by volunteers receiving film-coated tablets of pivmecillinam hydrochloride. Chemotherapy 25:1–4
Andrews J, Kendall MJ, Mitchard M (1976) Factors influencing the absorption and disposition of mecillinam and pivmecillinam in man. Br J Clin Pharmacol 3:627–632
Andriole VT (1978) Pharmacokinetics of cephalosporins in patients with renal failure or reduced renal function. J Infect Dis 1375:S88–97
Aoki N, Sekine O, Usuda Y, Shimizu T, Hirasawa Y, Aoki T (1980) Serum, urine, and bile levels of cefoperazone (T-1551). In: Nelson JD, Grassi C (eds) Current chemotherapy

of infectious diseases: proceedings of the 11th international congress of chemotherapy – 1979. American Society for Microbiology, Washington, DC, pp 159–161
Apicella MA, Perkins RL, Saslaw S (1966) Cephaloridine treatment of bacterial infections. Am J Med Sci 251:266–276
Appel GB, Neu HC, Parry MF, Goldberger MJ, Jacob GB (1976) Pharmacokinetics of cefamandole in the presence of renal failure and in patients undergoing hemodialysis. Antimicrob Agents Chemother 10:623–625
Applestein JM, Crosby EB, Johnson WD, Kaye D (1968) In vitro antimicrobial activity and human pharmacology of cephaloglycin. Appl Microbiol 16:1006–1010
Arancibia A, Guttman J, Gonzalez G, Gonzalez C (1980) Absorption and disposition kinetics of amoxicillin in normal human subjects. Antimicrob Agents Chemother 17:199–202
Archer GL, Polk RE, Duma RJ, Lower R (1978) Comparison of cephalothin and cefamandole prophylaxis during insertion of prosthetic heart valves. Antimicrob Agents Chemother 13:924–929
Armbruster C, Fuellhaas J, Groetzinger M (1980) Concentrations of CGP-9000 in plasma and wound secretions. In: Nelson JD, Grassi C (eds) Current chemotherapy of infectious diseases: proceedings of the 11th international congress of chemotherapy – 1979. American Society for Microbiology, Washington, DC, pp 217–218
Arvidsson A, Borga O, Alvan G (1979) Renal excretion of cephapirin and cephaloridine: Evidence for saturable tubular reabsorption. Clin Pharmacol Ther 25:870–876
Arvidsson A, Borga O, Alvan G (1980) Renal excretion and reabsorption processes of cephapirin, cephaloridine, cephalexin and cefoxitin. In: Nelson JD, Grassi C (eds) Current chemotherapy and infectious disease: proceedings of the 11th international congress of chemotherapy – 1979. American Society for Microbiology, Washington, DC, pp 567–568
Asscher AW, Johnson SE, Simon DA (1970) Effect of urinary pH on the renal clearance of cephaloridine. Postgrad Med J 46S:56–57
Assael BM, Como ML, Miraglia M, Pardi G, Sereni F (1979) Ampicillin kinetics in pregnancy. Br J Clin Pharmacol 8:286–288
Axelrod JL, Kochman RS (1978) Cefamandole levels in primary aqueous humor in man. Am J Ophthalmol 85:342–348
Axelrod JL, Kochman RS (1980) Cefaclor levels in human aqueous humor. Arch Ophthalmol 98:740–742
Axline SG, Yaffe SJ, Simon HJ (1967) Clinical pharmacology of antimicrobials in premature infants: II. Ampicillin, methicillin, oxacillin, neomycin, and colistin. Pediatrics 39:97–107
Ayliffe GAJ, Davies A (1965) Ampicillin levels in human bile. Br J Pharmacol 24:189–193
Aziz NS, Gambertoglio JG, Lin ET, Benet LZ (1977) Multicompartmental kinetics of cephalothin and its less active desacetyl metabolite using a specific chemical assay. Clin Res 25:267A
Aziz NS, Gambertoglio JG, Lin ET, Grausz H, Benet LZ (1978) Pharmacokinetics of cefamandole using a HPLC assay. J Pharmacokinet Biopharm 6:153–164
Baier R, Zelder O, Bode JC (1980) Epicillin – Konzentrationen in Galle und Serum nach parenteraler Gabe. Arzneimittelforsch 30:109–113
Bailey K, Cruickshank JG, Bisson PG, Radford BL (1980) Mecillinam in patients on hemodialysis. Br J Clin Pharmacol 10:177–180
Bailey RR, Gower PE, Dash CH (1970) The effect of impairment of renal function and haemodialysis on serum and urine levels of cephalexin. Postgrad Med J 46(S):60–64
Baker LH, Gerjarusak P, Hinthorn DR, Romig DA, Harms J, Liu C (1975) Effect of probenecid on human CSF cephalosporin concentration. In: Day RA (ed) Fifteenth interscience conference on antimicrobial agents and chemotherapy. American Society for Microbiology, Washington DC, Abst. 85
Baker S, Wise R, Gillett AP, Andrews JM (1980) Tissue penetration, as measured by a blister technique, and pharmacokinetics of CGP 7174/E compared with carbenicillin. In: Nelson JD, Grassi C (eds) Current chemotherapy infectious diseases: proceedings of the 11th international congress of chemotherapy – 1979. American Society for Microbiology, Washington, DC, pp 647–649

Balant L, Dayer P, Rudhardt M, Allaz AF, Fabre J (1980) Cefoperazone: pharmacokinetics in humans with normal and impaired renal function and pharmacokinetics in rats. Clin Ther 3:50–59
Ball AP, Viswan AK, Mitchard M, Wise R (1978a) Plasma concentrations and excretion of mecillinam after oral administration of pivmecillinam in elderly patients. J Antimicrob Chemother 4:241–246
Ball P, Barford T, Gilbert J, Johnson T, Mitchard M (1978b) Prolonged serum elimination half-life of amoxycillin in the elderly. J Antimicrob Chemother 4:385–386
Ball AP, Davey PG, Geddes AM, Farrell ID, Brookes GR (1980) Clavulanic acid and amoxycillin: a clinical, bacteriological, and pharmacological study. Lancet 1:620–623
Ballard BE (1966) Effect of physical activity on the absorption rates of procaine penicillin G implants. J Pharm Sci 55:515–516
Banner Jr W, Gooch III WM, Burckart G, Korones SB (1980) Pharmacokinetics of nafcillin in infants with low birth weights. Antimicrob Agents Chemother 17:691–694
Barbhaiya R, Thin RN, Turner P, Wadsworth J (1979) Clinical pharmacology studies of amoxycillin: Effect of probenecid. Br J Vener Dis 55:211–213
Barnett HL, McNamara H, Shultz S, Tompsett R (1949) Renal clearance of sodium penicillin G, procaine penicillin G, and insulin in infants and children. Pediatrics 3:418–422
Barr W, Graham RM (1967) Placental transmission of cephaloridine. J Obstet Gynaecol Br Commonw 74:739–745
Barrios S, Sorensen JH, Spickett RGW (1975) Bioavailability of cephalexin after intramuscular injection of its lysine salt. J Pharm Pharmacol 27:711–712
Bartolozzi G, Cocchi P, Princi P (1967) Serum levels of methicillin in premature infants. Chemotherapia 12:146–154
Barza M, Miao PVW (1977) Antimicrobial spectrum, pharmacology and therapeutic use of antibiotics. Part 3: Cephalosporins. Am J Hosp Pharm 34:621–629
Barza M, Weinstein L (1974) Penetration of antibiotics into fibrin loci in vivo. I. Comparison of penetration of ampicillin into fibrin clots, abcesses, and "interstitial fluid." J Infect Dis 129:59–65
Barza M, Weinstein L (1976) Pharmacokinetics of the penicillin in man. Clin Pharmacokinet 1:297–308
Barza M, Melethil S, Berger S, Ernst EC (1976) Comparative pharmacokinetics of cefamandole, cephapirin, and cephalothin in healthy subjects and effect of repeated dosing. Antimicrob Agents Chemother 10:421–425
Basch H, Erickson R, Gadebusch H (1971) Epicillin: in vitro laboratory studies. Infec Immun 4:44–49
Bassaris HP, Quintiliani R, Maderazo EG, Tilton RC, Nightingale CH (1976) Pharmacokinetics and penetration characteristics of cefazolin into human spinal fluid. Curr Ther Res 19:110–120
Bastert G, Muller WG, Wallauser H (1975) Pharmacokinetische Untersuchungen zum Übertritt von Antibiotika in das Fruchtwasser am Ende der Schwangerschaft. 3. Teil: Oxacillin. Z Geburtshilfe Perinatol 179:346–355
Batra VK, Morrison JA, Lasseter KC, Joy VA (1979) Piperacillin kinetics. Clin Pharmacol Ther 26:41–53
Bax R, White L, Reeves D, Ings R, Bywater M, Holt H (1980) Pharmacokinetics of cefotaxime and its desacetyl metabolite. In: Nelson JD, Grassi C (eds) Current chemotherapy of infectious diseases: proceedings of the 11th international congress of chemotherapy – 1979. American Society of Microbiology, Washington, DC, pp 155–157
Bechtel TP, Slaughter RL, Moore TD (1980) Seizures associated with high cerebrospinal fluid concentrations of cefazolin. Am J Hosp Pharm 37:271–273
Begue P, Befekadu E, Laplane R (1977) Pharmacokinetic and clinical study of cefazoline in children. Sem Hop Paris 53:1633–1136
Belohradsky BH, Geiss D, Marget W, Bruch K, Kafetzis D, Peters G (1980) Intravenous cefotaxime in children with bacterial meningitis. Lancet 1:61–63
Bengtsson S, Lindholm CE, Osterman K (1979) Azidocillin levels in tracheo bronchial secretions. Scand J Respir Dis 60:225–229
Bennett JV, Kirby WMM (1965) A rapid, modified ultrafiltration method for determining serum protein binding and its application to new penicillins. J Lab Clin Med 66:721–732

Bergan T (1977) Comparative pharmacokinetics of cefazolin, cephalothin, cephacetril, and cephapirine after intravenous administration. Chemotherapy 23:389–404
Bergan T (1978a) Pharmacokinetic comparison of oral becampicillin and parenteral ampicillin. Antimicrob Agents Chemother 13:971–974
Bergan T (1978b) Pharmacokinetics of mezlocillin in healthy volunteers. Antimicrob Agents Chemother 14:801–806
Bergan T (1978c) Penicillins. In: Schonfeld H (ed) Pharmacokinetics. Karger, Basel (Antibiot Chemother 25:1–122)
Bergan T (1980) Pharmacokinetics of a new cephalosporin, CGP 9000 (cefroxadine), in healthy volunteers. Chemotherapy 26:225–230
Bergan T, Michalsen H (1979) Pharmacokinetics of azlocillin in children with cystic fibrosis. Arzneimittelforsch 29(II):1955–1957
Bergan T, Midtvedt T, Erikssen J (1970) Human pharmacokinetics of cephalexin. Pharmacology 4:264–272
Bergan T, Berdal BO, Holm V (1976) Relative bioavailability of phenoxymethyl penicillin preparations in cross-over study. Acta Pharmacol Toxicol 38:308–320
Bergan T, Brodwall EK, Orjavik O (1977) Pharmacokinetics of cefazolin in patients with normal and impaired renal function. J Antimicrob Chemother 3:435–443
Bergan T, Bratlid D, Brondbo A (1978a) Pharmacokinetics of becampicillin in infants. J Antimicrob Chemother 4:79–84
Bergan T, Digranes A, Schreiner A (1978b) Absorption, distribution and elimination of cefazolin in patients with normal renal function. Chemotherapy 24:277–282
Bergan T, Brodwall EK, Wiik-Larsen E (1979) Mezlocillin pharmacokinetics in patients with normal and impaired renal functions. Antimicrob Agents Chemother 16:651–654
Bergholz H, Erttmann RR, Damm KH (1980) Effects of probenecid on plasma/tissue distribution of ^{14}C-benzylpenicillin in rats. Experientia 36:333–334
Bergogne E, Lambert N, Rouvillois JL (1976) Pharmacokinetics of cephradine. In: Williams JD, Geddes AM (eds) Chemotherapy 5. Plenum, New York, pp 259–262
Bergogne-Berezin E, Morel C, Benard Y, Berthelot G, Kafe H (1978) Pharmacokinetic study of β-lactam antibiotics in bronchial secretions. Scand J Infect Dis [Suppl] 14:267–273
Bergogne-Berezin E, Morel C, Kafe H, Berthelot G, Benard Y, Lambert-Zechovsky N, Rouvillois JL (1979a) Etude pharmacocinetique chez l'homme de la cefoxitine. Diffusion intrabronchique et transplacentaire. Therapie 34:345–354
Bergogne-Berezin E, Lambert-Zechovsky N, Rouvillois JL (1979b) Etude du passage transplacentaire des beta-lactamines. J Gynecol Obstet Biol Reprod (Paris)8:359–364
Bergogne-Berezin E, Pierre J, Berthelot G, Kafe J, Morel C (1979c) Pharmacokinetics of cephalosporins in human bronchial secretions. Drugs Exp Clin Res 5:159–165
Berman SJ, Boughton WH, Sugihara JG, Wong EGC, Sato MM, Siemsen AW (1978) Pharmacokinetics of cefaclor in patients with end stage renal disease and during hemodialysis. Antimicrob Agents Chemother 14:281–283
Bernard B, Thielen P, Garcia-Cazares SJ, Ballard CA (1977a) Maternal-fetal pharmacology of cefatrizine in the first 20 weeks of pregnancy. Antimicrob Agents Chemother 12 2:231–236
Bernard B, Barton L, Abate M, Ballard CA (1977b) Maternal-fetal transfer of cefazolin in the first twenty weeks of pregnancy. J Infect Dis 136:377–382
Berte F, Arrigoni E, Benzi G (1972) Plasma, urine and bile levels of ampicillin after i.m. treatment with ampicillin sodium salt and/or benzathineampicillin, in dog and man. Farmaco [Prat] 27:205–213
Beyer KH, Russo HF, Tillson EK, Miller AK, Verway WF, Gass SR (1951) "Benemid" p-(di-n-propylsulfamyl)benzoic acid: its renal affinity and its elimination. Am J Physiol 166:625–640
Binderup E, Godtfredsen WO, Roholt K (1971) Orally active cephaloglycin esters. J Antibiot 24:767–773
Bird AE, Marshall AC (1967) Correlation of serum binding of penicillins with partition coefficients. Biochem Pharmacol 16:2275–2290
Birner J (1970) Determination of phenoxymethyl penicilloic acid and phenoxyethyl penicilloic acid in urine in the presence of the parent penicillins. J Pharm Sci 59:757–760

Biro L, Ivan E, Arr M, Foldi (1972) Klinisch-pharmakologische Untersuchung des Ampicillins (Beziehungen zwischen Blut- und Gewebekonzentration). Int J Clin Pharmacol 6:342–345
Bloch R, Szwed JJ, Sloan RS, Luft FC (1977) Pharmacokinetics of cefaclor in normal subjects and patients with chronic renal failure. Antimicrob Agents Chemother 12:730–732
Bodey GP, Vallejos C, Stewart D (1972) Flucloxacillin: a new semisynthetic isoxazolyl penicillin. Clin Pharmacol Ther 13:512–515
Bodin N-O, Ekström B, Forsgren U, Jalar L-P, Magni JL, Ramsay C-H, Sjöberg (1975) Becampicillin: a new orally well-absorbed derivative of ampicillin. Antimicrob Agents Chemother 8:518–525
Bodine JA, Strausbaugh LJ, Sande MA (1976) Ampicillin and an ester in experimental hemophilus influenzae meningitis. Clin Pharmacol Ther 20:727–732
Bodner SJ, Koenig MG (1972) Clinical and in vitro evaluation of cephapirin: A new parenteral cephalosporin. Am J Med Sci 263:43–51
Boe RW, Williams CPS, Bennett JV, Oliver TK Jr (1967) Serum levels of methicillin and ampicillin in newborn and premature infants in relation to postnatal age. Pediatrics 39:194–201
Bolme P, Eriksson M (1976) The bioavailability of oral penicillin V. A comparative study of the absorption of different salts of penicillin V in children. Acta Pediatr Scand 65:253–256
Bolme P, Eriksson M (1978) Absorption of phenoxymethylpenicillin in children. Scand J Infect Dis 10:223–227
Bolme P, Eriksson M, Stintzing G (1977) The gastrointestinal absorption of penicillin V in children with suspected coeliac disease. Acta Pediatr Scand 66:573–578
Bond JM, Lightbrown JW, Barber M, Waterworth PM (1963) A comparison of four phenoxypenicillins. Br Med J 2:956–951
Boothman R, Kerr MM, Marshall MJ, Burland WL (1973) Absorption and excretion of cephalexin by the newborn infant. Arch Dis Child 48:147–150
Boreus LO (1971) Placental transfer of ampicillin in man. Acta Pharmacol Toxicol [Suppl] 3:250–254
Bourreille J, Lebihan G, Beau B, Leroy A, Humbert G, Barthes P-X (1979) Etude du passage transperitoneal de la cefoxitine chez le cirrhotique ascitique. Med Chir Dig 8:667–670
Boyle GL, Hein HF, Leopold IH (1970) Intraocular penetration of cephalexin in man. Am J Ophthalmol 69:868–872
Brisson AM, Fourtillan JB, Barthes D, Courtois P, Becq-Giraudon B (1980) Comparison des profils pharmacocinetiques de la cefazoline et de la cefoxitine chez l'homme. Therapie 35:209–220
Brodwall EK, Bergan T, Orjavik O (1977) Kidney transport of cefazolin in normal and impaired renal function. J Antimicrob Chemother 3:585–592
Brogard JM, Haegele P, Kohler JJ, Dorner M, Lavillaureix J, Stahl J (1973) The biliary excretion of cephalothin. Chemotherapy 18:212–221
Brogard JM, Haegele P, Dorner M, Lavillaureix J (1974) Biliary levels of carbenicillin. J Int Med Res 2:142–148
Brogard JM, Pinget M, Dorner M, Lavillaureix J (1975a) Determination of cefalexin pharmacokinetics and dosage adjustments in relation to renal function. J Clin Pharmacol 15:666–673
Brogard JM, Dorner M, Pinget M, Adloff M, Lavillaureix J (1975b) The biliary excretion of cefazolin. J Infect Dis 131:625–633
Brogard JM, Dorner M, Brandt C, Lavillaureix J (1976a) Cephacetrile – Application of pharmacokinetic data to dosage determination. Int J Clin Pharmacol Biopharm 13:168–176
Brogard JM, Brandt C, Dorner M, Dammron A (1976b) Adjustment of cephaloridine (Keflodin®) dosage according to its pharmacokinetics. Chemotherapy 22:1–11
Brogard JM, Pinget M, Comte F, Lavillaureix J (1977a) Cefamandole: Bacteriological study and pharmacokinetic data. Drugs Exp Clin Res 3:39–49

Brogard JM, Pinget M, Brandt C, Lavillaureix J (1977 b) Pharmacokinetics of cefazolin in patients with renal failure, special reference to hemodialysis. J Clin Pharmacol 17:225–230
Brogard JM, Pinget M, Meyer C, Dorner M, Lavillaureix J (1977 c) Biliary excretion of ampicillin: experimental and clinical study. Chemotherapy 23:213–226
Brogard JM, Comte F, Pinget M (1978) Pharmacokinetics of cephalosporin antibiotics. In: Schonfeld H (ed) Pharmacokinetics. Karger, Basel (Antibiot Chemother 25:123–162)
Brogard JM, Kopferschmitt J, Spach MO, Grudet O, Lavillaureix J (1979 a) Cefamandole pharmacokinetics and dosage adjustments in relation to renal function. J Clin Pharmacol 19:366–377
Brogard JM, Kopferschmitt J, Spach MO, Lavillaureix J, Grudet O (1979 b) Cefuroxime pharmacokinetics in subjects with normal and impaired renal function. Prediction of serum concentrations and dosage adjustments. Drugs Exp Clin Res 5:427–443
Brogard JM, Pinget M, Doffoel M, Adloff M, Lavillaureix J (1979 c) Evaluation of the biliary excretion of penicillin G. Chemotherapy 25:129–139
Brogden RN, Heel RC, Speight TM, Avery GS (1979) Cefuroxime: a review of its antibacterial activity, pharmacological properties and therapeutic use. Drugs 17:233–266
Brown AG, Butterworth D, Cole M, Hanscomb G, Hood JD, Reading C, Rolinson GN (1976) Naturally occurring β-lactamase inhibitors with antibacterial activity. J Antibiot 29:668–669
Brown DM, Hannan DP, Langley PF (1969) Biotransformation of hetacillin to ampicillin in man. Toxicol Appl Pharmacol 15:136–142
Brumfitt W, Kosmidis J, Hamilton-Miller JMT, Gilchrist JNG (1974) Cefoxitin and cephalothin: antimicrobial activity, human pharmacokinetics, and toxicology. Antimicrob Agents Chemother 6:290–299
Buchanan N, Mithal Y, Witcomb M (1980) Cefoxitin: Intravenous pharmacokinetics and intramuscular bioavailability in kwashiorkor. Br J Clin Pharmacol 9:623–627
Buck RE, Price KE (1977) Cefadroxil, a new broad-spectrum cephalosporin. Antimicrob Agents Chemother 11:324–330
Buckingham M, Welply G, Miller JF, Elstein M (1975) Gastro-intestinal absorption and transplacental transfer of amoxycillin during labour and the influence of metoclopramide. Curr Med Res Opin 3:392–396
Buhs RP, Maxim TE, Allen N, Jacob TA, Wolf FJ (1974) Analysis of cefoxitin, cephalothin and their deacylated metabolites in human urine by high-performance liquid chromatography. J Chromatogr 99:609–618
Bullen BR, Ramsden CH, Kester RC (1979) Evaluation of tissue levels of cefamandole in severely ischaemic lower limbs using two regimens of dosage. Curr Med Res 6:244–248
Bunn PA, Knight R, Anberg J (1960) Some notes about a new synthetic penicillin for staphylococcal disease. NY State J Med 60:3074
Burch KH, Pohlod D, Savalatz LD, Madhavan T, Kiani D, Quinn EL, DelBusto R, Cardenas J, Fisher EJ (1979) Ceforanide: in vitro and clinical evaluation. Antimicrob Agents Chemother 16:386–391
Burns LE, Hodgman JE, Wehrle PF (1965) Treatment of premature infants with oxacillin. In: Hobby GL (ed) Antimicrobial agents and chemotherapy – 1964. American Society for Microbiology, Bethesda, pp 192–199
Bustrack JA, Lawson LA, Bauer LA, Wilson HD, Foster TS (1980) A comparative pharmacokinetic and safety study of an investigational oral cephalosporin, RMI 19,592. Curr Ther Res 28:208–217
Butler K (1971) Metabolism and laboratory studies with indanyl carbenicillin. Del Med J 43:366–375
Butler K, English AR, Riggs B, Gralla E, Stebbius RB, Hobbs (1973) Indanyl carbenicillin: chemistry and laboratory studies with a new semisynthetic penicillin. J Infect Dis 127 [Suppl]: 97–104
Cabana BE, Van Harken DR, Hottendorf GH, Doluisio JT, Griffen Jr WO, Bourne DWA, Dittert LW (1975) The role of the kidney in the elimination of cephapirin in man. J Pharmacokinet Biopharmacol 3:419–437

Cabana BE, Van Harken DR, Hottendorf GH (1976) Comparative pharmacokinetics and metabolism of cephapirin in laboratory animals and humans. Antimicrob Agents Chemother 10:307–317

Cahn MM, Levy EJ, Actor P, Pauls JF (1974) Comparative serum levels and urinary recovery of cefazolin, cephaloridine, and cephalothin in man. J Clin Pharmacol 14:61–66

Campillo JA, Lanao JM, Dominguez-Gil A, Tabernero JM, Rubio F (1979) Pharmacokinetics of cefamandole in patients undergoing hemodialysis. Int J Pharmacol Bio-Pharmacol 17:416–420

Carter MJ, Brumfitt W (1962) Bacteriological and clinical studies with phenoxybenzylpenicillin. Br Med J 1:80–82

Chang CT, Khan AJ, Agbayani MM, Jhaveri R, Amin I, Evans HE (1978) Pharmacokinetics and safety of cefamandole in infants and children. Antimicrob Agents Chemother 14:838–841

Ceccarelli G, Ciampini M (1979) Blood levels, transplacental passage, tissue distribution and clinical activity of a new prodrug of ampicillin, becampicillin. Survey of some Italian data. Drugs Exp Clin Res 5:201–205

Chalas J, Laboyle D, Macarrio J, Barraud D, Lindenbaum A, Buffet C, Chaput JC (1980) Metabolism and kinetics of ampicillin elimination in cirrhosis. Sem Hop Paris 56:464–469

Chelvan P, Hamilton-Miller JMT, Brumfitt W (1979) Pharmacokinetics of parenteral amoxycillin, biliary excretion and effect of renal failure. J Antimicrob Chemother 5:232–233

Chisholm DR, Leitner F, Misiek M, Wright GE, Price KE (1970) Laboratory studies with a new cephalosporanic acid derivative. In: Hobby GL (ed) Antimicrobial agents and chemotherapy – 1969. American Society for Microbiology, Bethesda, pp 244–246

Cho K, Takimoto M, Yoshida H, Nanbo H (1979a) Pharmacokinetics and results of clinical administration of CS-1170. I. Pharmacokinetics of CS-1170. Jpn J Antibiot 32:1–5

Cho N, Uehara K, Sugizaki K, Suzuki H, Takenouchi T, Kimura S, Kunii K (1979b) Clinical studies on cefmetazole (CS-1170) in the field of obstetrics and gynecology. Chemother (Tokyo) 27:900–906

Chow M, Quintiliani R, Cunha BA, Thompson M, Finkelstein E, Nightingale CH (1979) Pharmacokinetics of high-dose oral cephalosporins. J Clin Pharmacol 19:185–194

Christophidis N, Dawborn JK, Vajda FJE (1978) Studies of intravenous cefoxitin (MK-306). Med J Aust 1:512–514

Clarke JT, Libke RD, Ralph ED, Luthy RP, Kirby WMM (1974) Human pharmacokinetics of BL-P1654 compared with ampicillin. Antimicrob Agents Chemother 6:729–733

Clayton JP, Cole M, Elson SW, Ferres H (1974) BRL 8988 (Talampicillin), a well-absorbed oral form of ampicillin. Antimicrob Agents Chemother 5:670–671

Clayton JP, Cole M, Elson SW, Hardy KD, Mizen LW, Sutherland R (1975) Preparation, hydrolysis, and oral absorption of α-carboxy esters of carbenicillin. J Med Chem 18:172–177

Clayton JP, Cole M, Elson SW, Ferres H, Hanson JC, Mizen LW, Sutherland R (1976) Preparation, hydrolysis, and oral absorption of lactonyl esters of penicillins. J Med Chem 19:1385–1391

Clumeck N, Thys JP, Vanhoof R, Vanderlinden MP, Butzler JP, Yourassowsky E (1978) Amoxicillin entry into human cerebrospinal fluid: comparison with ampicillin. Antimicrob Agents Chemother 14:531–532

Colburn WA, Gibaldi M, Yoshioka H, Takimoto M, Riley HD Jr (1976) Pharmacokinetic model for serum concentration of ampicillin in the newborn infant. J Infect Dis 134:67–69

Cole DR, Pung J (1977) Penetration of cefazolin into pleural fluid. Antimicrob Agents Chemother 11:1033–1035

Cole M, Ridley B (1978) Absence of bioactive metabolites of ampicillin and amoxycillin in man. J Antimicrob Chemother 4:580–582

Cole M, Kenig MD, Hewitt VA (1973) Metabolism of penicillins to penicilloic acids and 6-aminopenicillanic acid in man and its significance in assessing penicillin absorption. Antimicrob Agents Chemother 3:463–468

Cooper MS, Anders MW, Mirkin BL (1973) Ion-pair extraction and high-speed liquid chromatography of cephalothin and desacetylcephalothin in human serum and urine. Drug Metab Dispos 1:659–662
Corbeel L, Van Acker G, Eeckels R, Vandepitte J, Verbist L (1979) Cefuroxime plasma and CSF levels in children with meningitis. Arch Dis Child 54:729–730
Craft I, Forster TC (1978) Materno-fetal cephradine transfer in pregnancy. Antimicrob Agents Chemother 14:924–926
Craig WA (1980) Single-dose pharmacokinetics of cefoperazone following intravenous administration. Clin Ther 3:46–49
Craig WA, Suh B (1978) Changes in protein binding during disease. Scand J Infect Dis [Suppl] 14:239–245
Craig WA, Welling PG, Jackson TC, Kunin CM (1973) Pharmacology of cefazolin and other cephalosporins in patients with renal insufficiency. J Infect Dis 128S:347–353
Currie JP (1976) Cephaloridine: pharmacology and toxicology. Postgrad Med J 43:S22:26
Curtis JR, Marshall MJ (1970) Cephaloridine serum levels in patients on maintenance hemodialysis. Br Med J 2:149–151
Cutler RE, Blair AD, Kelly MR (1979) Cefadroxil kinetics in patients with renal insufficiency. Clin Pharmacol Ther 25:514–521
Czerwinski AW, Pederson JA (1979) Pharmacokinetics of cefamandole in patients with renal impairment. Antimicrob Agents Chemother 15:161–164
Czerwinski AW, Pederson JA, Barry JP (1974) Cefazolin plasma concentrations and urinary excretion in patients with renal impairment. J Clin Pharmacol 14:560–566
Daikos GK, Kosmidis J, Stathakis C, Anyfantis A, Plakoutsis T, Papathanassiou B (1977a) Bioavailability of cefuroxime in various sites including bile, sputum and bone. Proc R Soc Med 70:S38–41
Daikos GK, Kosmimdis JC, Stathakis C, Giamarellou H (1977b) Cefuroxime: antimicrobial activity, human pharmacokinetics and therapeutic efficacy. J Antimicrob Chemother 3:555–562
Daikos GK, Giamarellou H, Hadjipolydorou K, Kanellakopaulou K (1979) Pseudomonas infections of the lung treated with azlocillin. Arzneimittelforsch 29 II:2001–2002
Daschner FD, Blume E, Langmaack H, Wolfart W (1979a) Cefamandole concentrations in pulmonary and subcutaneous tissue. J Antimicrob Chemother 5:474–475
Daschner FD, Langmaack H, Spillner G, Ahmadi A, Schlosser V (1979b) Penetration of cephradine into heart valves, subcutaneous tissue and muscle of patients undergoing open heart surgery. J Antimicrob Chemother 5:711–715
Davies JA, Holt JM (1972) Clinical pharmacology of cephalexin administered by intravenous injection. J Clin Pathol 25:518–510
Davies JA, Holt JM (1975) Absorption of cephalexin in diseased and aged subjects. J Antimicrob Chemother 1 (Suppl):9–70
Davies JA, Strangeways JEM, Holt JM (1970) Absorption of cephalexin from the gastrointestinal tract in disease subjects. Postgrad Med J 46S:16–19
Davis AE, Pirola RC (1968) Absorption of phenoxymethylpenicillin in patients with steatorrhoea. Australas Ann Med 17:63–65
Dean S, Harding LK, Wise R, Wright N (1979) Absorption and excretion of cephalexin in health and acute illness. Eur J Clin Pharmacol 16:73–74
De Felice EA (1967) Serum levels, urinary recovery, and safety of dicloxacillin, a new semisynthetic penicillin, in normal volunteers. J Clin Pharmacol 7:275–277
Dekel A, Elian I, Gibor Y, Goldman JA (1980) Transplacental passage of cefazolin in the first trimester of pregnancy. Eur J Obstet Gynecol Reprod Biol 10:303–307
Del Busto R, Haas E, Madhaven T, Burch K, Cox F, Fisher E, Quinn E, Pohlod D (1976) In vitro and clinical studies of cefatrizine, a new semisynthetic cephalosporin. Antimicrob Agents Chemother 9:397–405
Dell D, Ings RMJ (1978) The liquid chromatographic analysis and pharmacokinetics of the semi-synthetic cephalosporin 3-methyl-7-[4-(1,4,5,6-tetrahydro-2-pyrimidyl)-phenylacetamido]-Δ^3-cephalosporanic acid (I). Arzneimittelforsch 28:940–944
DeMaine JB, Kirby WMM (1971) Clinical pharmacology of cephalexin administered intravenously. In: Hobby GL (ed) Antimicrobial agents and chemotherapy – 1970. American Society for Microbiology, Bethesda, pp 190–194

Depp R, Kind AC, Kirby WMM, Johnson WL (1970) Transplacental passage of methicillin and dicloxacillin into the fetus and amniotic fluid. Am J Obstet Gynec 107:1054–1957
DeSchepper P, Harvengt C, Vranckx C, Boon B, Lamy F (1973) Pharmacologic study of cefazolin in volunteers. J Clin Pharmacol 13:83–88
Dettli L, Spring P, Lomar AV (1976) Über die Pharmakokinetik der Cephalosporine im Liquor cerebrospinalis. Infection 4:S195–202
Diaz CR, Kane JG, Parker RH, Pelsor FR (1977) Pharmacokinetics of nafcillin in patients with renal failure. Antimicrob Agents Chemother 12:98–101
Dittert LW, Griff WO Jr, LaPiana JC, Shainfeld FJ, Doluisio JT (1970) Pharmacokinetic interpretation of penicillin levels in serum and urine after intravenous administration. In: Hobby GL (ed) Antimicrobial agents and chemotherapy – 1969. American Society for Microbiology, Bethesda, pp 42–48
Dolan MM, Rhodes RE, Steelman RL, Stewart RC, Ferlauto RJ (1962) A new semisynthetic penicillin, SK&F 12141 II. Pharmacological Studies. In: Finland M, Savage GM (eds) Antimicrobial agents and chemotherapy – 1961. American Society for Microbiology, Bethesda, pp 655–660
Doluisio JT, LaPiana JC, Wilkinson GR, Dittert LW (1970) Pharmacokinetic interpretation of dicloxacillin levels in serum after extravascular administration. In: Hobby GL (ed) Antimicrobial agents and chemotherapy – 1969. American Society for Microbiology, Bethesda, pp 49–55
Doluisio JT, LaPiana JC, Dittert LW (1971) Pharmacokinetics of ampicillin trihydrate, sodium ampicillin, and sodium dicloxacillin following intramuscular injection. J Pharm Sci 60:715–719
Dorhofer G, Faigle JW (1976) Beitrag zur Biotransformation von Cephacetril im Menschen. Infection 4:S188–194
Dornbusch K, Hugo H, Lidstrom A (1980) Antibacterial activity of cefuroxime in human bone. Scand J Infect Dis 12:49–53
Douglas JG, Bax RP, Munro JF (1980) The pharmacokinetics of cefuroxime in the elderly. J Antimicrob Chemother 6:543–551
Duval J, Mora M, Chartier M, Mansour N (1972) La cephalexine: son transfert placentaire. Nouv Presse Med 1:1419–1420
Duval J, Mora M, Soussy CJ (1974) Pharmacocinetique d'une nouvelle cephalosporine: la cephacetrile taux seriques et urinaires chez l'adulte et le premature. Diffusion menengee et passage transplacentaire. Med Malad Infect 4:221–229
Dvoracek K, Modr Z, Schmidt O, Necaskova A (1974) Contribution to the pharmacokinetics of a new cephalosporin derivative. Arzneimittelforsch 24:1468–1470
Ehrnebo M (1978) Distribution of ampicillin in human whole blood. J Pharm Pharmacol 30:730–731
Ehrnebo M, Nilsson S-O, Boreus LO (1979) Pharmacokinetics of ampicillin and its prodrugs bacampicillin and pivampicillin in man. J Pharmacokinet Biopharm 7:429–451
Eickhoff TC, Kislak JW, Finland M (1965) Sodium ampicillin: absorption and excretion of intramuscular and intravenous doses in normal young men. Am J Med Sci 249:163–171
Elek E, Ivan E, Arr M (1972) Passage of penicillins from mother to foetus in humans. Int J Clin Pharmacol 6:223–228
Elias W, Price AH, Merrion HJ (1951) N, N[1]-Dibenzylethylenediamine penicillin: a new repositiory from of penicillin. Antibiot Chemother 1:491–498
Ellis CJ, Geddes AM, Davey PG, Wise R, Andrews JM, Grimley RP (1979) Mezlocillin and azlocillin: an evaluation of two new β-lactam antibiotics. J Antimicrob Chemother 5:517–525
English AR, McBride TJ (1962) Bacteriological comparison of 1- and d-phenethicillin. In: Finland M, Savage GM (eds) Antimicrobial agents and chemotherapy – 1961. American Society for Microbiology, Bethesda, pp 636–641
English AR, Huang HT, Sobia BA (1960)6-Amino-penicillanic acid in urine after oral administration of penicillins. Proc Soc Exp Biol Med 104:405–406
English AR, Retsema JA, Ray VA, Lynch JE (1972) Carbenicillin indanyl sodium, an orally active derivative of carbenicillin. Antimicrob Agents Chemother 1:185–191
Eshelman FN, Spyker DA (1978) Pharmacokinetics of amoxicillin and ampicillin: crossover study of the effect of food. Antimicrob Agents Chemother 14:539–543

Esumi Y, Otsuki T, Nanpo T (1979a) Studies on absorption, distribution, and excretion of cefadroxil. Jpn J Antibiot 32:1350–1355
Esumi Y, Otsuki M, Miwa A, Nanpo T (1979b) Absorption, distribution, metabolism, and excretion of ^{14}C-cefadroxil (^{14}C-BL-S 578) in rats. Jpn J Antibiot 32:1335–1349
Evans MAL, Wilson P, Leung T, Williams JD (1978) Pharmacokinetics of piperacillin following intravenous administration. J Antimicrob Chemother 4:255–261
Evans MAL, Leung T, Wilson P, Williams JD (1979) Pharmacokinetics of intravenously administered antibiotics: a study of piperacillin, a new semi-synthetic penicillin. Drugs Exp Clin Res 5:111–116
Fabre J, Burgy C, Rudhardt M, Herrera A (1972) The behavior in man of C.P. 15,464, a carbenicillin absorbed following oral administration. Chemotherapy 17:334–343
Fabre J, Allaz AF, Rudhardt M, Dayer P, Balant L (1980) Pharmacokinetics of cephalosporin T-1551 (Cefoperazone) in normal men and in men with renal failure, and behavior in tissues of rats. In: Nelson JD, Grassi C (eds) Current chemotherapy of infectious diseases: proceedings of the 11th international congress of chemotherapy – 1979. American Society for Microbiology, Washington, DC, pp 171–172
Farquhar JD, Dolan MM, Dorman MG, Ziv DS, Ferlauto RJ (1962) A new semi-synthetic penicillin, SK&F 12141 III. Laboratory and clinical evaluation. In: Finland M, Savage GM (eds) Antimicrobial agents and chemotherapy – 1961. American Society for Microbiology, Bethesda, pp 661–665
Feldman WE, Nelson JD, Stanberry LR (1978) Clinical and pharmacokinetic evaluation of nafcillin in infants and children. J Pediatr 93:1029–1033
Feldman WE, Moffitt S, Sprow N (1980) Clinical and pharmacokinetic evaluation of parenteral cefoxitin in infants and children. Antimicrob Agents Chemother 17:669–674
Fernandez CA, Menezes JP, Ximenes J (1973) The effect of food on the absorption of pivampicillin and a comparison with the absorption of ampicillin potassium. J Int Med Res 1:530–533
Ferrara A, Zanon P (1979) Pharmacokinetics of bacampicillin administered orally. Drug Exp Clin Res 5:189–195
Fiegel P, Becker K (1978) Pharmacokinetics of azlocillin in persons with normal and impaired renal functions. Antimicrob Agents Chemother 14:288–291
Fillastre JP, Leroy A, Godin M, Oksenhendler G, Humbert G (1978) Pharmacokinetics of cefoxitin sodium in normal subjects and in uraemic patients. J Antimicrob Chemother [Suppl B] 4:B79–83
Fillastre JP, Leroy A, Humbert G, Godin M (1980) Cefaclor pharmacokinetics and renal impairment. J Antimicrob Chemother 6:155–156
Finkelstein E, Quintiliani R, Lee R, Bracci A, Nightingale CH (1978) Pharmacokinetics of oral cephalosporins: Cephradine and cephalexin. J Pharm Sci 67:1447–1450
Fitzgerald Jr RH, Kelly PJ, Snyder RJ, Washington JA II (1978) Penetration of methicillin, oxacillin, and cephalothin into bone and synovial tissues. Antimicrob Agents Chemother 14:723–726
Flippin HF, Matteucci WV, Schimmel NH, Bartholomeu LE, Roger WP (1952) The hydroiodide of diethylaminoethyl ester of penicillin G, Neoperil I. A comparative study of plasma concentration and urinary recoveries with procaine penicillin. Antibiot Chemother 2:208–214
Foglesong MA, Lamb JW, Dietz JV (1978) Stability and blood level determinations of cefaclor, a new oral cephalosporin antibiotic. Antimicrob Agents Chemother 13:49–52
Foley TH, Jones NF, Barraclough MA, Cranston WI (1967) The renal excretion of cephaloridine in man. Postgrad Med J 43(S):85–87
Foltz EL, Graves BS, Rosenblatt A (1962) Comparison of two new derivatives of 6-aminopenicillanic acid with methicillin. In: Finland M, Savage GM (eds) Antimicrobial agents and chemotherapy – 1961. American Society for Microbiology, Bethesda, pp 568–574
Foltz EL, West JW, Brelow IH, Wallick H (1971) Clinical pharmacology of pivampicillin. In: Hobby GL (ed) Antimicrobial agents and chemotherapy – 1970. American Society for Microbiology, Bethesda, pp 442–454
Fong IW, Ralph ED, Engelking ER, Kirby WMM (1976) Clinical pharmacology of cefamandole as compared with cephalothin. Antimicrob Agents Chemother 9:65–69

Foord RD (1976) Cefuroxime: human pharmacokinetics. Antimicrob Agents Chemother 9:741–747
Fossieck JR BE, Kane JG, Diaz CR, Parker RH (1977) Nafcillin entry into human cerebrospinal fluid. Antimicrob Agents Chemother 11:965–967
Foster TS, Shrewsbury RP, Coonrod JD (1980) Bioavailability and pain study of cefamandole nafate. J. Clin Pharmacol 20:526–533
Franchi R, Perraro F (1967) Studio dell assorbiments e dell'eliminozione di un nuovo antibiotico a largo spetto (melampicillina). Atti Accad Med Lomb 22:543–553
Francke EL, Appel GB, Neu HC (1979a) Kinetics of intravenous amoxicillin in patients on long-term dialysis. Clin Pharmacol Ther 26:31–35
Francke EL, Mehta S, Neu HC, Appel GB (1979b) Kinetics of intravenous mezlocillin in chronic hemodialysis patients. Clin Pharmacol Ther 26:228–231
Francke EL, Appel GB, Neu HC (1979c) Pharmacokinetics of intravenous piperacillin in patients undergoing chronic hemodialysis. Antimicrob Agents Chemother 16:788–791
Friedman LA, Lewis PJ (1980) The effect of semisynthetic penicillins on the binding of bilirubin by neonatal serum. Br J Clin Pharmacol 9:61–65
Friedrich H, Haensel-Friedrich G, Langmaak H, Daschner F-D (1980) Investigations of cefuroxime levels in the cerebrospinal fluid of patients with and without meningitis. Chemother 26:92–97
Friedrich H, Pelz K, Hansel-Friedrich G (1979) Lack of penetration of cephacetril into the cerebro-spinal fluid of patients without meningitis. Infection 7:41–44
Fry W, Ximenes J, Siskin DB (1980) Concentrations of cephapirin sodium in plasma and gynecologic tissue after a single preoperative dose. Int J Clin Pharmacol Ther Toxicol 18:92–96
Fu KP, Aswapokee P, Ho I, Matthijssen C, Neu HC (1979) Pharmacokinetics of cefotaxime. Antimicrob Agents Chemother 16:592–597
Fujimoto M, Sakai K, Shiraha Y, Kawabata N, Doi S, Sawada A, Sasaki T, Maeda S, Masada A (1978) A clinical trial of CS-1170 in the field of surgery. Chemotherapy (Tokyo) 26(S-5):410–419
Fukaya K, Kitamoto O (1971) Pharmacokinetics of antimicrobial agents – on sulfobenzylpenicillin. Chemotherapy 19:910–919
Gadebusch HH, Miraglia GJ, Basch HI, Goodwin C:2Pan S, Renz K (1972) Cephradine – A new orally absorbed cephalosporin antibiotic. In: Hejzlar M, Semonsky M, Masak S (eds) Advances in antimicrobial and antineoplastic chemotherapy, vol 1. Proceedings of the VII international congress of chemotherapy – 1971. Urban and Schwarzenberg, Berlin, pp 1059–1062
Galvao PAA, Lomar AV, Francisco W, DeGodoy CVF, Norrby R (1980) Cefoxitin penetration into cerebrospinal fluid in patients with purulent meningitis. Antimicrob Agents Chemother 17:526–529
Gambertoglio JG, Aziz NS, Lin ET, Grausz H, Naughton JL, Benet LZ (1979) Cefamandole kinetics in uremic patients undergoing hemodialysis. Clin Pharmacol Ther 26:592–599
Gambertoglio JG, Barriere SL, Lin ET, Conte JE Jr, Benet LZ (1980) Pharmacokinetics of mecillinam in normals utilizing a specific high-pressure liquid chromatographic assay. Clin Pharmacol Ther 27:255–256
Garcia MJ, Dominguez-Gil A, Tabernero JM, Tomero JAS (1979a) Pharmacokinetics of cefoxitin in patients with normal or impaired renal function. Eur J Clin Pharmacol 16:119–124
Garcia MJ, Dominguez-Gil A, Tabernero JM, Roman AB (1979b) Pharmacokinetics of cefoxitin in patients undergoing hemodialysis. Int J Clin Pharmacol Biopharma 17:366–370
Garcia MJ, Dominguez-Gil AA, Cepeda M, Dominguez-Gil A (1980) Influence of experimental renal impairment in the pharmacokinetics of cefoxitin after intravenous administration to rabbits. Int J Pharm Amst 5:117–125
Gardner ME, Fritz WL, Hyland RN (1978) Antibiotic-induced seizures – a case attributed to cefazolin. Drug Intell Clin Pharmacol 12:268–271
Gau W, Horster FA (1979) Hochdruckflüssigkeits-chromatographische Analyse von Azlocillin und seinem Penicilloat im Urin. Arzneimittelforsch 29 II:1941–1943

Gaver RC, Deeb G (1980) Disposition of ^{14}C-cefatrizine in man. Drug Metab Dispos 8:157–162
Geddes AM, Schnurr LP, Ball AP, McGhie D, Brookes GR, Wise R, Andrews J (1977) Cefoxitin: a hospital study. Br Med J 1:1126–1128
Geddes AM, McGhie D, Ball AP, Gould I (1978) Studies with cefuroxime and cefoxitin. Scand J Infect Dis [Suppl] 13:78–81
Gibaldi M, Schwartz MA (1968) Apparent effect of probenecid on the distribution of penicillins in man. Clin Pharmacol Ther 9:345–349
Gibaldi M, Davidson D, Plaut ME, Schwartz MA (1970) Modification of penicillin distribution and elimination by probenecid. Int J Clin Pharmacol 3:182–189
Giebel W, Schonleber KH, Breuninger H, Ullman U (1978) A comparison of the pharmacokinetics in serum and nasal secretions after oral becampicillin and ampicillin. Scand J Infect Dis [Suppl] 14:285–287
Gillett AP, Wise R (1978) Penetration of four cephalosporins into tissue fluid in man. Lancet 1:962–964
Ginsburg CM, McCracken Jr GH (1979) Pharmacokinetics of cephradine suspension in infants and children. Antimicrob Agents Chemother 16:74–76
Ginsburg CM, McCracken GH Jr, Clahsen JC, Thomas ML (1978) Clinical pharmacology of cefadroxil in infants and children. Antimicrob Agents Chemother 13:845–848
Ginsburg CM, McCracken Jr GH, Thomas ML, Clahsen J (1979) Comparative pharmacokinetics of amoxicillin and ampicillin in infants and children. Pediatrics 64:627–631
Glynne A, Goulbourn A, Ryden R (1978) A human pharmacology study of cefaclor. J Antimicrob Chemother 4:343–348
Goodwin CS, Raftery EB, Goldberg AD, Skeggs H, Till AE, Martin CM (1974) Effects of rate of infusion and probenecid on serum levels, renal excretion, and tolerance of intravenous doses of cefoxitin in humans: Comparison with cephalothin. Antimicrob Agents Chemother 6:338–346
Goodwin CS, Dash CH, Hill JP, Goldberg AD (1977) Cefuroxime: pharmacokinetics after a short infusion, and in vitro activity against hospital pathogens. J Antimicrob Chemother 3:253–261
Gordon RC, Barrett FF, Clark DJ, Yow MD (1971) Laboratory and pharmacologic studies of BL-P-1322 (cephapirin sodium) in children. Curr Ther Res 13:398–406
Gordon RC, Regamey C, Kirby WMM (1972) Comparative clinical pharmacology of amoxicillin and ampicillin administered orally. Antimicrob Agents Chemother 1:504–507
Goto S (1977) The in vitro and in vivo antibacterial activity of cefuroxime. Proc R Soc Med [Suppl 9] 70:56–62
Gourevitch A, Wolfe S, Lein J (1962) Effects of side chain configuration on the activity of certain semisynthetic penicillins. In: Finland M, Savage GM (eds) Antimicrobial agents and chemotherapy – 1961. American Society for Microbiology, Bethesda, pp 576–580
Gower PE, Dash CH (1969) Cephalexin: human studies of absorption and excretion of a new cephalosporin antibiotic. Br J Pharmacol 37:738–747
Gower PE, Dash CH (1977) The pharmacokinetics of cefuroxime after intravenous injection. Eur J Clin Pharmacol 12:221–227
Gower PE, Dash CH, O'Callaghan CH (1973) Serum and blood concentration of sodium cephalexin in man given single intramuscular and intravenous injections. J Pharm Pharmacol 25:376–381
Gower PE, Kennedy MRK, Dash CH (1977) The effect of renal failure and dialysis on the pharmacokinetics of cefuroxime. Proc R Soc Med [Suppl 9] 70:150–157
Graber H, Perenyi T, Arr M, Ludwig E (1976) On human biotransformation of some penicillins. Int J Clin Pharmacol 14:284–289
Granetek ES (1963) N-Methylol-α-amino-benzylpenicillin. U.S. Patent No. 3,198,788
Grassi GG, Dionigi R, Ferrara A, Pozzi E (1980) Penetration of HGR-756 (cefotaxime) in lung tissue and bronchial secretions. In: Nelson JD, Grassi C (eds) Current chemotherapy of infectious diseases: proceedings of the 11th international congress of chemotherapy – 1979. American Society for Microbiology, Washington, DC, pp 120–121
Greene DS, Tice AD (1977) Effect of hemodialysis on cefazolin protein binding. J Pharm Sci 66:1508–1510

Greene DS, Flanagan DR, Quintiliani R, Nightingale CH (1976) Pharmacokinetics of cephalexin: An evaluation of one- and two-compartment model pharmacokinetics. J Clin Pharmacol 16:257–264
Greene DS, Quintiliani R, Thompson MA, Nightingale CH (1977) Effect of probenecid on the renal clearance of cefamandole. Curr Ther Res Clin Exp 22:737–740
Griffith RS, Black HR (1964) Cephalothin – a new antibiotic. JAMA 189:823–828
Griffith RS, Black HR (1971) Blood, urine and tissue concentrations of the cephalosporin antibiotics in normal subjects. Postgrad Med J [Suppl] 32–40
Griffith RS, Black HR, Brier GL, Wolny JD (1976) Cefamandole: in vitro and clinical pharmacokinetics. Antimicrob Agents Chemother 10:814–823
Grose WE, Bodey GP, Stewart D (1976) Observations in man on some pharmacologic features of cefamandole. Clin Pharmacol Ther 20:579–584
Grossman M, Ticknor W (1966) Serum levels of ampicillin, cephalothin, cloxacillin, and nafcillin in the newborn infant. In: Hobby GL (ed) Antimicrobial agents and chemotherapy – 1965. American Society for Microbiology, Bethesda, pp 214–219
Halprin GM, McMahon SM (1973) Cephalexin concentrations in sputum during acute respiratory infections. Antimicrob Agents Chemother 3:703–707
Haginaka J, Nakagawa T, Uno T (1979) Acidic degradation of cephaloglycin and high performance liquid chromatographic determination of deacetylcephaloglycin in human urine. J Antibiot 32:462–467
Haginaka J, Nakagawa T, Uno T (1980) Chromatographic analysis and pharmacokinetic investigation of cephaloglycin and its metabolites in man. J Antibiot 33:236–243
Hamilton-Miller JMT, Brumfitt W (1979) The bioavailability of four commercially available brands of ampicillin compared with that of talampicillin. J Antimicrob Chemother 5:699–704
Hansson E, Magni L, Wahlguist S (1968) α-Azidobenzylpenicillin II. Preliminary clinical pharmacol. In: Hobby GL (ed) Antimicrobial agents and chemotherapy – 1967. American Society for Microbiology, Bethesda, pp 568–572
Harada Y, Matsubara S, Kamimoto M, Noto T, Nehashi T, Kimura T, Suzuki S, Ogawa H, Koyama K (1976) Ceftezole, a new cephalosporin C derivative II. Distribution and excretion in parenteral administration. J Antibiot 29:1071–1082
Harding SM (1980) Cefuroxime: therapeutic success – clinical experience. Praxis 69:729–741
Harding SM, Eilon LA, Harris AM (1979) Factors affecting the intramuscular absorption of cefuroxime. J Antimicrob Chemother 5:87–93
Hartstein AI, Patrick KE, Jones SR, Miller MJ, Bryant RE (1977) Comparison of pharmacological and antimicrobial properties of cefadroxil and cephalexin. Antimicrob Agents Chemother 12:93–97
Harvengt C, De Schepper P, Lamy F, Hansen J (1973) Cephradine absorption and excretion in fasting and nonfasting volunteers. J Clin Pharmacol 13:36–40
Harvengt C, Meunier H, Lamy F (1977) Pharmacokinetic study of cefazaflur compared to cephalothin and cefazolin. J Clin Pharmacol 17:128–133
Hattori M, Nishi K, Miyabayashi T (1977) Metabolites of pivmecillinam in human urine. Chemotherapy (Tokyo) 25:123–126
Heathcote AGJ, Nassau E (1951) Concentration of penicillin in the lungs: effects of two penicillin esters in chronic pulmonary infection. Lancet 1:1255–1256
Heimann G, von Heereman B, Gladtke E (1979) Pharmacokinetik von Azlocillin bei Früh- und Neugeborenen. Arzneimittelforsch 29(II):1949–1951
Hekster YA, Vree TB, Von Dalen R, Van der Kleijn E (1980) Pharmacokinetics of cefuroxime and cefoxitin in normal, impaired and probenecid functionally impaired kidney function. In: Nelson JD, Grassi C (eds), Current chemotherapy and infectious disease: proceedings of the 11th international congress of chemotherapy – 1979. American Society for Microbiology, Washington DC, pp 570–572
Hellström K, Rosen A, Swahn Å (1974a) Fate of oral ^{35}S-cloxacillin in man. Europ J Clin Pharmacol 7:125–131
Hellström K, Rosen A, Swahn Å (1974b) Absorption and decomposition of potassium ^{35}S-phenoxymethyl penicillin. Clin Pharmacol Ther 16:826–833

Henegar GC, Silverman M, Gardner RJ, Kukral JC, Preston FW (1962) Excretion of methicillin in human bile. In: Finland M, Savage GM (eds) Antimicrobial agents and chemotherapy – 1961. American Society for Microbiology, Bethesda, pp 348–351

Henness DM, Richards D, Santella PF, Rubinfeld F (1978) Oral bioavailability of cefadroxil, a new semisynthetic cephalosporin. Clin Ther 1:263–273

Hertz CG (1973) Serum and urinary concentrations of cyclacillin in humans. Antimicrob Agents Chemother 4:361–365

Hess JR, Berman SJ, Boughton WH, Sugihara JG, Musgrave JE, Wong EGC, Siemsen AM (1980) Pharmacokinetics of ceforanide in patients with end stage renal disease on hemodialysis. Antimicrob Agents Chemother 17:251–253

Hey H, Matzen P, Andersen JT (1979) A gastroscopic and pharmacological study of the disintegration time and absorption of pivampicillin capsules and tablets. Br J Clin Pharmacol 8:237–242

Hierholzer G, Linzenmeier G, Kleining R, Horster G (1974) Vergleichende Untersuchungen über die Konzentration von Cephacetril und Cephalotin im normalen und chronisch entzündeten Knochengewebe. Arzneimittelforsch 24:1501–1504

Hineno T, Yamaguchi K, Itoh N, Mita T, Ishigami J (1978) Laboratory and clinical studies on CS-1170 for urinary tract infection. Chemotherapy (Tokyo) 26(S-5):487–500

Hiner LB, Baluarte HJ, Polinsky MS, Gruskin AB (1980) Cefazolin in children with renal insufficiency. J Pediatr 96:335–339

Hinthorn DR, Liu C, Hodges GR, Dworzack DL, Rosett W, Harms J (1978) Cefoxitin. Cerebrospinal fluid penetration of cefoxitin and experience in treatment of bacterial infections. In: Siegenthaler W, Luthy R (eds) Current chemotherapy: proceedings of the 10th international congress of chemotherapy, 1977. American Society for Microbiology, Washington, DC, vol 2, pp 757–758

Hirabayashi K, Okada E, Okamoto T, Fukunaga M (1978) Fundamental and clinical studies on CS-1170 in the field of obstetrics and gynecology. Chemotherapy (Tokyo) 26(S-5):575–581

Hirsch HA, Herbst S, Lang R, Dettli L, Gablinger A (1974) Transfer of a new cephalosporin antibiotic to the foetus and the amniotic fluid during a continuous infusion (steady state) and single repeated intravenous injections to the mother. Arzneimittelforsch 24:1474–1478

Hirtz J, Lecaillon J-B, Gerardin A, Schoeller J-P, Humbert G, Guibert J (1980) Pharmacokinetics of a new cephalosporin, CGP 9000, in humans. In: Nelson JD, Grassi C (eds) Current chemotherapy of infectious diseases: proceedings of the 11th international congress of chemotherapy – 1979. American Society for Microbiology, Washington, DC, pp 211–213

Hitzenberger G, Jaschek I (1974) Comparative studies on the absorption of ampicillin trihydrate and potassium ampicillin. Int J Clin Pharmacol 9:114–119

Hitzenberger G, Jaschek I (1980) Pharmacokinetics and tolerance of cefazedone compared with cefazolin. Wien Med Wochenschr 130:135–142

Hobbs DC (1972) Metabolism of indanyl carbenicillin by dogs, rats, and humans. Antimicrob Agents Chemother 2:272–275

Hodges GR, Liu C, Hinthorn DR, Harms JL, Dworzack DL (1978) Pharmacological evaluation of cefaclor in volunteers. Antimicrob Agents Chemother 14:454–456

Hoehn MM, Pugh CT (1968) Method for the detection and quantitative assay of cephaloglycin and its biologically active metabolites. Appl Microbiol 16:1132–1133

Hoehn MM, Murphy HW, Pugh CT, Davis NE (1970) Paper chromatographic techniques for the determination of cephalothin and desacetylcephalothin in body fluids. Appl Microbiol 20:734–736

Hoffler D, Dalhoff A (1980) Pharmacokinetics of clavulanic acid in patients with normal and impaired renal function. In: Nelson JD, Grassi C (eds) Current chemotherapy of infectious diseases: proceedings of the 11th international congress of chemotherapy – 1979. American Society for Microbiology, Washington, DC, pp 322–323

Hoffler D, Koeppe P (1975) Zur Pharmakokinetik intravenös applizierten Cefradins. Muench Med Wochenschr 117:1169–1173

Hoffler D, Moecke D, Sassmann M (1978) Cefamandol: Pharmacokinetics with normal and impaired renal function. Dtsch Med Wochenschr 103:1334–1338
Hoffman TA, Cestero R, Bullock WE (1970) Pharmacokinetics of carbenicillin in patients with hepatic and renal failure. J Infect Dis [Suppl] 122:75–77
Holt HA, Broughall JM, Fullhaas J, Bint AJ, Reeves DS (1978) Multidose human pharmacology of CGP 9000 in volunteers. In: Siegenthaler W, Luthy R (eds) Current Chemotherapy: proceedings of the 10th international congress of chemotherapy – 1977. American Society for Microbiology, Washington, DC, pp 829–830
Hottendorf GH, Price KE, Van Harken DR (1975) Comparative plasma bactericidal activity of cephapirin and cefazolin. Curr Ther Res 18:364–370
Howell A, Sutherland R, Rolinson CN (1972) Penetration of ampicillin and cloxacillin into synovial fluid and the significance of protein binding on drug distribution. Ann Rheum Dis 31:538–540
Hughes SPF, Benson MKD, Dash CH, Field CA (1975) Cephaloridine penetration into bone and synovial capsule of patients undergoing hip joint replacement. J Antimicrob Chemother [Suppl] 1:41–46
Hultberg ER, Backelin B (1972) Studies on the absorption of pivampicillin and ampicillin. Scand J Infect Dis 4:149–153
Humbert G, Fillastre J-P, Leroy A (1975) La demi-vie plasmatique de la cefazoline. Nouv Med 4:2525–2526
Humbert G, Fillastre JP, Leroy A, Godin M, Van Winzum C (1979a) Pharmacokinetics of cefoxitin in normal subjects and in patients with renal insufficiency. Rev Infect Dis 1:118–125
Humbert G, Leroy A, Fillastre JP, Godin M (1979b) Pharmacokinetics of cefadroxil in normal subjects and in patients with renal insufficiency. Chemotherapy 25:189–195
Humbert G, Spyker D, Fillastre JP, Leroy A (1979c) Pharmacokinetics of amoxicillin: dosage nomogram for patients with impaired renal function. Antimicrob Agents Chemother 15:28–33
Humbert G, Leroy A, Rogez J-P, Cherubin C (1980) Cefoxitin concentrations in the cerebrospinal fluids of patients with meningitis. Antimicrob Agents Chemother 17:675–678
Husson GS (1947) Oral penicillin in infants. J Pediatr 31:651–657
Indelicato JM, Wilham WL, Cerimele BJ (1976) Conversion of cefamandole nafate to cefamandole sodium. J Pharm Sci 65:1175–1178
Ingold A (1976) Conversion of benzylpenicillin to penicilloic acid in patients with chronic bronchial infections. Chemotherapy 22:88–96
Intoccia AP, Walkenstein SS, Jospeh G, Wittendorf R, Girman C, Walz DT, Actor P, Weisbach J (1978) Distribution in normal and inflammatory tissue of a new semisynthetic cephalosporin SK&F 75073. J Antibiot 31:1188–1194
Irmer W, Lubach D, Sucker U (1971) Cephalexin determination in serum, urine, bile, peritoneal exudate, and marrow. Dtsch Med Wochenschr 96:464–468
Ishii T, Yokoyama T, Kishi D, Ichikawa T, Takeda M, Furomoto F (1978) Fundamental and clinical studies on CS-1170 in surgical field. Chemotherapy (Tokyo) 26(S-5):420–424
Ishiyama S, Nakayama I, Imamoto H, Iwai S, Okui M, Matsubara T (1971) Absorption tissue concentration, and organ distribution of cefazolin. In: Hobby GL (ed) Antimicrobial agents and chemotherapy – 1970. American Society for Microbiology, Bethesda, pp 476–480
Ishiyama S, KawakamiI, Nakayama I, Iwamoto H, Iwai S, Oshima T, Takatori M, Kawabe T, Suzuki K, Murakami F (1971) Laboratory and clinical evaluation of sulfobenzylpenicillin (SB-PC). Chemotherapy 19:988–998
Ishiyama S, Nakayama I, Iwamoto H, Iwai S, Sakata I, Murata I, Mizuashi H (1976) A comparative study of ceftezol (demethyl-cefazolin) and cefazolin: absorption, distribution, and metabolism. In: Williams JD, Geddes AM (eds) Chemotherapy, vol 5. Plenum, New York, pp 241–246
Ishiyama S, Nakayama I, Iwamoto H, Iwai S, Takotori M, Kawabe T, Akieda Y, Ohashi M, Murata I, Mizuashi H (1978) Studies on CS-1170 in surgery – antibacterial activity, pharmacokinetics, tissue distribution, metabolism and its clinical application. Chemotherapy (Tokyo) 26(S-5):381–393

Israel KS, Black HR, Griffith RS, Birer GL, Wolvy JD (1980) Pharmacology of LY 127935 (Shionogi compound 6059-S) in humans. In: Nelson JD, Grassi C (eds) Current chemotherapy of infectious diseases: proceedings of the 11th international congress of chemotherapy – 1979. American Society for Microbiology, Washington, DC, pp 107–108

Issell BF, Bodey GP, Weaver S (1978) Clinical pharmacology of mezlocillin. Antimicrob Agents Chemother 13:180–183

Ivan E, Arr M, Földi (1972) The change in serum, urine and renal tissue levels after administration of various doses of carbenicillin. Int J Clin Pharmacol 6:320–323

Iwai N, Sasaki A, Miyazu M, Osuga T, Inokuma K (1980) A study of cefotaxime in the field of pediatrics. Chemotherapy (Tokyo) [Suppl] 28:509–534

Janssen FW, Young EM, Ruelius HW (1976) Effect of sex hormones on the disposition in rats of 1-aminocyclohexane carboxylic acid, a metabolite of a semisynthetic penicillin. Drug Metab Dispos 4:540–546

Jeffery DJ, Jones KH, Langley PF (1978) The metabolism of talampicillin in rat, dog and man. Xenobiotica 8:419–427

Jensen KA, Dragsted PJ, Kiaer I, Neilsen EJ, Fredericksen E (1951) Leocillin (benzylpenicillin β-diethylaminoethyl ester hydroiodide). Acta Pathol Microbiol Scand 28:407–414

Johnson BE, Sabath LD (1979) Effect of pH on the protein binding of penicillins and cephalosporins. Clin Res 27:718A

Johnson WP, Applestein JM, Kaye D (1968) Cephaloglycin. JAMA 206:2698–2702

Jolly ER, Henness DM, Richards D (1977) Human safety, tolerance, and pharmacokinetic studies of cefadroxil, a new cephalosporin antibiotic for oral administration. Curr Ther Res Clin Exp 22:727–736

Jones KH, Langley PF, Lees LJ (1978) Bioavailability and metabolism of talampicillin. Chemotherapy 24:217–226

Jordan MC, DeMaine JB, Kirby WMM (1971) Clinical pharmacology of pivampicillin as compared with ampicillin. In: Hobby GL (ed) Antimicrobial agents and Chemotherapy – 1970. American Society for Microbiology, Bethesda, pp 438–441

Jusko WJ, Gibaldi M (1972) Effect of change in elimination on various parameters of the two-compartment open model. J Pharm Sci 61:1270–1273

Jusko WJ, Lewis GP (1972) Precaution in pharmacokinetic evaluation of ampicillin precursors. Lancet 1:690–691

Jusko WJ, Lewis GP (1973) Comparison of ampicillin and hetacillin pharmacokinetics in man. J Pharm Sci 62:69–76

Jusko WJ, Lewis GP, Schmitt GW (1973) Ampicillin and hetacillin pharmacokinetics in normal and anephric subjects. Clin Pharmacol Ther 14:90–99

Jusko WJ, Mosovich LL, Gerbracht LM, Mattar ME, Yaffe SJ (1975) Enhanced renal excretion of dicloxacillin in patients with cystic fibrosis. Pediatrics 56:1038–1044

Kabins SA, Cohen S (1966) Cephaloridine therapy as related to renal function. In: Hobby GL (ed) Antimicrobial agents and chemotherapy – 1965. American Society for Microbiology, Bethesda, pp 922–932

Kampffmeyer HG, Hartmann I, Metz H, Breault GO, Skeggs HR, Till AE, Weidner L (1975) Serum concentrations of ampicillin and probenecid and ampicillin excretion after repeated oral administration of a pivampicillin-probenecid salt (MK-356). Eur J Clin Pharmacol 9:125–129

Kampmann J, Molholm Hansen J, Siersbaek-Nielsen K, Laursen H (1972) Effect of some drugs on penicillin half-life in blood. Clin Pharmacol Ther 13:516–519

Kampmann J, Lindahl F, Molholm Hansen J, Siersbaek-Nielsen K (1973) Effect of probenecid on the excretion of ampicillin in human bile. Br J Pharmacol 47:782–786

Kawada Y (1979) Profile of cefmetazole. II. Absorption, excretion, distribution and metabolism. Kansenshogaku Zasshi 53:66–74

Kawada Y (1980) Pharmacokinetic studies on cefmetazole, a new cephamycin derivative. In: Nelson JD, Grassi C (eds) Current chemotherapy of infectious diseases: proceedings of the 11th international congress of chemotherapy – 1979. American Society for Microbiology, Washington, DC, pp 231–232

Kawamura N, Sameshima M, Murakami Y, Ohkoshi M (1978) Study on CS-1170 in the field of urology. Chemotherapy (Tokyo) 26(S-5):457–461

Kaye D, Wenger N, Agarwal B (1978) Pharmacology of intraperitoneal cefazolin in patients undergoing peritoneal dialysis. Antimicrob Agents Chemother 14:318–321
Kemmerich B, Lode H, Gruhlke G, Dzwillo G, Koeppe P, Wagner I (1980) Clinical pharmacology of cefotaxime in bronchopulmonary infections. In: Nelson JD, Grassi C (eds) Current chemotherapy of infectious diseases: proceedings of the 11th international congress of chemotherapy – 1979. American Society for Microbiology, Washington, DC, pp 130–132
Kester RC, Ramsden CH, Matharu SS (1979) The penetrability of cephazolin into the subcutaneous fat and skeletal muscle of ischaemic lower limbs with atherosclerotic disease. Curr Med Res Opin 6:44–49
Kienel VG (1976) Vergleich der Pharmakokinetik von Epicillin und Ampicillin. Arzneimittelforsch 26:781–789
Kikuchi H, Seno T, Tamura S, Yamamoto T, Nabeshima K, Sugimoto T, Otsuru N, Horai Z, Sumi K (1980) Studies on ceftezole in human sputum. Jpn J Antibiot 33:554–557
Kind AC, Kestle DG, Standiford HC, Kirby WMM (1969) Laboratory and clinical experience with cephalexin. In: Hobby GL (ed) Antimicrobial agents and Chemotherapy – 1968. American Society for Microbiology, Bethesda, pp 361–365
KindAC, Tupasi TE, Standiford HC, Kirby WMM (1970) Mechanisms responsible for plasma levels of nafcillin lower than those of oxacillin. Arch Intern Med 125:685–690
Kirby WMM, Kind AC (1967) Clinical pharmacology of ampicillin and hetacillin. Ann NY Acad Sci 145:291–297
Kirby WMM, Regamey C (1973) Pharmacokinetics of cefazolin compared with four other cephalosporins. J Infect Dis 128:S341–346
Kirby WMM, DeMaine JB, Serrill WC (1971) Pharmacokinetics of the cephalosporins in healthy volunteers and uremic patients. Postgrad Med J S41–46
Kishi H, Miyamura R, Nishimura Y, Koiso K, Niijima T (1978) Laboratory and clinical evaluations of CS-1170 in the field of urology. Chemotherapy (Tokyo) 26(S-5):447–456
Kislak JW, Steinhauer BW, Finland M (1966) Cephaloridine activity in vitro and absorption and urinary excretion in normal young men. Am J Med Sci 251:433–447
Kiss J, Farago E, Fabian E (1974) Study of oxacillin levels in human serum and lung tissue. Ther Hung 22:55–59
Kiss JI, Farago E, Comory A, Kiss B, Varhelyi I (1977) Human pharmacokinetics of cephacetrile (Celospor). Curr Chemother 1:392–393
Kjaer TB, Welling PG, Madsen PO (1977) Pharmacokinetics of ampicillin and the methoxymethyl ester of hetacillin in dogs. J Pharm Sci 66:345–347
Klein JO, Eickhoff TC, Tilles JG, Finland M (1964) Cephalothin: activity in vitro, absorption and excretion in normal subjects and clinical observations on 40 patients. Am J Med Sci 248:640–656
Klein JO, Finland M (1963a) Ampicillin activity in vitro and absorption and excretion in normal young men. Am J Med Sci 245:544–555
Klein JO, Finland M (1963b) Nafcillin; antimicrobial action in vitro and absorption and excretion in normal young men. Am J Med Sci 246:10–26
Knirsch AK, Hobbs DC, Korst JJ (1973) Pharmacokinetics, toleration, and safety of indanyl carbenicillin in man. J Infect Dis [Suppl] 127:105–108
Knudsen ET, Rolinson GN, Stevens Å (1961) Absorption and excretion of "penbritin". Br Med J 2:198–200
Kobyletzki von D, Reither K, Gellen J, Kanyo A, Glocke M (1974) Pharmakokinetische Untersuchungen mit Cefazolin in Geburtshilfe und Gynäkologie. Infection [Suppl 1] 2:60–67
Kobyletzki von D, Sas M, Dingeldein E, Wahlig H, Wiemann H (1979) Pharmacokinetic investigations of cefazedone in gynaecology and obstetrics. Arzneimittelforsch 29:1763–1768
Koerner F, Jaeschke B (1974) A preliminary report of the estimation of cephalexin in human serum, fat tissue, muscle tissue and epididymis. Int J Clin Pharmacol Ther Toxicol [Suppl] 8:42–43
Kohonen A, Paavolainen M, Renkoven OV (1975) Concentration of cephalexin in maxillary sinus mucosa and secretion. Ann Clin Res 7:50–53

Kornguth ML, Kunin CM (1976a) Uptake of antibiotics by human erythrocytes. J Infect Dis 133:175–184
Kornguth ML, Kunin CM (1976b) Binding of antibiotics to the human intracellular erythrocyte proteins hemoglobin and carbonic anhydrase. J Infect Dis 133:185–193
Korzeniowski OM, Scheld WM, Sande MA (1977) Comparative pharmacology of cefaclor and cephalexin. Antimicrob Agents Chemother 12:157–162
Korzeniowski OM, Carvalho Jr EM, Rocha H, Sande MA (1978) Evaluation of cefamandole therapy of patients with bacterial meningitis. J Infect Dis 137:S169–179
Kosmidis J, Stathakis C, Anyfantis A, Daikos GK (1977) Cefuroxime in renal insufficiency: therapeutic results in various infections and pharmacokinetics including the effects of dialysis. Proc Soc Med [Suppl 9] 70:139–143
Kosmidis J, Pragastis D, Athanassiou A, Daikos GK (1978) Cefatrizine: clinical efficacy, human pharmacokinetics, and in vitro activity. In: Siegenthaler W, Luthy R (eds) Current chemotherapy: proceedings of the 10th international congress of chemotherapy – 1977. American Society for Microbiology, Washington, DC, pp 750–752
Kosmidis J, Doundoulaki P, Stathakis Ch, Zerefos N, Bounia A, Daikos GK (1979) Elimination kinetics of mezlocillin in normal and impaired renal function including the effects of dialysis. Arzneimittelforsch 29 II:1960–1962
Kratochvil P, Brandstatter G, Adam D, Koch E (1979) Biliare Elimination von Cefazedon. Muench Med Wochenschr 121:497–498
Kunin CM (1966) Therapeutic implications of serum protein binding of new semi-synthetic penicillins. In: Hobby GL (ed) Antimicrobial agents and chemotherapy – 1965. American Society for Microbiology, Bethesda, pp 1025–1033
Kunin CM (1966a) Clinicalpharmacology of the new penicillins. I. The importance of serum protein binding in determining antimicrobial activityand concentration in serum. Clin Pharmacol Ther 7:166–179
Kunin CM (1966b) Clinical pharmacolgy of the new penicillins. II. Effect of drugs which interfere with binding to serum proteins. Clin Pharmacol Ther 7:180–188
Kurihara J, Matsumoto K, Uzuka Y, Shishido H, Nagatake T, Yamada H, Yoshida T, Oguma T, Kimura Y, Tochino Y (1980) Human pharmacokinetics of 6059-S. In: Nelson JD, Grassi C (eds) Current chemotherapy of infectious diseases: proceedings of the 11th international congress of chemotherapy – 1979. American Society for Microbiology, Washington, DC, pp 110–111
Kuzemko JA, Walker SR (1979) Cefuroxime plasma and CSF levels in children with meningitis. Arch Dis Child 54:235–236
Landesman SH, Corrado ML, Cherubin CC, Gombert M, Cleri D (1980) Diffusion of a new beta-lactam (LY 127935) into cerebrospinal fluid. Am J Med 69:92–98
Lane AZ, Chudzik GM, Siskin SB (1977) Comparative pharmacokinetic studies of cephapirin and cephalothin following intravenous and intramuscular administration. Curr Ther Res Clin Exp 21:117–127
Lecaillon JB, Hirtz JL, Schoeller JP, Humbert G, Vischer W (1980) Pharmacokinetic comparison of cefroxadin (CGP 9000) and cephalexin by simultaneous administration to humans. Antimicrob Agents Chemother 18:656–660
Lee CC, Anderson RC (1962) Absorption, distribution, and excretion of L-α-phenoxypropyl, D-α-phenoxypropyl, DL-α-phenoxyethyl, and phenoxymethyl penicillins. In: Finland M, Savage GM (eds) Antimicrobial agents and chemotherapy – 1961. American Society for Microbiology, Bethesda, pp 555–567
Lee CC, Herr EB, Anderson RC (1963) Pharmacological and toxicological studies on cephalothin. Clin Med 70:1123–1138
Lee FH, Pfeffer M, Van Harken DR, Smyth RD, Hottendorf GH (1980) Comparative pharmacokinetics of ceforanide (BL-S786R) and cefazolin in laboratory animals and humans. Antimicrob Agents Chemother 17:188–192
Lee RD, Brusch JL, Barza MJ, Weinstein L (1975) Effect of probenecid on penetration of oxacillin into fibrin clots in vitro. Antimicrob Agents Chemother 8:105–106
Leitner F, Buck RE, Misiek M, Pursiano T, Price KE (1975) BL-S640, a cephalosporin with a broad spectrum of antibacterial activity: properties in vitro. Antimicrob Agents Chemother 7:298–305

Leopold G, Ungethüm W, Pabst J, Dingeldein E (1977) Pharmacokinetics of cefazedone, a new cephalosporin antibiotic, in humans. Curr Chemother 2:831–832
Lerner PI (1969) Penetration of cephalothin and lincomycin into the cerebrospinal fluid. Am J Med Sci 257:125–131
Lerner PI (1971) Penetration of cephaloridine into cerebrospinal fluid. Am J Med Sci 262:321–326
Leroy A, Canonne MA, Fillastre JP, Humbert G (1974) Pharmacokinetics of cefazolin, a new cephalosporin antibiotic in normal and uraemic patients. Curr Ther Res Clin Exp 16:878–889
Leroy A, Fillastre JP, Oksenhendler G, Humbert G (1977) Pharmacokinetics of cefamandole in normal subjects and in uraemic patients. Drugs Exp Clin Res 3:51–59
Leroy A, Humbert G, Godin M, Fillastre JP (1980) Pharmacokinetics of azlocillin in subjects with normal and impaired renal function. Antimicrob Agents Chemother 17:344–349
Lev-El A, Newby J, Dubna J, Katznelson A, Rubinstein E (1980) Cefuroxime concentrations in blood and joint fluid. In: Nelson JD, Grassi C (eds) Current chemotherapy of infectious diseases: proceedings of the 11th international congress of chemotherapy – 1979. American Society for Microbiology, Washington, DC, pp 664–665
Levison ME, Levison SP, Ries K, Kaye D (1973) Pharmacology of cefazolin in patients with normal and abnormal renal function. J Infect Dis 128:S354–357
Levison ME, Santoro J, Agarwal BN (1979) In vitro activity and pharmacokinetics of cefaclor in normal volunteers and patients with renal failure. Postgrad Med J [Suppl 4] 55:12–16
Levy G (1967) Effect of bed rest on distribution and elimination of drugs. J Pharm Sci 56:928–929
Libke RD, Clarke JT, Ralph ED, Luthy RP, Kirby WMM (1975) Ticarcillin vs carbenicillin: clinical pharmacokinetics. Clin Pharmacol Ther 17:441–446
Litvak AS, Franks CS, Vaught SK, McRoberts JW (1976) Cefazolin and cephalexin levels in prostatic tissue and sera. Urology 7:497–499
Little PJ, Peddie BA (1974) Absorption and excretion of amoxycillin and pivampicillin, two new semisynthetic pivampicillins. Med J Aust 2:598–600
Llorens-Terol J, Lobato A, Adam D (1979) Treatment of childhood meningitis with mezlocillin. Arzneimittelforsch 29 II:2001–2002
Lode H, Janisch P, Küpper, Weuta H (1974) Comparative clinical pharmacology of three ampicillins and amoxicillin administered orally. J Infect Dis [Suppl] 127:156–168
Lode H, Gebert S, Hendrischk A (1975) Comparative pharmacokinetics and clinical experience with a new cephalosporin derivative: cefazolin. Chemotherapy 21:19–32
Lode H, Niestrath U, Koeppe P, Langmaack H (1977) Azlocillin und Mezlocillin: zwei neue semisynthetische Acylureidopenicilline. Infection 5:163–169
Lode H, Stahlmann R, Koeppe P (1979) Comparative pharmacokinetics of cefalexin, cefaclor, cefadroxil, and CGP 9000. Antimicrob Agents Chemother 16:1–6
Lode H, Kemmerich B, Koeppe P, Belmega D, Jendroschek H (1980 a) Comparative pharmacokinetics of cefoperazone and cefotaxime. Clin Ther 3:80–88
Lode H, Tomas W, Koeppe P, Wagner J (1980 b) Clinical pharmacology of a new uriedopenicillin: Bay k 4999. Chemotherapy 26:81–90
Lode H, Stahlmann R, Dzwillo G, Koeppe P (1980 c) Vergleichende Pharmakokinetik oraler Cephalosporine: Cephalexin, Cefaclor und Cefadroxil. Arzneimittelforsch 30:505–509
Logan MN, Wise R, Grimley RP (1979) Biliary levels of cefoxitin. J Antimicrob Chemother 5:620–621
Loo JCK, Foltz EL, Wallick H, Kwan KC (1974) Pharmacokinetics of pivampicillin and ampicillin in man. Clin Pharmacol Ther 16:35–43
Lukash WM, Frank PF (1963) The effects of physical activity and site of injection on penicillinemia following administration of 1.2 million units of benzathine penicillin G. Am J Med Sci 246:429–438
Lund B, Mogensen C, Molholm-Hansen J, Kampmann J, Siersbaek-Nielsen K (1974) Ampicillin in portal and peripheral blood and bile after oral administration of ampicillin and pivampicillin. Eur J Clin Pharmacol 7:133–135

Lund B, Kampmann JP, Lindahl F, Hansen JM (1976a) Pivampicillin and ampicillin in bile, portal and peripheral blood. Clin Pharmacol Ther 19:587–591
Lund F, Roholt K, Tybring L, Godtfredsen WO (1976b) Mecillinam and pivmecillinam – new beta-lactam antibiotics with high activity against gram-negative bacilli. In: Williams JD, Geddes AM (eds) Chemotherapy, vol 5. Plenum, New York, pp 159–165
Luscombe DK, Nicholls PJ, Owens DR, Russell AD (1974) Pharmacokinetic studies in animals and humans of a new cephalosporin, the sodium salt of 7-cyanacetyl-amino-cephalosporanic acid. Arzneimittelforsch 24:1478–1481
Luthy R, Munch R, Blaser J, Bhend H, Siegenthaler W (1979) Human pharmacology of cefotaxime (HR 756), a new cephalosporin. Antimicrob Agents Chemother 16:127–133
MacAulay MA, Berg SR, Charles D (1968) Placental transfer of dicloxacillin at term. Am J Obstet Gynecol 102:1162–1168
MacAulay MA, Molloy WB, Charles D (1973) Placental transfer of methicillin. Am J Obstet Gynecol 115:58–65
Mad'acsy L, Bokor M, Matusovits L (1975) Penicillin clearance in diabetic children. Acta Paediatr Acad Sci Hung 16:139–142
Mad'acsy L, Bokor M, Kozocsa G (1976) Carbenicillin half-life in children with early diabetes mellitus. Int J Clin Pharmacol 14:155–158
Maddocks JL (1975) Absorption of ampicillin from the human lung. Thorax 30:68–71
Madhavan T, Quinn EL, Freimer E, Fisher E, Cox F, Burch K, Pohlod D (1973) Clinical studies of cefazolin and comparison with other cephalosporins. Antimicrob Agents Chemother 4:525–531
Madhavan T, Yaremchuk K, Levin N, Fisher E, Cox F, Burch K, Haas E, Pohlod D, Quinn EL (1975a) Effects of renal failure and dialysis on cefazolin pharmacokinetics. Antimicrob Agents Chemother 8:63–66
Madhavan T, Block M, Quinn EL, Cox F, Fisher EJ, Burch KH, Haas EJ (1975b) Comparative biliary concentrations of cephazolin and cephalothin in patients with biliary tract disease. Scott Med J 20:255–258
Madhavan T, Pohlod D, Saravolatz L, Cardenas J (1980) Simultaneous salivary and serum concentrations of cefamandole in human volunteers and efficacy in pharyngeal gonorrhea. In: Nelson JD, Grassi C (eds) Current chemotherapy and infectious disease: proceedings of the 11th international congress of chemotherapy – 1979. American Society for Microbiology, Washington, DC, pp 1262–1263
Magni L, Sjovall J (1972) Absorption of ampicillin and pivampicillin in relation to food intake. Farm Fidende 32:645–648
Malandain H, Humbert G, Fillastre J-P, Acar J, Dubois D, Leroy J, Robert M, Daufresne M-F (1973) Administration parenterale d'une nouvelle cephalosporine chez les malades insuffisants renaux chroniques. Pathol-Biol 21:233–239
Marget W, Hopner F, Roos R, Belohradsky BH (1979) Die Behandlung von Neu- und Frühgeborenen mit Cefoxitin. Infection 7:110–112
Maroske D, Knothe H, Rox A (1976) Die Lebergewebekonzentration von Cephradin und Cephracetril sowie deren Gallenausscheidung. Infection 4:159–165
Marshall II JP, Salt WB, Elam RO, Wilkinson GR, Schenker S (1977) Disposition of nafcillin in patients with cirrhosis and extrahepatic biliary obstruction. Gastroenterology 73:1388–1392
Marty JJ, Hersey JA (1975) Absorption of phenethicillin from oral pediatric formulations. Med J Aust 1:382–384
Masada M, Nakagawa T, Uno T (1979) A new metabolite of ampicillin in man. Chem Pharmacol Bull 27:2877–2878
Mashimo K, Kato Y, Saito A, Matoumoto Y, Sakuraba T, Tanaka K, Matsuui K, Ideuchi H, Yajima O, Tomisawa M, Nakayama I (1970) Laboratory and clinical studies on aminocyclohexylpenicillin. Jpn J Antibiot 23:47
Mashimo K, Kato Y, Yajima O, Nakayama I, Tomizawa M, Ideuchi H, Matsumoto Y, Matsui K (1971) Basic and clinical evaluation of sulfobenzylpenicillin. Chemotherapy 19:881–886
Mashimo K, Kunii O, Fukaya K, Tani S, Haranaka K, Watanabe M, Komatsu T, Satomi N (1978) Studies on CS-1170. Chemotherapy (Tokyo) 26(S-5):193–202

Matharu SS, Ramsden CH, Kester RC (1978) A study on tissue concentrations of cephradine achieved in patients with peripheral vascular disease. Curr Med Res Opin 4:427–432

Mathews DD (1975) Cephaloridine serum levels after intravenous injection. J Antimicrob Chemother [Suppl] 1:37–40

Matsen JM (1971) Cephaloglycin in pediatric patients. Am J Dis Child 121:38–42

Matsuda S, Kiyota A, Tanno M, Kashiwagura T (1978) Fundamental and clinical studies of CS-1170 in the field of obstetrics and gynecology. Chemotherapy (Tokyo) 26(S-5):550–557

Matsuda S, Fanno M, Kashiwagura T, Furuya H (1980) Placental transfer of cefoperazone (T-1551) and a clinical study of its use in obstetrics and gynecological infections. In: Nelson JD, Grasse C (eds) Current chemotherapy of infectious diseases: Proceedings of the 11th international congress of chemotherapy – 1979. American Society for Microbiology, Washington, DC, pp 168–169

Matsumoto K, Uzuka Y, Nagatake T, Shishido H (1980) Clinical evaluation of 6059-S, a new active oxacephem. In: Nelson JD, Grassi C (eds) Current chemotherapy of infectious diseases: proceedings of the 11th international congress of chemotherapy – 1979. American Society for Microbiology, Washington, DC, pp 112–113

Matsuzaki M, Matsumoto H, Ochiai K, Hirata Y, Hino M (1976a) Absorption and excretion of cefatrizine (S-640P). Jpn J Antibiot 29:83–89

Matsuzaki M, Ohtawa M, Akiyama I, Yamamato M, Tomioka J, Kiyohara M, Mabuchi T (1976b) Metabolism of cefatrizine (S-640P) in rat, rabbit, dog, monkey, and human. Jpn J Antibiot 29:90–106

McCarthy CG, Finland M (1960) Absorption and excretion of four penicillins. New Engl J Med 263:315–326

McCloskey RV, Terry EE, McCracken AW, Sweeney MJ, Forland MF (1972) Effect of hemodialysis and renal failure on serum and urine concentrations of cephapirin sodium. Antimicrob Agents Chemother 1:90–93

McCracken Jr GH, Ginsburg CM, Chrane DF, Thomas MCL, Horton LJ (1973) Clinical pharmacology of penicillin in the newborn infants. J Pediatr 82:692–698

McCracken Jr GH, Ginsburg CM, Clahsen JC, Thomas ML (1978a) Pharmacologic evaluation of orally administered antibiotics in infants and children: effect of feeding on bioavailability. Pediatrics 62:738–743

McCracken Jr GH, Ginsburg CM, Clahsen JC, Thomas ML (1978b) Pharmacokinetics of cefaclor in infants and children. J Antimicrob Chemother 4:515–521

McKendrick MW, Geddes AM, Wise R (1980) Clinical experience with cefotaxime (HR-756). In: Nelson JD, Grassi C (eds) Current chemotherapy of infectious diseases: proceedings of the 11th international congress of chemotherapy – 1979. American Society for Microbiology, Washington, DC, pp 123–125

McLeish AR, Strachan CJL, Powis SJA, Wise R, Bevan PG (1977) The influence of biliary disease on the excretion of cefazolin in human bile. Surgery 81:426–430

Mellin H-E, Welling PG, Madsen PO (1977) Pharmacokinetics of cefamandole in patients with normal and impaired renal function. Antimicrob Agents Chemother 11:262–266

Meyer-Brunot HG, Randazzo D, Spring P, Theobald W (1976) Zur Kenntnis der Pharmakokinetik von Cephalosporinen. Infection 4:S181–187

Meyers BR, Hirschman SZ (1977) Pharmacokinetics of cefamandole in patients with renal failure. Antimicrob Agents Chemother 11:248–250

Meyers BR, Hirschman SZ, Nicholas P (1972) Cephanone: in vitro antibacterial activity and pharmacology in normal human volunteers. Antimicrob Agents Chemother 2:250–254

Meyers BR, Ribner B, Yancovitz S, Hirschman SZ (1976) Pharmacological studies with cefamandole in human volunteers. Antimicrob Agents Chemother 9:140–144

Meyers BR, Hirschman SZ, Wormser G, Gartenberg G, Srulevitch E (1978) Pharmacologic studies with cefaclor, a new oral cephalosporin. J Clin Pharmacol 18:174–179

Meyers BR, Hirschman SZ, Strougo L, Srulevitch E (1980) Comparative study of piperacillia, ticarcillin, and carbenicillin pharmacokinetics. Antimicrob Agents Chemother 17:608–611

Miki F, Higashi T, Iwasaki T, Akao M, Ozaki T, Sugiyama H, Hara M (1970) Fundamental and clinical studies on aminocyclohexylpenicillin. Jpn J Antibiot 23:59
Miller AK, Celozzi E, Kong Y, Pelak BA, Hendlin D, Stapley EO (1974) Cefoxitin, a semi-synthetic cephamycin antibiotic: in vivo evaluation. Antimicrob Agents Chemother 5:33–37
Miller KW, Chan KKH, McCoy HG, Fischer RP, Lindsay WG, Zaske DE (1979) Cephalothin kinetics: before, during, and after cardiopulmonary bypass surgery. Clin Pharmacol Ther 26:54–62
Miller KW, McCoy HG, Chan KKH, Fischer RP, Lindsay WG, Seifert R, Zaske DE (1980) Effect of cardiopulmonary bypass on cefazolin disposition. Clin Pharmacol Ther 27:550–556
Miller RP (1962) A paper chromatographic assay for cephalosporins. Antibiot Chemother 12:689–693
Minamitani M, Hayashi H, Tohma T, Kojima T, Sahashi Y, Terao T (1980) Studies on the shift of cefmetazole into the gastrointestinal tract. Jpn J Antibiot 33:10–17
Mischler TW, Corson SL, Bolognese RJ, Letocha MJ, Neiss ES (1974a) Presence of cephradine in body fluids of lactating and pregnant women. Clin Pharmacol Ther 15:214
Mischler TW, Sugerman AA, Willard DA, Brannick LJ, Neiss ES (1974b) Influence of probenecid and food on the bioavailability of cephradine in normal male subjects. J Clin Pharmacol 14:604–611
Mitchard M, Andrews J, Kendall MJ, Wise R (1977) Mecillinam serum levels following intravenous injection: a comparison with pivmecillinam. J Antimicrob Chemother [Suppl B] 3:83–88
Miyake Y, Ebata M (1976) Binding of cephalothin, cephaloridine and cefazolin to human serum proteins. J Antibiot 29:667
Miyamoto S, Nishio A, Kumamoto Y (1978) Experimental and clinical studies on CS-1170. Chemotherapy (Tokyo) 26(S-5):435–446
Moatti N, Fournial G, Berthoumieu F, Gaillard J (1978) Etude, chez l'homme, des concentrations pulmonaires et seriques de la cefradine. Pathol Biol (Paris) 26:577–580
Modai J, Pierre J, Bergogne-Berezia E, Avril MF (1979a) Cerebrospinal fluid penetration of mezlocillin. Arzneimittelforsch 29(II):1927–1969
Modai J, Pierre J, Bergogne-Berezin E, Avril MF (1979b) Cerebrospinal fluid penetration of cefuroxime. Drugs Exp Clin Res 5:455–458
Modr Z, Dvoracek K (1970) Pharmacokinetics of ampicillin and hetacillin. Rev Czech Med 16:84–95
Modr Z, Dvoracek K, Krebs V, Janku I (1975) Farmakokinetika amoxycilinu, pivampicilinu a ampicilinu. Cas Lek Cesk 114:611–615
Modr Z, Dvoracek K, Janku I, Krebs V (1977) Pharmacokinetics of carfecillin and carindacillin. Int J Clin Pharmacol 15:81–83
Moellering Jr RC, Swartz MN (1976) The newer cephalosporins. N Engl J Med 294:24–28
Moll TB, Crawford JR, McPherson SD (1971) Ocular penetrance of cephaloridine after subconjunctival injection. Am J Ophthalmol 71:992–996
Morehead CD, Shelton S, Kusmiesz H, Nelson JD (1972) Pharmacokinetics of carbenicillin in nonates of normal and low birth weight. Antimicrob Agents Chemother 2:267–271
Morrison JA, Batra VK (1979) Pharmacokinetics of piperacillin sodium in man. Drugs Exp Clin Res 5:105–110
Morrow S, Palmisano P, Cassady G (1968) The placental transfer of cephalothin. J Pediatr 73:262–264
Moskowitz B, Somani SM, McDonald RH (1973) Salicylate interaction with penicillin and secobarbital binding sites on human serum albumin. Clin Toxicol 6:247–256
Motomura R, Nakajima H, Kawano M, Yamabe T (1978) Fundamental and clinical studies on CS-1170 in the field of obstetrics and gynecology. Chemother (Tokyo) [S-5] 26:582–587
Muggleton PW, O'Callaghan CH, Stevens WK (1964) Laboratory evaluation of a new antibiotic-cephaloridine (Ceporin). Br Med J 2:1234–1237
Muller C, Netland A, Dawson AF, Andrew E (1980) The penetration of cefuroxime into the cerebrospinal fluid through inflamed and non-inflamed meninges. J Antimicrob Chemother 6:279–283

Munch R, Luthy R, Blaser J, Sugenthaler W (1980) Clavulanic acid: human pharmacokinetics and penetration into cerebrospinal fluid. In: Nelson JD, Grassi C (eds) Current chemotherapy of infectious Diseases: proceedings of the 11th international congress of chemotherapy – 1979. American Society for Microbiology, Washington, DC, pp 345–347
Murai Y, Nakagawa T, Uno T (1980) GC-MS identification of active metabolite of oxacillin in man. Chem Pharm Bull 28:362–364
Murakawa T, Kono Y, Nishida M (1972) Studies on the formation and activity of the transformation product of ampicillin. II. J Antibiot 25:421–426
Murakawa T, Sakamoto H, Fukada S, Nakamoto S, Hirose T, Itoh N, Nishida M (1980) Pharmacokinetics of ceftizoxime in animals after parenteral dosing: Antimicrob Agents Chemother 17:157–164
Murdoch JM, Speirs CF, Geddes AM, Wallace ET (1964) Clinical trial of cephaloridine (Ceporin), a new broad-spectrum antibiotic derived from cephalosporin C. Br Med J 2:1238–1240
Murray BE, Moellering RC (1979) The cephalosporin and cephamycin antibiotics: a status report. Clin Ther 2:155–179
Naber KG, Meyer-Brunot HG, Reitz I (1976) Cephacetrile: plasma concentrations during and after constant infusion. In: Williams JD, Geddes AM (eds) Chemotherapy, vol 5. Plenum, New York, pp 223–226
Nakagawa K (1977) Phase one clinical study on cefuroxime. Proc R Soc Med [Suppl 9] 70:22–24
Nakai Y, Shirakawa Y, Fujita T, Suzuoki Z (1972) The metabolic fate of α-sulphobenzylpenicillin in rats. Xenobiotica 2:147–157
Nakano H, Sasaki K, Mizoguchi M, Ishibe T, Nihira H (1977) Absorption and excretion of carbenicillin indanyl sodium in patients with reduced kidney function. Chemotherapy 23:299–308
Nakashima M (1980) Clinical pharmakocinetics and safety of FK-749 in healthy volunteers. In: Nelson JD, Grassi C (eds) Current chemotherapy of infectious diseases: proceedings of the 11th international congress of chemotherapy – 1979. American Society for Microbiology, Washington, DC, pp 259–261
Nakatomi M, Nasu M, Saito A, Mori N, Hayashi T, Shigeno Y, Tomonaga A, et al. (1978) Fundamental and clinical studies on a new semisynthetic cephamycin CS-1170. Chemotherapy (Tokyo) 26(S-5):350–367
Nakatomi M, Nasu M, Nagasawa T, Shigeno V, Saito A, Hara K (1980) Cefsulodin in treatment of chronic bronchitis due to *Pseudomonas aeruginosa*. In: Nelson JD, Grassi C (eds) Current chemotherapy of infectious diseases: proceedings of the 11th international congress of chemotherapy – 1979. American Society for Microbiology, Washington, DC, pp 204–205
Nakayama I, Iwamoto H, Iwai S, Mizuashi H, Ishiyama S (1978) Comparative study of CS-1170 and cefoxitin: absorption, distribution and metabolism. In: Siegenthaler W, Luthy R (eds) Current chemotherapy: proceedings of the 10th international congress of chemotherapy, Zurich, 18–23 Sept 1977. American Society for Microbiology, Washington, DC, pp 851–852
Nakayama I, Kawaguchi H, Ishiyama S (1980 a) Comparative study on different assays of CGP-9000 and CGP-3940. In: Nelson JD, Grassi C (eds) Current chemotherapy infectious diseases: proceedings of the 11th international congress of chemotherapy – 1979. American Society for Microbiology. Washington, DC, pp 209–211
Nakayama I, Akieda Y, Kawamura H, Kawaguchi H, Mizuashi H, Sakao K, Nishimoto A, Ishiyama S (1980 b) Studies on cefotaxime in surgery: antibacterial activity, absorption, excretion, metabolism, tissue distribution and clinical use. Chemotherapy (Tokyo) [Suppl 1] 28:606–622
Naumann P (1967) Kinetik der Cephalosporine im menschlichen Organismus. Int J Clin Pharmacol Ther Toxicol 2:113–115
Nauta EH, Mattie H (1975) Pharmacokinetics of flucloxacillin and cloxacillin in healthy subjects and patients on chronic intermittent haemodialysis. Br J Clin Pharmacol 2:111–121

Nauta EH, Mattie H (1976) Dicloxacillin and cloxacillin: pharmacokinetics in healthy and hemodialysis subjects. Clin Pharmacol Ther 20:98–108
Nauta EH, Mattie H, Goslings WRO (1973) Pharmacokinetics of cloxacillin in patients on chronic intermittent haemodialysis and in healthy subjects. Chemotherapy 19:261–271
Nayler JHC, Long AAW, Brown TM, Acred P, Rolinson GN, Batchelor FR, Stevens S, Sutherland R (1962) Chemistry, toxicology, pharmacology, and microbiology of new acid-stable penicillin, resistant to penicillinase (BRL 1621). Nature 195:1264–1267
Neiss ES (1973) Cephradine – a summary of preclinical studies and clinical pharmacology. J Ir Med Assoc [Suppl] 66:1–12
Neu HC (1974) Antimicrobial activity and human pharmacology of amoxicillin. J Infect Dis [Suppl] 129:123–131
Neu HC (1978) Comparison of the pharmacokinetics of cefamandole and other cephalosporin compounds. J Infect Dis 137:S80–87
Neu HC, Aswapokee N, Aswapokee P, Fu KP (1979a) HR 756, a new cephalosporin active against gram-positive and gram-negative aerobic and anaerobic bacteria. Antimicrob Agents Chemother 15:, 73–281
Neu HC, Kung K, Aswapokee N, Fu KP (1979b) The comparative in vitro activity and β-lactamase stability of a new ureido penicillin. J Antibiot 32:148–155
Neu HC, Aswapokee P, Fu KP, Ho I, Matthijssen C (1980) Cefotaxime kinetics after intravenous and intramuscular injection of single and multiple doses. Clin Pharmacol Ther 27:677–685
Neuvonen PJ, Elonen E, Pentikainen PJ (1977) Comparative effect of food on absorption of ampicillin and pivampicillin. J Int Med Res 5:71–76
Nielsen RL, Wolen R, Luft FC, Ozawa T (1979) Hydrolysis of cefamandole nafate in dialysis patients. Antimicrob Agents Chemother 16:683–685
Nightingale CH, Bassaris H, Tilton R, Quintiliani R (1975a) Changes in pharmacokinetics of cefazolin due to stress. J Pharm Sci 64:712–714
Nightingale CH, Greene DS, Quintiliani R (1975b) Pharmacokinetics and clinical use of cephalosporin antibiotics. J Pharm Sci 64:1899–1927
Nilsson-Ehle I, Nilsson-Ehle P (1979) Pharmacokinetics of cephalothin: accumulation of its deacetylated metabolite in uremic patients. J Infect Dis 139:712–716
Nishida M, Matsubara T, Murakawa T, Mine Y, Yokota Y, Kuwahara S, Goto S (1970) In vitro and in vivo evaluation of a new cephalosporin C derivative. In: Hobby GL (ed) Antimicrobial agents and chemotherapy – 1969. American Society of Microbiology, Bethesda, pp 236–243
Nishida M, Matsubara T, Murakawa T, Mine Y, Yokata Y, Goto S, Kuwahara S (1970) Cefazolin, a new semisynthetic cephalosporin antibiotic. III. Absorption, excretion, and tissue distribution in parenteral administration. J Antibiot 23:184–194
Nishida M, Murakawa T, Mine Y, Fukada S, Kono Y, Sueda Y (1971) Studies on the formation and activity of the transformation product of ampicillin. J Antibiot 24:641–645
Nishida M, Murakawa T, Kamimura T, Okada N, Sakamoto H, Fukada S, Nakamoto S, Yokota Y, Miki K (1976a) In vitro and in vivo evaluation of ceftezole, a new cephalosporin derivative. Antimicrob Agents Chemother 10:1–13
Nishida M, Murakawa T, Kamimura T, Okada N, Sakamoto H, Fukada S, Nakamoto S, Yokota Y, Miki K (1976b) Laboratory evaluation of FR 10612, a new oral cephalosporin derivative. J Antibiot 29:444–459
Nishikata E (1978) Clinical investigations of CS-1170 in surgical field. Chemotherapy (Tokyo) 26(S-5):430–434
Nishimura T, Hiromatsu K, Takashima T, Tabuki K, Kotani Y (1979a) Laboratory and clinical studies on cefuroxime. Jpn J Antibiot 32:1211–1218
Nishimura T, Kotani Y, Takashima T, Hiromatsu K (1979b) Pharmacokinetics and clinical studies on CS-1170. Jpn J Antibiot 32:221–227
Nissenson AR, Levin NW, Parker RH (1972) Effect of renal failure and hemodialysis on cephacetrile pharmacokinetics. Clin Pharmacol Ther 13:887–894
Nolan CM, Ulmer Jr WC (1978) Measurement of cephalothin and desacetylcephalothin in CSF in experimental meningitis. Clin Res 26:29A

Nolan CM, Ulmer WC (1980) A study of cephalothin and desacetylcephalothin in cerebrospinal fluid in therapy for experimental pneumococcal meningitis. J Infect Dis 141:326–330
Norrby R, Foord RD, Price JD, Hedlund P (1977a) Pharmacokinetic and clinical studies on cefuroxime. Proc R Soc Med [Suppl 9] 70:25–32
Norrby R, Foord RD, Hedlund P (1977b) Clinical and pharmacokinetic studies on cefuroxime. J Antimicrob Chemother 3:355–362
Nunes HL, Pecora CC, Judy K, Rosenman SB, Warren GH, Martin CM (1965) Turnover and distribution of nafcillin in tissues and body fluids of surgical patients. In: Hobby GL (ed) Antimicrobial agents and chemotherapy – 1964. American Society for Microbiology, Bethesda, pp 237–249
O'Callaghan CH, Harding SM (1977) The pharmacokinetics of cefuroxime in man in relation to its antibacterial activity. Proc R Soc Med [Suppl 9] 70:4–10
O'Callaghan CH, Tootill JPR, Robinson WD (1971) A new approach to the study of serum concentrations of orally administered cephaloxin. J Pharm Pharmacol 23:50–57
O'Callaghan CH, Sykes RB, Ryan DM, Foord RD, Muggleton PW (1976) Cefuroxime – a new cephalosporin antibiotic. J Antibiot 29:29–37
O'Callaghan CH, Acred P, Harper PB, Ryan DM, Kirby SM, Harding SM (1980) GR 20263, a new broad-spectrum cephalosporin with anti-pseudomonal activity. Antimicrob Agents Chemother 17:876–883
O'Connor WJ, Warren GH, Mandala PS, Edrada LS, Rosenman SB (1965) Serum concentrations of nafcillin in new born infant and children. In: Hobby GL (ed) Antimicrobial agents and Chemotherapy – 1964. American Society for Microbiology, Bethesda, pp 188–191
O'Connor WJ, Warren GH, Edrada LS, Mandala PS, Rosenman SB (1966) Serum concentrations of sodium nafcillin in infants during the perinatal period. In: Hobby GL (ed) Antimicrobial agents and Chemotherapy – 1965. American Society for Microbiology, Bethesda, pp 220–222
Oe PL, Simonian S, Verhoef J (1973) Pharmacokinetics of the new penicillins. Chemotherapy 19:279–288
Ohkawa M, Kuroda K (1980) Pharmacokinetics of ceftezole in patients with normal and impaired renal function. Chemotherapy 26:242–247
Ohkawa M, Shimamura M, Sawaki M, Nakashita E, Naito K, Kuroda K (1978) Experimental and clinical studies of CS-1170 in complicated urinary tract infections. Chemother (Tokyo) 26(S-5):467–472
Ohkawa M, Orito M, Sugata T, Shimamura M, Sawaki M, Nakashita E, Kuroda K, Sasahara K (1980) Pharmacokinetics of cefmetazole in normal subjects and in patients with impaired renal function. Antimicrob Agents Chemother 18:386–389
Oishi M, Nishizuka K, Motoyama M, Ogawa T (1976) Ocular penetration and clinical evaluation of ceftezole for ocular infections. In: Williams JD, Geddes AM (eds) Chemotherapy, vol 5. Plenum, New York, pp 293–298
Oishi M, Nishizuka K, Motoyama M, Ogawa T (1979) Experimental and clinical investigations with mezlocillin in ophthalmology. Arzneimittelforsch 29 II:1989–1992
Okamoto Y, Okubo H, Go K, Ueda Y, Maehara K, Makino J (1978) Basic and clinical studies on CS-1170. Chemotherapy (Tokyo) 26(S-5):303–312
Okubo H, Fujimmoto Y, Okamoto Y, Tsukada J, Makino J (1970) Fundamental and clinical studies on aminocyclohexyl penicillin. Jpn J Antibiot 23:60–68
Olegard R, Jodal U, Brorsson JE, Jonsson J, Lincoln P, Bjure J, Norrby R (1980) Pharmacokinetics of cefoxitin. In: Nelson JD, Grassi C (eds) Current chemotherapy and infectious disease: proceedings of the 11th international congress of chemotherapy – 1979. American Society for Microbiology, Washington, DC, pp 1152–1154
Onsrud M, Gjonnaess H, Bergan T (1979) Amoxycillin absorption and penetration in pelvic inflammatory disease. Acta Obstet Gynecol 58:401–403
Orsolini P (1970) Tissue distribution and serum levels of cephalexin in man. Postgrad Med J 46S:13–16
Orsolini P, Xerri L, Vallaperta P (1979) Cefuroxime: pharmacokinetics after intravenous injection. Drugs Exp Clin Res 5:423–426

Pabst J, Leopold G, Ungethum W, Dingeldein E (1979) Clinical pharmacology phase I of cefazedone, a new cephalosporin, in healthy volunteers. Arzneimittelforsch 29:437–443

Palatsi I, Kaipainen W (1971) A comparative study of blood concentrations after peroral benzathine (DBED) penicillin V and potassium penicillin V. Scand J Infect Dis 3:71–74

Palmu A, Jarvinen H, Hallynck T, Pyck P (1980) Cefadroxil levels in bile in biliary infection. In: Nelson JD, Grassi C (eds) Current chemotherapy of infectious diseases: proceedings of the 11th international congress of chemotherapy – 1979. American Society for Microbiology, Washington, DC, pp 643–644

Pancoast SJ, Neu HC (1978) Kinetics of mezlocillin and carbenicillin. Clin Pharmacol Ther 24:108–116

Paradelis AG, Stathopoulos G, Trianthaphyllidis C, Logaras G (1977) Pharmacokinetics of five cephalosporins in healthy male volunteers. Arzneimittelforsch 27:2167–2170

Paradisi F, Cioffi R (1979) Blood levels and urinary elimination after administration of bacampicillin and amoxicillin in patients with liver or kidney impairment. Drugs Exp Clin Res 5:207–214

Parsons JN, Romano JM, Levison ME (1980) Pharmacology of a new L-oxa-β-lactam (LY 127935) in normal volunteers. Antimicrob Agents Chemother 17:226–228

Parsons RL, Beavis JP, Paddock GM, Hossack GM (1976a) Cephradine bone concentrations during total hip replacement. In: Williams JD, Geddes AM (eds) Chemotherapy, vol 1. Plenum, New York, pp 201–211

Parsons RL, Hossack GM, Paddock GM (1976b) Plasma profile and urinary excretion of mecillinam after pivmecillinam. In: Williams JD, Geddes AM (eds) Chemotherapy, vol 5. Plenum, New York, pp 173–181

Patel D, Moellering RC, Thrasher K, Fahmy NR, Harris WH (1979) The effect of hypotensive anesthesia on cephalothin concentrations in bone and muscle of patients undergoing total hip replacement. J Bone Joint Surg 61-A:531–538

Pazin GJ, Schwartz SN, Ho M, Lyon JA, Pasculle AW (1979) Treatment of septicemic patients with cefoxitin: pharmacokinetics in renal insufficiency. Rev Infect Dis 1:189–194

Perkins RL, Saslaw S (1966) Experiences with cephalothin. Ann Intern Med 64:13–24

Perkins RL, Smith ES, Saslaw S (1969) Cephalothin and cephaloridine: comparative pharmacodynamics in chronic uremia. Am J Med Sci 257:116–124

Peterson LR, Gerding DN, Zinneman HH, Moore BM (1977) Evaluation of three newer methods for investigating protein interactions of penicillin G. Antimicrob Agents Chemother 11:993–998

Pfeffer M, Jackson A, Ximenes J, De Menezes JP (1977) Comparative human oral clinical pharmacology of cefadroxil, cephalexin, and cephradine. Antimicrob Agents Chemother 11:331–338

Pfeffer M, Gaver RC, Van Harken DR (1980) Human pharmacokinetics of a new broad-spectrum parenteral cephalosporin antibiotic, ceforanide. J Pharm Sci 69:398–402

Philipson A (1978) Plasma levels of ampicillin in pregnant women following administration of ampicillin and pivampicillin. Am J Obstet Gynecol 130:674–683

Philipson A, Sabath LD, Rosner B (1975) Sequence effect on ampicillin blood levels noted in an amoxicillin, ampicillin, and epicillin triple crossover study. Antimicrob Agents Chemother 8:311–320

Pitkin DH, Actor P, Alexander F, Dubb J, Stote R, Weisbach JA (1980a) Cefonicid (SK&F 75073) serum levels and urinary recovery after intramuscular and intravenous administration. In: Nelson JD, Grassi C (eds) Current chemotherapy of infectious diseases. proceedings of the 11th international congress of chemotherapy – 1979. American Society for Microbiology, Washington, DC, pp 252–254

Pitkin DH, Actor P, Weisbach JA (1980b) Serum protein binding alterations of selected cephalosporin antibiotics by fatty acids and their derivatives. J Pharm Sci 69:354–356

Plaue R, Fabricius K, Wysocki S (1974) Cephalothinspiegel-Bestimmungen an menschlichen Geweben. Chirurg 45:274–278

Plaue UR, Muller O, Fabricius K, Bethke RO (1978) Untersuchungen über die Diffusionsrate von Cefamandol in verschiedene menschliche Gewebe. Arzneimittelforsch 28:2343–2349

Plaue R, Muller O, Fabricius K, Bethke O (1979a) Serum- und Gewebespiegel nach einmaliger Cefaclorgabe. Infection 7:252–255
Plaue UR, Muller O, Jenne V, Fabricius K, Bethke RO (1979b) Experimentelle Untersuchungen über die Diffusionsrate von Cefoxitin in verschiedene menschliche Gewebe. Med Klin 74:481–487
Plaut ME, O'Connell CJ, Pabico RC, Davidson DD (1969) Penicillin handling in normal and azotemic patients. J Lab Clin Med 74:12–18
Polk RE, Archer GL, Lower R (1978) Cefamandole kinetics during cardiopulmonary bypass. Clin Pharmacol Ther 23:473–480
Pollard JP, Hughes SPF, Evans MJ, Scott JE, Benson MKD (1979) Concentration of flucloxacillin in femoral head and joint capsule in total hip replacement. J Antimicrob Chemother 5:721–726
Poole JW, Owen G, Silverio J, Freyhoff JN, Rosenman SB (1968) Physiochemical factors influencing the absorption of anhydrous and trihydrate forms of ampicillin. Curr Ther Res 10:292–303
Prakesh A, Chalmers JA, Onojobi OIA (1970) Transfer of limecycline and cephaloridine from mother to fetus – a comparative study. J Obstet Gynaecol Br Commenw 77:247–252
Prenna M, Ripa S (1980) Serum levels and urinary excretion in humans of BL-S 578 (cefadroxil), a new semisynthetic cephalosporin. Chemotherapy 26:98–102
Price KE, Leitner F, Misiek M, Chisholm DR, Pursiano TA (1971) BL-P 1654, a new broad-spectrum penicillin with marked antipseudomonal activity. In: Hobby GL (ed) Antimicrobial agents and Chemotherapy – 1970. American Society for Microbiology, Bethesda, pp 17–29
Price KE (1977a) Structure-activity relationships of semisynthetic penicillins. In: Perlman D (ed) Structure-activity relationships among the semisynthetic antibiotics. Academic, New York, pp 1–59
Price KE (1977b) Structure-activity relationships of semisynthetic penicillins (supplement). In: Perlman D (ed) Structure-activity relationships among the semisynthetic antibiotics. Academic, New York, pp 61–86
Prigot A, Froix CJ, Rubin E (1963) Absorption, diffusion, and excretion of a new penicillin, oxacillin. In: Sylvester JC (ed) Antimicrobial agents and chemotherapy – 1962. American Society for Microbiology, Bethesda, pp 402–410
Pryor JS, Joekes AM, Foord JD (1967) Cephaloridine excretion in patients with normal and impaired renal function. Postgrad Med J 43:S82–85
Quinn EL, Madhaven T, Wixson R, Guise E, Levin N, Block M, Burch K, Fisher E, Suarez A, DelBusto R (1978) Cefamandole: observations on its spectrum, concentration in bone and bile, excretion in renal failure, and clinical efficacy. In: Siegenthaler W, Luthy R (eds) Current chemotherapy – proceedings of the 10th international congress of chemotherapy. American Society for Microbiology, Washington, DC, pp 803–804
Ram MD, Watanatittan S (1974) Cephalothin levels in human bile. Arch Surg 108:187–189
Ram MD, Watanatittan S (1976) Biliary excretion and concentration of cefazolin. Am J Gastroenterol 66:540–545
Rammelkamp CH, Keefer CS (1943) The absorption, excretion, and distribution of penicillin. J Clin Invest 22:425–437
Ramsay CH, Bodin NO, Hansson E (1972) Absorption, distribution, biotransformation, and excretion of azidocillin, a new semi-synthetic penicillin, in mice, rats, and dogs. Arzneimittelforsch 22:1962–1970
Rattie ES, Ravin LJ (1975) Pharmacokinetic interpretation of blood levels and urinary excretion data for cefazolin and cephalothin after intravenous and intramuscular administration in humans. Antimicrob Agents Chemother 7:606–613
Rattie ES, Bernardo PD, Ravin LJ (1976) Pharmacokinetic interpretation of cephradine levels in serum after intravenous and extravascular administration in humans. Antimicrob Agents Chemother 10:283–287
Ratzan KR, Ruiz C, Irvin GL III (1974) A comparison of the biliary tract excretion of cefazolin, cephalothin, and cephaloridine. Clin Res 22:37A

Ratzan KR, Baker HB, Lauredo I (1978) Excretion of cefamandole, cefazolin, and cephalothin into T-tube bile. Antimicrob Agents Chemother 13:985–987
Records RE (1966) The human intraocular penetration of methicillin. Arch Ophthalmol 76:720–722
Records RE (1967) Human intraocular penetration of sodium oxacillin. Arch Ophthalmol 77:693–695
Records RE (1968) Intraocular penetration of cephalothin II. Human studies. Am J Ophthalmol 66:441–443
Records RE (1969) Intraocular penetration of cephaloridine. Arch Ophthalmol 81:331–335
Regamey C, Kirby WMM (1973) Pharmacokinetics of cephanone in healthy adult volunteers. Antimicrob Agents Chemother 4:589–592
Regamey C, Libke RD, Clarke JT, Kirby WMM (1974) Pharmacokinetic of parenteral sodium cephalexin in comparison with cephalothin and cefazolin. Infection 2:132–136
Rein MF, Westervelt FB, Sande MA (1973) Pharmacodynamics of cefazolin in the presence of normal and impaired renal function. Antimicrob Agents Chemother 4:366–371
Renlund M, Pettay O (1977) Pharmacokinetics and clinical efficacy of cefuroxime in the newborn period. Proc R Soc Med [Suppl 9] 70:179–182
Reutter F, Maurice NP (1974) Serum half-lives and elimination rates of a new semi-synthetic cephalosporin, cephacetrile, in nephrectomized patients and in patients with impaired or normal renal function. Arzneimittelforsch 24:1466–1467
Richards AB, Bron AJ, McLendon B, Kennedy MRK, Walker SR (1979) The intraocular penetration of cefuroxime after parenteral administration. Br J Ophthalmol 63:687–689
Richter I (1980) Amoxicillin in pediatrics, with special reference to its excretion into bronchial secretion. Int J Clin Pharmacol Ther Toxicol 18:185–189
Riley FC, Boyle GL, Leopold IH (1968) Intraocular penetration of cephaloridine in humans. Am J Ophthalmol 66:1042–1049
Rizzo M, DeCarlo G, Amato M, Parri F, Lamanna S, Mini E, Mazzei T (1979) Cefamandole pharmacokinetics in man. Drugs Exp Clin Res 5:141–152
Robertson CE (1980) The pharmacokinetics of cefuroxime lysine in the elderly. Methods Find Exp Clin Pharmacol 2:167–170
Robinson OPW (1968) Human pharmacology of carbenicillin, a semi-synthetic penicillin active against *Pseudomonas aeruginosa*. In: Hobby GL (ed) Antimicrobial agents and chemotherapy – 1967. American Society for Microbiology, Bethesda, MD, pp 614–618
Robinson OPW, Sutherland R (1967) Absorption and excretion studies of a new penicillin BRL 2064 (carbenicillin) in man. Vth international congress of chemotherapy, vol 6. Verlag der Wiener Medizinischen Academie, Vienna, pp 525–529
Rodriguez V, Inagaki J, Bodey GP (1973) Clinical pharmacology of ticarcillin (α-carboxyl-3-thienylmethyl penicillin, BRL-2228). Antimicrob Agents Chemother 4:31–36
Rodriguez WJ, Ross S, Khan WN, Goldenberg R (1978) Clinical and laboratory evaluation of cefamandole in infants and children. J Infec Dis 137:S150–154
Rogers HJ, James CA, Morrison PJ, Bradbrook ID (1980) Effect of cimetidine on oral absorption of ampicillin and cotrimoxazole. J Antimicrob Chemother 6:297–300
Roholt K (1977) Pharmacokinetic studies of mecillinam and pivmecillinam. J Antimicrob Chemother [Suppl B] 3:71–81
Roholt K, Nielsen B, Kristensen E (1975) Pharmacokinetic studies with mecillinam and pivmecillinam. Chemotherapy 21:146–166
Rolewicz TF, Mirkin BL, Cooper MJ, Anders MW (1977) Metabolic disposition of cephalothin and deacetylcephalothin in children and adults: comparison of high-performance liquid chromatographic and microbial assay procedures. Clin Pharmacol Ther 22:928–935
Rolinson GN (1974) Laboratory evaluation of amoxicillin. J Infect Dis [Suppl] 129:139–145
Rolinson GN, Batchelor FR (1963) Penicillin metabolites. In: Sylvester JC (ed) Antimicrobial agents and chemotherapy – 1962. American Society for Microbiology, Bethesda, pp 654–660
Rolinson GN, Sutherland R (1965) The binding of antibiotics to serum protein. Br J Pharmacol 25:638–650

Rolinson GN, Sutherland R (1968) Carbenicillin, a new semisynthetic penicillin active against *Pseudomonas aeruginosa*. In: Hobby GL (ed) Antimicrobial agents and chemotherapy – 1967. American Society for Microbiology, Bethesda, pp 609–613

Rolinson GN, Sutherland R (1973) Semisynthetic penicillins. Adv Pharmacol Chemother II:151–220

Rollag H, Midtvedt T, Wetterhus S (1975) Serum levels of penicillin V after oral administration of pediatric preparations to healthy subjects. Acta Pediatr Scand 64:421–424

Rollo LM, Somers GF, Burley DM (1962) Bacteriological and pharmacological properties of phenoxybenzylpenicillin. Br Med J 1:76–80

Roos R, Von Hattingberg HM, Belohradsky GH, Marget W (1980) Pharmacokinetics of cefoxitin in premature and newborn babies. In: Nelson JD, Grassi C (eds) Current chemotherapy and infectious disease: proceedings of the 11th international congress of chemotherapy – 1979. American Society for Microbiology, Washington, DC, pp 1159–1161

Rosenblatt JE, Kind AC, Brodie JL, Kirby WMM (1968) Mechanisms responsible for the blood level differences of isoxazolyl penicillins. Arch Intern Med 121:345–348

Rosenman SB, Weber LS, Owen G, Warren GH (1968) Antimicrobial activity and pharmacological distribution of Wy-4508, an aminoalicylic penicillin. In: Hobby GL (ed) Antimicrobial agents and chemotherapy – 1967. American Society for Microbiology, Bethesda, pp 590–596

Rubi R, Galan HM (1979) Cephapirin concentrations in prostatic and seminal vesicle tissues. Int J Clin Pharmacol Biopharmacol 17:87–89

Rudoy RC, Goto N, Pettit D, Uemura H (1979) Pharmacokinetics of intravenous amoxicillin in pediatric patients. Antimicrob Agents Chemother 15:628–629

Ruedy J (1967) The use of cephaloridine in adult patients with renal failure. Postgrad Med J 43(S):87–89

Rylander M, Mannheimer C, Brorson J-E (1979) Penetration of cephradine and cefazolin into ulcers of patients suffering from peripheral arterial circulatory insufficiency. Scand J Infect Dis 11:281–286

Ryrfeldt Å (1971) Biliary excretion of penicillins in the rat. J Pharm Pharmacol 23:460–464

Ryrfeldt Å (1973) Uptake and degradation of ^{3}H-phenoxymethyl-penicillin in rat liver slices. Acta Pharmacol Suec 10:161–170

Sabath LD, Postic B, Finland M (1962) Laboratory studies on methicillin. Am J Med Sci 244:484–500

Sabath LD, Klein JO, Finland M (1963) Ancillin (2-biphenylpenicillin): antibacterial activity and clinical pharmacology. Am J Med Sci 246:129–146

Saikawa I, Takai A, Nakashima Y, Yoshida C, Yasuda T, Shimizu E, Sakai H, Taki H, Tai M, Takashita Y (1977) 6-[D(-)-α-(4-ethyl-2,3-dioxo-1-piperazinecarboxamido)phenylacetamido]penicillanic. J Pharmacol Soc Jpn 97:705–826

Saikawa I, Nakashima Y, Sakai H, Momonoi K, Ikegami T, Minami H, Hayakawa H, Ochiai H, Todo Y (1980) Studies on β-lactam antibiotics for medicinal purpose. XI. Studies on the metabolism of sodium 7-[D(-)-α-(4-ethyl-2,3-dioxo-1-piperazinecarboxamido-α-(4-hydroxyphenyl)acetamido]-3-[(1-methyl-1*H*-tetrazol-5-yl)thiomethyl]-3-cephem-4-carboxylate (T-1551). Yakugaku Zasshi 100:625–640

Sailer H, Diekmann HW, Faro H-P, Garbe A (1979) Pharmacokinetics and metabolism of cefazedone in wistar rat, beagle dog and rhesus monkey. Arzneimittelforsch 29:404–411

Saito A, Kato Y, Ishikawa K, Uremura H, Tomizawa M, Nakayama I, Sakurabe T, Matsui K, Yajima O (1978) CS-1170: Pharmacokinetics and clinical evaluation. Chemotherapy (Tokyo) 26(S-5):145–154

Sakai S, Kuriyama M, Kawada Y, Nishiura T (1978) Bacteriological and clinical studies on CS-1170. Chemotherapy (Tokyo) 26(S-5):473–481

Sakatsuge F, Aikawa N, Ishibiki K (1978) Experimental and clinical studies on CS-1170 in surgical field. Chemotherapy (Tokyo) 26(S-5):473–481

Sales JEL, Rimmer DMD (1977) Biliary tract excretion of cefuroxime. Proc R Soc Med [Suppl 9] 70:95–97

Sales JEL, Sutcliffe M, O'Grady F (1972) Cephalexin levels in human bile in presence of biliary tract disease. Br Med J 3:441–443

Santoro J, Agarwal BN, Martinelli R, Wenger N, Levison ME (1978) Pharmacology of cefaclor in normal volunteers and patients with renal failure. Antimicrob Agents Chemother 13:951–954
Sassiver ML, Lewis A (1977) Structure-activity relationships among semisynthetic cephalosporins. I. The first geoneration compounds. In: Perlman D (ed) Structure-activity relationships among the semisynthetic antibiotics. Academic Press, New York, pp 87–160
Saunders JH, McPherson Jr SD (1980) Ocular penetration of cefazolin in humans and rabbits after subconjunctival injection. Am J Ophthalmol 89:564–566
Schreinger A, Hellum KB, Digranes A, Bergman I (1978) Transfer of penicillin G and ampicillin into human skin blisters induced by suction. Scand J Infect Dis [Suppl] 14:233–238
Schrogie JJ, Davies RO, Yeh KC, Rogers D, Holmes GI, Skeggs H, Martin CM (1978) Bioavailability and pharmacokinetics of cefoxitin sodium. J Antimicrob Chemother [Suppl B] 4:69–78
Schrogie JJ, Rogers JD, Yeh KC, Davies RO, Holmes GI, Skeggs H, Martin CM (1979) Pharmacokinetics and comparative pharmacology of cefoxitin and cephalosporins. Rev Infect Dis 1:90–97
Schurig R, Kampf D, Becker H, Forster D (1979) Pharmacokinetik von Azlocillin bei Niereninsuffizienz und Hämodialyse. Arzneimittelforsch 29 II:1944–1948
Schurman DJ, Burton DS, Kajiyama G, Moser K, Nagel DA (1976) Sodium cephapirin disposition and distribution into human bone. Curr Ther Res 20:194–203
Schurman DJ, Hirschman HP, Kajiyama G, Moser K, Burton DS (1978) Cefazolin concentrations in bone and synovial fluid. J Bone Joint Surg 60-A:359–362
Schurman DJ, Hirschman HP, Burton DS (1980) Cephalothin and cefamandole penetration into bone, synovial fluid, and wound drainage fluid. J Bone Joint Surg 62-A:981–985
Schwartz MA, Hayton WL (1972) Relative stability of hetacillin and ampicillin in solution. J Pharm Sci 61:906–909
Seddon M, Wise R, Gillett AP, Livingston R (1980) Pharmacokinetics of Ro 13-9904, a broad-spectrum cephalosporin. Antimicrob Agents Chemother 18:240–242
Severn M, Powis SJA (1979) Biliary excretion and tissue levels of cefuroxime. J Antimicrob Chemother 5:183–188
Shah PM, Helm EG, Stille W (1979) Klinische Erfahrungen mit Cefotaxim, einem neuen Cephalosporin-derivat. Med Welt 30:298–301
Shemonsky NK, Carrizosa J, Levison ME (1975) In vitro activity and pharmacokinetics of cefamandole, a new cephalosporin antibiotic. Antimicrob Agents Chemother 8:679–683
Shibata K, Yura K, Shinagawa N, Suzuki Y, Doi T, Ishikawa S, Takaoka T (1978) Fundamental and clinical studies on CS-1170 in surgical field. Chemotherapy (Tokyo) 26/S-5):403–409
Shimada J, Ueda Y, Yamaji T, Abe Y, Nakamura M (1980) Renal excretion of 6059-S, a new semisynthetic beta-lactam antibiotic. In: Nelson JD, Grassi C (eds) Current chemotherapy of infectious diseases: proceedings of the 11th international congress of chemotherapy – 1979. American Society for Microbiology, Washington, DC, pp 109–110
Shimizu K (1980) Cefoperazone: absorption, excretion, distribution, and metabolism. Clin Ther 3:60–79
Shimizu K, Kuni O (1971) Basic and clinical studies on sulfobenzylpenicillin. Chemotherapy 19:905–909
Shimizu K, Nishimura H (1970) Problems in the bio-assay of orally administered cephaloglycin in biological fluids and method for the detection of its metabolite, desacetylcephaloglycin. J Antibiot 23:216–222
Shiobara Y, Tachibana A, Sasaki H, Watanabe T, Sado T (1974) Phthalidyl D-α-aminobenzylpenicillinate hydrochloride (PC-183), a new orally active ampicillin ester. J Antibiot 27:665–673
Silverstein H, Bernstein JM, Lerner PI (1966) Antibiotic concentrations in middle ear effusions. Pediatrics 38:33–39
Simon C (1980a) Zur Pharmakokinetik von Cefadroxil, einem neuen Ora-Cephalosporin. Arzneimittelforsch 30-I:503–504
Simon C (1980b) Pharmakokinetik von Cefuroxim in Vergleich zu Cefalothin. Praxis 69:870–874

Simon C, Gatzemeier U (1979) Serum and sputum levels of cefaclor. Postgrad Med J [Suppl 4] 55:30–34
Simon C, Malerczyk V (1977) Serum and skin blister concentrations of cefuroxime in relation to dose and in comparison to cephalothin. Proc R Soc Med [Suppl 9] 70:19–21
Simon C, Bekesch M, Malerczyk V (1972) Zur Pharmakokinetik von Penicillin V im Kindesalter (insbesondere bei Neugeborenen). Med Welt 23:1717–1720
Simon C, Malerczyk V, Brahmstaedt E, Toeller W (1973) Cefazolin, ein neues Breitspektrum-antibiotikum. Dtsch Med Wochenschr 98:2448–2450
Simon C, Malerczyk V, Von Wulffen CG (1976a) In vitro-Aktivität und Pharmakokinetik von Propicillin, Penicillin V and Phenethicillin. Med Welt 27:2476–2481
Simon C, Malerczyk V, Tenschert B, Mohlenbeck F (1976b) Die geriatrische Pharmakologie von Cefazolin, Cefradin und Sulfisomidin. Arzneimittelforsch 26:1377–1381
Simon C, Malerczyk V, Klaus M (1978a) Absorption of bacampicillin and ampicillin and penetration into body fluids (skin blister fluid, saliva, tears) in healthy volunteers. Scand J Infect Dis [Suppl] 14:228–232
Simon C, Meyer E, Malerczyk V (1978b) Cefoxitin, ein neues β-Lactamasestabiles Antibiotikum. Arzneimittelforsch 28:1541–1545
Sinagowitz E, Pelz K, Burgert A, Kaczkowski W (1976a) Concentration of cefazolin in human skeletal muscle. Infection 4:192–195
Sinagowitz E, Pelz K, Burgert A, Kaczkowski W, Sommerkamp H, Westenfelder SR (1976b) Tissue concentrations of cefazolin in man. Chemotherapy 5:305–310
Singhvi SM, Heald AF, Gadebusch HH, Resnick ME, DiFazio LT, Leitz MA (1977) Human serum protein binding of cephalosporin antibiotics in vitro. J Lab Clin Med 89:414–420
Singhvi SM, Heald AF, Schreiber EC (1978) Pharmacokinetics of cephalosporin antibiotics: protein-binding considerations. Chemotherapy 24:121–133
Sitka U, Weingärtner, Patsch R, Richter I (1980) Pharmacokinetics of azlocillin in neonates. Chemotherapy 26:171–176
Sjoberg B, Ekstrom B, Forsgren U (1968) α-Azidobenzylpenicillin. I. Chemistry, bacteriology, and experimental chemotherapy. In: Hobby GL (ed) Antimicrobial agents and chemotherapy – 1967. American Society for Microbiology, Bethesda, pp 560–567
Sjövall J, Magni L, Bergan T (1978) Pharmacokinetics of becampicillin compared with those of ampicillin, pivampicillin, and amoxycillin. Antimicrob Agents Chemother 13:90–96
Smyth RD, Pfeffer M, Glick A, Van Harken DR, Hottendorf GH (1979) Clinical pharmacokinetics and safety of high doses of ceforanide (BL-S786R) and cefazolin. Antimicrob Agents Chemother 16:615–621
Solomon AE, Briggs JD, McGeachy R, Sleigh JD (1975) The administration of cephradine to patients in renal failure. Br J Clin Pharmacol 2:443–448
Sonneville PF, Kartodirdjo RR, Skeggs H, Till AE, Martin CM (1976) Comparative clinical pharmacology of intravenous cefoxitin and cephalothin. Eur J Clin Pharmacol 9:397–403
Sonneville PF, Albert KS, Skeggs H, Gentner H, Kwan KC, Martin CM (1977) Effect of lidocaine on the absorption, disposition and tolerance of intramuscularly administered cefoxitin. Eur J Clin Pharmacol 12:273–279
Sorin M, Ghnassia JC, Demerleire F, Saudubray JM (1977) Pharmacokinetic and clinical study of cefuroxime in infants. Proc R Soc Med [Suppl 9] 70:175–178
Spector R, Lorenzo AV (1974) The effects of salicylate and probenecid on the cerebrospinal fluid transport of penicillin, aminosalicylic acid and iodidie. J Pharmacol Exp Ther 188:55–65
Speer ME, Taber LH, Clark DB, Rudolph AJ (1977) Cerebrospinal fluid levels of benzathine penicillin G in the neonate. J Pediatrics 91:996–997
Spring Von P, Raber J, Reber H, Dettli L (1974) Die Elimination des Antibiotikums Cephacetril bei Patienten mit eingeschränkter Nierenfunktion. Arzneimittelforsch 24:1462–1466
Spyker DA, Rugloski RJ, Vann RL, O'Brien WM (1977) Pharmacokinetics of amoxicillin: dose dependence after intravenous, oral, and intramuscular administration. Antimicrob Agents Chemother 11:141–143

Spyker DA, Thomas BL, Sande MA, Bolton WK (1978) Pharmacokinetics of cefaclor and cephalexin: dosage nomograms for impaired renal function. Antimicrob Agents Chemother 14:172–177

Stein GH, Pickering MJ, Johnson III JE (1974) Cephaloglycin studies in patients with varying renal impairment. Clin Med 81:36–38

Steinberg EA, Overturf GD, Baraff LJ, Wilkins J (1977) Penetration of cefamandole into spinal fluid. Antimicrob Agents Chemother 11:933–935

Stewart GT, Harrison M (1961) Excretion and re-excretion of a broad-spectrum penicillin in bile. Br J Pharmacol 17:414–419

Stewart GT, Coles HMT, Nixon HH, Holt RJ (1961) "Penbritin": an oral penicillin with broad-spectrum activity. Br Med J 2:200–206

Stewart KS, Shafi M, Andrews J, Williams JD (1973) Distribution of parenteral ampicillin and cephalosporins in late pregnancy. J Obstet Gynecol Br Commonw 80:902–908

Strausbaugh LJ, Girgis NI, Mikhail LA, Edman DC, Miner WF, Yassin MW (1978) Penetration of amoxicillin into cerebrospinal fluid. Antimicrob Agents Chemother 14:899–902

Strojny N, DeSilva JAF (1980) Determination of mecillinam in urine by reversed-phase high-performance liquid chromatography. J Chromatog 181:272–281

Stuflesser H, Walker N, Meyer-Brunot HG, Theobald W (1978) Microbiological assessment of the concentration of cephacetrile in plasma and cancellous bone of femoral heads. J Antimicrob Chemother 4:188

Sullivan HR, McMahon RE (1967) Metabolism of oral cephalothin and related cephalosporins in the rat. Biochem J 102:976–982

Sullivan HR, Billings RE, McMahon RE (1969a) Metabolism of D-cephaloglycin-^{14}C and L-cephaloglycin-^{14}C in the rat. J Antibiot 22:27–33

Sullivan HR, Billings RE, McMahon RE (1969b) Metabolism of cephalexin-^{14}C in mice and in rats. J Antibiot 22:195–200

Sullivan HR, Due SL, Kau DKL, Quay JF, Miller WM (1976) Metabolism of [^{14}C]-cefaclor, a cephalosporin antibiotic, in three species of laboratory animals. Antimicrob Agents Chemother 10:630–638

Sullivan HR, Due SL, Kau DLK, Quay JF, Miller WM (1977) Metabolic fate of [^{14}C]cefamandole, a parenteral cephalosporin antibiotic, in rats and dogs. Antimicrob Agents Chemother 12:73–79

Sullivan NP, Symmes AT, Miller HC, Rhodehammel HW (1948) A new penicillin for prolonged blood levels. Science 107:169–170

Sutherland R, Wise PJ (1971) α-Carboxy-3-thienylmethylpenicillin (BRL 2288), a new semisynthetic penicillin: absorption and excretion in man. In: Hobby GL (ed) Antimicrobial agents and chemotherapy – 1970. American Society for Microbiology, Bethesda, pp 402–406

Sutherland R, Burnett J, Rolinson GN (1971) α-Carboxy-3-thienylmethylpenicillin (BRL 2288), a new semisynthetic penicillin: in vitro evaluation. In: Hobby GL (ed) Antimicrobial agents and chemotherapy – 1970. American Society for Microbiology, Bethesda, pp 390–395

Sutherland R, Croydon EAP, Rolinson GN (1970) Flucloxacillin, a new isoxazolyl penicillin, compared with oxacillin, cloxacillin, and dicloxacillin. Br Med J 4:455–460

Sutherland R, Elson S, Croydon EAP (1972) Metampicillin. Chemotherapy 17:145–160

Swahn Å (1975) On the absorption and metabolism of ^{35}S-ampicillin. Eur J Clin Pharmacol 9:117–124

Symes JM, Jarvis JD, Tresidder GC (1974) An appraisal of cephalexin monohydrate levels in semen and prostatic tissue. Chemotherapy 20:257–262

Szabo JL, Edwards CD, Bruce NF (1951) N,N^1-Dibenzylethylenediamine penicillin: preparation and properties. Antibiot Chemother 1:499–503

Takamoto H, Kamata H, Hirano M, Kondo K, Araki T, Matsumura Y, Ohmori H, Kondo A, Nanba K, Katayama Y (1978) Clinical and experimental studies on CS-1170 in urological fields. Chemotherapy (Tokyo) 26(S-5):501–514

Takase Z, Shirafuji H, Uchida M (1978) Fundamental and clinical studies of CS-1170 in field of obstetrics and gynecology. Chemotherapy (Tokyo) 26(S-5):566–574

Tally FP, Jacobus NV, Barza M (1979) In vitro activity and serum protein-binding of cefaclor. J Antimicrob Chemother 5:159–165
Tan JS, Salstrom SJ (1977) Levels of carbenicillin, ticarcillin, cephalothin, cefazolin, cefamandole, gentamicin, tobramycin, and amikacin in human serum and interstitial fluid. Antimicrob Agents Chemother 11:698–700
Tan JS, Salstrom SJ (1979) Bacampicillin, ampicillin, cephalothin, and cephapirin levels in human blood and interstitial fluid. Antimicrob Agents Chemother 15:510–512
Tan JS, Trott A, Phair JP, Watanakunakorn C (1972) A method of measurement of antibiotics in human interstitial fluid. J Infect Dis 126:492–497
Tan JS, Bannister T, Phair JP (1974) Levels of amoxicillin and ampicillin in human serum and interstitial fluid. J Infect Dis [Suppl] 129:146–148
Tanayama S, Yoshida K, Kanai Y (1978) Metabolic fate of SCE-129, a new anti pseudomonal cephalosporin, after parenteral administration in rats and dogs. Antimicrob Agents Chemother 14:137–143
Tetzlaff TR, McCracken Jr GH, Thomas ML (1978) Bioavailability of cephalexin in children: relationship to drug formulations and meals. J Pediatr 92:292–294
Thijssen HHW (1978) Physico-chemical properties of the active metabolites of the isoxazolylpenicillins as deduced from their chromatographic behaviour. Drug Res 28:1065–1067
Thijssen HHW (1979) Identification of the active metabolites of the isoxazolyl-penicillins by means of mass-spectrometry. J Antibiot 32:1033–1037
Thijssen HHW, Mattie H (1976) Active metabolites of isoxazolylpenicillins in humans. Antimicrob Agents Chemother 10:441–446
Thornhill RS, Levison ME, Johnson WD, Kaye D (1969) In vitro antimicrobial activity and human pharmacology of cephalexin, a new orally absorbed cephalosporin C antibiotic. Appl Microbiol 17:457–461
Thys JP, Vanderkelen B, Klastersky J (1976) Pharmacological study of cefazolin during intermittent and continuous infusion: a crossover investigation in humans. Antimicrob Agents Chemother 10:395–398
Tjandramaga TB, Mullie A, Verbesselt R, DeSchepper PJ, Verbist L (1978) Piperacillin: human pharmacokinetics after intravenous and intramuscular administration. Antimicrob Agents Chemother 14:829–837
Tsuchiya K, Yamazaki T, Kuchimura A, Fugono T (1972) Absorption, excretion and tissue distribution of sulfocillin administered parenterally in mice, rats, rabbits, and dogs. J Antibiot 25:336–342
Tsuji A, Miyamoto E, Terasaki T, Yamana T (1979) Physiological pharmacokinetics of β-lactam antibiotics: penicillin V distribution and elimination after intravenous administration in rats. J Pharma Pharmacol 31:116–119
Tuano SB, Johnson LD, Brodie JL, Kirby WMM (1966) Comparative blood levels of hetacillin, ampicillin and penicillin G. N Engl J Med 275:635–639
Tuano SB, Brodie JL, Kirby WMM (1967) Cephaloridine versus cephalothin: relation of the kidney to blood level differences after parenteral administration. In: Hobby GL (ed) Antimicrobial agents and chemotherapy – 1966. American Society for Microbiology, Bethesda, pp 101–106
Turner JR, Preston DA, Wold JS (1977) Delineation of the relative antibacterial activity of cefamandole and cefamandole nafate. Antimicrob Agents Chemother 12:67–72
Ueda Y, Matsumoto F, Nakamura N, Saito A, Noda K, Furuya C, Omori M, Shimojyo S, Hanaoka H, Utsunomiya M, Fujinoki T (1970) A study on cyclacillin. Jpn J Antibiot 23:48–53
Ueda Y, Matsumoto F, Saito A, Noda K, Shimada J, Kobayashi C, Omori M, Shiba K, Yamaji T (1971) Studies on sulfobenzylpenicillin. Chemotherapy 19:920–926
Ueda Y, Matsumoto F, Saito A, Ohomori M, Shiba K, Yamaji T, Ihara H (1978) Clinical studies on CS-1170. Chemotherapy (Tokyo) 26(S-5):203–209
Ullmann U, Wurst W (1979) Antibacterial active components in human urine after administration of penicillins. Infection 7:187–189
Ungethüm, Pabst J, Dingeldein E, Leopold G (1979) Clinical pharmacology of cefazedone, a new cephalosporin, in healthy volunteers. Arzneimittelforsch 29:443–448

Uwaydah MW, Faris BM, Samara IN, Shammas HF, To'mey KF (1976) Cloxacillin penetration. Am J Ophthalmol 82:114–116
Valdivieso RF-C, Flores-Mercado F, Estopier-Jauregui C, Galindo-Hernandez E, Diaz-Gonzales C (1977) Farmacologia clinica del cefadroxil y la cefalexina. Invest Med Int 4:3–9
Vanderhaeghe H, Van Dijck P, Claesen M, DeSomer P (1962) Preparation and properties of 3,4-dichloro-α-methoxybenzylpenicillin. In: Finland M, Savage GM (eds) Antimicrobial agents and chemotherapy – 1961. American Society for Microbiology, Bethesda, pp 581–587
Vanderhaeghe H, Parmentier G, Evrard E (1963) Identification of p-hydroxy phenoxymethyl penicillin as a metabolite of phenoxymethyl penicillin. Nature 200:891
Van Dijck PJ, Claesen M, Vanderhaeghe H, De Somer P (1962) Laboratory studies of 3,4-dichloro-α-methoxybenzylpenicillin. Antibiot Chemother 12:192–203
Van Harken DR, Dixon CW, Essery JM (1970) An active metabolite of dicloxacillin. Pharmacologist 12:220
Vent J (1979) Mezlocillin-Konzentrationen im menschlichen Knochen. Arzneimittelforsch 29 II:1969–1971
Venuto RC, Plaut ME (1971) Cephalothin handling in patients undergoing hemodialysis. In: Hobby GL (ed) Antimicrobial agents and chemotherapy – 1970. American Society for Microbiology, Bethesda, pp 50–52
Verbist L (1974) Triple crossover study on absorption and excretion of ampicillin, pivampicillin, and amoxycillin. Antimicrob Agents Chemother 6:588–593
Verbist L (1976) Triple crossover study on absorption and excretion of ampicillin, talampicillin, and amoxycillin. Antimicrob Agents Chemother 10:173–175
Verbist L, VanderHeyden JS (1980) Penetration of cefuroxime into uterine and ovarian tissue. In: Nelson JD, Grassi C (eds) Current chemotherapy of infectious diseases: proceedings of the 11th international congress of chemotherapy – 1979. American Society for Microbiology, Washington, DC, pp 1170–1171
Verbist L, Tjandramaga TB, Verbessett R, DeSchepper PJ (1979) Mezlocillin pharmacokinetics. Arzneimittelforsch 29 II:1962–1966
Verhoef J, Oe PL, Simonian S (1973) The clearance of antibiotics by the artificial kidney. Chemotherapy 19:272–278
Veronese FM, Bevilacqua R, Boccu E, Benassi CA (1977) Drug-protein interaction: The binding of cephalosporins to albumins. Farmaco [Sci] 32:303–310
Verway WF, Williams Jr HR (1963) Relationships between the concentrations of various penicillins in plasma and peripheral lymph. In: Sylvester JC (ed) Antimicrobial agents and chemotherapy – 1962. American Society for Microbiology, Bethesda, pp 476–483
Vianna NJ, Kaye D (1967) Penetration of cephalothin into the spinal fluid. Am J Med Sci 254:216–220
Viek P (1963) Concentration of sodium nafcillin in pathological synovial fluid. In: Sylvester JC (ed) Antimicrobial agents and chemotherapy – 1962. American Society for Microbiology, Bethesda, pp 379–383
Vitti TG, Gurwith MJ, Ronald AR (1974) Pharmacologic studies of amoxicillin in nonfasting adults. J Infect Dis [Suppl] 129:149–153
Vlasses PH, Holbrook AM, Schrogie JJ, Rogers JD, Ferguson RK, Abrams WB (1980) Effect of orally administered probenecid on the pharmacokinetics of cefoxitin. Antimicrob Agents Chemother 17:847–855
Von Daehne W, Godtfredsen WO, Roholt K, Tyboing L (1971) Pivampicillin, a new orally active ampicillin ester. In: Hobby GL (ed) Antimicrobial agents and chemotherapy – 1970. American Society for Microbiology, Bethesda, pp 431–437
Von Daehne W, Frederiksen E, Gundersen E, Lund F, Morch P, Petersen HJ, Rohalt K, Tybring L, Godtfredsen WO (1970) Acyloxymethyl esters of ampicillin. J Med Chem 13:607–612
Vukovich RA, Brannick LJ, Sugerman AA, Neiss ES (1975a) Sex differences in the intramuscular absorption and bioavailability of cephradine. Clin Pharmacol Ther 18:215–220

Vukovich RA, Sugerman AA, Fields LA (1975b) Effect of 2% procaine hydrochloride solution on the bioavailability of cephradine after intramuscular injection. Curr Ther Res 18:711–719
Wagner ES, Lindley B, Talbert M (1977) Benzylpenicillin migrates irreversibly into human erythrocytes. J Antibiot 30:1115–1118
Wagner JG, Leslie LG, Gove RS (1969) Relative absorption of both tetracycline and penicillin G administered rectally and orally in aqueous solution. Int J Clin Pharmacol 2:44–51
Wahlig H, Dingeldein E, Mitsuhashi S, Kawabe A (1979) Cefazedone: microbiological evaluation in comparison with cephalothin and cefazolin. Arneimittelforsch 29:369–378
Walkenstein SS, Kuna M, Seifter J (1954a) Fate and sojourn of C^{14}-dibenzylethylenediamine (DBED) and C^{14}-DBED dipenicillin G (Bicillin) following oral and intramuscular injection. Antibiot Chemother 4:700–706
Walkenstein SS, Chumakow N, Seifter J (1954b) Fate and sojourn of dibenzylethylenediamine C^{14}-dipenicillin G and C^{14}-penicillin G following oral and intramuscular injection. Antibiot Chemother 4:1245–1250
Walkenstein SS, Wiser R, Leboutillier E, Gudmundsen C, Kimmel H (1963) Absorption, metabolism, and excretion of the semisynthetic penicillin 6-(2-ethoxy-1-naphthamido)-penicillanic acid (nafcillin). J Pharm Sci 52:763–767
Walker SH, Gahol VP (1978) Pharmacokinetics of cefamandole in infants and children. Antimicrob Agents Chemother 14:315–317
Warren S, Bryan C, Glazer J, Arbeter A, Plotkin SA (1980) Clinical and pharmacologic studies of cefoxitin in children. In: Nelson JD, Grassi C (eds) Current chemotherapy and infectious disease: proceedings of the 11th international congress of chemotherapy – 1979. American Society for Microbiology, Washington, DC, pp 1150–1151
Wasz-Hockert O, Nummi S, Vuspala S, Jarviren (1970) Transplacental passage of azidocillin, ampicillin, and penicillin G during early and late pregnancy. Acta Pediatr Scand 206:109–110
Watanabe Y, Hayashi T, Takada R, Yasuda T, Saikawa I, Shimizu K (1980) Studies on protein binding of antibiotics. I. Effect of cefazolin on protein binding and pharmacokinetics of cefoperazone. J Antibiot 33:625–635
Watanakunakorn C (1977) Absorption of orally administered nafcillin in normal healthy volunteers. Antimicrob Agents Chemother 11:1007–1009
Waterman NG, Eickenberg HU, Scharfenberger L (1976) Concentration of cefamandole in serum interstitial fluid, bile, and urine. Antimicrob Agents Chemother 10:733–735
Webber JA, Ott JL (1977) Structure-activity relationships in the cephalosporins. II. Recent developments. In: Perlman D (ed) Structure-activity relationships among the semisynthetic antibiotics. Academic, New York, pp 161–237
Weingarten L, Sitka U, Patsch R, Richter I, Thiemann HH (1979) Zur Frage der Ausscheidung von Azlocillin in das Bronchialsekret im Kindesalter. Arzneimittelforsch 29 II:1952–1954
Weinstein AJ (1980) The cephalosporins: activity and clinical use. Drugs 19:137–154
Weliky I, Leitz M (1976) Effect of serum protein binding on the comparative bioavailability of cephradine and cefazolin. Clin Res 24:514A
Weliky I, Gadebusch HH, Kripalani K, Arnow P, Schreiber EC (1974) Cephradine: absorption, excretion, and tissue distribution in animals of a new cephalosporin antibiotic. Antimicrob Agents Chemother 5:49–54
Welling PG, Huang H, Koch PA, Craig WA, Madsen PO (1977) Bioavailability of ampicillin and amoxicillin in fasted and non-fasted subjects. J Pharm Sci 66:549–552
Welling PG, Dean S, Selen A, Kendall MJ, Wise R (1979) The pharmacokinetics of the oral cephalosporins cefaclor, cephradine, and cephalexin. Int J Clin Pharmacol Biopharma 17:397–400
Westenfelder SR, Naber KG, Madsen PO (1974) Pharmacokinetics of a new cephalosporin, cephacetrile, in patients with normal and impaired renal function. Arzneimittelforsch 24:1481–1485
Westerman G, Pearl MA, Dykyj R, Mapp Y, Winstin D, Nodine JH (1965) Human in vivo kinetics of penicillinase activity against penicillin G, methicillin, and nafcillin. In: Syl-

vester JC (ed) Antimicrobial agents and chemotherapy – 1964. American Society for Microbiology, Bethesda, pp 321–328
Whelton A, Sapir DG, Carter GG, Garth MA, Walker WG (1972) Intrarenal distribution of ampicillin in the normal and diseased human kidney. J Infect Dis 125:466–470
Whelton A, Carter GG, Bryant HH (1973) Carbenicillin concentrations in normal and diseased kidneys. A therapeutic consideration. Ann Intern Med 78:659–662
Whelton A, Blanco LJ, Carter GG, Craig TJ, Bryant HH, Herbst DV, King TM (1980) Therapeutic implications of doxycycline and cephalothin concentrations in the female genital tract. Obstet Gynecol 55:28–32
Wick WE (1966) In vitro and in vivo laboratory comparison of cephalothin and desacetylcephalothin. In: Hobby GL (ed) Antimicrobial agents and chemotherapy – 1965. American Society for Microbiology, Bethesda, pp 870–875
Wick WE (1967) Cephalexin, a new orally absorbed cephalosporin antibiotic. Appl Microbiol 15:765–769
Wick WE, Boniece WS (1965) In vitro and in vivo laboratory evaluation of cephaloglycin and cephaloridine. Appl Microbiol 13:248–253
Wick WE, Preston DA (1972) Biological properties of three 3-heterocyclicthiomethyl cephalosporin antibiotics. Antimicrob Agents Chemother 1:221–234
Wick WE, Streightoff F, Boniece WS (1962) Evaluation of the biological activities of alphaphenoxypropyl penicillin. In: Finland M, Savage GM (eds) Antimicrobial agents and chemotherapy – 1961. American Society for Microbiology, Bethesda, pp 588–593
Wick WE, Wright WE, Kuder HV (1971) Cephaloglycin and its biologically active metabolite desacetylcephaloglycin. Appl Microbiol 21:426–434
Widholm O, Renkonen O-V (1973) Placental transfer of a cephalosporin derivative (C 36'278-Ba). Ann Med Exp Biol Fenn 51:155–157
Williams JD, Andrews J, Mitchard M, Kendall MJ (1976) Bacteriology and pharmacology of the new amidino penicillin-mecillinam. J Antimicrob Chemother 2:61–69
Wilkinson PJ, Reeves DS, Wise R, Allen JT (1975) Volunteer and clinical studies with carfecillin: a new orally administered ester of carbenicillin. Br J Med 2:250–252
Wilkinson PJ, Coddington CAM, Noblett HR, Turner A (1979) Perioperative use of cefoxitin in children. Res Clin Forums 1:97–102
Windorfer A, Gasteiger U (1977) Studies on serum and cerebrospinal fluid levels of cephacetrile in neonates. Infection 5:242–247
Winley CL, Spears JC, Scott JK (1979) Comparison of cefamandole nafate to cefamandole by microbiological assay. Antimicrob Agents Chemother 16:424–426
Wirth K, Schomerus M, Hengstmann JH (1976a) Zur Pharmakokinetik von Azlocillin, einem neuen halbsynthetischen Breitspektrumantibiotikum. Infection 4:25–30
Wirth K, Hengstmann JH, Langebartels FH, Träger (1976b) Zur Kinetik von Ampicillin, Oxacillin und Carbenicillin nach intravenöser Kurzinfusion beim Menschen. Arzneimittelforsch 26:1709–1714
Wirz H, Vischer WA, Fullhaas J, Imhof (1978) Pharmacokinetics of CGP 9000, a new orally active cephalosporin, in healthy volunteers. In: Siegenthaler W, Lutley R (eds) Current chemotherapy proceedings of the 10th international congress of chemotherapy – 1977. American Society for Microbiology, Washington, DC, pp 827–830
Wise R, Reeves DS (1975) Two aspects of the availability of cephalosporins after intramuscular injection. J Antimicrob Chemother 1:S47–52
Wise R, Reeves DS, Parker AS (1974) Administration of ticarcillin, a new antipseudomonal antibiotic, in patients undergoing dialysis. Antimicrob Agents Chemother 5:119–120
Wise R, Cadge B, Gillett AP, Bhamjee A (1979a) The pharmacology of cefoxitin and the comparison of two human tissue models. Infection [Suppl 1] 1:49–56
Wise R, Cadge B, Gillett AP, Bhamjee A, Livingston R, Welling PG, Thornhill DP (1979b) Pharmacokinetics of Bay K 4999, a new broad-spectrum penicillin. Antimicrob Agents Chemother 15:670–673
Wise R, Andrews JM, Hammond D, Wills PJ, Geddes AM, McKendrick MW (1980a) Comparison of the activity of the desacetyl metabolite of cefotaxime (HR-756) with that of cefotaxime and other cephalosporins. In: Nelson JD, Grassi C (eds) Current chemotherapy of infectious diseases: proceedings of the 11th international congress of chemotherapy – 1979. American Society for Microbiology, Washington, DC, pp 118–119

Wise R, Baker S, Livingston R (1980b) Comparison of cefotaxime and moxalactam pharmacokinetics and tissue levels. Antimicrob Agents Chemother 18:369–371
Wise R, Baker S, Wright N, Livingston R (1980c) The pharmacokinetics of LY 127935, a broad spectrum oxa-β-lactam. J Antimicrob Chemother 6:319–322
Wise R, Wills PJ, Andrews JM, Bedford KA (1980d) Activity of the cefotaxime (HR 756) desacetyl metabolite compared with those of cefotaxime and other cephalosporins. Antimicrob Agents Chemother 17:84–86
Wise R, Gillett AP, Cadge B, Durham SR, Baker S (1980e) The influence of protein binding upon tissue fluid levels of six β-lactam antibiotics. J Infect Dis 142:77–82
Wittke RR, Adam D (1980) Diffusion of cefsulodin (CGP 7174/E) into human tissues. In: Nelson JD, Grassi C (eds) Current chemotherapy of infectious diseases: proceedings of the 11th international congress of chemotherapy – 1979. American Society for Microbiology, Washington, DC, pp 197–199
Wittmann DH, Schassan H-H, Welter J, Seidel H (1980) Verfügbarkeit von Cefotaxim. Muench Med Wochenschr 122:637–641
Wold JS, Joost RR, Black HR, Griffith RS (1978) Hydrolysis of cefamandole nafate to cefamandole in vivo. J Infect Dis 137:S17–24
Wright N, Wise R (1980) Cefotaxime elimination in patients with renal and liver dysfunction. In: Nelson JD, Grassi C (eds) Current chemotherapy of infectious diseases: proceedings of the 11th international congress of chemotherapy – 1979. American Society for Microbiology, Washington, DC, pp 133–134
Wright WE, Frogge JA (1980) Hydrolysis of 3-acetoxymethyl cephalosporins by lysed whole blood. Antimicrob Agents Chemother 17:99–100
Yaffe SJ, Gerbracht LM, Mosovich LL, Mattar ME, Danish M, Jusko WJ (1977) Pharmacokinetics of methicillin in patients with cystic fibrosis. J Infect Dis 135:828–831
Yamada N, Kido K, Uchida H, Yano J, Sagawa N, Hayashi S (1980) Application of cephalosporins to obstetrics and gynecology: transfer of cefazolin and cephalothin to uterine tissue. Am J Obstet Gynecol 136:1036–1040
Yamamoto T, Kitaura S, Kato M, Nagasaka H, Kan S, Takeuchi T (1978a) Laboratory and clinical studies on CS-1170. Chemotherapy (Tokyo) 26(S-5):275–282
Yamamoto Y, Furuhara K, Shimura H (1978b) Clinical studies on CS-1170 in surgical field. Chemotherapy (Tokyo) 26(S-5):425–429
Yamaoka K, Narita S, Nakagawa T, Uno T (1979) High-performance liquid chromatographic analyses of sulbenicillin and carbenicillin in human urine. J Chromatog 168:187–193
Yamasaku F, Suzuki Y (1978) Pharmacokinetics of CS-1170. Chemotherapy (Tokyo) 26(S-5):264–267
Yoshioka H, Takimoto M, Riley Jr HD (1974) Pharmacokinetics of ampicillin in the newborn infant. J Infect Dis 129:461–464
Yoshioka H, Takimoto M, Shimizu T, Haga H (1979a) Pharmacokinetics of intramuscular carbenicillin in the newborn. Infection 7:27–29
Yoshioka H, Cho K, Takimoto M, Maruyama S, Shimizu T (1979b) Transfer of cefazolin into human milk. J Pediatr 94:151–152
Zaki A, Schreiber EC, Weliky I, Knill JR, Hubsher (1974) Clinical pharmacology of oral cephradine. J Clin Pharmacol 14:118–126
Zech P, Pozet N, Monnier JC, Beruard M, Traeger J (1974) Etude du metabolisme renal d'un sel sodique de l'acide cephalosporanique. Pathol Biol 22:365–370
Ziv G, Sulman FG (1974) Effects on probenecid on the distribution, elimination, and passage into milk of benzylpenicillin, ampicillin, and cloxacillin. Arch Int Pharmacodyn 207:373–382

CHAPTER 16

Toxicology of β-Lactam Antibiotics

M. C. BROWNING and B. M. TUNE

A. Introduction

One of the most important qualities of the animal and human pharmacology of the first penicillins has been a remarkably favorable chemotherapeutic index. Aside from problems of local irritation and of neurotoxicity with extremely large doses, these antibiotics have minimal direct toxicity. For nearly 20 years, allergic or immune-mediated reactions represented the only common complications of the use of penicillins. However, the development of the newer penicillins and the cephalosporins, although providing some of the safest and most important antibiotics in current use, has introduced new problems in direct, nonallergic toxicity.

This discussion summarizes a large and widely dispersed literature on the toxic effects of the various penicillins and cephalosporins. Where there is adequate experience with a problem in both animals and humans, an effort has been made to discuss toxicity separately for both groups. Wherever possible, a discussion of the mechanisms of toxicity is also included.

B. Local Reactions to Parenteral Administration

Pain and sterile inflammatory reactions at the site of intramuscular injection are among the most common local effects of therapy with the penicillins and cephalosporins. With benzylpenicillin these reactions appear to be related to the concentration of the antibiotic, and this may also be the case for the other penicillins (MANDELL and SANDE 1980).

Phlebitis develops in many patients receiving intravenous penicillins or cephalosporins (SVEDHEM et al. 1980). The relative risk of phlebitis among the different cephalosporins is unsettled (CARRIZOSA et al. 1973; BERGER et al. 1976; TROLLFORS et al. 1979). Cephalothin has the reputation for being more irritative than many (MANDELL and SANDE 1980), but comparative clinical trials have reported conflicting results (BRAN et al. 1972; LIPMAN 1974; SHEMONSKY et al. 1975; BERGERON et al. 1976). The variations in outcome of these studies may be the result of differences in experimental design or the small numbers of patients involved.

C. Gastrointestinal Side Effects

Gastrointestinal side effects are among the most common adverse reactions to oral treatment with the β-lactam antibiotics. Some degree of gastric irritation is reported in 2%–7% of patients (BERGAN 1979). The discomfort occasionally results in discontinuation of the drug, but serious consequences are rare.

Diarrhea is also a relatively common problem, which may be of mild or life-threatening severity. At least three types are distinguishable: (1) nonspecific diarrhea, (2) pseudomembranous colitis, and (3) presumed ischemic colitis.

I. Nonspecific Diarrhea

The frequency of nonspecific diarrhea varies from one drug to another, being as high as 20%–35% in humans taking ampicillin (BASS et al. 1967, 1973; TEDESCO 1975). Parenterally administerd agents or those which are well absorbed after oral dosage have been associated with low rates of diarrhea (BERGAN 1979).

The etiology of this process has not been determined. Speculation centers on an alteration in gut flora (ABRAMOWITZ 1981), with a resulting predominance of bacterial species which elaborate a locally acting irritant. However, no pathogenic bacterium, toxin, or irritant has been identified, and a direct effect of the drug or a metabolite on susceptible intestinal mucosa cannot be excluded.

II. Pseudomembranous Colitis

The association of a lethal cecitis with penicillin administration to hamsters and guinea pigs has been known for some time (BARTLETT et al. 1978). Pseudomembranous colitis, a similar disease in humans, has also been associated with benzylpenicillin, ampicillin, cephalothin, cephaloridine, cefazolin, cephalexin, and cefoxitin (CHRISTIE and AMENT 1975; BARTLETT et al. 1978, 1979; HUTCHEON et al. 1978; NEWMAN and MCCOLLUM 1979; DONTA et al. 1980; SCHWARTZ et al. 1980).

Evidence that a microbial organism was involved was the early observation that germ-free guinea pigs tolerated penicillin well (NEWTON et al. 1964). There is now considerable evidence, in both animals and humans, that pseudomembranous colitis is caused by intestinal overgrowth of an enterotoxigenic clostridial species. BARTLETT et al. (1978) reported that the stools of hamsters dying of cecitis after cephalothin, cephalexin, or ampicillin administration contained *Clostridium difficile* and its toxin. Reports in humans have also implicated this species or its toxin in histologically confirmed pseudomembranous colitis (BARTLETT et al. 1979; DONTA et al. 1980; SCHWARTZ et al. 1980).

Antibiotic susceptibility testing reveals that the clostridia are generally resistant to the cephalosporins (GEORGE et al. 1978), but may be sensitive to ampicillin (SCHWARTZ et al. 1980). The diarrhea associated with antibiotic-sensitive enterotoxigenic clostridia may follow discontinuation of the offending drug (CHRISTIE and AMENT 1975; HUTCHEON et al. 1978; SCHWARTZ et al. 1980), and may be due to an overgrowth of these organisms during recolonization of the intestine. Both animals and humans respond to therapy directed at the *Clostridium* (vancomycin) or its toxin (cholestyramine) (BARTLETT et al. 1979; NEWMAN and MCCOLLUM 1979; SCHWARTZ et al. 1980).

III. Ischemic Colitis

TOFFLER et al. (1978) reported five distinctive cases involving patients receiving a penicillin. They interpreted the findings as consistent with bowel ischemia and speculated that the ischemia might be immunologically mediated. Another case with strikingly similar features has been reported (FOX 1979). All cases recovered shortly after withdrawal of the antibiotic.

D. Immunologically Mediated Toxicity

I. Human Toxicity

Some of the most important reactions to β-lactam antibiotics result from the involvement of humoral or cellular immunity. Almost all patients receiving benzylpenicillin develop antibodies to it (PETZ 1976; MANDELL and SANDE 1980). Few go on to develop allergic complications, but in those who do the clinical manifestations include examples of the entire spectrum of immune-mediated reactions. Whether this breadth of reaction is so for other β-lactam antibiotics remains to be determined.

The frequency of allergic reactions to penicillins has been reported as 0.7%–10% (STEWART 1973; MANDELL and SANDE 1980), and that to cephalosporins has been estimated to be 0.8%–7.5% (PETZ 1978, MANDELL and SANDE 1980).

Humoral hypersensitivity produces some of the most serious adverse effects, including urticaria, angioedema, bronchospasm, and anaphylaxis. The frequency of anaphylactic reactions to penicillin has been estimated to be 0.015% (MANDELL and SANDE 1980) to 0.045% (PORTER and JICK 1977). A history of previous exposure to penicillin is common but not invariable (MANDELL and SANDE 1980). Skin testing may be helpful in distinguishing those patients at risk for anaphylaxis, especially if testing is conducted with both major and minor antigenic determinants of the penicillin (LEVINE and ZOLOV 1969; PETZ 1978).

Skin rashes during the administration of a penicillin or cephalosporin are relatively common, occurring in approximately 2% of cases (VAN WINZUM 1978; BERGAN 1979; AHLSTEDT et al. 1980). Contact dermatitis may also be a problem for individuals preparing penicillin solutions or given penicillin in a topical ointment (MANDELL and SANDE 1980). An erythematous, macular or maculopapullar rash may occur in as many as 9% of patients receiving aminopenicillins such as ampicillin (BERGAN 1979; AHLSTEDT et al. 1980; MANDELL and SANDE 1980). The rates may be higher still when these penicillins are given to patients with infectious mononucleosis (Epstein–Barr virus or cytomegalovirus), viral infections of the respiratory tract, or chronic lymphatic leukemia (AHLSTEDT et al. 1980; MANDELL and SANDE 1980). It is unclear whether these skin reactions represent an immunologic or toxic phenomenon.

II. Sensitization Process

The β-lactam antibiotics are low-molecular weight, variably substituted bicyclic compounds. By themselves, they have little direct immunogenicity. However, they are potentially reactive compounds, and by binding covalently to carrier structures may form hapten-carrier compounds of significant antigenicity. The macromolecular carriers for β-lactam-derived haptens are chiefly proteins and carbohydrates capable of nucleophilic attack on various positions of the core structure or side groups. β-Lactam polymers may form by a similar mechanism if the antibiotic contains a side-chain amino group or if a decomposed structure with a free thiazolidine or dehydrothiazine amino group is present (Dewdney et al. 1971; Stewart 1973).

A variety of antigenic determinants may thus be formed, either as a direct result of these reactions or after secondary structural rearrangement within the altered molecule. At least eight determinants are known to be derived from benzylpenicillin (Ahlstedt et al. 1980).

In contrast to what has been shown with the penicillins, less is known of hapten type or carrier conjugation of the cephalosporins. The similarity of the chemical structure might lead one to expect that similar reactions and determinants should be produced by these drugs. However, this assumption is unlikely to be entirely true. β-Lactamase hydrolysis of the cephalosporins results in unstable intermediates and potential fragmentation of the molecule (Newton and Hamilton-Miller 1967; Flynn 1967), and chemical degradation of the cephalosporins does not yield analogs of penicillamine, penicilloates, or penicillenates (Abraham 1965). As further circumstantial evidence of a fundamental difference from the penicillins, antibodies to different cephalosporins do not cross-react as well as do antibodies to different penicillins (Stewart 1973). Nevertheless, the cephalosporins are susceptible to nucleophilic attack (Indelicato et al. 1974, 1977) and may conjugate to proteins in a manner similar to that seen with the penicillins (Mashimo et al. 1967).

The immunogenic potency of a hapten-host macromolecular conjugate is low unless a large number of hapten determinants are bound to the carrier, an unlikely occurrence in most therapeutic situations (Ahlstedt et al. 1980). Thus, the role of in vivo coupling of a β-lactam hapten to a host carrier in the primary induction of immunity may be minor. A more likely inducer of the primary response may be exogenous protein impurities retained during the manufacturing process (Ahlstedt et al. 1980). Lower rates of allergic reactions with more purified penicillin preparations lend support to this hypotheses (Ahlstedt and Kristofferson 1979; Kristofferson et al. 1979). Once the host is sensitized, however, the hapten-autologous carrier is probably as effective as an equivalently substituted foreign molecule in eliciting a secondary immune response or allergic reaction.

The issue of immunologic cross-reactivity between penicillins and cephalosporins is complex. It seems clear that cross-reactivity does occur between these two groups (Mashimo et al. 1967; Petz 1978; Delafuente et al. 1979), but it is also apparent that an immune response specific to cephalosporins may occur (Abraham et al. 1968; De Weck and Schneider 1980). Conceivably, the cephalosporin nucleus may be sufficiently similar to the penicillin-derived antigen to elicit a hypersensitivity reaction in a sensitized individual, even where it cannot induce the same antibody in a nonsensitized person. However, the clinical importance of a history of a specific β-lactam allergy or the presence of cross-reacting antibodies remains unclear.

E. Immune Hemolytic Anemia

Benzylpenicillin is one of the drugs most frequently associated with hemolytic anemia (GARRATTY and PETZ 1975; PETZ 1976). Two mechanisms have been delineated.

In the majority of cases, the process involves three steps: (1) covalent binding of a penicillin-derived hapten to the surface of the red blood cell, (2) fixation of immunoglobulin, usually IgG, directed against the penicillin hapten, and (3) extravascular (reticuloendothelial) removal of the erythrocyte (SPATH et al. 1971a; SWISHER 1974; GARRATTY and PETZ 1975; PETZ 1976). About 3% of patients receiving high-dose penicillin therapy progress through the second step to develop a positive direct antiglobulin (Coomb's) test (PETZ 1976). However, only a fraction of these develop overt hemolysis (GARRATTY and PETZ 1975). Although most cases of hemolysis are associated with high-dose therapy (10–20 million units per day), this is not invariable (DOVE et al. 1975). Antibody titers to penicillin determinants are commonly high, often greater than 1:1,000 (PETZ 1976). An occasional patient will fix complement with the immunoglobulin on the red cell membrane, and a brisk, intravasuclar hemolysis may ensue (RIES et al. 1975; PETZ 1980).

In a few cases, a second mechanism, the "innocent bystander" process, may contribute to hemolysis (RIES et al. 1975). In such instances, circulating immune complexes associate reversibly with the erythrocyte membrane, fixing complement at the same time. The antigen–antibody complex then dissociates from the red cell, leaving the complement in place, and repeats the process at another site (GARRATTY and PETZ 1975). In this way, small numbers of circulating complexes may initiate significant complement-mediated hemolysis.

A number of cephalosporins have been found to cause hemolysis by the first mechanism, albeit much less frequently than does benzylpenicillin (JEANNET et al. 1976; PETZ 1980). Nevertheless, a positive direct antiglobulin test is not uncommon, being seen in 3%–4% of patients receiving cephalothin (SPATH et al. 1971b; SWISHER 1974; SCHWARZ et al. 1975). Individuals with severe illnesses or renal insufficiency may have even higher rates (SPATH et al. 1971b; GARRATTY and PETZ 1975).

Some instances of a positive direct antiglobulin test may result from the nonspecific adsorption of serum proteins to the red cell membrane. In vitro incubation of normal erythrocytes with cephalothin produces a cell which relatively firmly binds a number of serum proteins, including IgG and complement (SPATH et al. 1971a, b; SWISHER 1974). The minimal concentration of cephalothin necessary to induce a positive direct antiglobulin test varies inversely with the concentration of gamma globulin (FERRONE et al. 1971a). The effect is not seen with penicillin-treated or isosensitized red blood cells (SPATH et al. 1971b).

Studies of erythrocyte metabolism after in vitro incubation with cephalothin (FERRONE et al. 1968) have shown several abnormalities similar to those seen in erythrocytes from patients with paroxysmal nocturnal hemoglobinuria. However, red cells from patients who develop a positive direct antiglobulin test while receiving cephalothin do not have the metabolic abnormalities exhibited by the cells incubated in vitro (FERRONE et al. 1971 b), and in vitro incubation of erythrocytes with cephalothin does not alter the red cell half-life in vivo (FERRONE and SIRCHIA 1968). Whether nonimmunologic adsorption of proteins to the erythrocyte surface contributes to a hemolytic process therefore remains to be determined.

F. Neutropenia

Neutropenia is an important adverse effect of therapy with the penicillins and cephalosporins. The most commonly implicated drugs have been nafcillin (FELDMAN et al. 1978; WILSON et al. 1979; CARPENTER 1980), methicillin (CARPENTER 1980), and oxacillin (LEVENTHAL and SIKEN 1976; CHU et al. 1977). Cephalothin (SANDERS et al. 1974; HOMAYOUNI et al. 1979), cefamandole (HOMAYOUNI et al. 1979), cephapirin (SANDERS et al. 1974), benzylpenicillin (HOMAYOUNI et al. 1979), and piperacillin (WILSON et al. 1979) have also been cited. The case frequency cannot be stated with certainty, but two series of pediatric patients receiving either nafcillin (FELDMAN et al. 1978) or methicillin (YOW et al. 1976) had reported frequencies of about 4%.

The fall in neutrophil count is usually abrupt, that is in the interval between consecutive counts. The neutropenia has appeared 9–28 days after beginning therapy, but the majority of cases occur after 3 weeks (FINCH 1977; CARPENTER 1980). A relative or absolute eosinophilia is an inconstant feature (FINCH 1977; WILSON et al. 1979; CARPENTER 1980). Most cases occur during parenteral administration of high doses, although neutropenia during a prolonged course of oral therapy has been reported (YOW et al. 1976). Aspiration of the bone marrow commonly shows maturational arrest of the granulocytic series at the myelocyte stage. Recovery after discontinuation of the drug is prompt, usually within 1 week and almost invariably within 2 weeks (CARPENTER 1980).

The clinical pattern is not always the same. Continuation of methicillin in the face of neutropenia did not prevent recovery of the white count in two cases (CARPENTER 1980), whereas rechallenge with the same drug or another β-lactam has produced mixed results in others (LEVENTHAL and SIKEN 1976; HOMAYOUNI et al. 1979; CARPENTER 1980).

Two possible mechanisms have been proposed to explain this phenomenon. A role of the immune system has been inferred from the duration of the latent period and the presence of eosinophilia (FINCH 1977; HOMAYOUNI et al. 1979). Examples of idiopathic antibody-mediated destruction of circulating neutrophils have been described (BOXER et al. 1975). However, there has been no evidence of tissue-bound drug-derived antigens, specific antibodies, circulating immune complexes, or an inflammatory or infiltrative process in the bone marrow in cases of β-lactam-induced neutropenia.

The evidence for a toxic mechanism is circumstantial and rests on interpreting the clinical syndrome as being a process most consistent with a direct effect on the granulocyte precursor (LEVENTHAL and SIKEN 1976; CHU et al. 1977; HOMAYOUNI et al. 1979). Indirect support for this hypothesis has been presented in two reports. In one, rechallenge of nine patients with the same antibiotic at a lower dose did not provoke a recurrence of the neutropenia (HOMAYOUNI et al. 1979). In the other, the investigators were unable to find evidence of rapid neutrophil turnover in a case of oxacillin-associated neutropenia and were able to demonstrate normal in vitro culture of the patient's bone marrow (CHU et al. 1977). However, these findings are open to different interpretations, and more direct evidence for a toxic mechanism is lacking.

G. Disorders of Hemostasis

Three types of hemostatic abnormalities have occurred with the penicillins and/or the cephalosporins: (1) thrombesthenia, (2) plasma factor coagulopathy, and (3) thrombocytopenia.

I. Thrombesthenia

Thrombesthenia has been the most intensively investigated abnormality of this group. Carbenicillin was the first penicillin reported to cause a platelet defect, and the clinical phenomenon seems to be largely confined to this and closely related penicillins (BROWN et al. 1974; STUART 1980; GENTRY 1981). However, laboratory evidence of platelet dysfunction in humans receiving high-dose methicillin, benzylpenicillin, or ampicillin and in platelets incubated in vitro with cefamandole has been described (BROWN et al. 1976b; ANDRASSY et al. 1976; CUSTER et al. 1979).

The typical clinical presentation is that of an abrupt onset of bleeding several days after the initiation of therapy with a high daily dose (300–400 mg/kg carbenicillin or ticarcillin) or with lower doses in patients with impaired renal function (STUART 1980). Withdrawal of the offending drug leads to resolution of the clinical picture, usually within 2 days, although laboratory evidence of abnormal platelet function may persist for a week or more.

The defect has been characterized in humans by BROWN (1974, 1975, 1976b) and by NATELSON (1976) and their associates, and in dogs by JOHNSON et al. (1978a, b). The most consistent effects of the penicillins are a dose-related decrease in ADP-induced platelet aggregation and a prolongation of template bleeding time. The impaired ADP-induced aggregation is the earlier effect and the most sensitive known measure of the antibiotic-related platelet defect. Other measures of platelet function, including epinephrine- or collagen-induced aggregation, are less consistently affected. Inhibition of platelet aggregation can be partially overcome with higher concentrations of the proaggregatory agent. In in vivo studies with cephalosporins, with the possible exception of cephalothin (NATELSON et al. 1976), no effect on platelet function is demonstrable (CUSTER et al. 1979).

Addition of carbenicillin, benzylpenicillin or cefamandole to normal platelets in vitro produces effects qualitatively similar to those seen in vivo (CAZENARE et al. 1973; CUSTER et al. 1979; SHATTIL et al. 1980). However, studies using in vitro incubation should be interpreted cautiously, first because the effect on the platelets is immediate, whereas it is delayed in vivo, and second because the in vitro drug concentrations necessary to induce the platelet dysfunction are much higher than those occurring in the intact animal.

The molecular basis of the thrombesthenic effect of the penicillins is unclear. They probably act independently of prostaglandin synthesis (JOHNSON et al.

1978a, b), of alterations in internal calcium flux or of changes in the platelet content of adenine nucleotides or serotonin (BROWN et al. 1976b; SHATTIL et al. 1980). Inasmuch as the laboratory abnormality in platelet function persists for a period consistent with platelet life span, the penicillin effect may be the result of a permanent change in the affected platelets (CAZENARE et al. 1973; BROWN et al. 1976b), or a transient alteration in the megakaryocytes (BROWN et al. 1975). A more speculative proposal has been that a direct, perhaps covalent, interaction between the penicillin and the platelet membrane reduces the affinity for or limits the availability of membrane receptors for proaggretory substances (CAZENARE et al. 1973; SHATTIL et al. 1980). However, JOHNSON et al. (1978a, b) believe the mechanism to be more complicated than membrane receptor inhibition would imply.

II. Plasma Factor Coagulopathy

Prolonged prothrombin, partial thromboplastin, and thrombin times have been associated with the therapeutic use of cefazolin (LERNER and LUBIN 1974), cefamandole (HOOPER et al. 1980), and cephalothin (NATELSON et al. 1976). Overt hemorrhage, when present, occurs 5–12 days after the initiation of treatment (LERNER and LUBIN 1974; HOOPER et al. 1980) and is reversed by either withdrawing the offending antibiotic (LERNER and LUBIN 1974) or by giving vitamin K (HOOPER et al. 1980). Rechallenge in one case provoked a recurrence of the abnormal clotting tests after 10 days of therapy (LERNER and LUBIN 1974). Factors which may have predisposed to the development of the coagulopathy were the presence of uremia in one case, and fasting for longer than 7 days in several others (HOOPER et al. 1980). The pathogenesis of these effects is unknown. However, HOOPER et al. (1980) speculated that the antibiotics affected vitamin K utilization or synthesis, possibly in part by altering gut flora.

III. Thrombocytopenia

Thrombocytopenia is a rare complication of β-lactam therapy (SCHIFFER et al. 1976). The etiology has been related to that discussed for neutropenia (CARPENTER 1980) or immunologic hemolytic anemia (SHEIMAN et al. 1968; GRALNICK et al. 1972; SCHIFFER et al. 1976), but has not been well studied. The reader is referred to sections E and F for the discussions of those phenomena.

H. Interstitial Nephritis and Cystitis

Drug-induced interstitial nephritis is a clinicopathological process of uncertain etiology for which there is no animal model. The presumption of immunologic mechanism(s) has been supported both by the constellation of findings associated with this diagnosis, and by the similarities between the disease in humans and immune-mediated interstitial nephritides in rats and guinea pigs (VAN ZWIETEN et al. 1977; APPEL 1980; LINTON et al. 1980). Nevertheless, in most human cases there is no clear evidence for a primary role of either humoral or cell-mediated immunity.

I. Clinical Picture

The frequency of antibiotic-associated interstitial nephritis is difficult to assess, both because of the variability of its signs and symptoms and because of the occurrence of a variety of other acute renal diseases in the patient groups receiving these drugs. The frequency of methicillin-associated interstitial nephritis has been reported to be 16%–17% (SANJAD et al. 1974; NOLAN and ABERNATHY 1977). This high rate seems peculiar to methicillin; the majority of β-lactam antibiotics in general use are not as commonly associated with interstitial nephritis.

The disease typically arises in patients being treated for a serious infection. The time from initiation of therapy to the appearance of urinary abnormalities ranges from 2 to 44 days, with a median of about 2 weeks. Several authors have commented upon a relationship between dosage and the occurrence of interstitial nephritis (BALDWIN et al. 1968; FEIGIN et al. 1974; SARFF and MCCRACKEN 1977). Both FEIGIN et al. (1974) and SARFF and MCCRACKEN (1977) suggested that administration of greater than 200 mg/kg per day increased the likelihood of interstitial nephritis. However, this assessment has been disputed by others (DITLOVE et al. 1977; APPEL 1980).

The clinical hallmark of interstitial nephritis has been hematuria, but fever, skin rash, eosinophilia, pyuria, and proteinuria are also frequently reported. The sequence of appearance and the severity of each symptom and sign is variable. Several authors have suggested that eosinophiluria may be an important finding (DITLOVE et al. 1977; GALPIN et al. 1978), but its diagnostic utility has yet to be established. Occasional patients have positive skin reactions to the penicillin (APPEL 1980) and/or elevated serum IgE concentrations. Renal insufficiency has occurred in 50% of reported cases (DITLOVE et al. 1977). Recovery of renal function is the rule, but prolonged or permanent impairment is possible (ENGLE et al. 1975; DITLOVE et al. 1977; GALPIN et al. 1978).

The renal biopsy characteristically shows a diffuse cortical mononuclear infiltrate, with occasional aggregations of plasma cells and eosinophils and a variable degree of tubular atrophy. The glomeruli and blood vessels are generally spared.

II. Immunofluorescence

Immunofluorescence of biopsies is generally negative or shows only scattered deposits of immunoglobulin or complement. However, dramatic cases of positive immunofluorescence have been described. In one case BALDWIN et al. (1968) demonstrated a linear pattern of immunofluorescent staining along the glomerular basement membrane (GBM) and, to a lesser extent, along the tubular basement membrane (TBM) with rabbit anti-dimethoxyphenylpenicilloyl-polylysine (DPO) antibody. The putative DPO hapten appeared bound to the tissue, as extensive washing did not elute the antigen. The patient had other evidence of both humoral and cell-mediated immunity against penicilloyl determinants. In another case, BORDER et al. (1974) found IgG, the third component of complement, and methicillin antigen in a linear pattern along the TBM. Using the same antiserum, they were unable to demonstrate the presence of DPO antigen in the kidneys of four patients receiving methicillin who had no interstitial nephritis.

However, the significance of these immunofluorescent findings may be argued. COLVIN et al. (1974) showed diffuse benzylpenicillin antigen binding to the interstitium, GBM and TBM of kidneys from patients who had received the antibiotic for several days before death but had no evidence of interstitial nephritis. Further, cases of interstitial nephritis without demonstrable β-lactam-related antigen or immunoglobulin deposition are not uncommon (SCULLY et al. 1975). It has been suggested that appearance of anti-TBM antibodies or tissue binding of the β-lactam antibiotic may therefore not be central to the pathogenesis of interstitial nephritis, but rather an epiphenomenon of the primary insult (COLVIN et al. 1974; APPEL 1980).

III. Cystitis

Several authors have suggested that some cases of β-lactam-associated urinary tract toxicity may in fact be instances of cystitis. SARFF and MCCRACKEN (1977) have reported a frequent association of dysuria with the hematuria in children with methicillin toxicity. Recurrent gross hematuria and dysuria were provoked in one child by each of three semisynthetic penicillins (CHUDWIN et al. 1979). Cystoscopic evidence of cystitis in patients receiving methicillin was provided by BRACIS et al. (1977), who described a diffuse hemorrhagic bladder wall in three patients. The bladder of the one patient biopsied was heavily infiltrated with eosinophils and lymphoid cells and had deposits of IgG and IgM. All patients improved after the penicillin was withdrawn.

I. Nephrotoxicity

Of the β-lactam antibiotics, several cephalosporins and a single penicillin, guanylureidopenicillin (WILLIAMS et al. 1974), have been reported to have direct or nonimmunologic nephrotoxic potential. Only the cephalosporins have been studied in detail (TUNE and FRAVERT 1980a, b), and they therefore provide the basis for the following discussion.

The nephrotoxic cephalosporins cause a selective proximal tubular necrosis in the rabbit, guinea pig, rat, and mouse (ATKINSON et al. 1966; WELLES et al. 1966), as well as in humans (FOORD 1975). In the rabbit and guinea pig development of necrosis has been quantitatively correlated with the renal accumulation of the antibiotic (TUNE et al. 1977a, b). This relationship apparently also holds for the rat and the mouse (TUNE 1975), although these species are so resistant to cephalosporin nephrotoxicity (ATKINSON et al. 1966; WELLES et al. 1966) that they have not been studied in detail. Renal cortical concentrations of cephalosporins have not been measured in humans, but parallells in the toxic process may be inferred from the similarities in their toxic histopathology (ATKINSON et al. 1966; FOORD 1970) and renal transport (BEYER et al. 1944; TUNE et al. 1974) in both humans and rabbits.

I. Human Toxicity

Review of the clinical reports of renal damage related to cephaloridine and cephalothin has revealed some cases of allergic interstitial nephritis, but also many instances of histologically documented acute tubular necrosis (FOORD 1970). Factors identified as contributing to the development of nephrotoxic renal failure (FOORD 1975) have included patient age greater than 50 years, pre-existing renal or prerenal azotemia, the use of potent diuretics, the administration of other potentially nephrotoxic antibiotics and, most importantly, the use of cephalosporin doses which are excessively large for the patient's renal function.

The renal failure may be oliguric or nonoliguric. Mortality rates have been 38%–47%, with a more favorable outcome reported in the nonoliguric cases. However, cephalosporin toxicity is restricted to the proximal tubule, which has a high potential for regeneration (ATKINSON et al. 1966). For this reason, the likelihood of recovery from cephalosporin-induced renal failure is probably better than reflected in the existing reports, except where there are nonrenal complicating features.

II. Cellular Mechanisms

The process of renal injury in the rabbit has thus far been correlated with three elements: (1) secretory uptake from blood-to-cell, (2) secretory efflux from cell-to-tubular fluid, and (3) molecular affinity or reactivity, i.e., the ability of the drug to participate in the toxic process at the subcellular level. The balance between the first two elements determines the extent and duration of the intracellular concentrations of the antibiotics. The third element determines the toxic potential of cephalosporins for which there is not substantial or prolonged intracellular accumulation.

1. Uptake

The penicillins and cephalosporins are variably secreted across the proximal renal tubule by the transport system for the organic anion para-aminohippurate (PAH) (TUNE and FERNHOLT 1973). The primary transport step occurs at the antiluminal (blood) side of the cell and results in an intracellular antibiotic concentration several-fold higher than that in the extracellular fluid. Other organic anions, such as probenecid, may inhibit uptake at this step, and tubular necrosis can be prevented to the extent that the reduction in cortical concentration is achieved and maintained (TUNE et al. 1977a, b).

The organic anion carrier may not, however, be the only route of access to the molecular target of the β-lactams. For example, the nephrotoxicity of guanylureidopenicillin (this laboratory, unpublished work) and that of very high-dose cephaloglycin (TUNE 1982) are not prevented by probenecid. Whether access to the molecular targets in these cases occurs at an extracellular site, by another active transport step or by passive entry into the cell, and whether this entry occurs from the luminal or antiluminal side remains to be determined.

2. Efflux: Cephaloridine

The other factor which influences the intracellular accumulation of the antibiotic is the movement from cell-to-tubular lumen (TUNE et al. 1974). Presumably, as is the case for PAH, the cephalosporins move passively down their concentration gradients from the tubular cell into the luminal fluid, and thus into the urine.

Among the cephalosporins, cephaloridine most strikingly exhibits the importance of efflux in the toxic process. Cephaloridine is trapped within the tubular cell because of a relative impermeability across the luminal membrane (TUNE et al. 1974). This diffusional block may be the result of the fixed positive charge on the pyridinium side-group of cephaloridine (TUNE and FRAVERT 1980b). The resulting intracellular concentrations are uniquely high among the cephalosporins, and are probably a major reason for the significant toxicity of this particular drug. Of further interest, inhibitors of the organic cation transport system, which is somehow involved in the limited efflux of cephaloridine from the cell (WOLD and TURNIPSEED 1980), increase its cortical concentrations and its toxicity (WOLD et al. 1979).

3. Reactivity or Receptor Affinity: Cephaloglycin

Cephaloglycin is normally secreted across the tubular cell, with limited and comparatively transient intracellular concentrations (TUNE and FRAVERT 1980a, b). The discovery of nephrotoxicity of cephaloglycin comparable to that of cephaloridine led to the development of the concept that there must be two potential determinants of the toxicity of a given cephalosporin. The first, as best represented by cephaloridine, is that of prolonged intracellular trapping, but with apparently limited affinity for or reactivity with its molecular target. The second, as best seen with cephaloglycin, is that of a toxin with relatively high affinity for or reactivity with its target, with comparable cytotoxicity despite significantly lower and less sustained intracellular concentrations.

Several observations lend support to the concept that cephaloridine does have the relatively low and cephaloglycin the relatively high affinity or reactivity properties suggested above (TUNE and FRAVERT 1980a, b). First, the nephrotoxicity of cephaloridine can be prevented by the intravenous infusion of a bolus of probenecid as late as 20 min after antibiotic infusion, while that of cephaloglycin cannot. Second, cephaloridine shows little or no cumulative toxicity when given in a series of marginally toxic doses, whereas cephaloglycin shows striking cumulative toxicity when given in a series of injections of even lower single-dose toxicity. Finally, although the cellular respiratory toxicity of a dose of cephaloridine appears to be significantly reversed during the process of renal cortical mitochondrial isolation and washing (TUNE et al. 1979), that of a comparably nephrotoxic dose of cephaloglycin is not.

It is not yet clear whether the molecular target(s) of cephaloridine and cephaloglycin is (or are) the same. However, the unique ability of nontoxic β-lactam antibiotics to protect against cephaloridine and cephaloglycin nephrotoxicity at the molecular level, i.e., without inhibition of cellular transport, may indicate that the two are toxic at a common molecular site (TUNE et al. 1982).

III. Less Toxic Cephalosporins

The fundamental differences between the patterns of toxicity of cephaloridine and cephaloglycin lead to concerns beyond the question of whether the two antibiotics act upon the same molecular target(s). Central to the problem of cephalosporin nephrotoxicity is whether the less toxic members of this class more closely resemble cephaloglycin or cephaloridine in their nephrotoxic properties. The study of two potentiating factors, that of combined use with aminoglycosides and that of acute obstruction of the urinary tract, has produced results which lead to the conclusion that there is probably a greater similarity of the less toxic cephalosporins to cephaloglycin than to cephaloridine.

1. Additive Aminoglycoside–Cephalosporin Toxicity

It has been difficult to demonstrate directly any cumulative toxicity of the less toxic cephalosporins. This is not surprising, because these drugs are not nearly as toxic as cephaloglycin. However, the aminoglycoside–cephalosporin interaction provides indirect evidence of cumulative toxicity and direct support for the conclusion that the less toxic cephalosporins may fit the cephaloglycin model better than that of cephaloridine.

Both the aminoglycosides (KOSEK et al. 1974) and cephaloglycin are cumulatively nephrotoxic in a series of limited doses, whereas cephaloridine is not. It was speculated that the mildly toxic cephalosporins, because they are normally secreted and do not undergo prolonged intracellular trapping, might resemble cephaloglycin in being cumulatively toxic and therefore additively toxic with the aminoglycosides (BENDIRDJIAN et al. 1981).

One early human survey had failed to demonstrate statistical significance of a trend toward additive toxicity of cephalothin and gentamicin (FANNING et al. 1976). However, there is a growing body of evidence that such an interaction does exist in human use (KLASTERSKY et al. 1975; EORTC GROUP 1978; WADE et al. 1978). Although the results of early studies of this interaction in laboratory animals were negative (HARRISON et al. 1975; DELLINGER et al. 1976; LUFT et al. 1976), these studies were done in the rat, which is unusually resistant to the cephalosporins (ATKINSON et al. 1966; WELLES et al. 1966).

Therefore, subsequent studies of the toxic interaction of cephaloridine and cephaloglycin, and the mildly toxic, normally secreted cephalosporins cefaclor and cefazolin, with several aminoglycosides were done in the rabbit. Combined treatment in this species produced no additive toxicity of cephaloridine and the aminoglycosides (DOLISLAGER et al. 1979). In contrast, combined treatment with the three secreted toxic cephalosporins and the different aminoglycosides resulted in almost consistently additive toxicity (BENDIRDJIAN et al. 1981).

This additive toxicity is almost certainly the result of a synergy at the molecular level. In animals given only a 3-day course of neomycin pretreatment (nontoxic), followed later by a single, mildly toxic dose of cephaloglycin (BENDIRDJIAN et al. 1981), severe toxicity was seen in the absence of an effect of the aminoglycoside on either the peak or the rate of decline of cortical or serum concentrations of the cephalosporin. Correlated studies of the mitochondrial toxicity of cephaloglycin revealed a potentiation of this respiratory toxicity by the aminoglycoside, within 1 h of administration of the cephalosporin. Thus, potentiation occurs very early, at the subcellular level, and is unrelated to any effect of the aminoglycoside on the renal transport or elimination of the cephalosporin.

2. Effects of Ureteral Obstruction

Ureteral ligation doubles the cortical concentrations of PAH (TUNE et al. 1974). Concentrations of PAH are increased in both tubular fluid and cell water after obstruction, because the exit of the anion from cell water to tubular fluid to urine is restricted, while active transport into the cell continues (TUNE et al. 1969). To the extent that the secreted cephalosporins undergo a similar elevation of intracellular concentrations during ureteral obstruction, their toxicity should be proportionately increased.

In studies of ureteral obstruction applied for 1–2 h shortly after the intravenous administration of mildly toxic doses of cephaloridine, cefazolin, cephaloglycin, and cefaclor, toxicity is significantly increased only with the last two, i.e., rapidly secreted cephalosporins (WANG et al. 1982). In correlated studies of uptake, ureteral ligation does not increase the cortical concentrations of cephaloridine, the cellular concentrations of which are already substantial because of its restricted efflux into the tubular fluid, but does increase both the degree and duration of cortical accumulation of cephaloglycin and cefaclor. It therefore appears that the less toxic cephalosporins more closely resemble cephaloglycin than cephaloridine in regard to the relationship between their transcellular movement and toxic potential, but only to the extent that they are rapidly secreted.

IV. Molecular Basis of Toxicity

Two potential mechanisms of toxicity at the subcellular level have been proposed: (1) the formation of a highly reactive metabolite, and (2) the production of mitochondrial respiratory inhibition. Clearly the two need not be mutually exclusive.

1. Metabolite Hypothesis

This hypothesis was proposed by MCMURTRY and MITCHELL (1977) on the basis of studies with cephaloridine in the mouse and the rat. Cobaltous chloride and piperonyl butoxide, substances which decrease the activity of cytochrome P-450-dependent mixed-function oxidase (MFO) activity, also reduce the toxicity of cephaloridine. A role of MFO activity in the production of a toxic alkylating metabolite, presumed to be an epoxide of the thiophene moiety, was therefore proposed.

The general significance of this hypothesis is in question, however, because of the absence of a thiophene side-ring in other nephrotoxic cephalosporins (e.g., cephaloglycin, cefaclor, cefazolin, and cefamandole) (TUNE and FRAVERT 1980b) and because of evidence in the rabbit which allows an alternative explanation for the effects of these MFO inhibitors (TUNE et al. 1983). In the rabbit, cobalt does not protect against cephaloridine. Moreover, although piperonyl butoxide protects, it substantially reduces cortical cephaloridine concentrations, possibly by an augmentation of cellular efflux of the cephalosporin. Finally, piperonyl butoxide has no protective effect against cephaloglycin in the rabbit.

2. Mitochondrial Respiratory Toxicity

Depression of mitochondrial respiration has been shown to be a very early and characteristic functional insult in the evolution of cephalosporin-induced toxicity. It has been demonstrated with both cephaloridine and cephaloglycin after in vivo administration, a finding which provides further evidence that the differences between the toxicity of these two cephalosporins may relate more to their affinity for or reactivity with their molecular target than to their being active at different sites.

The features of respiratory toxicity in mitochondria isolated from drug-treated animals (in vivo exposure) are: (a) a correlation between the toxic potential of a cephalosporin and the extent of the respiratory depression that it produces (TUNE and FRAVERT 1980a); (b) a gradual progression of mitochondrial toxicity, over 0.5–2 h, as intracellular antibiotic concentrations have substantially declined (TUNE and FRAVERT 1980a, b); (c) the later development, between 1 and 5 h, of the first evidence of ultrastructural damage (SILVERBLATT et al. 1970); and (d) an early augmentation of mitochondrial toxicity after a nontoxic but potentiating regimen of neomycin (BENDIRDJIAN et al. 1981).

Whereas the time of evolution and the correlations between the development of mitochondrial respiratory inhibition and tubular cell toxicity (necrosis) are consistent with a pathogenic relationship, these findings do not establish the precise role of the mitochondrial insult in the events leading to cell death, nor do they define the mechanism by which the toxic cephalosporins cause this mitochondrial damage.

J. Hepatic Toxicity

Hepatic injury has been seen with the use of some cephalosporins and semisynthetic penicillins. In humans, the most common manifestation is an elevation in serum transaminase levels (BINT et al. 1978). Rarely are there symptoms. Isolated cases of anicteric hepatitis (WILSON et al. 1975) and intrahepatic cholestasis (TEN PAS and QUINN 1965; GOLDSTEIN and ISHAK 1974) have been described, but the assumption of a causal relationship between the antibiotic and the hepatic injury has been questioned (POLLACK et al. 1978).

The frequency of elevated serum transaminases has been reported to be approximately 3% with cefoxitin (VAN WINZUM 1978) and may be higher with large doses of dicloxacillin (KOHLER et al. 1975) or cloxacillin (POLLACK et al. 1978). Of interest, the substitution of nafcillin or benzylpenicillin for oxacillin has been followed by a return of serum transaminase levels to normal (OLANS and WEINER 1976).

The acid-stable esters of the penicillins are a group for which the risk of hepatotoxicity may be of special concern. Hydrolysis of the ester linkage by nonspecific esterases widely distributed in mammalian tissues (SWAHN 1976) produces potentially toxic products (BINT 1980). In the dog, where measurable amounts of intact talampicillin and pivampicillin enter the portal circulation, chronic administration of these drugs has produced liver damage (MASUDA et al. 1974; MAWDESLEY-THOMAS et al. 1977; JEFFERY et al. 1978; BINT 1980). In contrast, rats, which do not have detectable levels of the intact drugs in portal vein blood, have not developed liver damage during chronic administration (JEFFERY et al. 1978).

The mechanism of hepatotoxicity of penicillins other than the esters of ampicillin is less clear. The work with the esters and the observation that resolution occurs despite the continued administration of another, hepatically excreted penicillin (WILSON et al. 1975; OLANS and WEINER 1976) support the importance of a distinctive side-chain or metabolic derivative. However, further work remains to be done to clarify the pathogenetic mechanism.

K. Neurotoxicity

I. Human Toxicity

The neurotoxicity of benzylpenicillin has been recognized for 35 years (WALKER et al. 1945) as one of the major limitations to high-dose penicillin therapy. However, with the dosages commonly employed in practice, the incidence of this complication is quite low [1.3/1,000 in one series (PORTER and JICK 1977)]. Benzylpenicillin is most often implicated, but oxacillin (MALONE et al. 1977; PORTER and JICK 1977), dicloxacillin (KOHLER et al. 1975), carbenicillin (FOSSIECK and PARKER 1974; NICHOLLS 1980), ticarcillin (KALLAY et al. 1979), and the cephalosporins cephaloridine (MURDOCH et al. 1964; GABRIEL et al. 1970) and cephalexin (SAKER et al. 1973) have also been associated with an encephalopathy.

The patient at risk is generally receiving more than 20 million units per day of penicillin, often in a continuous infusion, and commonly has another predisposing factor (CONWAY et al. 1968; FOSSIECK and PARKER 1974; NICHOLLS 1980), such as renal insufficiency (FOSSIECK and PARKER 1974). Most cases of encephalopathy occur within 12–72 h of instituting therapy, although cases have been reported as early as 8 h or as late as 9 days (CONWAY et al. 1968; FOSSIECK and PARKER 1974). When cerebrospinal fluid (CSF) penicillin concentrations have been measured, they have been elevated, and there is a progressive increase in concentration as sampling moves in a cephalad direction (FOSSIECK and PARKER 1974).

The symptoms and signs of the encephalopathy include drowsiness, hallucinations, asterixis, hyperreflexia, myoclonic twitches, focal or generalized seizures and coma (CONWAY et al. 1968; FOSSIECK and PARKER 1974; NICHOLLS 1980). Of these, myoclonus and generalized convulsions are the most frequently described (FOSSIECK and PARKER 1974). They may arise with or without a prodrome of the less severe manifestations (CONWAY et al. 1968). The electroencephalogram shows diffuse slow and sharp wave forms in all leads (FOSSIECK and PARKER 1974). Resolution usually occurs within 12–72 h of discontinuation of the antibiotic (FOSSIECK and PARKER 1974).

II. Animal Toxicity

Experience with the animal toxicity of the penicillins has largely come from their use as convulsants in the study of epileptogenesis. Vertebrates and invertebrates appear to respond similarly (HOCHNER et al. 1976; PELLMAR and WILSON 1977; PRINCE 1978; KINNES et al. 1980). Topical application of the penicillin to a selected region of the central nervous system is commonly employed in the intact mammal, but parenteral or intrathecal administration will also provoke seizures in the same species (O'BRIEN and MC LAURIN 1968; GUTNICK and PRINCE 1971; WEIHRAUCH et al. 1975; GUTNICK et al. 1976). In the cat neocortex, recordings from the affected neurons show increased amplitude, prolonged depolarization and high-frequency bursts of spikes at the same time that interictal paroxysmal discharges appear in the electroencephalogram (AYALA et al. 1970; PRINCE 1978). As in human neurotoxicity, most experience has been with benzylpenicillin, but nearly all of several penicillins and a few cephalosporins tested have produced similar effects (WEIHRAUCH et al. 1975; GUTNICK et al. 1976; SAFANDA and SOBOTKA 1976).

III. Mechanism

Although penicillin has been widely used in the investigation of animal models of epilepsy, the understanding of the cellular or molecular basis of its neurotoxicity remains incomplete. Three hypotheses have been formulated: (1) interference with gamma-aminobutyric acid-mediated (GABA-ergic) neural transmission, (2) reduction of chloride conductance of the neuronal cell membrane; and (3) reduction of the activity of the sodium-potassium exchange pump on the neuronal cell membrane.

1. Effects on Gamma-Aminobutyric Acid (GABA)-Mediated Transmission

Evidence for this possibility was introduced by DAVIDOFF (1972a, b) with the demonstration that penicillin blocks primary afferent depolarization induced by dorsal root stimulation or external application of GABA. Since then, studies using several systems have shown that the inhibitory responses elicited by or attributed to GABA are attenuated by penicillin (HOCHNER et al. 1976; MACDONALD and BARKER 1977, 1978; PELLMAR and WILSON 1977; DEISZ et al. 1979). It has been presumed that this reduction of inhibitory input produces seizure activity by enhancing neuronal responsiveness to excitatory stimuli, including positive feedback and the recruitment of neurons not in the original focus (HOCHNER et al. 1976; PELLMAR and WILSON 1977; PRINCE 1978).

The mechanism by which penicillin interferes with GABA-ergic transmission is unclear. Several groups have found evidence for competitive inhibition by penicillin at the GABA receptor (CURTIS et al. 1972; MACDONALD and BARKER 1977, 1978; PELLMAR and WILSON 1977). MACDONALD and BARKER (1977, 1978) showed that penicillin rapidly produces a specific, dose-dependent, and reversible inhibition of the voltage and conductance changes evoked by GABA in spinal cord cell cultures.

In related work with benzodiazepine receptors, ANTONIADIS et al. (1980) demonstrated that epileptogenic concentrations of penicillin inhibit benzodiazepine binding to rat brain homogenate in a dose-dependent fashion. Because benzodiazepine receptors are thought to be part of a system that facilitates GABA-ergic transmission, they concluded that the penicillin-benzodiazepine receptor interaction contributes to the attenuation of the GABA-mediated inhibitory response.

2. Effects on Chloride Conductance

HOCHNER et al. (1976) and others (PELLMAR and WILSON 1977, PRINCE 1978; DEISZ et al. 1979) found a noncompetitive component of the penicillin effect and an ability of penicillin to antagonize the inhibitory effects of several other neurotransmitters. They proposed that the effects of penicillin are not the result of direct GABA antagonism, but are instead mediated by a reduction in chloride conductance at sites in the synapse or elsewhere along the neuronal cell membrane. In addition to the reduction in inhibitory input, reduced chloride conductance might produce a depolarization shift, a phenomenon known to exist in penicillin-induced epilepsy (Hochner et al. 1976; Prince 1978).

3. Effects on the Sodium–Potassium Exchange Pump

Ayala et al. (1970) found that penicillin increases the excitability of the crayfish stretch receptor. They attributed this finding to an increase in extracellular potassium concentration resulting from poisoning of the sodium–potassium exchange pump. Significant elevations of extracellular potassium have been documented during epileptic discharges (Prince 1978). However, it remains to be established whether the elevated potassium concentration is a primary event, due to inhibition of the pump, and whether this altered microenvironment affects the activity of cortical neurons (Futamachi and Prince 1975; Prince 1978).

IV. Structure–Activity Relationships

Although Curtis et al. (1972) have called attention to configurational correspondences between the penicillins and GABA, a full understanding of the correlation between structure and convulsant potency has not been attained. Studies have shown, however, that penicillin epileptogenesis depends upon (a) the presence of the β-lactam ring (Gutnick and Prince 1971; Safanda and Sobotka 1976), (b) the relative lipophilicity of the penicillin (Weihrauch et al. 1975; Safanda and Sobotka 1976; Antoniadis et al. 1980), (c) the amidic character of the C-6 carbon (Safanda and Sobotka 1976), and (d) the type of substitution of the 6-aminopenicillanic acid nucleus (Safanda and Sobotka 1976).

The presence of the β-lactam bond appears to be an absolute requirement. In an interesting demonstration of this, Gutnick and Prince (1971) shortened the time course of established penicillin-evoked convulsions in the cat by infusing penicillinase.

Two groups (Weihrauch et al. 1975; Safanda and Sobotka 1976) have reported a strong correlation between high lipid-water partition coefficient and epileptogenic potency. The strength of this relationship is unlikely to rest solely on an enhanced ability to penetrate the blood–brain barrier, because results obtained using systemic administration (Gutnick and Prince 1971; Weihrauch et al. 1975), topical application (Gutnick and Prince 1971; Safanda and Sobotka 1976), and binding studies with whole brain homogenate (Antoniadis et al. 1980) are similar.

Finally, a greater activity for penicillins with aliphatic compared to those with aromatic substitutions has been described. The lower activity of the aromatic penicillins is independent of lipophilicity, and has been attributed to steric hindrance at the β-lactam bond (Safanda and Sobotka 1976).

Although a few cephalosporins have been shown to be convulsants (O'BRIEN and MC LAURIN 1968; GUTNICK et al. 1976; SAFANDA and SOBOTKA 1976), the bearing of the above-mentioned variables on the neurotoxic potency of the cephalosporins has not been established.

V. Regulation of Penicillin Concentration in the Central Nervous System

Under normal circumstances, the blood–brain barrier effectively restricts penicillin entry to the CNS (BARZA and WEINSTEIN 1976; NICHOLLS 1980). Access is further limited by the binding of penicillins to serum proteins. In addition, the choroid plexus actively secretes these antibiotics out of the CSF (BARZA and WEINSTEIN 1976). The overall effect of these factors is that CSF concentrations of benzylpenicillin are only 0.5%–2.1% of plasma levels under normal steady-state conditions (BARZA and WEINSTEIN 1976).

Abnormal conditions may alter either entry into or removal from the CNS (HARTER and PETERSDORF 1960; DOBELL et al. 1966; SPECTOR and SNODGRASS 1976). In bacterial meningitis, there is both an increase in permeability of the blood–brain barrier (HARTER and PETERSDORF 1960) and reduced transport of penicillin by the choroid plexus (SPECTOR and LORENZO 1974). Likewise, in the presence of renal insufficiency there are alterations in both entry and removal of substances from the CSF (SPECTOR and SNODGRASS 1976). The latter effect appears to be due to competition between weak organic acids, which accumulate in uremia, and penicillin for the choroid plexus transport system (BARZA and WEINSTEIN 1976).

VI. Nonspecific Neurotoxic Reactions

The inadvertent injection of penicillin into a peripheral nerve, most commonly the sciatic nerve, is followed by severe pain and dysfunction in the area of distribution of the nerve. The discomfort and loss of function may persist for weeks (MANDELL and SANDE 1980).

Transverse myelitis has been described as a complication of presumed intra-arterial injection of penicillin in the gluteal region (SHAW 1966; ATKINSON 1969). The effect appears to be rapid in onset and largely irreversible, leading to a flaccid paralysis of the lower extremities and loss of bowel and bladder sphincter tone. The spinal cord lesion has been attributed to local ischemia produced by vascular injury (SCHANZER et al. 1979) and has not been considered to represent a specific reaction of the neural tissue (SHAW 1966; ATKINSON 1969).

L. Disulfiram-Like Reactions

Two of the newer cephalosporins, moxalactam (NEU and PRINCE 1980) and cefaperazone (MC MAHAN 1980; REEVES and DAVIES 1980), have been implicated in the production of a disulfiram-like reaction to alcohol ingestion. The effect is transient, but may produce significant symptoms for 2–3 days after the agent has been stopped. Presumably, the drug or a metabolite prevents the complete oxidation of alcohol, and the toxic intermediate acetaldehyde accumulates. However, documentation for this is lacking at this time.

M. Newer β-Lactams

It is too early to say whether the several new β-lactam antibiotics under development (Brown et al. 1976a; Kahan et al. 1978; Butterworth et al. 1979; Sakamoto et al. 1979; Kropp et al. 1980) will be as free of toxicity as most of the penicillins and cephalosporins. Unfortunately, studies of animal toxicity are published late, if at all, in the process of drug development and testing. The accumulation of experience in human therapy requires even longer.

For these reasons, it is not appropriate to review the toxicology of these new drugs at this time. However, experience with certain toxic effects of some of the newer penicillins and of the cephalosporins indicates that it is unwise to assume that the new β-lactam antibiotics will necessarily be as free of toxicity as a drug like benzylpenicillin.

Acknowledgment. Supported in part by a grant from the American Heart Association (No. 81–910) with Funds contributed by the Northern California Heart Association. Dr. Browning is a recipient of fellowship funding under National Institutes of Health grant number AM-07357.

References

Abraham EP (1965) The chemistry of new antibiotics. Am J Med 39:692–707
Abraham GN, Petz LD, Fudenberg HH (1968) Cephalothin hypersensitivity associated with anticephalothin antibodies. Int Arch Allergy Appl Immunol 34:65–74
Abramowitz M (ed) (1981) Bacampicillin hydrochloride (Spectro bid). Med Lett 23:49–50
Ahlstedt S, Kristofferson A (1979) Experimental evidence of a decreased incidence of penicillin allergy through use of pure penicillins. Infection [Suppl] 7:S499–S502
Ahlstedt S, Ekstrom B, Svard PO, Sjoberg B, Kristofferson A, Ortengren B (1980) New aspects on antigens in penicillin allergy. CRC Crit Rev Toxicol 7:219–277
Andrassy K, Ritz E, Hasper B (1976) Penicillin-induced coagulation disorder. Lancet 2:1039–1041
Antoniadis A, Muller WE, Wollert U (1980) Benzodiazepine receptor interactions may be involved in the neurotoxicity of various penicillin derivatives. Ann Neurol 8:71–73
Appel GB (1980) A decade of penicillin related acute interstitial nephritis – more questions than answers. Clin Nephrol 13:151–154
Atkinson JP (1969) Transverse myelopathy secondary to injection of penicillin. J Pediatr 75:867–869
Atkinson RM, Currie JP, Davis B, Pratt DAH, Sharpe HM, Tomich EG (1966) Acute toxicity of cephaloridine, an antibiotic derived from cephalosporin C. Toxicol Appl Pharmacol 8:398–406
Ayala GF, Lin S, Vasconetto C (1970) Penicillin as epileptogenic agent: its effect on an isolated neuron. Science 167:1257–1260
Baldwin DS, Levine BB, Mc Cluskey RT, Gallo GR (1968) Renal failure and interstitial nephritis due to penicillin and methicillin. N Engl J Med 279:1245–1252
Bartlett JG, Chang FW, Moon N, Onderdonk AB (1978) Antibiotic induced lethal enterocolitis in hamsters: studies with eleven agents and evidence to support the pathogenic role of toxin-producing clostridia. Am J Vet Res 39:1525–1530

Bartlett JG, Willey SH, Chang TW, Lowe B (1979) Cephalosporinassociated pseudomembranous colitis due to *Clostridium difficile*. JAMA 243:2683–2685
Barza M, Weinstein L (1976) Pharmacokinetics of the penicillins in man. Clin Pharmacokinet 1:297–308
Bass JW, Cohen SH, Corless JD, Mamunes P (1967) Ampicillin compared to other antimicrobials in acute otitis media. JAMA 202:137–142
Bass JW, Crowley DM, Steele RW, Young FSH, Harden LB (1973) Adverse effects of orally administered ampicillin. J Pediatr 83:106–108
Bendirdjian J-P, Prime DJ, Browning MC, Hsu C-Y, Tune BM (1981) Additive nephrotoxicity of cephalosporins and aminoglycosides in the rabbit. J Pharmacol Exp Ther 218:681–685
Bergan T (1979) Aminopenicillins: concluding remarks. Infection [Suppl] 7:507–512
Berger S, Ernst EC, Barza M (1976) Comparative incidence of phlebitis due to buffered cephalothin, cephapirin and cefamandole. Antimicrob Agents Chemother 9:575–579
Bergeron MG, Brusch JL, Barza M, Weinstein L (1976) Significant reduction in the incidence of phlebitis with buffered versus unbuffered cephalothin. Antimicrob Agents Chemother 9:646–648
Beyer KH, Woodward F, Peters L, Verwey WF, Mattis PA (1944) Prolongation of penicillin retention in body by means of para-aminohippuric acid. Science 100:107–108
Bint AJ (1980) Esters of penicillins – are they hepatotoxic? J Antimicrob Chemother 6:697–699
Bint AJ, Holt HA, Reeves DS, Stocks PJ (1978) Clinical experience with cefoxitin. In: Siegenthaler W, Luthy R (eds) Current chemotherapy. American Society for Microbiology, Washington, DC, p 783
Border WA, Lehman PH, Egan JD, Sass HJ, Glode JE, Wilson CB (1974) Antitubular basement membrane antibodies in methicillin-associated interstitial nephritis. N Engl J Med 291:381–384
Boxer LA, Greenberg MS, Boxer GJ, Stossel TP (1975) Autoimmune neutropenia. N Engl J Med 293:748–753
Bracis R, Sanders CV, Gilbert DN (1977) Methicillin hemorrhagic cystitis. Antimicrob Agents Chemother 12:438–439
Bran JL, Levison ME, Kaye D (1972) Clinical and *in vitro* evaluation of cephapirin, a new cephalosporin antibiotic. Antimicrob Agents Chemother 1:35–41
Brown AG, Butterworth D, Cole M, Hanscomb G, Hood JD, Reading C (1976a) Naturally occurring β-lactamase inhibitors with antibacterial activity. J Antibiot 29:668–669
Brown CH III, Natelson EA, Bradshaw MW, Williams TW Jr, Alfrey CP Jr (1974) The hemostatic defect produced by carbenicillin. N Engl J Med 291:265–270
Brown CH III, Natelson EA, Bradshaw MW, Alfrey CP Jr, Williams TW Jr (1975) Study of the effects of ticarcillin on blood coagulation and pletelet function. Antimicrob Agents Chemother 7:652–657
Brown CH III, Bradshaw MW, Natelson EA, Alfrey CP Jr, Williams TW Jr (1976b) Defective platelet function following the administration of penicillin compounds. Blood 47:949–956
Butterworth D, Cole M, Hanscomb G, Rolinson GN (1979) Olivanic acids, a family of β-lactam antibiotics with β-lactamase inhibitory properties produced by streptomyces species. I. Detection, properties and fermentation studies. J Antibiot 32:287–294
Carpenter J (1980) Neutropenia induced by semisynthetic penicillin. South Med J 73:745–748
Carrrizosa J, Levison ME, Kaye D (1973) Double-blind controlled comparison of phlebitis produced by cephapirin and cephalothin. Antimicrob Agents Chemother 3:306–307
Cazenare J-P, Packham MA, Guccione MA, Mustard JF (1973) Effects of penicillin G on platelet aggregation, release and adherence to collagen. Proc Soc Exp Biol Med 142:159–166
Christie DL, Ament ME (1975) Ampicillin-associated colitis. J Pediatr 87:657–658
Chu J-Y, O'Connor DM, Schmidt RR (1977) The mechanism of oxacillin-induced neutropenia. J Pediatr 90:668–669

Chudwin DS, Chesney PJ, Mischler EH, Chesney RW (1979) Hematuria associated with carbenicillin and other semisynthetic penicillins. Am J Dis Child 133:98–99
Colvin RB, Burton JR, Hyslop NE Jr, Spitz L, Lichtenstein NS (1974) Penicillin-associated interstitial nephritis. Ann Intern Med 81:404–405
Conway N, Beck E, Sommerville J (1968) Penicillin encephalopathy. Postgrad Med J 44:891–897
Curtis DR, Game CJA, Johnston GAR, Mc Culloch RM, Mac Lachlan RM (1972) Convulsive action of penicillin. Brain Res 43:242–245
Custer GM, Briggs BR, Smith RE (1979) Effect of cefamandole nafate on blood coagulation and platelet function. Antimicrob Agents Chemother 16:869–872
Davidoff RA (1972a) Penicillin and presynaptic inhibition in the amphibian spinal cord. Brain Res 36:218–222
Davidoff RA (1972b) Penicillin and inhibition in the cat spinal cord. Brain Res 45:638–642
Deisz RA, Aickin C, Lux HD (1979) Decrease of inhibitory driving force in crayfish stretch reception: a mechanism of the convulsant action of penicillin. Neurosci Lett 11:347–352
Delafuente JC, Panush RS, Caldwell JR (1979) Penicillin and cephalosporin immunogenicity in man. Ann Allergy 43:337–340
Dellinger P, Murphy T, Pinn V, Barza M, Weinstein L (1976) Protective effect of cephalothin against gentamicin-induced nephrotoxicity in rats. Antimicrob Agents Chemother 9:172–178
Dewdney JM, Smith H, Wheeler AW (1971) The formation of antigenic polymers in aqueous solutions of beta-lactam antibiotics. Immunology 21:517–525
De Weck AL, Schneider CH (1980) Allergic and immunological aspects of therapy with cefotaxime and other cephalosporins. J Antimicrob Chemother [Suppl] 6:161–168
Ditlove J, Weidmann P, Bernstein M, Massry SG (1977) Methicillin nephritis. Medicine 56:483–491
Dobell ARC, Wyant JD, Seamans KB, Gloor P (1966) Penicillin epilepsy: studies on the blood-brain barrier during cardiopulmonary bypass. J Thorac Cardiovasc Surg 52:469–475
Dolislager D, Fravert D, Tune BM (1979) Interaction of aminoglycosides and cephaloridine in the rabbit kidney. Res Commun Chem Pathol Pharmacol 26:13–23
Donta ST, Lamps GM, Summer RW, Wilkins TD (1980) Cephalosporinassociated colitis and *Clostridium difficile*. Arch Intern Med 140:574–576
Dove AF, Thomas DJB, Aronstam A, Chant RD (1975) Hemolytic anaemia due to penicillin. Br Med J 3:684
Engle JE, Drago J, Carlin B, Schoolwerth AC (1975) Reversible acute renal failure after cephalothin. Ann Intern Med 83:232–233
EORTC International Antimicrobial Therapy Project Group (1978) Three antibiotic regimens in the treatment of infection in febrile granulocytopenic patients with cancer. J Infect Dis 137:14–29
Fanninng WL, Gump D, Jick H (1976) Gentamicin and cephalothin associtated rises in blood urea nitrogen. Antimicrob Agents Chemother 10:80–82
Feigin RD, Van Reken DE, Pickering LK (1974) Dosage in methicillin-associated nephropathy. J Pediatr 85:734–735
Feldman WE, Nelson JD, Stanberry CR (1978) Clinical and pharmacokinetic evaluation of nafcillin in infants and children. J Pediatr 93:1029–1033
Ferrone S, Sirchia G (1968) Survival of cephalothin-treated erythrocytes. JAMA 206:378
Ferrone S, Zanella F, Mercuriali F, Pizzi C (1968) Some enzymatic and metabolic activities of normal human erythrocates treated in vitro with cephalothin. Eur J Pharmacol 4:211–214
Ferrone S, Mercuriali F, Scalamogna M (1971a) Cephalothin positive direct Coomb's test. Relationship to serum immunoglobulin concentration. Experienta 27:193–194
Ferrone S, Zanella A, Scalamogna M (1971b) Red cell metabolism in positive direct Coomb's test after cephalothin therapy. Experientia 27:194–195
Finch SC (1977) Granulocyte disorders – benign, quantitative abnormalities of granulocytes. In: Williams WJ, Beutler E, Erslev AJ, Rundles RW (eds) Hematology, 2nd edn. McGraw-Hill, New York, p 717

Flynn EH (1967) Biological and chemical studies of the cephalosporins. Antimicrob Agents Chemother 1966:715–726

Foord RD (1970) Cephaloridine and the kidney. In: Progress in antimicrobial and anticancer chemotherapy. Proceedings of the 6th international congress chemotherapy, vol 1. University Park Press, Baltimore, p 597

Foord RD (1975) Cephaloridine, cephalothin and the kidney. J Antimicrob Chemother 1:119–133

Fossieck B Jr, Parker RH (1974) Neurotoxicity during intravenous infusion of penicillin: a review. J Clin Pharmacol 14:504–512

Fox VL (1979) Gastrointestinal bleeding due to oral dicloxacillin therapy for osteomyelitis. Pediatrics 63:676–677

Futamachi KJ, Prince DA (1975) Effect of penicillin on an excitatory synapse. Brain Res 100:589–597

Gabriel R, Foord RD, Joekes AM (1970) Reversible encephalophathy and acute renal failure after cephaloridine. Br Med J 4:283–284

Galpin JE, Shinaberger JH, Stanley TM et al. (1978) Acute interstitial nephritis due to methicillin. Am J Med 65:756–765

Garratty G, Petz LD (1975) Drug-induced immune hemolytic anemia. Am J Med 58:398–407

Gentry LO, Jemsek JG, Natelson EA (1981) Effects of sodium piperacillin on platelet function in normal volunteers. Antimicrob Agents Chemother 19:532–533

George WL, Sutter VL, Finegold SM (1978) Toxigenicity and antimicrobial susceptibility of *Clostridium difficile*, a cause of antimicrobial agent-associated colitis. Curr Microbiol 1:55–58

Goldstein LI, Ishak KG (1974) Hepatic injury associated with penicillin therapy. Arch Pathol 98:114–117

Gralnick HR, Mc Ginniss M, Halterman R (1972) Thrombocytopenia with sodium cephalothin therapy. Ann Intern Med 77:401–404

Gutnick MJ, Prince DA (1971) Penicillinase and the convulsant action of penicillin. Neurology 21:759–764

Gutnick MJ, van Duijn H, Citri N (1976) Relative convulsant potencies of structural analogues of penicillin. Brain Res 114:139–143

Harrison WO, Silverblatt FJ, Turck M (1975) Gentamicin nephrotoxicity: failure of the three cephalosporins to potentiate injury in rats. Antimicrob Agents Chemother 8:209–215

Harter DH, Petersdorf RG (1960) A consideration of the pathogenesis of bacterial meningitis: review of experimental and clinical studies. Yale J Biol Med 32:280–309

Hochner B, Spira ME, Werman R (1976) Penicillin decreases chloride conductance in crustacean muscle: a model for the epileptic neuron. Brain Res 107:85–103

Homayouni H, Gross PA, Setia U, Lynch TJ (1979) Leukopenia due to penicillin and cephalosporin homologues. Arch Intern Med 139:827–828

Hooper CA, Haney BA, Stone HH (1980) Gastrointestinal bleeding due to vitamin K deficiency in patients on parenteral cefamandole. Lancet 1:39

Hutcheon DF, Milligan FD, Yardley JH, Hendrix TR (1978) Cephalosporin-associated pseudomembranous colitis. Am J Dig Dis 23:321–326

Indelicato JM, Norvilas TT, Pfeiffer RR, Wheeler WJ, Wilham WL (1974) Substituent effects upon base hydrolysis of penicillins and cephalosporins. J Med Chem 17:523–527

Indelicato JM, Dinner A, Peters LR, Wilham WL (1977) Hydrolysis of 3-chloro-3-cephems. Intramolecular nucleophilic attack in cefaclor. J Med Chem 20:961–963

Jeannet M, Bloch A, Dayer JM, Farquet JJ, Girard JP, Cruchaud A (1976) Cephalothin-induced immune hemolytic anemia. Acta Haematol (Basel) 55:109–117

Jeffery DJ, Jones KH, Langley PF (1978) The metabolism of talampicillin in rat, dog and man. Xenobiotica 8:419–427

Johnson GJ, Leis LA, Rao GHR, White JG (1978a) Prostaglandin synthesis remains intact in non-aggregating carbenicillin treated platelets. Circulation 58:II 125

Johnson GJ, Rao GHR, White JG (1978b) Platelet dysfunction induced by parenteral carbenicillin and ticarcillin. Am J Pathol 91:85–106

Kahan JS, Kahan FM, Goegelman R et al. (1978) Thienamycin, a new β-lactam antibiotic. I. Discovery, taxonomy, isolation and physical properties. J Antibiot 32:1–12
Kallay MC, Tebechian H, Riley GR, Chessin LN (1979) Neurotoxicity due to ticarcillin in patient with renal failure. Lancet I:608–609
Kinnes CG, Connors B, Somjen G (1980) The effects of convulsant doses of penicillin on primary afferents, dorsal root ganglion cells and on presynaptic inhibition in the spinal cord. Brain Res 192:495–512
Klastersky J, Hensgens C, Debusscher L (1975) Empiric therapy for cancer patients: comparative study of ticarcillin-tobramycin, ticarcillin-cephalothin, and cephalothin-tobramycin. Antimicrob Agents Chemother 7:640–645
Kohler H, Weihrauch TR, Prellwitz W, Hoffler D (1975) Side effects of high-dose dicloxacillin therapy. In: Williams JD, Geddes AM (eds) Chemotherapy, vol 4. Plenum, New York, p 333
Kosek JC, Mazze RI, Cousins MJ (1974) Nephrotoxicity of gentamicin. Lab Invest 30:48–57
Kristofferson A, Ahlstedt S, Hall E (1979) Antigens in penicillin allergy. Int Arch Allergy Appl Immunol 60:295–301
Kropp H, Sundelof JG, Kahan JS, Kahan FM, Birnbaum J (1980) MK0787 (N-formimidoyl thienamycin): Evaluation of in vitro and in vivo activities. Antimicrob Agents Chemother 17:993–1000
Lerner PI, Lubin A (1974) Coagulopathy with cefazolin in uremia. N Engl med 290:1324
Leventhal JM, Siken AB (1976) Oxacillin-induced neutropenia in children. J Pediatr 89:769–771
Levine BB, Zolov DM (1969) Prediction of penicillin allergy by immunological tests. J Allergy 43:231–244
Linton AL, Clark WF, Driedger AA, Turnbull DI, Lindsay RM (1980) Acute interstitial nephritis due to drugs. Ann Intern Med 93:735–741
Lipman AG (1974) Effect of buffering on the incidence and severity of cephalothin-induced phlebitis. Am J Hosp Pharm 31:266–288
Luft FC, Patel V, Yum MN, Kleit SA (1976) Nephrotoxicity of cephalosporin-gentamicin combinations in rats. Antimicrob Agents Chemother 9:831–839
MacDonald RL, Barker JL (1977) Pentylenetetrazol and penicillin are selcetive antagonists of GABA-mediated post-synaptic inhibition in culutred mammalian neurones. Nature 267:720–721
MacDonald RL, Barker JL (1978) Spoecific antagonism of GABA-mediated post-synaptic inhibition in cultured mammalian spinal cord neurones: a common mode of convulsant action. Neurology 28:325–330
Malone AJ Jr, Field S, Rosman J, Shemerdiak WP (1977) Neurotoxic reaction to oxacillin. N Engl J Med 296:453
Mandell GL, Sande MA (1980) Penicillins and cephalosporins. In: Gilman AG, Goodman LS, Gilman A (eds) The pharmacologic basis of therapeutics. Macmillan, New York, p 1126
Mashimo K, Horiuchi Y, Atsumi T, Shibata K (1967) Immunological cross reactivities of cephalothin with penicillin G. In: Spitzy KH, Haschek H (eds) Fifth international congress of chemotherapy, vol 5. Wiener Medizinische Akademie, Vienna, p 81
Masuda Y, Suzuki U, Okonogi T (1974) Toxicity test of pivampicillin with experimental animals. Chemotherapy (Tokyo) 22:357–373
Mawdesley-Thomas LE, Noel PRB, Worden AN (1977) The oral administration of pivampicillin to beagle dogs for fourteen weeks. Toxicol Lett 1:17–20
McMahan FG (1980) Disulfiram-like reaction to a cephalosporin. JAMA 243:2397
McMurtry RJ, Mitchell JR (1977) Renal and hepatic necrosis after metabolic activation of 2-substituted furans and thiophenes, including fuurosemide and cephaloridine. Toxicol Appl Pharmacol 42:285–300
Murdoch JM, Speirs CF, Geddes AM, Wallace ET (1964) Clinical trial of cephaloridine (Ceporin), a new broadspectrum antibiotic derived from cephalosporin C. Br Med J 2:1238–1240

Natelson EA, Brown CH III, Bradshaw MW, Alfrey CP Jr, Williams TW Jr (1976) Influence of cephalosporin antibiotics on blood coagulation and platelet function. Antimicrob Agents Chemother 9:91–93
Neu HC, Prince AS (1980) Interaction between moxalactam and alcohol. Lancet I:1422
Newman RJ, McCollum CM (1979) Pseudomembranous colitis due to cephradine. Br J Clin Pract 33:32–33
Newton GGF, Hamilton-Miller JMT (1967) Cephaloridine: chemical and biochemical aspects. Postgrad Med J [Suppl] 43:10–17
Newton WL, Steinman HG, Brandriss MW (1964) Absence of lethal effect of penicillin in germ-free guinea pigs. J Bacteriol 88:537–538
Nicholls PJ (1980) Neurotoxicity of penicillin. J Antimicrob Chemother 6:161–165
Nolan CM, Abernathy RL (1977) Nephropathy associated with methicillin therapy. Arch Intern Med 137:997–1000
O'Brien MS, McLaurin RL (1968) Tolerance of the central nervous system to the local instillation of cephalothin. Surg Forum 19:435–437
Olans RN, Weiner LB (1976) Reversible oxacillin hepatotoxicity. J Pediatr 89:835–838
Pellmar TC, Willson WA (1977) Penicillin effects on iontophoretic responses in Aplysia californica. Brain Res 136:89–101
Petz LD (1976) Autoimmune and drug-immune hemolytic anemias. In: Rose NR, Friedman HH (eds) Manual of clinical immunology. American Society of Microbiology, Washington DC, p 527
Petz LD (1978) Immunologic cross-reactivity between penicillins and cephalosporins. J Infect Dis [Suppl] 134:S74–S78
Petz LD (1980) Drug induced immune hemolytic aenemia. Clin Haematol (Basel) 9:455–482
Pollack AA, Berger SA, Simberkoff MS, Rahal JJ Jr (1978) Hepatitis associated with high-dose oxacillin therapy. Arch Intern Med 138:915–917
Porter J, Jick H (1977) Drug-induced anaphylaxis, convulsions, deafness and extrapyramidal symptoms. Lancet I:587–588
Prince DA (1978) Neurophysiology of epilepsy. Annu Rev Neurosci 1:395–415
Reeves DS, Davies AJ (1980) Antabuse effect with cephalosporins. Lancet 2:540
Ries CA, Rosenbaum TJ, Garratty G, Petz LD, Fudenberg HH (1975) Penicillin-induced immune hemolytic anemia. JAMA 233:432–435
Safanda J, Sabotka PP (1976) Structural dependence of epileptogenic action of penicillins. Experientia [Suppl] 23:145–148
Sakamoto M, Iguchi H, Okamura K, Hori S, Fukugawa Y, Ishikura T (1979) PS-5, a new β-lactam antibiotic. II. Antimicrobial activity. J Antibiot 32:272–279
Saker BM, Musk AW, Haywood EF, Hurst PE (1973) Reversible toxic psychosis after cephalexin. Med J Aust 1:497–498
Sanders WE Jr, Johnson JE III, Taggart JG (1974) Adverse reactions to cephalothin and cephapirin. N Engl J Med 290:424–429
Sanjad SA, Haddad GG, Nassar VH (1974) Nephropathy, an underestimated complication of methicillin therapy. J Pediatr 84:873–877
Sarff LD, Mc Cracken GH (1977) Methicillin-associated nephropathy or cystitis. J Pediatr 90:1031–1032
Schanzer H, Gribetz I, Jacobson JH II (1979) Accidental intraarterial injection of penicillin G. JAMA 242:1289–1290
Schiffer CA, Weinstein HJ, Wiernik PH (1976) Methicillin-associated thrombocytopenia. Ann Intern Med 85:338–339
Schwartz JN, Hamilton JP, Fekety R et al. (1980) Ampicillin-induced enterocolitis: implication of toxigenic Clostridium perfringens type C. J Pediatr 97:661–663
Schwarz S, Gabi F, Huber H, Spath P (1975) Positive direct antiglobulin (Coomb's) test caused by cephalexin administration in humans. Vox Sang 29:59–65
Scully RE, Galdabini JJ, Mc Neely BU (eds) (1975) Case records of the Massachusetts General Hospital (case 49-1975). N Engl J Med 293:1308–1316
Shattil SJ, Bennett JS, Mc Donough M, Turnbull J (1980) Carbenicillin and penicillin G inhibit platelet function *in vitro* by impairing the interaction of agonists with the platelet surface. J Clin Invest 65:329–337

Shaw EB (1966) Transverse myelitis from injection of penicillin. Am J Dis Child 111:548–551
Sheiman L, Spielvogel AR, Horowitz HI (1968) Thrombocytopenia caused by cephalothin sodium. JAMA 203:601–603
Shemonsky NK, Carrizosa J, Kaye D, Levison ME (1975) Doubleblind comparison of phlebitis produced by cefazolin versus cephalothin. Antimicrob Agents Chemother 7:481–482
Silverblatt F, Turck M, Bulger R (1970) Nephrotoxicity due to cephaloridine: a light- and electron-microscopic study in rabbits. J Infect Dis 122:33–44
Spath P, Garratty G, Petz L, (1971 a) Studies on the immune response to penicillin and cephalothin in humans. J Immunol 107:854–859
Spath P, Garraty G, Petz L (1971 b) Studies on the immune response to penicillin and cephalothin in humans. II. Immunohematologic reactions to cephalothin administration. J Immunol 107:860–869
Spector R, Lorenzo AV (1974) Inhibition of penicillin transport from the cerebrospinal fluid after intracisternal inoculation of bacteria. J Clin Invest 54:316–325
Spector R, Snodgrass SR (1976) The effect of uremia on penicillin flux between blood and cerebrospinal fluid. J Lab Clin Med 87:749–759
Stewart GT (1973) Allergy to penicillin and related antibiotics: antigenic and immunochemical mechanism. Annu Rev Pharmacol 13:309–324
Stuart JJ (1980) Ticarcillin-induced hemorrhage in a patient with thrombocytosis. South Med J 73:1084–1085
Svedhem A, Alestig K, Jertborn M (1980) Phlebitis induced by parenteral treatment with flucloxacillin and cloxacillin: a double blind study. Antimicrob Agents Chemother 18:349–352
Swahn A (1976) Gastrointestinal absorptions and metabolism of two ^{35}S-labelled ampicillin esters. Eur J Clin Pharmacol 9:299–306
Swisher SN (1974) Antibiotics and red blood cells. In: Dimitrov NV, Nodine JH (eds) Drugs and hematologic reactions. Grune & Stratton, New York, p 123
Tedesco JF (1975) Ampicillin-associated diarrhea – a prospective study. Am J Dig Dis 20:295–297
Ten Pas A, Quinn EL (1965) Cholestatic hepatitis following the administration of sodium oxacillin. JAMA 191:674–675
Toffler RB, Pingoud EG, Burrell MI (1978) Acute colitis related to penicillin and penicillin derivatives. Lancet 2:707–709
Trollfors B, Alestig K, Norrby R (1979) Local gastrointestinal reactions to intravenously administered cefoxitin and cefuroxime. Scand J Infect Dis 11:315–316
Tune BM (1975) Relationship between the transport and toxicity of cephalosporins in the kidney. J Infect Dis 132:189–194
Tune BM (1982) Cephalosporin nephrotoxicity. Mechanisms and modifying factors. In: Porter G (ed) Nephrotoxic mechanisms of drugs and environmental toxins. Plenum, New York, p 151
Tune BM, Fernholt M (1973) Relationship between cephaloridine and p-aminohippurate transport in the kidney. Am J Physiol 225:1114–1117
Tune BM, Fravert D (1980 a) Cephalosporin nephrotoxicity. Transport, cytotoxicity and mitochondrial toxicity of cephaloglycin. J Pharmacol Exp Ther 215:186–190
Tune BM, Fravert D (1980 b) Mechanisms of cephalosporin nephrotoxicity. A comparison of cephaloridine and cephaloglycin. Kidney Int 18:591–600
Tune BM, Burg MB, Patlak CS (1969) Characteristics of p-aminohippurate transport in proximal renal tubules. Am J Physiol 217:1057–1063
Tune BM, Fernholt M, Schwartz A (1974) Mechanism of cephaloridine transport in the kidney. J Pharmacol Exper Therap 191:311–317
Tune BM, Wu KY, Kempson RL (1977 a) Inhibition of transport and prevention of toxicity of cephaloridine in the kidney. Dose-responsiveness of the rabbit and the guinea pig to probenecid. J Pharmacol Exp Ther 202:466–471

Tune BM, Wu KY, Longerbeam DF, Kempson RL (1977b) Transport and toxicity of cephaloridine in the kidney. Effect of furosemide, p-aminohippurate and saline diuresis. J Pharmacol Exp Ther 202:472–478
Tune BM, Wu KY, Fravert D, Holtzman D (1979) Effect of cephaloridine on respiration by renal cortical mitochondria. J Pharmacol Exp Ther 210:98–100
Tune BM, Browning MC, Hsu C-Y, Fravert D (1982) Prevention of cephalosporin nephrotoxicity by other cephalosporins and by penicillins without significant inhibition of renal cortical uptake. J Infect Dis 145:174–180
Tune BM, Kuo C-H, Hook JB, Hsu C-Y, Fravert D (1983) Effects of piperonyl butoxide on cephalosporin nephrotoxicity in the rabbit. An effect on cephalosporidine transport. I Pharmacol Exp Ther 224:520–524
van Winzum C (1978) Clinical safety and tolerance of cefoxitin sodium: on overview. J Antimicrob Chemother [Suppl] 4:91–104
van Zwieten MJ, Leber PD, Bhan AK, Mc Cluskey RT (1977) Experimental cell-mediated interstitial nephritis induced with exogenous antigens. J Immunol 118:589–593
Wade JC, Petty BG, Conrad G et al. (1978) Cephalothin plus an aminoglycoside is more nephrotoxic than methicillin plus an aminoglycoside. Lancet 2:604–606
Walker AE, Johnson HC, Funderburk WH (1945) Convulsive factor in commercial penicillin. Arch Surg 50:69–73
Wang PL, Prime DJ, Hsu C-Y, Tune BM (1982) Effects of ureteral obstruction on the nephrotoxicity of cephalosporins in the rabbit kidney. J Infect Dis 145:574–581
Weihrauch TR, Kohler H, Hoffler D, Rieger H, Krieglstein J (1975) Neurotoxicity of different penicillins and the effect of diazepam and phenytoin on penicillin-induced convulsions. In: Williams JJD, Geddes AM (eds) Chemotherapy, vol 4. Plenum, New York, p 339
Welles JS, Gibson WR, Harris PN, Small RM, Anderson RC (1966) Toxicity, distribution, and excretion of cephaloridine in laboratory animals. Antimicrob Agents Chemother 1965:863–869
Williams BB, Cushing RD, Lerner AM (1974) Severe combined nephrotoxicity of BL-P1654 and gentamicin. J Infect Dis 130:694–695
Wilson FM, Belamaric J, Lauter CB, Lerner AM (1975) Anicteric carbenicillin hepatitis. JAMA 232:818–821
Wilson G, Greenhood G, Remington JS, Vosti KL (1979) Neutropenia after consecutive treatment courses with nafcillin and piperacillin. Lancet 1:1150
Wold JS, Turnipseed SA (1980) The effect of renal cation transport inhibitors on the *in vivo* and *in vitro* accumulation and efflux of cephaloridine. Life Sci 27:2559–2564
Wold JS, Turnipseed SA, Miller BL (1979) The effect of renal cation transport inhibition on cephaloridine nephrotoxicity. Toxicol Appl Pharmacol 47:115–122
Yow MD, Taber LH, Barrett FF, Mintz AA et al. (1976) A ten-year assessment of methicillin-associated side effects. Pediatrics 58:329–334

CHAPTER 17

Therapeutic Application of β-Lactam Antibiotics

J.V. URI and P. ACTOR

A. Introduction

Since the first successful parenteral treatment of patients with very crude penicillin preparations, produced on a small laboratory scale, in early 1941 (FLOREY et al. 1949), the various β-lactam antibiotics, natural and semisynthetic, virtually revolutionized infectious diseases, research and treatment alike. A new chapter of pharmacology and therapeutics was born and the era of antibiotics was suddenly with us. In the broad field of antibiotics, the β-lactams are of paramount importance. In this chapter are covered the clinical application of all β-lactams: penicillins, cephalosporins, cephamycins and the newer atypical compounds which possess the β-lactam structure. We intend to place emphasis on therapeutic uses, the ultimate reasons for their paramount importance, since other aspects are treated in considerably greater detail in other chapters.

We will concentrate and center on the well-established β-lactams; however, since the development and introduction into therapy of new β-lactams – especially cephalosporins – are still continuing with great intensity all over the world, it seems prudent to summarize these new members, even though the clinical trials of many of them are not completed. It is generally accepted that among the newer β-lactams, especially the third-generation penicillins and cephalosporins, there are potentially new therapeutic applications, including the treatment of infections caused by such microbes as are not controlled by earlier β-lactams. The future holds even more possibilities, with fourth- and fifth-generation cephalosporins and β-lactams.

Although most of the chapter will concentrate on the use of β-lactams in human medicine, a brief reference will be made to their application in dental medicine and veterinary practice. In addition to treatment of existing infections, certain β-lactams are increasingly used for the prevention of infections. Consequently, a section will deal with their prophylactic use. Adverse reactions will be mentioned where it is felt to be necessary to lay a particular emphasis. A separate chapter of the book is devoted entirely to the toxicity of β-lactams. The mechanism(s) of action, the structure–activity relationships and other therapeutically important correlates like enzymatic influences and pharmacokinetics will be treated briefly, only to focus on the importance of new developments relevant to certain compounds (BAX et al. 1981). These subjects are also discussed in greater detail in these volumes.

We will follow the historical classification of the material; first the clinical use of penicillins, followed by the cephalosporins and cephamycins. The newer "structurally unusual or atypical" β-lactams will offer present therapeutic endeavor and future possibilities. Since the literature, especially that of the older β-lactams, is immense, no attempt will be made to list them individually; we will instead draw upon review articles and monographs in which the interested reader can find the original papers. Only those publications will be listed which are not contained in the summary papers and those which are of particular interest and historical importance.

With the development and introduction into therapy of newer β-lactams, more and more bacterial infections become amenable to treatment with the highly effective and nontoxic β-lactams. However, the era is not yet with us when all bacterial infections are safely and surely treatable with β-lactams. We have summarized (Table 1) the β-lactams presently used (or to be used in the very near future) against infections caused by various bacteria, together with other antibacterial antibiotics which fill the gaps where potent β-lactams are not available. This table should provide a quick orientation to the groups or individual antibiotics to be employed in specific infections, placing greater emphasis on the β-lactam antibiotics.

We have made every effort to cover all useful β-lactam antibiotics. However, the intention is to deal with the therapeutically important ones which are now used in the treatment of bacterial infections.

The chapter is not intended to provide a detailed encyclopedic knowledge of all clinical aspects of these antibiotics. It does highlight the basic principles of the therapeutic uses of β-lactams and provides the most important relevant data necessary for effective use of these drugs.

B. Penicillins in the Therapy of Human Infections

Benzylpenicillin or penicillin G was the first antibiotic introduced into the therapy of bacterial infections in humans, with great success. It was used predominantly by the parenteral routes. Soon it was followed by phenoxymethyl-penicillin or penicillin V which, being acid-stable, can be taken orally. Both of these penicillins are produced by fermentation; therefore, they are often referred to as natural penicillins (URI 1964c). The discovery and isolation on a large scale of 6-aminopenicillanic acid (6-APA) by BATCHELOR et al. in 1959 opened the way for the preparation of the semisynthetic penicillins. All the subsequent penicillins (penams) introduced into therapy are semisynthetic preparations. They are grouped partly by

Table 1. Antibacterial drugs of choice with particular reference to the β-lactam antibiotics. [Modified, with permission, from *The Medical Letter*, Vol. 22, No. 2 (Issue 549), January 25, 1980]

Infecting organism	Drug of first choice	Alternative drugs
Gram-positive cocci		
Staphylococcus aureus		
non-penicillinase-producing	Penicillin G or V	A cephalosporin; clindamycin; vancomycin
penicillinase-producing	A penicillinase-resistant penicillin	A cephalosporin; vancomycin; clindamycin

Table 1 (continued)

Infecting organism	Drug of first choice	Alternative drugs
Streptococcus pyogenes (Group A) and Groups C and G	Penicillin G or V	An erythromycin; a cephalosporin
Streptococcus, Group B	Penicillin G or ampicillin streptomycin	Chloramphenicol; an erythromycin; a cephalosporin
Streptococcus, viridans group	Penicillin G with or without streptomycin	A cephalosporin; vancomycin
Streptococcus bovis	Penicillin G or V	A cephalosporin; vancomycin
Streptococcus, Enterococcus group:		
endocarditis or other severe infection	Ampicillin or penicillin G with gentamicin or streptomycin	Vancomycin with gentamicin or streptomycin
uncomplicated urinary tract infection	Ampicillin or amoxicillin	Nitrofurantoin
Streptococcus, anaerobic	Penicillin G or V	Clindamycin; a tetracycline; an erythromycin; chloramphenicol; a cephalosporin
Streptococcus pneumoniae (pneumococcus)	Penicillin G or V	An erythromycin; a cephalosporin; chloramphenicol; vancomycin
Gram-negative cocci		
Neisseria gonorrhoeae	Penicillin G or amoxicillin or a tetracycline	Ampicillin; spectinomycin; a cephalosporin
Neisseria meningitidis	Penicillin G	Chloramphenicol; a sulfonamide; a cephalosporin
Gram-positive bacilli		
Bacillus anthracis (anthrax)	Penicillin G	An erythromycin; a tetracycline
Clostridium perfringens (welchii)	Penicillin G	Chloramphenicol; clindamycin; a cephalosporin; a tetracycline
Clostridium difficile	Vancomycin	
Clostridium tetani	Penicillin G	A tetracycline; a cephalosporin
Corynebacterium diphtheriae	An erythromycin	Penicillin G
Listeria monocytogenes	Ampicillin or penicillin G with or without gentamicin	Chloramphenicol; a tetracycline; a cephalosporin
Enteric gram-negative bacilli		
Bacteroides		
oropharyngeal strains	Penicillin G	Clindamycin; an erythromycin; a tetracycline
gastrointestinal strains	Clindamycin	Chloramphenicol; cefoxitin; metronidazole; a tetracycline; a cephalosporin
Enterobacter	Gentamicin or tobramycin	Carbenicillin or ticarcillin; amikacin; cefamandole; chloramphenicol; a tetracycline

Table 1 (continued)

Infecting organism	Drug of first choice	Alternative drugs
Escherichia coli	Gentamicin or tobramycin; a cephalosporin	Ampicillin; carbenicillin or ticarcillin; a cephalosporin; kanamycin; amikacin; a tetracycline; trimethoprim-sulfamethoxazole; chloramphenicol
Klebsiella pneumoniae	Gentamicin or tobramycin; a cephalosporin	Kanamycin; amikacin; a tetracycline; trimethoprim-sulfamethoxazole; chloramphenicol
Proteus mirabilis	Ampicillin; a cephalosporin	Gentamicin or tobramycin; carbenicillin or ticarcillin; amikacin; trimethoprim-sulfamethoxazole; chloramphenicol
other *Proteus*	Gentamicin or tobramycin; a cephalosporin	Carbenicillin or ticarcillin; amikacin; a tetracycline; trimethoprim-sulfamethoxazole; chloramphenicol
Providencia (*Proteus inconstans*)	Amikacin	Gentamicin or tobramycin; carbenicillin or ticarcillin; trimethoprim-sulfamethoxazole; chloramphenicol; cefoxitin or cefamandole
Salmonella typhi	Chloramphenicol	Ampicillin; amoxicillin; trimethoprim-sulfamethoxazole
other *Salmonella* spp.	Ampicillin or amoxicillin	Chloramphenicol; trimethoprim-sulfamethoxazole
Serratia spp.	A cephalosporin; gentamicin	Amikacin; trimethoprim-sulfamethoxazole; carbenicillin or ticarcillin
Shigella spp.	Trimethoprim-sulfamethoxazole; a cephalosporin	Chloramphenicol; a tetracycline; ampicillin
Other gram-negative bacilli		
Acinetobacter (Mima, Herellea)	Gentamicin or tobramycin; a cephalosporin	Kanamycin; amikacin; minocycline; doxycycline; trimethoprim-sulfamethoxazole
Bordetella pertussis (whooping cough)	An erythromycin	
Brucella (brucellosis)	A tetracycline with or without streptomycin	Chloramphenicol with or without streptomycin; trimethoprim-sulfamethoxazole
Calymmatobacterium granulomatis (granuloma inguinale)	A tetracycline	Streptomycin
Campylobacter (*Vibrio*) *fetus*	An erythromycin	A tetracycline; gentamicin; chloramphenicol
Francisella tularensis (tularemia)	Streptomycin	A tetracycline; chloramphenicol
Haemophilus ducreyi (chancroid)	Trisulfapyrimidines	A tetracycline

Table 1 (continued)

Infecting organism	Drug of first choice	Alternative drugs
Haemophilus influenzae		
Meningitis, epiglottitis and other life-threatening infections	A cephalosporin; chloramphenicol	Ampicillin; a tetracycline
Other infections	Ampicillin or amoxicillin	A tetracycline; trimethoprim-sulfamethoxazole; a sulfonamide; streptomycin; cefaclor; cefamandole
Corynebacterium vaginale (Formerly: *Haemophilus vaginalis*)	Metronidazole	–
Legionella pneumophila	An erythromycin with or without rifampin	A tetracycline
Leptotrichia buccalis (Vincent's infection)	Penicillin G	A tetracycline; an erythromycin
Pasteurella multocida	Penicillin G	A tetracycline; a cephalosporin
Pittsburgh Pneumonia Agent	An erythromycin with or without rifampin	Trimethoprim-sulfamethoxazole; a tetracycline
Pseudomonas aeruginosa		
Urinary tract infection	Carbenicillin or ticarcillin	Tobramycin; gentamicin; amikacin; a polymyxin; a cephalosporin
Other infections	Tobramycin or gentamicin with carbenicillin or ticarcillin	Amikacin with carbenicillin or ticarcillin; a cephalosporin
Pseudomonas (Actinobacillus) mallei (glanders)	Streptomycin with a tetracycline	Streptomycin with chloramphenicol
Pseudomonas pseudomallei (melioidosis)	A tetracycline with or without chloramphenicol	Trimethoprim-sulfamethoxazole; a sulfonamide
Spirillum minor (rat bite fever)	Penicillin G	A tetracycline; streptomycin
Streptobacillus moniliformis (rat bite fever; Haverhill fever)	Penicillin G	A tetracycline; streptomycin
Vibrio cholerae (cholera)	A tetracycline	Trimethoprim-sulfamethoxazole
Yersinia pestis (plague)	Streptomycin	A tetracycline; chloramphenicol
Actinomycetes		
Actinomyces israelii (actinomycosis)	Penicillin G	A tetracycline
Nocardia	Trisulfapyrimidines	Trimethoprim-sulfamethoxazole; trisulfapyrimidines with minocycline or ampicillin or erythromycin; cycloserine
Spirochetes		
Borrelia recurrentis (relapsing fever)	A tetracycline	Penicillin G
Leptospira	Penicillin G	A tetracycline
Treponema pallidum (syphilis)	Penicillin G	A tetracycline; an erythromycin
Treponema pertenue (yaws)	Penicillin G	A tetracycline

the chemical nature of the substituents attached to the 6-APA nucleus and partly on the basis of their biological properties. Thus it is customary to speak of the natural penicillins, the acid-stable penicillins, the penicillinase-resistant penicillins, the ampicillin group or aminopenicillins with broader antibacterial spectra, the antipseudomonas penicillins, some of them with extended spectra, the amidinopenicillins and, recently, the "atypical" penicillin-like β-lactams such as oxapenams, carbapenems, and the monocyclic β-lactams.

Table 2 lists the compounds with therapeutic potentials.

Although they have many properties in common, and, in several instances they can substitute for one another in the therapy, they all contain the common nucleus (6-APA). Their mechanisms of action are fundamentally the same: the inhibition of the synthesis of the bacterial cell wall peptidoglycan with consequent death and in most cases lysis of the cell. Their affinities to the penicillin-binding proteins of the cell membrane have much in common, but there are variations with the different penicillins. The most common cause of resistance to certain penicillins is the production by the bacteria of β-lactamase(s), which hydrolytically cleaves the β-lactam ring with loss of antibacterial activity. In this respect, gram-positive and gram-negative bacterial species may differ substantially. Non-β-lactamase-producing bacteria can be resistant to penicillins most probably because the penicillin cannot reach the receptor site. These are the so-called permeability mutants. In the case of methicillin-resistance other, as yet unknown, factors are in operation.

As a rule, penicillins can be given orally, but the absorption from the gastrointestinal tract varies widely; many of them are preferably applied parenterally. There are long-acting penicillins, mostly intramuscular "repository" or "depot" preparations. Their reversible binding (association) to serum proteins (albumin) varies from 15% to 98%. They distribute well in body fluids and organs and readily reach antibacterial concentrations. The main excretory organ for penicillins is the kidney with consequent high urinary concentrations. Biliary excretion (10%–100%) is known for certain penicillins which may be of importance in certain localized infections. Since the main mechanism of renal elimination is tubular secretion (e.g., as much as 4 g benzylpenicillin per hour), probenecid, with similar excretary properties, is able to increase serum levels and to prolong serum half-life as well as decrease serum binding. Because of these excretory mechanisms, renal impairment and liver dysfunction should be considered as dose-limiting circumstances. Penicillins are fundamentally safe drugs with the exception of the unpredictable non-dose-related hypersensitivity (allergic) reactions which vary from simple rash to immediate, life-threatening anaphylaxis. The major haptenic determinant of penicillin allergy is the penicilloic acid that avidly and covalently binds to proteins, serving as immunogen. Minor untoward reactions occur in rare cases with various penicillins, but they are seldom, if ever, severe enough to discontinue therapy. Penicillins, because of their unique mode of action, do not need much help from the host's immune system, although they do not appear to have any immunomodulating effect (FINCH 1980).

In the following pages, the clinical use of the individual pencillins will be discussed. To avoid unnecessary repetitions, the list of authors of books, monographs and review articles upon which we have drawn most often and widely are given herewith: URI and VALU (1963); URI (1964a); URI (1966); HOEPRICH (1968);

PLEMPEL and OTTEN (1969); THRUPP (1974); GARROD (1974); WEINSTEIN (1976); KUCERS and BENNETT (1977); SMITH (1977); NEU (1977); BALL et al. (1978); WISE (1978a); ASSCHER (1978); CSÁKY (1979); HAMILTON-MILLER and SMITH (1979); NEU (1979a); MEYERS et al. (1980); SELWYN (1980). The individual compounds will be discussed under the headings of penams, penems, oxapenams, carbapenems, and monocyclic β-lactams.

Table 2. β-Lactams with therapeutic potentials (penams, oxapenams, carbapenems, and monocyclic β-lactams)

Compound	Routes of use
Benzyl (G)-penicillin	
Sodium or potassium salt	IM, IV, (PO)
Procaine	IM
Benzathine	IM
Phenoxymethyl (V)-penicillin	
Free acid	PO
Potassium or sodium salt	PO, IM, IV
Phenethicillin	PO
Propicillin	PO
Methicillin	IM, IV
Nafcillin	IM, IV, (PO)
Oxacillin	PO, IM, IV
Cloxacillin	PO, IM, IV
Dicloxacillin	PO
Flucloxacillin	PO, IM, IV
Ampicillin	IM, IV, PO
Bacampicillin	PO
Pivampicillin	PO
Talampicillin	PO
Hetacillin	PO
Amoxicillin	PO, IM, IV
Epicillin	PO, IM, IV
Cyclacillin	PO
Carbenicillin	IM, IV
Indanyl carbenicillin	PO
Phenyl carbenicillin	PO
Ticarcillin	IM, IV
Temocillin	IM, IV
Azlocillin	IM, IV
Furazlocillin	IM, IV
Mezlocillin	IM, IV
Piperacillin	IM, IV
Mecillinam (amdinocillin)	IM, IV
Pivmecillinam	PO
Bacmecillinam	PO
Clavulanic acid	PO
Thienamycin	IM, IV
Formimidoylthienamycin	IM, IV
Nocardicin A	?
Sulfazecin	?
Azthreonam	IM, IV
Penems	PO, IM, IV

I. The Penams: The Biosynthetic or Natural Penicillins

Penicillin G or benzylpenicillin, its salts and repository forms as well as penicillin V or phenoxymethylpenicillin belong to this group. There are minor differences in the antibacterial spectrum and depth of activity but the major difference between the two natural penicillins is in their dosage forms. Basically penicillin G is a parenteral and penicillin V is an oral antibiotic. In the treatment of many infections they are interchangeable.

1. Penicillin G (Benzylpenicillin)

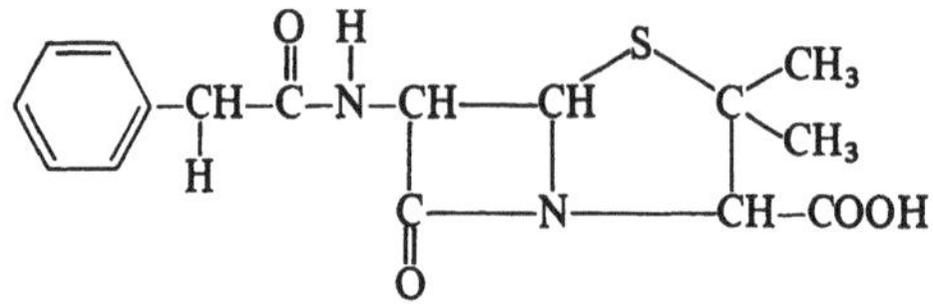

Penicillin G (benzylpenicillin)

Penicillin G is the antibiotic of choice in the treatment of a large number of infections (Table 1) caused by certain gram-positive pathogenic bacteria such as *Streptococcus pneumoniae*, *β*-hemolytic streptococci, *Streptococcus viridans*, gram-negative cocci such as *Neisseria meningitidis* and *Neisseria gonorrhoeae;* and many anaerobic infections produced by various *Clostridium* spp. (with the exception of *Bacteroides fragilis*), *Actinomyces israeli*, *Bacillus anthracis*, *Treponema pallidum* and other *Treponema* spp. Other bacteria sensitive to penicillin G include: *Erysipelothrix rhusiopathiae*, *Streptococcus agalactiae*, *Listeria monocytogenes*, *Leptotrichia buccalis*, *Streptobacillus moniliformis*, *Spirillum minor*, *Mima polymorpha*, and *Pasteurella multocida* (the only *Pasteurella* species sensitive to penicillin). Enterococci (*Streptococcus faecalis*) are not sensitive to most *β*-lactams, but infections (endocarditis) caused by them can be managed with the combination of two antibiotics, i.e. penicillin G (or ampicillin) and an aminoglycoside. The therapeutic effect of the combination of penicillin and gentamicin is synergistic for the majority of the enterococcus strains.

Staphylococcus aureus strains formerly extremely sensitive to penicillin G are now generally (60%–90%) resistant, and infections caused by penicillinase-producing resistant strains in hospitals should be treated with penicillinase-resistant penicillins or certain cephalosporins. Penicillin G is still the drug of choice for non-*β*-lactamase producing strains because of its high degree of therapeutic usefulness and low cost. The majority of streptococci (except enterococci) are very sensitive to penicillin G. *T. pallidum*, *B. anthracis* and *Corynebacterium diphtheriae* are also always sensitive to benzylpenicillin.

The Enterobacteriaceae (*Escherichia coli*, *Klebsiella*, *Salmonella*, *Shigella*, *Enterobacter*, *Proteus* spp.) and other gram-negative bacilli (*Vibrio cholerae*, *Pseudomonas aeruginosa*, *Brucella* spp., *Yersinia* spp., *Bacteroides* spp., *Hemophilus influenzae*, *Bordatella pertussis* and others) are usually not sensitive to penicillin G, at least not at therapeutic levels. Mycobacterial, rickettsial, chlamydial and protozoal infections or infestations are resistant to penicillin G treatment and so are, naturally, the mycoplasmal infections (the organism having no cell wall).

It is customary to express the minimum inhibitory concentrations (MIC) of penicillin G in μg/ml, but it is still traditionally prescribed in most parts of the world in units. One international unit of activity of the sodium benzylpenicillin is equal to 0.6 μg of the pure salt. The potency, or unit of activity was established in 1944 and intentionally discontinued in 1968 by the World Health Organization (WHO). The discontinuation was justifiable, since today's preparations are of such a degree of purity that their activity can be expressed on a weight basis, as is the situation with other penicillins and all other widely used antibiotics. It is hoped that the traditional designation will gradually fade away and the usage of unitage will be abandoned.

In the following infections penicillin G alone or sometimes in combination with another antibiotic is highly effective.

Respiratory tract infections in adults and in children (lobar pneumonia, bronchitis, empyema, croup) especially those caused by *S. pneumoniae* and group A β-hemolytic streptococcus are very reactive to penicillin G. If *H. influenzae* type b and/or *S. aureus* are also involved as the causative agents, penicillin G alone may not be sufficient, and comcomitant administration of other antibiotics is necessary.

Meningitis caused by pneumococcus, meningococcus or *L. monocytogenes* responds well to penicillin G, but large doses and prolonged (2 weeks) treatment is recommended. Intrathecal administration is completely abandoned. In mixed or undiagnosed infections, the combination of penicillin G and chloramphenicol is a satisfactory treatment. Chloramphenicol should be discontinued if the pathogens are found to be sensitive to penicillin G. In the meningococcal carrier state, penicillin G is ineffective.

Streptococcal pharyngitis, septic throat, scarlet fever, septicemia and cellulitis respond very well to penicillin G, although oral penicillin V is more often used. The incidence of rheumatic fever following streptococcal pharingitis is significantly reduced by penicillin, but less so that of the subsequent glomerulonephritis.

Infectious endocarditis caused by *S. viridans*, or by non-β-lactamase producing *S. aureus*, responds favorably to high doses and at least 2 weeks' duration of treatment with penicillin G alone or in combination with an aminoglycoside. Enterococcal endocarditis always requires this kind of combination therapy.

Otitis media and sinusitis of pneumonococcal and streptococcal origin are responsive to penicillin G (or V) in the majority of infections. In children, *H. influenzae* is often present as a pathogen or co-pathogen and penicillin G will not be satisfactory.

Gonococcal infections respond, in general, promptly and satisfactorily to penicillin G administration. Today higher doses are required than in the early years of the penicillin era, but still penicillin is the best antigonococcal agent. The emergence of penicillinase-producing *N. gonorrhoeae* strains creates an alarming therapy problem in certain parts of the world. It is expected that such strains will spread all over the world, although at present their incidence remains low in the United States. Infections caused by resistant strains require treatment with other antibiotics (certain new cephalosporins, tetracyclines and spectinomycin). Simple, uncomplicated urethritis in adults is treated with a single large dose of penicillin G (or oral ampicillin and/or amoxicillin) in combination with probenecid. Gonococcal arthritis and tenosynovitis, pelvic inflammations, disseminated gonococcal infections often with skin lesions, gonococcemia and the rare gonococcal endocarditis usually need very large doses of and long treatment with penicillin G, preferably intravenously, often with hospitalization. Ophthalmia neonatorum is usually readily treated with aqueous penicillin G.

The therapy of syphilis with penicillin G continues to be highly successful. For the treatment of primary, secondary, and latent syphilis the "single-session treatment" is extensively and successfully used with high doses of the long-acting benzathine penicillin G. Tertiary syphilis, today rare, requires prolonged treatment. Neuro- and cardiovascular syphilis can be brought to stagnation with extremely large and prolonged doses but is never cured by penicillin G, since the nature of the disease is progressive to death.

Syphilis during pregnancy, as well as the congential syphilis without neurological involvement, should be treated either with aqueous penicillin G for many days or with a single dose of benzathine penicillin G.

The anaerobic spore-forming bacilli are sensitive to penicillin G, therefore, the treatment of tetanus, gas gangrene and anthrax can be started as early as possible with moderate or high doses of penicillin G. It is also used, with not completely established value, to eradicate *Clostridium botulinum* from the bowel to prevent eventual toxin production. However, concomitant administration of specific antitoxins and/or human immunoglobulins and necessary debridement are required. Penicillin G is the drug of choice for the therapy of the various forms of actinomycosis. The gram-negative *B. fragilis* shows irregular sensitivity to penicillin G (infections above the diaphragm are more sensitive) and about 20%–50% of the strains may be insensitive even to high concentrations; therefore, the administration of other more potent antiinfective drugs is highly advisable.

The incidence of complications of diphtheria can be reduced by penicillin G or even better by erythromycin, but specific antitoxin remains the effective treatment.

Puerperal infections react well to penicillin G treatment, but usually the infection is caused by a mixture of bacteria (aerobes and anaerobes), so the use of other antibacterial agents is usually necessary.

A great diversity of other infections, like the fusospirochetal infections, erysipeloid, listerosis, rat-bite fever and certain gram-negative infections (mainly urinary tract infections) can very often successfully be treated with penicillin G.

Penicillin G is available as the sodium or potassium salt in aqueous solutions for intravenous or intramuscular injection. Intrathecal injection is rarely, if ever, used today. The potassium salt is also available in tablet form for oral administration, but it is rarely used now and not recommended. Similarly, the use of suppositories (rectal, vaginal) is not advised because of the unreliable absorption. The same relates to preparations designed for inhalation therapy and topical use. The only exception may be the neonatal eye-drop for prevention of gonococcal ophthalmitis. The repository long-acting preparations of procaine penicillin G and benzathine penicillin G are for intramuscular use to obtain prolonged (days or weeks) action. The tablets of benzathine penicillin are rarely used today.

The dosage and frequency of application and the duration of treatment with penicillin G depend on many factors. Among these the most important are the causative agent and its susceptibility to penicillin G. Also important are the severity and location as well as the natural course and probable duration of infection, the nature of mixed infections, the expected therapeutic outcome, the possible superinfection(s) and the patient's drug tolerance. There exists no standard dose regimen. The dose may vary from 100,000 units to many millions of units as a single dose or application for weeks, months and even for the purpose of continuous prophylaxis for years (life) to obtain objective cure or subjective improvement depending on the nature of infection. Fortunately, the extremely low incidence of direct dose-related toxicity of penicillin G permits large variations in dosage and duration of treatment.

The route of administration of penicillin G varies not only according to the disease but also to the preparation itself. The crystalline potassium or sodium salts of penicillin G are almost exclusively injected intramuscularly or intravenously. Their oral application is not practicable because of acid-lability. Procaine penicillin G, preferably as the aqueous suspension, must be injected only intramuscularly. This is less painful than the water-soluble crystalline salts. It should never be given intravenously. Utmost care must be taken to avoid such accidental injection. Benzathine penicillin as a suspension is only for intramuscular use. There are vials for intramuscular injection containing, in addition to benzathine penicillin G, procaine penicillin G and/or potassium penicillin G – to combine prompt action with prolonged effects. The oral application of benzathine penicillin G is rarely, if ever, used. Penicillin G preparations can be used to treat infections of newborns, infants and children with adjustment of dosages.

The clinical use of penicillin G was intentionally discussed at considerable length not only because of its historical significance but also because of its extremely wide and successful usage in a very large number of infections. This also serves as a basis for comparison with the use of other penicillins and cephalosporins to avoid much repetition.

2. Penicillin V and the Acid-Stable Phenoxypenicillins

Phenoxymethylpenicillin or penicillin V is a widely used "oral penicillin" since it is acid-stable and resists inactivation by gastric juice. Penicillin V is available as the potassium or sodium salt in the forms of tablets, capsules and oral suspension. The adult dose is 125–500 mg (250 mg) taken 4–6 hourly. The infant dose is 50 mg/kg per day in three divided doses. Basically, it can be substituted for penicillin G in the majority of indications when oral treatment of infections is reasonable. Serum levels of oral penicillin V are equal to or sometimes even higher than those of the intramuscular penicillin G. Its pharmacokinetics are quite similar to those of penicillin G. Gram-positive cocci and bacilli are almost equally sensitive to the natural penicillins although penicillin G is still somewhat more active. Penicillin V is less active than penicillin G against certain gram-negative cocci, like *N. gonorrhoeae* and *N. meningitidis*. *H. influenzae* is the pathogen least sensitive to penicillin V and the other gram-negative bacilli are almost completely insensitive to it. This insensitivity is not related to an ability to enzymatically degrade penicillin G. Penicillin V is equally often used in adult and pediatric practice as an oral replacement for penicillin G in upper respiratory tract infections caused by streptococci or pneumococci.

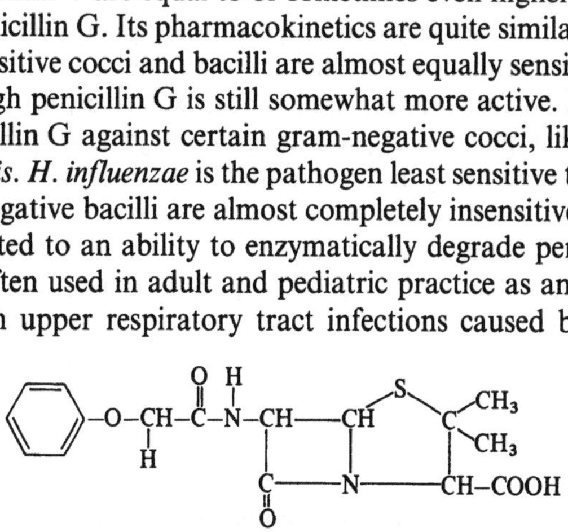

Penicillin V (phenoxymethylpenicillin)

The other members of the phenoxypenicillins (phenethicillin, propicillin and phenbencillin) are semisynthetic in their origin with similar therapeutic application and no clear practical advantage over penicillin V.

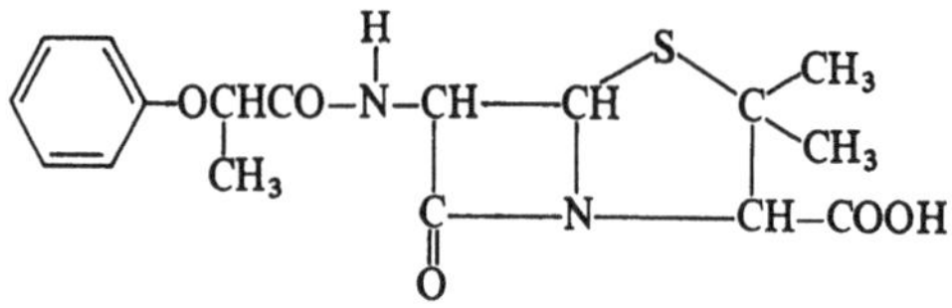

Phenethicillin

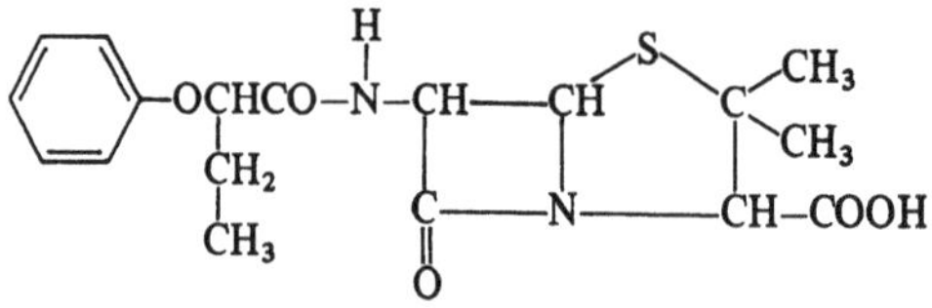

Propicillin

II. The Penicillinase-Resistant Penicillins

The discovery of acid-stable penicillins was later followed by the synthesis of derivatives of 6-APA that were resistant to the hydrolytic degradation of staphylococcal β-lactamase. The treatment of infections caused by β-lactamase-producing staphylococcal strains gradually became a serious problem in therapy. It became evident that certain groups added to the penicillin nucleus can protect the β-lactam ring from enzymatic degradation. Xylocaine-penicillin (VÁCZI and URI 1954) was the first with weak staphylococcal β-lactamase stability which may be considered as a structural prototype showing that ortho-ortho substituted bulky side chains attached to 6-APA can protect the β-lactam ring. It was weak clinically, but a most exciting beginning. Soon, several 6-APA derivatives were prepared, based on this structure–activity concept, with therapeutically useful β-lactamase stability. These semisynthetic penicillins are often referred to as the "antistaphylococcal penicillins" because they are used almost exclusively for the treatment of infections caused by staphylococci producing the enzyme. At present, almost all of the hospital strains and many in the community produce β-lactamase. Along with gain in β-lactamase stability was some loss in potency and spectrum of activity. Many of the *Staphylococcus epidermidis* strains are insensitive to the penicillinase-stable penicillins and also to many cephalosporins, despite some in vitro susceptibility. The penicillinase-resistant penicillins include: methicillin, nafcillin and the isoxazolyl penicillins (oxacillin, cloxacillin, dicloxacillin, flucloxacillin).

1. Methicillin

Methicillin was the first semisynthetic penicillin highly effective in penicillinase-producing staphylococcal infections.

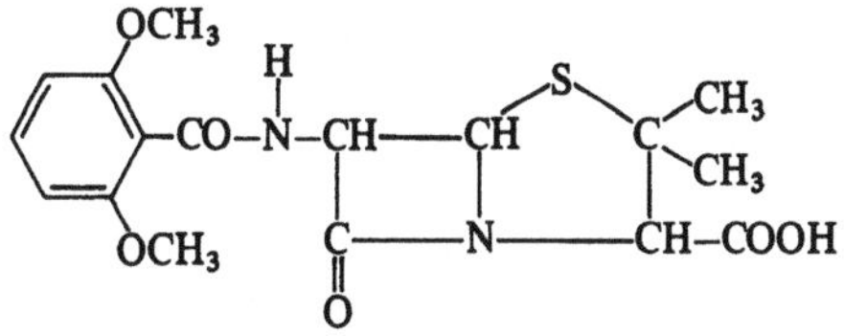

Methicillin

As a sodium salt, it is water soluble, stable in the dry state but unstable in solution, especially under acidic conditions. At pH 2 it is quickly inactivated, therefore cannot be given orally. It is administered intramuscularly or more often intravenously.

Although the antibacterial spectrum of methicillin is similar to that of penicillin G, its general potency is lower. Most *S. aureus* strains are inhibited by 1–4 μg/ml, including the penicillinase-producing strains. It inhibits *S. pneumoniae* and *S. pyogenes* (0.2–0.5 μg/ml) but not *S. faecalis* and gram-negative bacilli. Its only therapeutic indication is the treatment of staphylococcal infections, especially when penicillinase production is suspected or proved. It can be given intramuscularly 1 g every 4 h for the treatment of moderately severe infections. The intramuscular injection can be painful. To avoid this and to be able to introduce larger amounts in severe infections, the intravenous injection (bolus or rapid infusion) is the preferred route of administration. For adults, the usual daily intravenous dose is 4–6 g preferably given every 4 h. In severe infections, the recommended serum levels should be 2–4 times greater than the minimal inhibitory concentration (MIC) values. For continuous intravenous infusion, only the buffered solutions are stable, but not for longer than 8 h at room temperature. Glucose solution is seldom, if ever, used as diluent for intravenous infusion. About 40% of methicillin is bound to plasma protein. It is excreted mainly by tubular secretion, consequently probenecid enhances the serum levels and prolongs the excretion time. Methicillin has a low level of toxicity although reversible untoward reactions such as neutropenia, bone marrow depression and nephropathy are observed on rare occasions. It can be administered in the regular dose to patients with mild or moderate renal failure.

Methicillin-resistant *S. aureus* strains have been reported, although less frequently in the United States than in other parts of the world. The mechanism of this resistance is not the enzymatic destruction of methicillin. It is probably due to alterations in the cell wall synthesis or cell envelope formation or other unknown (mostly permeability) factors. The methicillin-resistant staphylococci represent not only basic theoretical interest but also a serious therapeutic problem. The treatment of infections due to these resistant bacteria may be difficult since they are resistant to all the other penicillinase-resistant penicillins, to cephalosporins and frequently to aminoglycosides, tetracyclines, chloramphenicol, erythromycin, lincomycin and clindamycin. In such serious infections the drug(s) of choice should be vancomycin, rifampicin or fusidic acid, alone or preferably in combination. Patients with methicillin-resistant strains should be kept isolated from other patients.

Although methicillin-resistant staphylococci are rare (about 2%), the severity of the therapeutic problem requires exact assessment of such strains. By routine laboratory susceptibility tests, the methicillin resistance is frequently overlooked as these strains grow more slowly than the sensitive strains. It is more easily detected by incubating cultures at 30 °C (preferably for 48 h) on an agar medium containing 5% sodium chloride. The pH of the medium is important. Acidity (pH 5.2) appears to abolish methicillin resistance (SABATH and WALLACE 1971). Not recognizing the importance of these cultural modifications may be the cause of differences in number and degree of the reported methicillin-resistance cases.

Newer compounds, synthesized following the same structure-activity consideration were found to have therapeutic advantages over methicillin. Nafcillin, oxacillin, cloxacillin, dicloxacillin and flucloxacillin are not only resistant to the degradation of staphylococcal penicillinase but they are acid-stable and well absorbed from the gastrointestinal tract (except nafcillin) and possess greater intrinsic activities.

2. Nafcillin

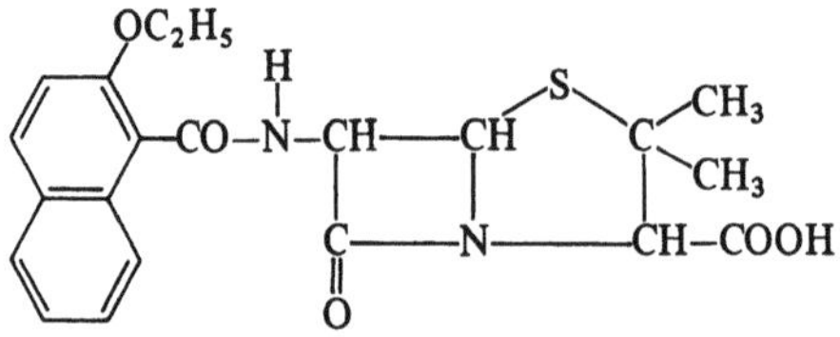

Nafcillin

The intrinsic activity of nafcillin is greater than that of methicillin against staphylococci, streptococci and pneumococci, but like all the other penicillins in this group, it has no activity against gram-negative microbes. It has wide clinical use in the United States in the treatment of serious infections caused by penicillinase-producing staphylococci, such as endocarditis, septicemia, osteomyelitis and pneumonia. Although it is highly bound to serum protein (about 90%), effective serum levels can be obtained after parenteral administration of 6–18 g/day, given in divided doses every 4 h to treat severe infections. Otherwise the dose should be 1 g intramuscularly with an average peak serum level of 8 μg/ml. To obtain high serum concentrations, the intravenous route is favored. Newborn infants and children tolerate it well with appropriately reduced doses. Only minor dose reduction is required for patients with renal failure since it is primarily excreted by the liver via the bile (bile concentrations being higher than those of serum) and a smaller portion by the kidney. Concomitant probenecid still increases the serum levels and elimination half-life. Its tissue penetration and distribution is good, and the concentrations in the cerebrospinal fluid are high enough to be curative in staphylococcal meningitis. It is partially inactivated in the liver. In addition to the parenteral injection (0.5-, 1-, 2-, and 4-g sterile vials of the sodium salt) it is available for oral administration in capsules (250 mg) and oral solution (200 mg/5 ml). The absorption after oral dosage is quite irregular (food intake impairs it), the serum peak level is usually low; therefore, this route of administration is not recommended. The reconstituted injections are stable for at least 4 h at room temperature. Many clinicians prefer nafcillin over methicillin mainly because it is believed to have a lower incidence of nephropathy, as is the case with the isoxazolyl penicillins.

3. Isoxazolyl Penicillins

The four commercially available and generally used members of this group of extremely effective antistaphylococcal penicillins are structurally closely related. The slight chemical differences in the congeners does not significantly influence their antimicrobial activities, but rather their pharmacokinetic profile. These semisynthetic compounds have excellent stability to β-lactamases and to gastric acid inactivation.

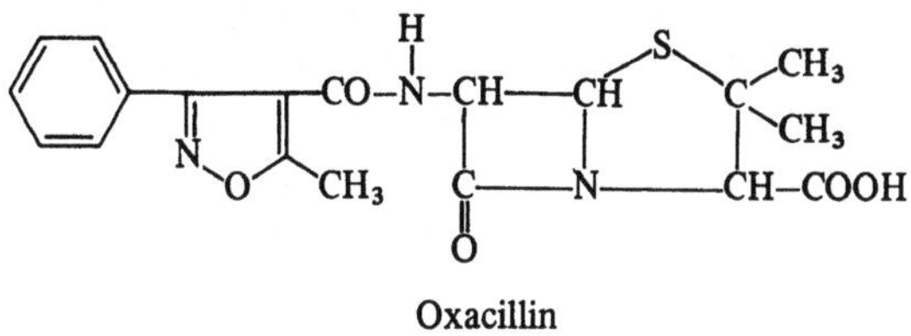

Oxacillin

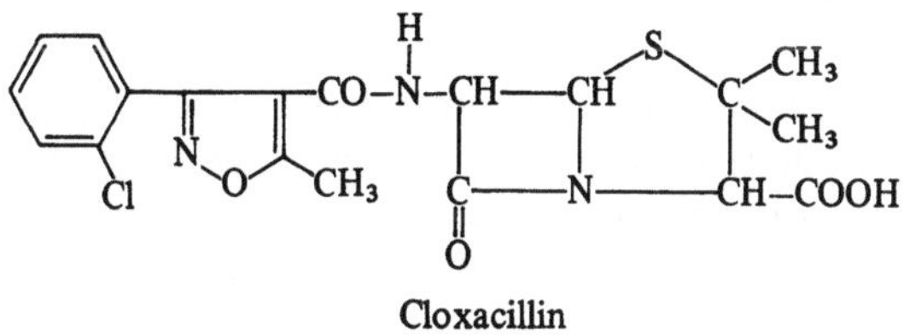

Cloxacillin

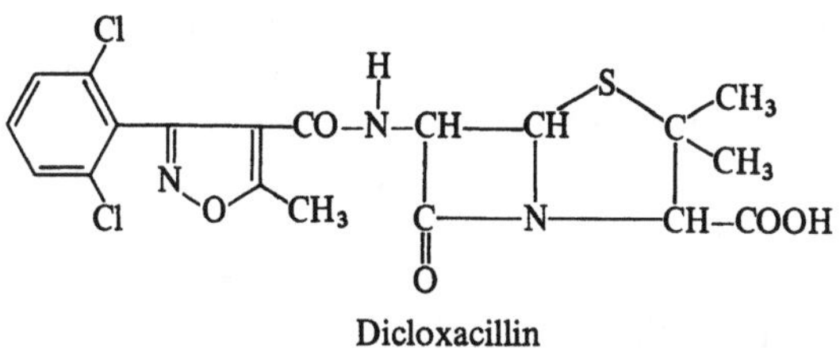

Dicloxacillin

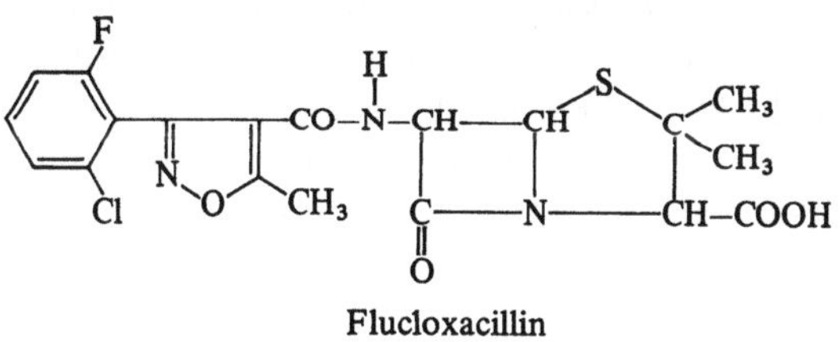

Flucloxacillin

The four congeners are: oxacillin, cloxacillin, dicloxacillin and flucloxacillin. Since they have many similarities and common features, they will be considered together. Their antibacterial spectra are similar, having activity against staphylococci, pneumonococci, streptococci (*S. faecalis* is an exception), other gram-positive bacilli and *Neisseria* spp. Cloxacillin has an interesting and not exploited activity against *Mycobacterium tuberculosis*. Again, the main therapeutic interest of these compounds rests on the fact that they are resistant to the staphylococcal penicillinase and are used successfully for the treatment of infections caused by such staphylococcal strains. They are all rapidly but variably absorbed from the gastrointestinal tract. There are important differences between them in the serum levels obtained, due to differences in absorption, rate of metabolism and elimination. Generally, flucloxacillin is best absorbed, followed by dicloxacillin, cloxacillin and oxacillin. Flucloxacillin appears to have the most favorable pharmacokinetics superseding cloxacillin and dicloxacillin for oral therapy. All four are highly bound to serum protein (about 93%–97%) but apparently this binding is reversible. In contrast to differences in their oral administration, they are, basically, therapeutically equal when administered parenterally. Dicloxacillin is available only for oral administration and is eliminated slowly. The other three are available for oral (capsules 250–500 mg and syrup) as well as parenteral (IM and IV) administration. Oral probenecid (2 g), as in the case with other penicillins, enhances serum levels. All are mainly excreted in the urine. Some biliary elimination is observed, especially with oxacillin and cloxacillin. The dosage of cloxacillin, dicloxacillin and flucloxacillin, but not that of oxacillin should be reduced if the patient has severe renal impairment. Infants and newborns tolerate the isoxazolyl penicillins well.

The antistaphylococcal, penicillinase-stable penicillins are extremely effective drugs. For oral treatment, the isoxazolyl penicillins are the most convenient antistaphylococcal penicillins. For parenteral use, it is difficult to establish a preference since in adequate doses they have the same therapeutic efficacy.

In closing this section, a few general remarks may be pertinent:

1. The antistaphylococcal penicillins should never be used to treat infections caused by bacteria sensitive to penicillin G since the latter is more potent and much cheaper.
2. For severe infections, the parenteral route of treatment is obligatory.
3. It should always be remembered that the methicillin-resistant *S. aureus* are also resistant to the other antistaphyloccal penicillins and to many other antibiotics. Susceptibility tests can guide the choice of an effective antibiotic (vancomycin, rifampicin, lincomycin, gentamicin) or combinations.
4. The combination of isoxazolyl penicillins with ampicillin or cephalosporins to protect the latter from the degradation of the β-lactamases of gram-negative bacteria was not very successful in human therapy. Newer extremely β-lactamase-stable cephalosporins and potent β-lactamase inhibitors like clavulanic acid, olivanic acids, PS-5, the penicillanic acid sulphones such as sulbactam or CP-45, 899 (RETSEMA et al. 1981) and its orally active dimethyloxopropoxymethyl ester, CP-47, 904, seem to be more promising for this kind of combination therapy.

III. The Broad-Spectrum Aminopenicillins

With the advent and availability on a large scale of 6-APA, a series of new penicillins were synthesized with the goal of overcoming the weaknesses of penicillin G. The previous compounds demonstrated the successes of two of these, mainly penicillinase- and acid-stabilities. The third defect of penicillin G is its low-degree and therapeutically insignificant activity against the great majority of gram-negative bacteria with the exception of *N. gonorrhoeae* and *N. meningitidis*. With the synthesis of the aminopenicillins (ampicillin and congeners), this weakness has also been overcome, to a certain extent (NEU 1975; REEVES and BULLOCK 1974). With the discovery of ampicillin, a new era of penicillin therapy was created; the extremely useful group of broad-spectrum penicillins enriched tremendously our armamentarium of antibiotics. These semisynthetic penicillins contain an amino group in the α-position of the side chain (α-aminobenzylpenicillins).

1. Ampicillin

Ampicillin was the first penicillin to which the term "broad-spectrum" was assigned. Amoxicillin and the other close congeners and esters of ampicillin have similar antibacterial spectrum with somewhat altered pharmacokinetics.

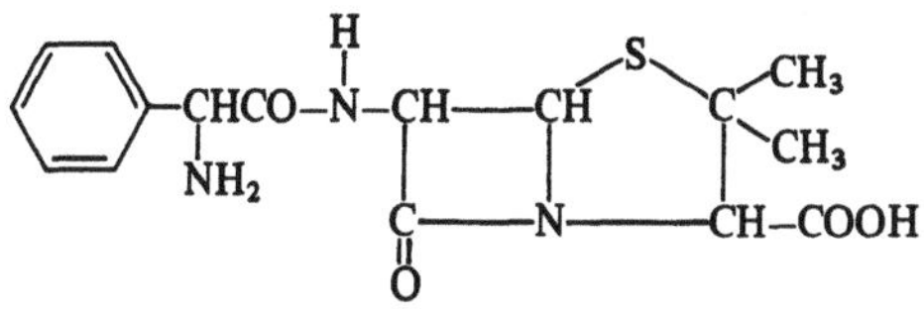

Ampicillin

Ampicillin and its congeners are today the most widely used semisynthetic penicillins for the therapy of infectious diseases. Activity is equal to or somewhat less than that of penicillin G, depending on the genus. *Streptococcus faecalis* and *Listeria monocytogenes* are exceptions, being more sensitive to ampicillin. Its antibacterial spectrum also includes (unlike the penicillins discussed earlier) many gram-negative bacilli, e.g., *E. coli, P. mirabilis, Haemophilus* spp., *Salmonella* and *Shigella* spp. Ampicillin is not stable to penicillinases and therefore, not indicated for use in infections caused by penicillinase-producing microorganisms. However, ampicillin (free acid or sodium salt)is acid-resistant and thus can be given orally. Because of the many favorable properties (penicillinase-sensitivity is a deficit) it has been widely used for the treatment of a great variety of infections which will be discussed in detail below.

Ampicillin and the other aminopenicillins are bactericidal compounds inducing lysis of the bacterial cells. In addition to the above-mentioned genera and species, activity of ampicillin includes: *Bordatella pertussis; Brucella* spp. and *H. influenzae*. Recently, a significant number of β-lactamase-producing ampicillin-resistant type b *H. influenzae* strains have been isolated from children with meningitis as well as from the nasopharynx of some children. Although at the beginning of the ampicillin era (early 1960s) most *E. coli, P. mirabilis, Shigella* and *Salmonella* spp. were ampicillin-sensitive, today many of these strains are resistant, most commonly through plasmid-mediated β-lactamase production. Most strains of *Pseudomonas, Serratia, Klebsiella, Acinetobacter, Enterobacter* and indole-positive *Proteus* as well as many strains of *Shigella* and *Salmonella* and *B. fragilis* are resistant, again because of episome-mediated β-lactamase production. The incidence of resistance is much higher among the hospital-isolated strains.

Ampicillin and amoxicillin have special therapeutic indications, in addition to those covered by the description of penicillin G, reflecting the broader antibacterial spectrum of these aminopenicillins. Their clinical uses include the following:

The bacteria responsible for upper respiratory infections (*H. influenza, S. pneumoniae, S. pyogenes*) are sensitive to ampicillin. These infections (otitis media, sinusitis, chronic bronchitis, bronchiolitis, croup and epiglottitis) can be effectively treated with oral ampicillin or preferably with amoxicillin in children and adults. These antibiotics are useful when administered in bronchiolitis and croup due to viral infection, by preventing the secondary supervening bacterial infections. Bacterial pharyngitis can be treated with penicillin G or V as well.

Uncomplicated acute urinary tract infections are most commonly caused by *E. coli*, *P. mirabilis* or *S. faecalis* and can be successfully treated with ampicillin. The drug is present in very high concentration in the urine, and therefore, the treatment is often successful despite the demonstrated in vitro resistance of the causative organism. Ampicillin can safely be given for the treatment of urinary tract infections during pregnancy and also to patients with renal failure. The treatment with ampicillin or amoxicillin of chronic urinary tract infections with underlying kidney disease is less successful because of relapse or reinfection most often with resistant *Enterobacter* or *Klebsiella* spp.

Of venereal diseases, gonococcal urethritis can be treated very successfully with oral ampicillin or amoxicillin. It should be given for 5–7 days. A single dose of 3.5 g orally together with 1 g of probenecid has been reported to be of use for the therapy of uncomplicated gonorrhoea. The penicillin G resistant *N. gonorrhoeae* strains are also usually resistant to ampicillin. Granuloma inguinale responds well to ampicillin treatment.

Meningitis caused by *H. influenzae* or *S. pneumoniae* in children responds favorably in the acute phase to large doses of ampicillin. Because of the increasing number of β-lactamase-producing *H. influenzae* strains (5%–30% today), the concurrent administration of chloramphenicol is recommended prior to the result of the sensitivity test.

Salmonella infections including typhoid fever respond favorably to ampicillin, but chloramphenicol is still the drug of choice or a combination of these two antibiotics. Ampicillin should be given in high doses. The typhoid carrier state without gallbladder disease and/or gallstones, a long-term problem, can be successfully eliminated by treatment for 1–3 months with large doses of ampicillin together with probenecid (MÜNNICH et al. 1964a, b). The gallstone-bearing carriers are best treated by a combination of surgery and prolonged ampicillin-probenecid administration.

Bacteremia and sepsis caused by gram-negative bacilli (*E. coli*, *P. mirabilis*) can be successfully treated with large parenteral doses of ampicillin. However, it is advisable to start therapy with a combination of ampicillin and gentamicin or another aminoglycoside prior to the result of the sensitivity test.

In cases of bacterial endocarditis, *S. faecalis* endocarditis can be treated very successfully with large parenteral doses of ampicillin alone. However, it is a general consensus that it should be given in combination with streptomycin. Gram-negative endocarditis is rare and the *E. coli* endocarditis should be treated with ampicillin combined with kanamycin.

In biliary tract infections, if the gallbladder and its ducts are intact, ampicillin can reach suitable concentration in the bile to be useful for treatment. In the case of biliary obstruction, the surgical solution has priority. Ampicillin undergoes enterohepatic circulation, consequently it appears in the bile and is excreted in the feces. It should be remembered, however, that in life-threatening infections caused by staphylococcal strains (often penicillinase-producing), parenteral rifampicin is the antibiotic of choice. It reaches therapeutic concentration not only in the lumen but most importantly in the wall of the gallbladder and biliary ducts.

Ampicillin has been useful in treating meningitis caused by *Listeria monocytogenes*. Penicillin G is a good alternative drug. Ampicillin has been also valuable for the treatment of neonatal listerosis.

Ampicillin is available for oral use in capsules as the sodium salt or as the trihydrate containing 125, 250 and 500 mg, or in 125-mg tablets and syrup containing 125 mg in 5 ml. The daily adult oral doses range from 2 to 6 g in divided doses and taken every 6 h. It may also be injected intramuscularly or intravenously, especially for the treatment of severe infections in doses ranging from 6 to 12 g per day. For parenteral use, the vials contain the sodium salt from 125 mg to 10 g. The serum protein binding of ampicillin is low, about 20%. Probenecid increases the concentration and persistance of ampicillin in the serum.

The adverse effects and untoward reactions observed with ampicillin are ususally the same as those caused by other penicillins. The only difference is that the incidence of rash is higher with ampicillin than with other penicillins and especially high (about 70%) in patients with infectious mononucleosis and some forms of leukemia. Sometimes this form of mononucleosis-ampicillin eruption may be a severe phenomenon with prolonged morbidity. Nausea and diarrhea after oral ampicillin are rarely serious enough to indicate discontinuation of therapy. Ampicillin sensitivity to penicillinases has restricted its application, although this can be overcome by administering it concomitantly with a β-lactamase inhibitor, such as clavulanic acid. The results are very good, especially in the urinary and respiratory tract infections.

2. Esters of Ampicillin

Pivampicillin, *Bacampicillin* and *Talampicillin*. These have no intrinsic antimicrobial activity; however, after absorption from the gastrointestinal tract they are rapidly hydrolysed by nonspecific esterases into ampicillin.

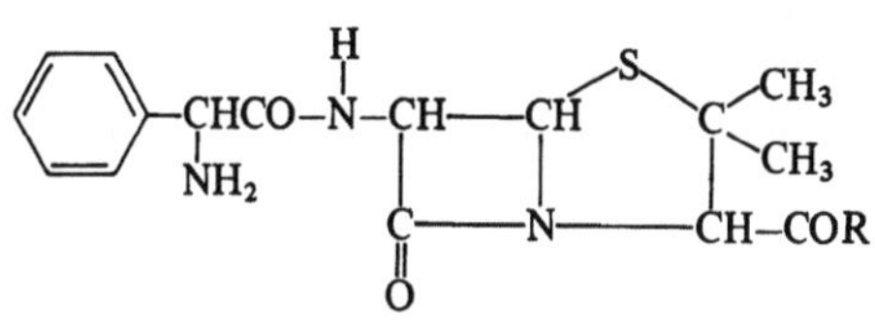

Ampicillin

	R
Bacampicillin	$-O.CH(CH_3).O.COO.C_2H_5$
Pivampicillin	$-O.CH_2.O.CO.C(CH_3)_3$
Talampicillin	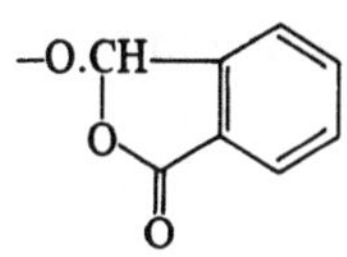

The only possible advantage these esters have over ampicillin is their more complete and faster absorption from the gastointestinal tract.

Talampicillin is claimed to be twice as well absorbed as is ampicillin and produces twice or three times the serum levels. In this respect it is similar to amoxicillin. In addition, it seems to cause less diarrhea than ampicillin. Pivampicillin, in contrast, causes more frequent gastrointestinal disturbances; it produces higher serum levels and urinary concentrations. Bacampicillin is similar to the other two esters.

3. Amoxicillin

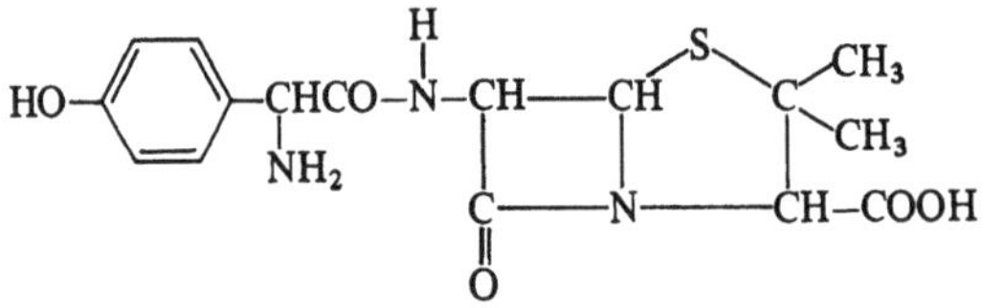

Amoxicillin

Amoxicillin, although closely related to ampicillin, is about twice as active against *S. faecalis* and *Salmonella* spp. and half as active against *Shigella* spp. *H. influenzae* appears to be slightly less sensitive to it. Amoxicillin is not converted into ampicillin in the body and it has its own intrinsic activity. It is more rapidly bactericidal and probably binds to different receptor proteins of gram-negative bacilli. Its only advantage over ampicillin is that it is more rapidly and efficiently absorbed after oral administration. Food does not diminish the absorption and the peak serum levels are about twice those achieved with an equivalent dose of oral ampicillin. In equivalent dose, oral amoxicillin produces serum levels similar to those obtained after intramuscular sodium ampicillin or ampicillin trihydrate. Its urinary excretion is also greater than that of ampicillin. Amoxicillin has a low serum binding (about 20%), similar to ampicillin. Amoxicillin has largely replaced oral ampicillin in the treatment of chronic bronchial infections (because of better absorption associated with better penetration into the bronchial secretions), urinary tract infections, typhoid and otitis media. Uncomplicated gonorrhoea responds satisfactorily to a "single dose" of 3 g oral amoxicillin without probenecid, which, however, may delay its excretion. It should never be used for the treatment of shigellosis.

Untoward reactions to amoxicillin are basically the same as to ampicillin, although rashes may be less common and diarrhea seems to be also less common, probably because of the more complete oral absorption.

Amoxicillin trihydrate is available in capsules (oral dose should be half that of ampicillin) of 250 and 500 mg, in oral suspension (125 and 250 mg/5 ml), and as pediatric drops (50 mg/ml). The recommended usual adult dose is 250 mg (or in serious infections 500 mg) three times a day (instead of four times for ampicillin). The usual dose for children is 20–40 mg/kg per day every 8 h. Recently, it became available for intramuscular and intravenous use (BRODGEN et al. 1979a).

For oral administration amoxicillin is becoming the preferred broad-spectrum aminopenicillin, not only in children but also in adults. Naturally, cost factors should not be neglected.

Like ampicillin, amoxicillin is liable to inactivation by β-lactamases and intensive effort has been made to eliminate this deficit. Combined administration with the β-lactamase inhibitor, clavulanic acid, appears to solve this important clinical problem. Augmentin, a fixed oral formulation containing amoxicillin and clavulanic acid in 2:1 ratio was reported to be successful in the treatment of urinary tract infections due to β-lactamase-producing pathogenic bacteria (COSMIDIS et al. 1980; LEIGH and BRADNOCK 1980; GOLDSTEIN et al. 1980). It is now available for general use (BROGDEN et al. 1981).

4. Epicillin and Cyclacillin

Epicillin and cyclacillin are newer members of the aminopenicillin group. They are in almost all respects similar to ampicillin. They do not seem to offer any practical advantage over ampicillin, and especially not over amoxicillin.

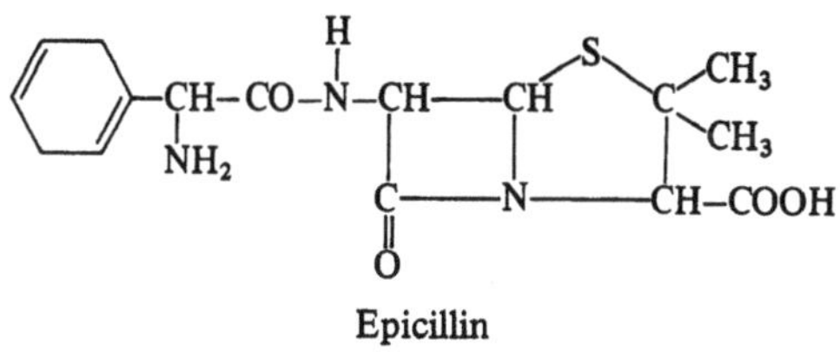

Epicillin

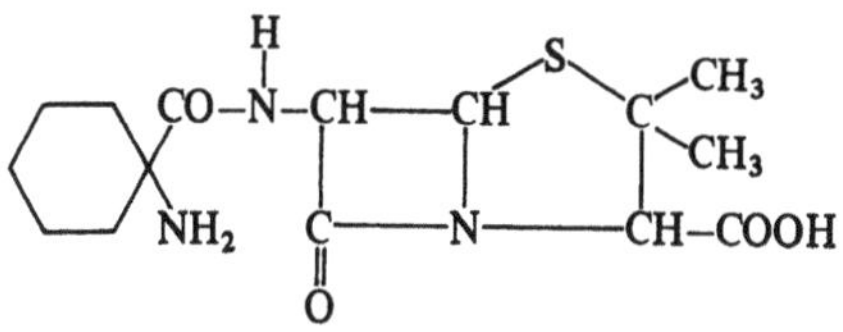

Cyclacillin

Epicillin can be given orally, intramuscularly or intravenously.

Cyclacillin is similar to but somewhat weaker than ampicillin in its antibacterial activity. Its chemical structure differs from the other aminopenicillins. It is more rapidly absorbed but also more rapidly excreted than ampicillin. Probenecid delays its excretion. It appears to be somewhat more stable to β-lactamase hydrolysis, and gives higher serum levels and greater urinary excretion after oral administration than ampicillin (WARREN 1976). Clinical trials in a variety of infections demonstrated its efficacy and safety although in the treatment of gonorrhoea and otitis media it is not as effective as ampicillin.

IV. The Antipseudomonal Penicillins

A group of semisynthetic penicillins, of which carbenicillin is the prototype, has the unique property of being active and clinically useful against *P. aeruginosa* and other gram-negative bacilli which are not usually sensitive to the broad spectrum aminopenicillins. Although they bear the name of antipseudomonal penicillins, in reality, they should be considered in a somewhat broader sense. Their main advantage is, undoubtedly, their practical usefulness in the various forms of pseudomonal infections. These compounds have many features in common. The newer antipseudomonal penicillins often referred to as the "acylureido" penicillins, have a more "extended" antibacterial spectrum than the carbenicillin-type compounds. The designation "acylureido" penicillins is correct chemically, in a broad sense, but they can also be considered as α-amino-substituted ampicillins. In addition, all these penicillins have many features in common with ampicillin although they are discussed separately because of their clinical usage. Their antibacterial spectra often cover more than just the pseudomonads. They can include indole-positive *Proteus* spp. and sometimes other gram-negative genera. In this respect, the individual compounds differ; some have broader spectrum including *Klebsiella* spp., *Enterobacter* spp., *Serratia* spp., *B. fragilis*, *E. coli*, *P. mirabilis* etc., while others have a more restricted spectrum. Their gram-positive activity is, as a rule, much weaker than that of the other penicillins and they can be sensitive to many β-lactamases. This liability should be kept in mind when therapy is considered with these penicillins.

The pharmacokinetics and human pharmacology of these penicillins are similar, with slight variations. They are basically safe compounds and are sometimes given in large doses. Consequently, dose-related reversible toxic signs or adverse reactions can be observed but overall, they are extremely useful and often life-saving antibiotics. Probenecid, as expected, augments their serum levels and delays their elimination from the circulation and from the body. For greater therapeutic benefit, they can be successfully administered in combination (but not in the same syringe or solution) with various aminoglycosides.

1. Carbenicillin

Carbenicillin, containing a carboxyl-group at the α-position of the side-chain was the first penicillin (β-lactam in general) used for the successful treatment of infections due to *P. aeruginosa*. Its primary use today is still in the therapy of serious *Pseudomonas* infections such as severe burns, sepsis, meningitis, osteomyelitis, urinary tract and pulmonary infections, especially in compromised and debilitated patients. In very serious infections, the concomitant administration of a potentially toxic aminoglycoside antibiotic is necessary for cure. For many years, carbenicillin was the only "safe" antibiotic with demonstrated satisfactory clinical efficacy in severe pseudomonal infections. In addition, for other severe infections caused by species of indole-positive *Proteus* or *Acetinobacter*, carbenicillin was the "safe" alternative alone or in combination to obtain reasonable clinical improvement or complete cure. Other gram-negative bacteria, e.g., *E. coli*, *P. mirabilis*, *Salmonella* and *Shigella* spp., *H. influenzae*, *N. gonorrhoeae* and *N. meningitidis* are almost as sensitive to carbenicillin as to ampicillin. *Klebsiella* spp., *S. marcescens* and *B. fragilis* are, unlike most clostridia, usually insensitive to carbenicillin. *Enterobacter* strains are variably inhibited. Against the gram-positive bacteria, penicillin G and ampicillin are much more effective. Carbenicillin is sensitive to β-lactamases and its binding to serum protein is about 50%.

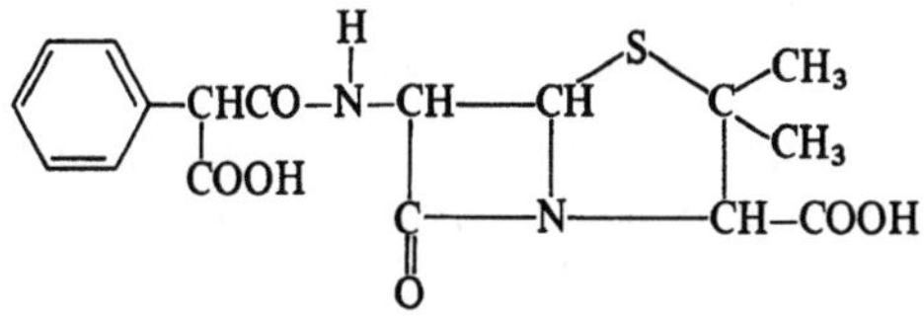

Carbenicillin

As mentioned above, its chief therapeutic indication is in the various forms of pseudomonas infections including children with respiratory infections associated with cystic fibrosis and chronic lung disease. Ampicillin-insensitive strains often react to carbenicillin and so do many other gram-negative bacteria. It is recommended that, for emergency treatment of neonatal infections before sensitivity data are available, carbenicillin should be used with an aminoglycoside instead of penicillin G or ampicillin.

Carbenicillin is not absorbed from the gastrointestinal tract and must be given either intramuscularly or intravenously, often in large doses. After the intramuscular injection of 1 g, the peak serum levels are about 20 μg/ml which is not adequate for the treatment of generalized infections (only for urinary tract infections). For this purpose, 100–150 μg/ml levels are needed and must be maintained longer. The intravenous infusion of 4–5 g over a 2-h period at 4-h intervals is required to achieve the serum levels necessary for treatment of serious infections. The daily intravenous dose may be 30–40 g of the disodium salt in life-threatening infections. In such cases, the pediatric doses should be 600–800 mg/kg.

Because very large quantities of carbenicillin are needed for therapy, the sodium overload may present a serious problem, not only for carbenicillin, but also, in general, with disodium salts of other β-lactams which have to be injected intravenously in large doses. In the case of carbenicillin, each gram disodium salt contains 4–7 mmol sodium which, on a daily basis, is 150 mmol sodium, equivalent of a 9 g sodium chloride diet. In patients with diminished cardiovascular reserve this sodium load may precipitate pulmonary edema and congestive heart failure. In addition, carbenicillin causes hypokalemia due to the load of nonresorbable anion in the distal tubule. For electrical neutrality, the kidney must excrete the carbenicillin anion in concert with cations (K^+, Na^+ and H^+). In the case of sodium retention (volume depletion, stress) K^+ or H^+ will be secreted in the distal tubule, leading to hypokalemic metabolic alkalosis with its seriuos consequences (ANDERSON et al. 1975).

High doses in patients with renal failure may cause bleeding disorders based on platelet dysfunction and/or inhibition of conversion of fibrinogen to fibrin (anticoagulant effect).

Carbenicillin is excreted by renal tubular secretion with a half-life of about 75 min. Probenecid increases the blood levels by about 50% and also delays excretion. Hepatic and renal dysfunctions require the appropriate adjustment of dose.

Carbenicillin is available as the disodium salt for parenteral injection in sterile vials containing 1, 2, 5, and 10 g. For systemic *Pseudomonas* infections, the usual intravenous dose is 400–600 mg/kg/day injected over 1–2 h, 6 times a day.

The indanyl (carindacillin) and phenyl (carfecillin) esters of carbenicillin are available for oral administration. Like the ampicillin esters, they do not have activity on their own but are hydrolyzed to free carbenicillin by nonspecific esterases after rapid absorption from the small intestine. The oral carbenicillins do not produce adequate serum levels for the treatment of systemic *Pseudomonas* infections. They should be used only for the treatment of urinary tract infections due to *P.*

aeruginosa. They may cause gastrointestinal irritation. The phenylester appears to be better tolerated because its taste is less bitter.

With the advent and increasing clinical use of the oral ampicillin and carbenicillin esters, the question emerged as to whether or not they exert hepatotoxic effects (cholestatic hepatitis) that were observed with erythromycin estolate, an ester of erythromycin. In contrast to results obtained from animal (dog) studies, in human beings there has been no reported incidence of functional or anatomic changes in the liver after short courses of these esters. However, it seems prudent to monitor liver functions in patients who receive prolonged oral treatment (BINT 1980).

Carbenicillin has been discussed in greater detail because of its historical background, its utility and also because all the newer anitpseudomonal β-lactams are compared with its efficacy.

2. Ticarcillin

Ticarcillin is very similar to carbenicillin, chemically, microbiologically, pharmacologically and in its therapeutic use.

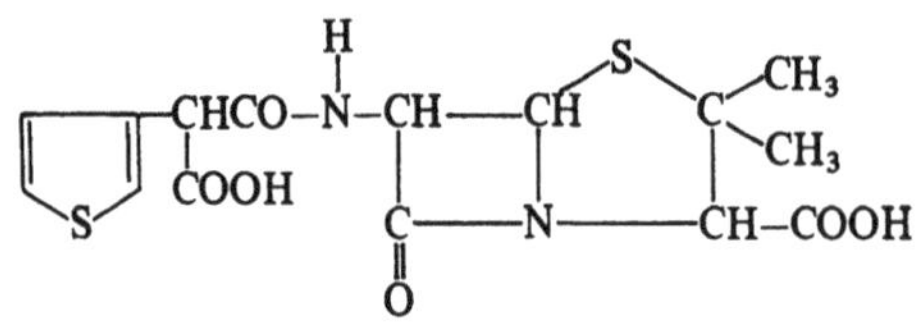

Ticarcillin

It has some potential advantages over carbenicillin. It is approximately twice as active against *P. aeruginosa* strains, therefore it can be used in lower doses, 200–300 mg/kg/day (12–24 g/day) versus 400–600 mg/kg per day (35–40 g/day) for carbenicillin. The reduced dosage of ticarcillin with the same clinical efficacy delivers lower sodium load, which may be beneficial in treating patients with borderline congestive cardiac failure. A slight advantage of ticarcillin may be that in equal doses it produces somewhat higher, more prolonged serum levels (WISE and REEVES 1974). Platelet dysfunctions are also recorded less frequently, probably as a consequence of reduced dose. It is available in vials of 1, 3, and 6 g for parenteral injection. Ticarcillin cresyl sodium showed no demonstrable clinical improvement. Its 6α-methoxy derivative (temocillin; BRL-17421) is the first β-lactamase stable penicillin with only gram-negative activity and with high and prolonged serum levels in man (SLOCOMBE et al. 1981), with a serum half-life of about 5 h after parenteral administration. Oral absorption is negligible, 85% is recovered in the urine in active form. The volunteers tolerated it well at I.M. or I.V. administration with no adverse side effects.

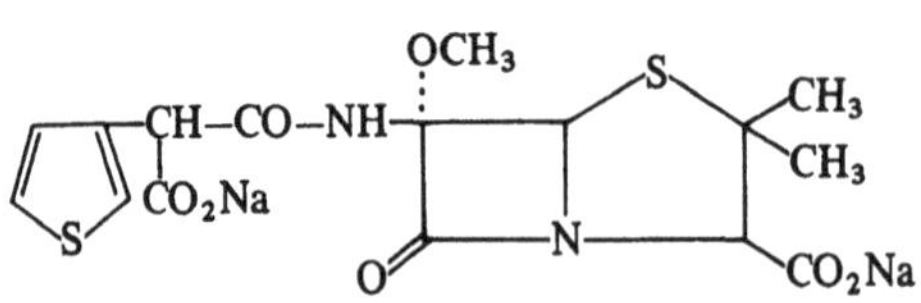

Temocillin

The Acylureido Antipseudomonal Penicillins. Several compounds have been synthesized and studied over the past 8–10 years by substituting the α-acyl amino group of ampicillin with moieties to obtain the ureido structure. The goal was to obtain antipseudomonal penicillins more potent than carbenicillin or ticarcillin. Many of the earlier compounds never reached the developmental stage. Although they were interesting and very potent antispeudomonal agents, they were abandoned because of their nephrotoxic side effects in experimental animals. However, three, namely azlocillin, mezlocillin, and piperacillin are very promising. Mezlocillin and piperacillin (but not azlocillin) possess extended antibacterial spectra in addition to their activity against *P. aeruginosa.* Usually they are more potent than carbenicillin. In contrast to carbenicillin, they do not produce the sodium overload with the electrolyte disorders and they are less liable to cause bleeding tendency. Overall, their favorable antimicrobial activity is accompanied by satisfactory pharmacologic and toxicologic picture. In addition, they require smaller doses and they could be useful antipseudomonal agents. Their clinical evaluation is being intensively pursued or completed in some countries and their potential usefulness will depend on further observation (SPITZY 1978; BINT and REEVES 1978; SCHACHT 1978; HUMBERT et al. 1979; ELLIS et al. 1979; FU and NEU 1978).

a) Azlocillin

Azlocillin's activity is similar to that of carbenicillin but it is 8–16 times more active against *P. aeruginosa* including the carbenicillin- and gentamicin-resistant strains, and this is its main advantage, although it has variable in vitro activity against the non-β-lactamase-producing cocci, *E. coli*, *Klebsiella*, *Enterobacter*, *Serratia*, *Proteus* and *Haemophilus* strains. Two grams of azlocillin is usually injected intravenously as a 10% solution in pyrogen-free, sterile water every 8 h for 5–10 days in severe infections. Good results were reported even in severe pseudomonal infections of the respiratory and urinary tract and other infections (KÖNIG et al. 1977; ALTHAN et al. 1979; MICHALSEN and BERGAN 1980; BAISCH et al. 1979; SCHACHT et al. 1979). It is sensitive to β-lactamases.

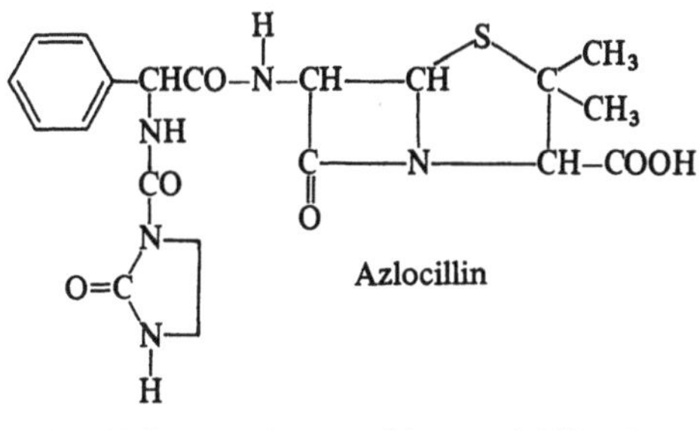

Azlocillin

Furazlocillin (Bay K 4999), another ureido penicillin, has similar antibacterial activity to other members of the group (VERBIST 1979) and, like piperacillin, binds specifically to penicillin-binding protein (PBP) 3 (BOTTA and PARK 1981).

b) Mezlocillin

Mezlocillin is under extensive clinical trial. It has a broader antibacterial spectrum (*S. faecalis*, group B of *S. agalactiae*, *Klebsiella* spp., *H. influenzae*, *N. gonorrhoeae*,

Proteus spp., other Enterobacteriacea as well as *B. fragilis*) than carbenicillin or ticarcillin, but it is less active against *P. aeruginosa*. Mezlocillin is unstable to β-lactamases although somewhat more stable than carbenicillin. It must be given parenterally, preferably intravenously. Its broader in vitro spectrum over that of ampicillin, carbenicillin and ticarcillin was confirmed in the therapy of serious infections (PANCOAST et al. 1979). Intramuscular injection of mezlocillin (1 g) was found to be less painful than that of 1 g ampicillin (BELLI et al. 1979). After intravenous injection of 2 g mezlocillin an average concentration of 20 μg/g was measured in the bone (VENT 1979).

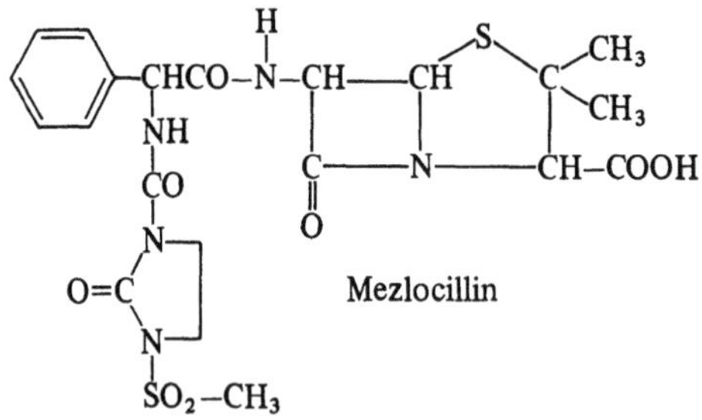

Mezlocillin

During intensive clinical trials, mezlocillin was found to be well-tolerated both systematically and locally. Therapeutically it was safe and efficacious in most aerobic, anaerobic and mixed infections. Mezlocillin was found in some pseudomonas infections more effective than carbenicillin, ticarcillin and piperacillin (THADEPALLI and RAO 1979; TETTENBORN et al. 1979). It showed high efficacy in several infections such as septicemia, endocarditis and purulent meningitis (FUJII 1979). The usual dose for the treatment of uncomplicated urinary and respiratory tract infections is 2 g every 6 h or 2 g every 8 h in 10% solution as a bolus injection but the dose can be raised up to 20 g per day (POPA et al. 1979; DE ALMEIDA et al. 1979). In another trial the predominant doses were between 6 and 15 g daily. It was administered as a slow intravenous injection (15–20 min) or short-term infusion three times daily. The reconstitution fluid is usually 5% dextrose. A single intravenous injection of 2 g mezlocillin produces a 95%–97% cure rate in the treatment of urogenital and pharyngeal gonorrhoea (FOWLER and KHAN 1979; LASSUS and RENKONEN 1979). Mezlocillin was found to be safe and highly effective in children treated for meningitis and pneumonia. The regular dose was 250 mg/kg per day divided into 3 portions and given intravenously. The duration of treatment varied between 5 and 7 days. Besides rash, no other side effects were reported (WEIPPL 1979; LLORRENS-TEROL et al. 1979).

c) Piperacillin

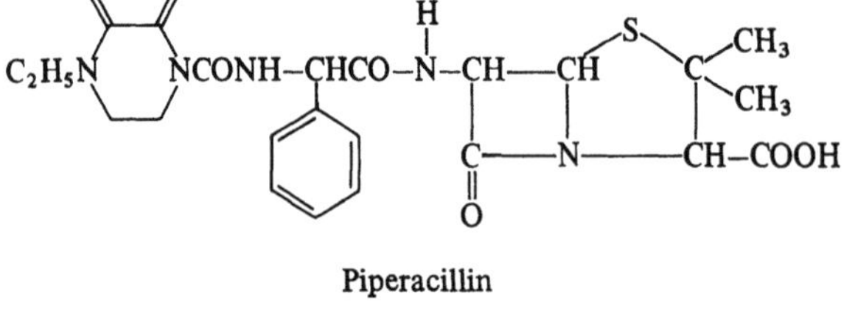

Piperacillin

Piperacillin has the best antipseudomonal activity of the three ureido penicillins. Only some newer members of the third generation cephalosporins, e.g., ceftazidime, have greater activity. Its activity against gram-positive bacteria is comparable to that of ampicillin and against gram-negative species to carbenicillin. Thus it has an unusually wide spectrum of activity. Piperacillin is the most potent penicillin against *B. fragilis* although it is hydrolyzed by β-lactamases both of gram-positive and gram-negative origin. It can be injected intramuscularly or intravenously up to 16 g per day, without toxic signs. Only about 20% is bound to serum proteins. Piperacillin is eliminated mainly by the kidney and partly with the bile during the first 6 h after injection (TJANDRAMAGA et al. 1978). Significant amounts are excreted via the biliary system (GIRON et al. 1981a; BAIER et al. 1981b; THOMPSON et al. 1981). The dose range varies according to the seriousness of disease. For the treatment of noncomplicated urinary tract infections, 1 g was used intramuscularly and dissolved immediately before use in 4 ml sterile water with 0.5% lidocaine. Dosage range was either 1 g every 6 h or 2 g every 12 h. Duration of treatment was 7 days. The results were satisfactory (SANDER et al. 1980). In another trial, it was used as a slow intravenous bolus injection (5 min in a dose of 2 g every 8 h for 4–29 days) with good success in various severe infections (LINGLOF et al. 1980) caused by *E. coli*, *Pseudomonas*, *Klebsiella*, *Enterobacter*, *Proteus*, *B. fragilis* or *Enterococcus*. Other dosage regimens included 3 g piperacillin every 4 h for a total daily amount of 18 g (SPICEHANDLER et al. 1980) or 100–500 mg/kg per day intravenously and 60–90 mg/kg per day intramuscularly. The higher doses (300–500 mg/kg per day) were used to treat serious pulmonary infections with cystic fibrosis and the lower doses for urinary tract infections (PRINCE et al. 1980). Others used 2 g intramuscularly every 12 h for 6–8 days for the treatment of urinary tract infections (SCHOUTENS et al. 1979). The therapeutic results with piperacillin to date show that it is a safe, potent, and promising new penicillin in the treatment of serious infections. It is particularly useful against *P. aeruginosa* including resistant strains.

V. The Amidinopenicillanic Acids – Amdinocillin

This is a new class of β-lactam antibiotics. At present amdinocillin (formerly mecillinam; BARRIERE et al. 1982) and its pivaloyloxymethyl ester (*pivmecillinam*) as well as ethoxycarbonyloxyethyl ester (*bacmecillinam*) belong to this class.

Amdinocillin is not a true penicillin, since by definition penicillins are *N*-acyl derivatives of 6-APA. Amdinocillin is a semisynthetic 6-amidino-penicillanic acid. Since it contains the β-lactam-thiazolidine fused structure, it can be considered as a close relative of the penicillins (ROLINSON 1979). This change in the chemical structure is associated with a marked alteration in its antibacterial spectrum and thus its clinical application.

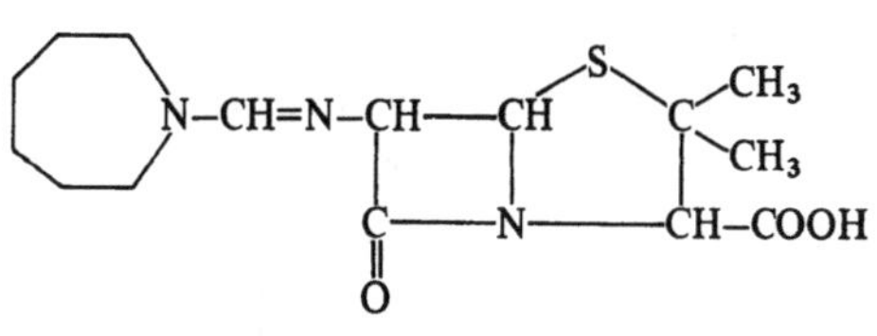

Amdinocillin

Amdinocillin is considerably more active against most gram-negative bacilli than against the gram-positive cocci. The reverse is true for the classic penicillins and cephalosporins. This same phenomenon is observed with some of the third-generation cephalosporins.

Amdinocillin is highly effective against such gram-negative bacilli as *E. coli* (including some β-lactamase-producing ampicillin resistant strains), *Klebsiella*, *Enterobacter*, *Citrobacter*, *Salmonella* and *Shigella* spp. Other gram-negative species, like *Haemophilus*,, *Neisseria*, *Serratia*, certain *Proteus* spp., *P. aeruginosa* and *B. fragilis* are insensitive to it. It has the disadvantage of being hydrolyzed by most β-lactamases. Amdinocillin is acid labile and is not absorbed when given orally. However, its esters, pivmecillinam, and bacmecillinam are well absorbed and quickly hydrolyzed giving rise to free amdinocillin in the serum and body. Amdinocillin is excreted in the urine, thus probenecid administration leads to higher serum levels. Biliary excretion also occurs. Amdinocillin sodium or free acid hydrochloride is injected intramuscularly or intravenously in doses of 200 or 400 mg, and the esters given orally in 400 mg (or as high as 1.2 g) doses every 6 or 8 h for many days. The esters can be combined with those of ampicillin which are similarly pro-drugs. Amdinocillin acts synergistically with ampicillin and other penicillins in the treatment of systemic infections because of the different modes of action by binding to different penicillin-binding proteins (LERVESTEDT et al. 1980; SPRATT 1977; PANCOAST et al. 1980). Amdinocillin appears to be promising in the management of urinary tract infections, including bacteriuria in pregnancy, enteric fever, respiratory and other infections caused by sensitive gram-negative organisms (GEDDES and CLARKE 1977; BINT and REEVES 1978; JONSSON and TUNEVALL 1975; ERNST and LORIAN 1980; NAJJAR et al. 1980). High concentrations are found in the urine and serum concentrations are adequate after injecting 10 mg/kg every 4 h (GAMBERTOGLIO 1980). According to ANDERSON (1977) resistance to amdinocillin can develop especially during the prolonged use needed in the management of *Salmonella* infections and the treatment of biliary typhoid carriers (TANPHAICHITRA et al. 1981).

VI. The Atypical β-Lactams

Recently several β-lactam structures have been isolated as fermentation products which have even less resemblance to the true penicillins than does mecillinam (amdinocillin).

All the penicillins which were discussed earlier, including amdinocillin, contain the 6-APA nucleus, acylated at the 6-*N* position (the "penam" β-lactam antibiotics). The new classes of β-lactams differ radically from the classic penams. Some of these have interesting and important new biological characteristics which may be exploited for useful therapeutic purposes.

1. The Monocyclic β-Lactams

Nocardicin A. The chemical structure of nocardicin A is shown here.

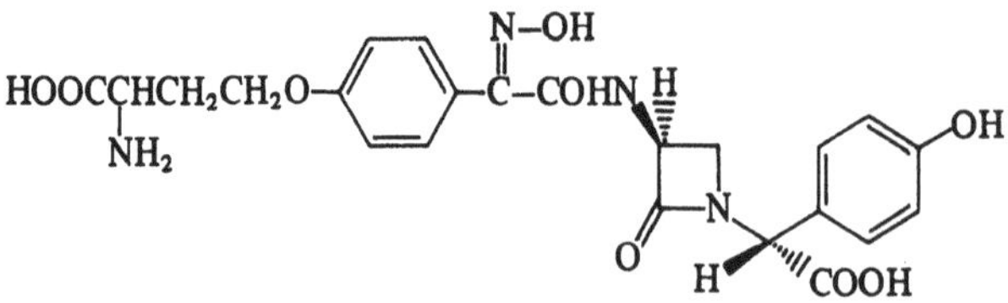

Nocardicin A

It is unique, because the phenylacylamino moiety contains at the α-position a hydroxyimino group (amino in ampicillin and carboxyl in carbenicillin). This natural product served as a prototype for the synthesis of alkoxyimino-substituted cephalosporins with great stability to β-lactamases. It has much better protective efficacy in experimental mouse infections than would be expected from the in vitro results. Time will tell its value (MINE et al. 1977).

The study of the mode of action of the monocyclic β-lactams including those of bacterial origin (LEISINGER and MARGRAFF 1979) and especially that of sulfazecin (IMADA et al. 1981 and those isolated by SYKES et al. 1981) led to the production of the novel nucleus, 3-aminomonobactamic acid (3-AMA) and made possible the preparation of a series of semisynthetic derivaties. Among them azthreonam (SQ 26,776) is a promising therapeutic agent (SYKES et al. 1982). It is produced by total synthesis and is highly stable to many β-lactamases and is specifically active against aerobic gram-negative bacteria, but has little activity against gram-positive cocci. Its mouse-protecting efficacy is comparable to that of cefotaxime and ceftadizime. In healthy volunteers it was infused in doses of 500, 1,000, and 2,000 mg with corresponding serum levels of 58, 125, and 242 μg/ml after 5 min. Serum half-life was found to be 1.66 h. Average urinary excretion was 68% of the administered dose. It was well tolerated with only mild rash in one patient. It may prove to be an effective new β-lactam in the treatment of infections caused by gram-negative bacteria (SWABB et al. 1981). This discovery supports the assumption that the β-lactam ring (azetidinone) is a universal pharmacophoric group.

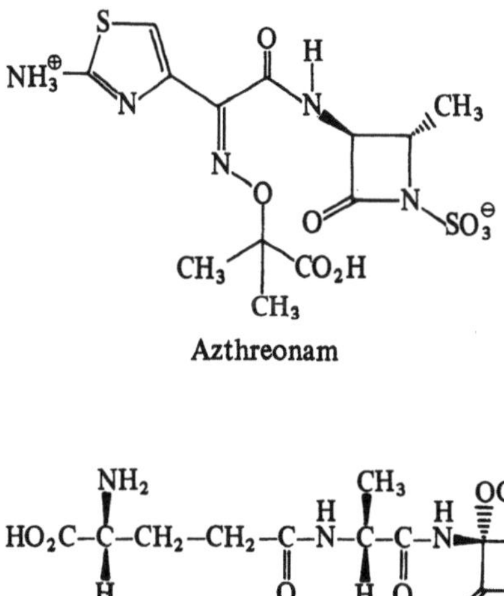

Azthreonam

Sulfazecin

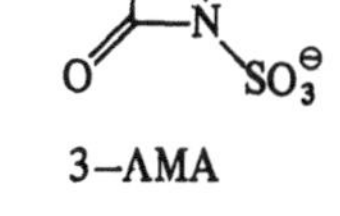

3–AMA

2. The Oxapenams

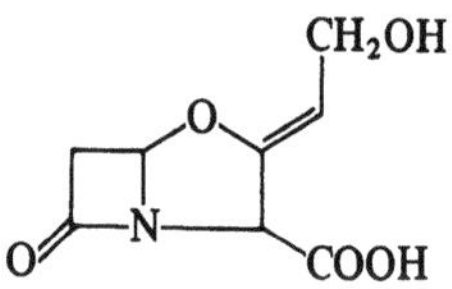

Clavulanic acid

Clavulanic Acid. Clavulanic acid, a natural product, has very weak antibacterial activity on its own; however, it functions as a potent irreversible (progressive) inhibitor of many β-lactamases (chromosomal and plasmid-mediated) produced by penicillin- and cephalosporin-resistant microbes (ROLINSON 1979). Clavulanic acid can be successfully combined with β-lactamase-sensitive penicillins such as ampicillin and amoxicillin. A combination preparation called augmentin proved to be useful in human therapy, as previously discussed in the section on amoxicillin (O'GRADY 1982). It is obvious that β-lactamase-insensitive potent β-lactams will have better therapeutic application than combination therapy (RICHMOND 1978).

3. The Carbapenems

Thienamycins. Thienamycin was the first of a series of atypical β-lactams whose structures are designated as "carbapenem" antibiotics. Other members of this family of naturally occurring β-lactams are the epithienamycins, olivanic acids, PS-5, and the carpetimycins. These compounds contain the fused β-lactam system in which the sulfur atom of the 5-membered ring is substituted by a carbon. They are also inhibitors of β-lactamases to some degree. Thienamycin, or rather its semisynthetic stable variant, formimidoylthienamycin (imipemide), is at present the most important in this series.

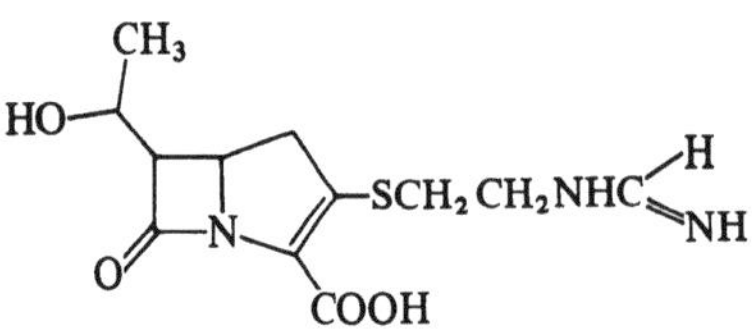

N–Formimidoylthienamycin
MK 0787

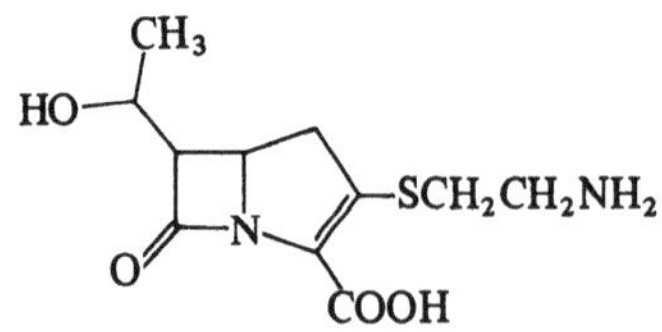

Thienamycin

They have a very wide spectrum of activity and excellent β-lactamase stability. Thienamycin and formimidoylthienamycin appear to be the most active of all the β-lactams known today. Only the more stable and somewhat more active formimidoyl derivative of thienamycin will be discussed here. Its antibacterial spectrum covers a great variety of gram-positive, gram-negative and anaerobic bacteria. The bactericidal activity appears to be the same as the bacteriostatic one. The β-lactamase resistance embraces enzymes of gram-positive and gram-negative origin, both chromosomal and plasmid-mediated.

The gram-positive cocci, *S. aureus* and *S. dermatitidis* as well as strepotococci are extremely sensitive to it. Thus, it resembles the classic natural penicillins with respect to gram-positive activity (KESADO et al. 1980; KROPP et al. 1980). It also has an expanded gram-negative antibacterial spectrum including almost all the *Enterobacteriaceae* and gram-negative cocci.

The anaerobic activity of formimidoylthienamycin is significant. *B. fragilis* and *C. difficile* are inhibited by 0.25–4 μg/ml concentrations. It also has activity against *H. influenzae* with MICs of 0.125–4 μg/ml. The only species intrinsically insensitive to MK 0787 is *P. maltophilia*, a strain nonsusceptible to many other antibiotics.

Formimidoylthienamycin appears to be the best and a very promising β-lactam antibiotic. It is currently under therapeutic evaluation in humans. It appears to be equi-nephrotoxic in rabbits (no human data) to cephaloridine. Another problem that has emerged is that it is extensively metabolized in the kidney, resulting in only 5%–30% recovery in the urine. Dipeptidases, especially dehydropeptidase I, localized in the basement membrane of the proximal tubules are responsible for this degradation. This fact may make its extensive application inadvisable, especially in the treatment of urinary tract infections. However, coadministration of potent dehydropeptidase inhibitors, rather than frequent dosages, may overcome this problem. These enzyme inhibitors were also reported to eliminate the nephrotoxic signs (KROPP et al. 1980b).

The evaluation of olivanic acids is at a very early stage (BASKER et al. 1980).

4. The Penems

The penems are synthetic penicillin analogs with a double bond in the thiazolidine ring and no substituent attatched to carbon 6 (BROWN 1981). They are more stable compounds than thienamycin, but are somewhat less resistant to β-lactamases and have a marginally narrower antibacterial spectrum. Before the description of the monobactams they were the simplest β-lactams with appreciable activity. The first members of this group had the disadvantage that they were eliminated from the animal body too fast. However, two promising derivatives (FCE 21420 and the orally active SCH 29482) have recently been reported (personal communication, 1982).

The number of new therapeutically useful penicillins has expanded tremendously since the introduction of penicillin G. FLOREY's prophecy, made in 1944, that "some day chemists will manipulate the penicillin molecule to improve its performance" has truly been fulfilled. This prediction is also true for the cephalosporin molecule.

C. Cephalosporins in the Therapy of Human Infections

The cephalosporins (cephems and oxacephems) have many features in common with the penicillins. Their close relationships include their chemistry, microbiology, pharmacology, mode of action, toxicology, as well as therapeutic and prophylactic uses. There is no naturally obtained cephalosporin used in therapy; cephalosporin C has weak activity but serves as a source of 7-aminocephalosporanic acid (7-ACA), a starting material for many of the semisynthetic cephalosporins. The nucleus, 7-ACA, provides more possibilities for chemical modifications than does 6-APA. The cephamycins contain a methoxy-group at the 7-position of the 7-ACA nucleus. The cephalosporins and the cephamycins form the large group of compounds collectively called the "cephems". As is the case of the penicillin molecule, selected chemical changes can be made in the nucleus. Replacing the sulfur with

Table 3. Clinically useful cephalosporins

Parenteral β-lactamase-susceptible – first-generation compounds
Cephalothin
Cephapirin
Cephacetrile
Cephaloridine
Cefazolin
Cephradine
Parenteral β-lactamase-resistant – second-generation compounds
Cefamandole
Cefoxitin[a]
Cefmetazole[a]
Cefuroxime
Ceforanide
Cefonicid
Parenteral β-lactamase-resistant antipseudomonal – third-generation compounds
Cefotaxime
Ceftizoxime
Moxalactam[b]
Cefoperazone
Ceftriaxon
Cefmenoxime
Ceftazidime
Cefotiam
Cefsulodin
Cefodizime (HR 221)
42480 RP
Oral β-lactamase-susceptible – first-generation compounds
Cephalexin
Cephradine
Cefatrizine
Cefaclor
Cefroxadine
Cefadroxil
Cephaloglycin

[a] Cephamycin
[b] Oxacephamycin

an oxygen atom in the nucleus results in a class of compounds, the "oxacephems", of which one, moxalactam has been approved for clinical use.

There are many semisynthetic derivatives. They have been classified on the basis of expansion of the antimicrobial spectrum (O'CALLAGHAN 1975, 1979). Other classifications based on therapeutic criteria have been described (WILLIAMS 1978; WINSTON and YOUNG 1980).

Although cephalosporins have been grouped into first, second and third generation products on the basis of their spectrum and β-lactamase stability, for certain compounds, this categorization is not clear-cut.

The compounds listed in Table 3 are covered by extensive clinical literature. As with the penicillins, all of the published papers will not be cited but rather a general description and discussion of the individual cephalosporins based on the data contained in selected articles, reviews and monographs will be used.

The review papers and monographs utilized in this section are the following: URI (1963, 1964b); O'CALLAGHAN (1975, 1979); PLEMPEL and OTTEN (1969); GRIFFITH (1974); OWENS et al. (1975); REGAMEY (1975); WEINSTEIN (1976); HÖFFLER and PALMER (1976); MOELLERING and SWARTZ (1976); SMITH (1977); BARZA and MIAO (1977); NORRBY (1978); FOSSATI (1978); BALL et al. (1978); WISE (1978); MANDELL (1979); WINSTON and YOUNG (1980); LODE et al. (1978); MANDELL and SANDE (1980); SELWYN (1980); WEINSTEIN (1980).

The cephalosporins are extremely effective therapeutic and prophylactic broad-spectrum antibiotics. They are relatively free from serious toxic side effects, although some may have nephrotoxic potential in man. Dose-related renal tubular necrosis caused by cephaloridine is well documented. In high doses cephalothin and cephalexin administration have rarely been implicated in kidney toxicity (interstitial nephritis and/or acute tubular necrosis). Concomitant administration of aminoglycosides appears to increase the incidence of nephrotoxicity. Allergic reactions and positive Coombs test may occur. A small percentage of patients allergic to penicillin cross-react with cephalosporins. Almost all cephalosporins produce thrombophlebitis with intravenous administration. The overall low level of adverse reactions is one of the reasons for the popularity of cephalosporins.

Cephalosporins are excreted mainly by the kidney. Probenecid generally increases serum levels and delays excretion. Patients with renal insufficiency need only moderate dose reduction. Some cephalosporins (cefazolin, cefamandole, cefmetazole) are also secreted into bile, reaching antibacterial levels as high as in serum. None of the presently used cephalosporins, with the exception of cefotaxime and other third-generation compounds, penetrate into the cerebrospinal fluid in therapeutic concentrations unless the meninges are inflamed. Penetration into other body cavities is variable but may reach antibacterial levels depending upon the susceptibility of the pathogen. Compounds containing the acetoxy group at the 3-position are metabolized in the body into the microbiologically less active desacetyl forms. Serum protein binding varies from 5%–95% and is generally rapidly reversible. The absorption of the oral cephalosporins is generally delayed by the presence of food, but the total quantity of drug absorbed is not affected. Peak serum concentrations are lower and duration in the serum is longer.

The mechanism of action of the cephalosporins is basically the same as that of the penicillins: inhibition of bacterial cell wall synthesis. They share membrane-binding protein sites with the penicillins but may also bind selectively. Their β-lactamase (both chromosomal and plasmid-mediated) susceptibility varies with the chemical structure.

The first and second generation cephalosporins are indicated as drugs of first choice only in infections caused by *Klebsiella* spp. (JAWETZ et al. 1980) or when patients are allergic to penicillins. Today the situation is changing and will continue to change with the introduction of the third-generation cephems and oxacephems.

The first-generation cephalosporins are similar in their antibacterial spectrum. This large group of compounds embraces cephalothin, cephapirin, cephaloridine, cefacetrile, cefadroxil, cefazolin, cephalexin, cephradine, and cefaclor. They are most active against many gram-positive cocci and bacteria. They are excellent antistaphylococcal agents. Penicillin-sensitive and -resistant strains alike of *S. aureus* are sensitive. *S. epidermidis* is more sensitive to them than to the antistaphylococcal penicillins. Methicillin-resistant strains are resistant to the cephalosporins. Almost all *S. pyogenes*, *S. pneumoniae*, *S. viridans* and *S. bovis* but not *S. faecalis* and *S. faecium*, are sensitive to these cephalosporins. Although *N. meningitidis* is very sensitive to the cephalosporins, the clinical results are not satisfactory, neither are those for cases of gonorrhoea. *Clostridium perfringens* (*welchii*), but not all other *Clostridium* spp. are sensitive to the cephalosporins. *B. fragilis* is not susceptible. *Listeria monocytogenes* is usually sensitive; and so are *Corynebacterium diphtheriae*, *B. subtilis* and *Actinomyces israeli*, but benzylpenicillin is more active against them.

Of the most common gram-negative bacilli, *K. pneumoniae* and other *Klebsiella*, most *E. coli*, *Proteus mirabilis*, *Salmonella*, and *Shigella* isolates are regularly sensitive to the first generation cephalosporins. The gram-negative species which are not sensitive to the first generation cephalosporins include: *P. aeruginosa*, indole positive *Proteus*, *E. cloacae*, *Citrobacter*, *Acinetobacter*, *Serratia* spp., and some strains of *H. influenzae*.

The second-generation cephalosporins (cefamandole, cefoxitin, cefuroxime, cefonicid, ceforanide and cefmetazole) have a somewhat more expanded spectrum of activity and higher resistance to β-lactamases than compounds of the first generation. They have gram-positive activity of the same range but less potent. Cefamandole has additional gram-negative activity against *Enterobacter* and indole-positive *Proteus* spp. as well as *H. influenzae*, but is not effective in the central nervous system infections. It has no activity against *B. fragilis*. Cefuroxime and ceforanide have additional action against *N. gonorrhoeae* and *H. influenzae*, including β-lactamase-producing strains. Cefoxitin is uniquely active against most *B. fragilis* strains and is also active against many strains of indole-positive *Proteus* spp., *Providencia stuartii* and *N. gonorrhoeae*. Some activity has been reported against a limited number of *S. marcescens* strains, but none against *Enterobacter*. Cefmetazole is similar to cefoxitin. It has increased resistance to gram-negative β-lactamases, similar to that of the other cephamycins.

The third-generation cephalosporins represent a therapeutic advance. They have a wide spectrum of activity against a gamut of gram-negative, gram-positive, and some anaerobic bacteria and, most importantly, varying activity against *P. aeruginosa* (SLACK 1981). While their in vitro activity against gram-positive microbes is somewhat weaker than that of the first and perhaps the second generation cephalosporins, they have an extremely high degree of potency against almost all gram-negative enteric bacilli. In addition, they have a very high degree of resistance to almost all forms of β-lactamases. It is worthwhile to consider those important infectious diseases where the presently available cephalosporins are clinically useful (OWENS et al. 1975; WISE 1978b; MANDELL and SANDE 1980).

At present, with the large number of parenteral cephalosporins available or soon to be available for general clinical use, many bacterial infections will be treatable with one or another of the cephalosporins. However, when an infection is expected to respond to penicillin, it should be considered as the drug of first choice, especially for the gram-positive organisms. Cephalosporins can be chosen in cases when the patient has a past history of penicillin hypersensitivity. For infections caused by *K. pneumoniae* a cephalosporin is the drug of first choice. In many surgical procedures, chemoprophylaxis with cephalosporins is effectively employed and will be used more extensively with the advent of the long-acting cephalosporins. Cephalosporins are widely used with good therapeutic successes in various infections of the urinary and respiratory tracts, bones and joints, skin and soft tissues. Various venereal diseases as well as infections in obstetrics and gynecology, pediatrics and ophthalmology are all indications for cephalosporin treatment. Gram-positive and gram-negative sepses react favorably to a well-selected cephalosporin. Infections caused by *P. aeruginosa* or other *Pseudomonas* spp. have been successfully and safely treated with high doses of several third generation cephalosporins, alone or in combination with an aminoglycoside.

I. Cephalothin

Cephalothin, the first cephalosporin for treatment of infectious diseases, was introduced in 1964. Originally it was approved by the U.S. Food and Drug Administration in doses of 0.5–1.0 g 6-hourly to treat severe infections (osteomyelitis, pneumonia, staphylococcal septicemia). The dose has subsequently been increased up to 12 g/day, a regimen which has been effective in the treatment of gram-negative sepsis and peritonitis following perforated viscus (GRIFFITH 1974). As much as 24 g per day has been administered to adults without side effects.

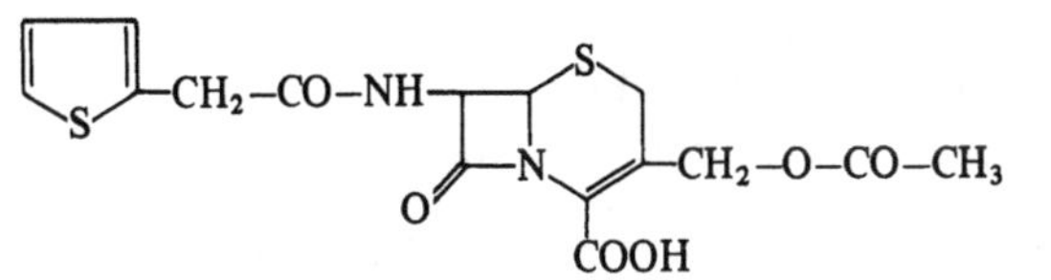

Cephalothin

The oral absorption of cephalothin is poor and the intramuscular injection is painful, therefore it is administered only intravenously. The adult dose varies with the severity of the infection, from 1 g every 6 h to 1 g every 2 h. Infants and children are treated with 40–100 mg/kg per day.

It is highly resistant to staphylococcal β-lactamases and considered by many to be the cephalosporin of choice in severe staphylococcal (*S. aureus*, *S. epidermidis*) infections, such as staphylococcal endocarditis. It is also effective in the treatment of infections caused by *S. pneumoniae*, group A streptococci and anaerobic streptococci as well as the gram-negative infections caused by sensitive *E. coli*, *P. mirabilis* and *K. pneumoniae* strains. It has a serum half-life of about 30–40 min and its binding to serum protein is about 60%. It distributes widely throughout the body tissues and fluids except the cerebrospinal fluid; therefore it cannot be used for the treatment of bacterial meningitis. It is mainly eliminated by the kidney and probenecid increases its half-life. About 20%–30% of cephalothin is metabolized into the weakly active desacetyl form. Phlebitis is an unpleasant side effect when the drug is given by intravenous drip.

Cephapirin and cephacetrile are two other similar parenteral cephalosporins.

II. Cephaloridine

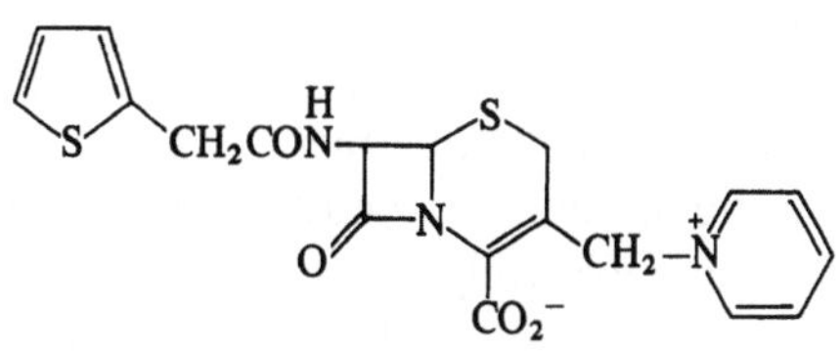

Cephaloridine

Cephaloridine differs from cephalothin in a number of biological aspects. It more frequently exhibits renal toxicity, especially when given in large doses. It is well tolerated by the tissues and can be injected intramuscularly without pain. It is a powerful bactericidal agent with a spectrum similar to that of cephalothin. It is less stable to β-lactamases than is cephalothin; therefore in severe infections due to penicillinase-producing staphylococci it should not be employed. It has been used with success and safety in patients with penicillin allergy. Its therapeutic uses include treatment of infections caused by sensitive strains of *Staphylococcus*, *Streptococcus*, pneumococcus, gonococcus and *C. diphtheriae*. *S. viridans* endocarditis in patients allergic to penicillin can be treated with cephaloridine. Syphilis, but not meningococcal meningitis, can also be treated. In infections due to *E. coli* or *P. mirabilis*, cephaloridine can be considered a suitable drug.

Cephaloridine is available in 250-, 500-, and 1,000-mg dosage forms. The usual intramuscular dose is 500 mg every 6 h up to 14 days, but 250 mg may be sufficient in less severe infections. The dose for intravenous drip infusion is 250 mg 6-hourly. The intramuscular dose in children is 10–30 mg/kg per day. An intrathecal dose above 50 mg may cause drowsiness and confusion and should be avoided. The adult daily dose should not exceed 4 g.

In addition to renal toxicity it may cause transient side-effects similar to other cephalosporins such as rash, neutropenia, alterations in liver function tests, and in elderly patients on larger doses, hemolytic anemia with positive Coombs test. As do other cephalosporins, it gives a false positive test for urinary glucose with Benedict's solution or with "Clinitest" (SMITH 1977).

III. Cefazolin

Cefazolin is the preferred parenteral first generation cephalosporin. It is metabolically stable and its spectrum is similar to that of cephalothin and cephaloridine; however it is additionally approved for use in *Enterobacter aerogenes* infections (URI et al. 1972). It can be injected intramuscularly, less frequently, and in smaller doses, since it produces higher and more prolonged serum levels (QUINTILIANI and NIGHTINGALE 1978).

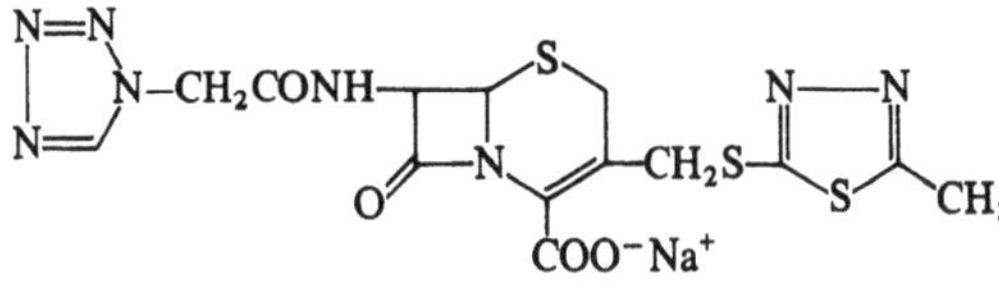

Cefazolin

It is active against *S. aureus* infections including the penicillin-resistant strains. In vitro it is somewhat less resistant to staphylococcal β-lactamase than is cephalothin, but this is not reflected in human therapy. Pneumonia caused by *S. pneumoniae* responds well to cefazolin treatment. Infections due to *P. mirabilis*, *K. pneumoniae*, *E. coli*, clostridia, and streptococci react very favorably to cefazolin treatment. Cefazolin produces relatively high concentrations in the bile and biliary tract; therefore it is particularly useful in the treatment of infections there. Hospital-acquired aspiration pneumonias are treated successfully with cefazolin.

Cefazolin has low nephrotoxic potential. Despite its high serum protein binding, it penetrates well into human tissues and body fluids (with the exception of cerebrospinal fluid). It is excreted mainly in the urine with some biliary excretion.

Cefazolin is available as the sodium salt in vials containing 250, 500, and 1,000 mg. In adults with mild infections, the dose is 150–500 mg every 8 h. In moderate or severe infections the usual adult dose is 0.5–1.0 g every 6–8 h, but daily doses as high as 6 g have been used intravenously in serious infections. The recommended daily dose for children is 25–50 mg/kg, but occasionally 100 mg/kg may be needed in severe infections.

Because of its favorable pharmacokinetic properties, cefazolin is extensively used for bacterial chemoprophylaxis, especially in surgery. Ceftezole (desmethylcefazolin) and cefazedon, although commercially available, have no therapeutic advantage over cefazolin.

IV. Cefamandole

Cefamandole together with cefoxitin, cefuroxime, cefonicid, ceforanide, and cefmetazole form the group designated as "second generation" cephalosporins. These cephalosporins have a more or less broadened antibacterial spectrum including more gram-negative genera and some are active against the anaerobic *B. fragilis*. Their gram-positive activity is generally poorer than that of the "first generation" cephalosporins and they have no activity against *P. aeruginosa*. Cefoxitin and cefmetazole are cephamycins. Cefamandole definitely has superior activity over cephalothin against *H. influenzae* strains but should not be used for meningeal infections (NEU 1980).

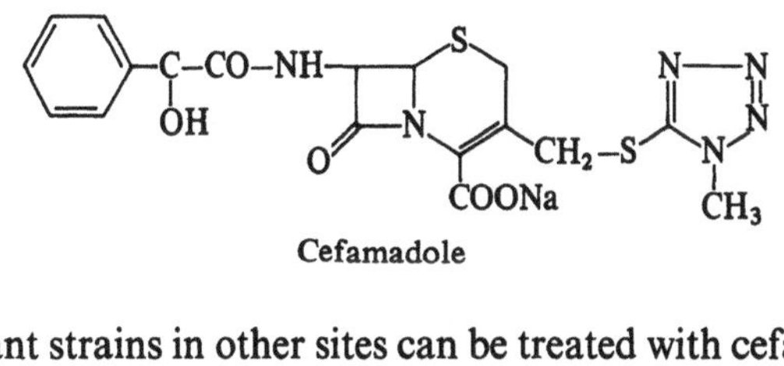

Cefamadole

Ampicillin-resistant strains in other sites can be treated with cefamandole (FRASER 1979; ROSETT et al. 1977; LITTLE et al. 1979). It also has increased activity against indole-positive *Proteus* spp., *E. coli*, *Citrobacter*, *Providencia*, *Klebsiella* and *Enterobacter* spp., but individual isolates should be tested for sensitivity before use of cefamandole. The gram-positive cocci are less sensitive to cefamandole than to cephalothin or cefazolin, and although therapeutic blood levels of cefamandole are achieved after high doses, it is not the cephalosporin of choice for the treatment of streptococcal and staphylococcal infections in patients allergic to penicillins.

A disulfiram-like reaction was observed with cefamandole (BUENING et al. 1981) similar to that of other methyltetrazolethiol-containing cephalosporins.

Cefamandole is available as the nafate in vials containing 0.5, 1, and 2 g for intravenous or intramuscular injections. Cefamandole nafate is converted in the body to cefamandole. The usual adult dose is 0.5–2 g every 4–6 h, up to 12 g per day in severe infections. The daily dose for children ranges from 50–150 mg/kg in 4 or 6 divided doses.

V. Cefoxitin

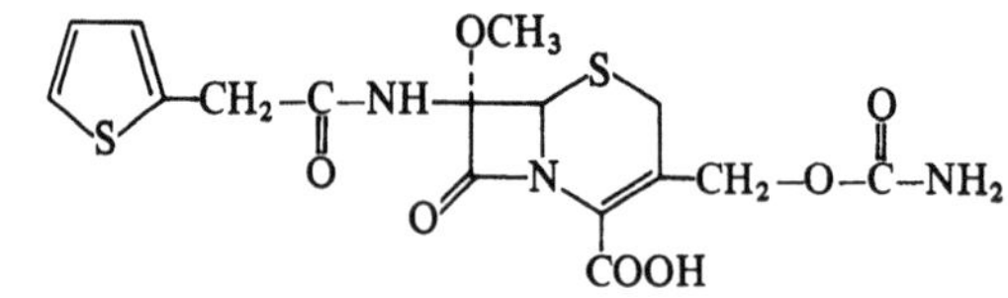

Cefoxitin

Cefoxitin is a cephamycin highly resistant to β-lactamases produced by gram-negative bacilli. It has a broad-spectrum activity against many aerobic and anaerobic gram-positive and gram-negative microbes; however, its activity against gram-positive bacteria is less than that of the first generation cephalosporins. It is also less active than cefamandole against *H. influenzae* and *Enterobacter* spp., but more active against indole-positive *Proteus* and *Serratia* spp. It is very active against *E. coli* and particularly against *B. fragilis* and other anaerobic bacteria. This latter activity makes it a viable choice in abdominal and gynecologic infections. Its activity includes the β-lactamase-producing strains, and its use is indicated for the treatment of serious infections of the respiratory and urinary tracts, and in septicemia, intra-abdominal, gynecological, bone, joint, skin, and soft tissue infections caused by susceptible strains. Cefoxitin is approved for the treatment of septicemias caused by *B. fragilis*. It has also been used for the treatment of gonorrhoea due to β-lactamase-producing *N. gonorrhoeae* strains.

Intramuscular injection is very painful and should only be given in 0.5% lidocaine solution. The peak serum level after 1 g intramuscular cefoxitin is approximately 20 μg/ml with a half-life of 40 min. It is excreted unchanged in the urine by both glomerular filtration and tubular secretion.

Cefoxitin is available in vials containing 1 or 2 g of the sodium salt for intravenous or intramuscular injection. The intravenous adult dose is 1–2 g every 6–8 h depending on the sensitivity of the causative organism and the general condition of the patient.

Additional references of interest include RIBNER et al. 1978b; BROGDEN et al. 1979a; WEBB et al. 1979; MOGABGAB et al. 1978.

VI. Cefmetazole

This semisynthetic cephamycin was recently marketed in Japan (Anonymous 1980). Like cefoxitin, it is very stable to β-lactamases (including those of indole-positive *Proteus* and *Serratia* spp.) and has broader spectrum and stronger activity against *E. coli* and *Klebsiella* spp.

At a dose of 1–4 g daily intramuscularly or intravenously, good therapeutic results were obtained in respiratory and urinary tract infections as well as gynecologic and hepatobiliary tract infections (MASHIMO 1980; OHKOSHI et al. 1980). The daily dose of cefmetazole for the treatment of serious infections of infants and children is 40–100 mg/kg either as a single intravenous injection or drip infusion (FUJII 1980). Cefmetazole reaches higher biliary levels than cefoxitin, otherwise the two compounds are expected to have similar clinical applications.

VII. Cefuroxime

This is the first semisynthetic cephalosporin containing the methoxy-(alkoxy) imino chain in the α-position of the 7-acylamino substituent. This structural configuration is reflected in its increased stability to β-lactamases and the broadened antibacterial spectrum, which is similar to that of cefamandole and cefoxitin. Cefuroxime is active against gram-positive cocci, including the penicillinase-producing and methicillin-sensitive strains, most gram-negative bacilli, including *Enterobacter* spp., indole-positive *Proteus* spp. and espcecially *Klebsiella* spp. (CARLONE et al. 1980). However, *S. marcescens*, *B. fragilis* and *P. aeruginosa* are not sensitive to it.

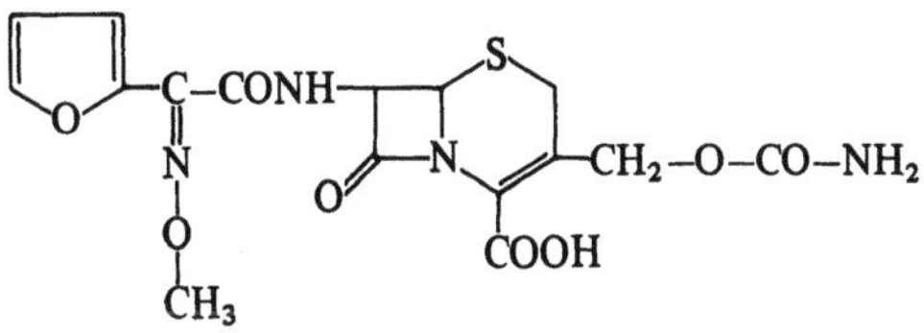

Cefuroxime

Cefuroxime is not metabolized and is excreted by tubular secretion (probenecid increases the serum levels and prolongs the elimination time). It can be found in the serum even at 8 h after administering 1 g intramuscularly. Its serum protein-binding is about 30%. It is well tolerated after intravenous injection. Usually it is given intramuscularly 1–2 g every 8 h, or 750 mg 3 times a day. Its therapeutic use is similar to that of cefamandole, over which it has no definite advantage (STONEY 1979; PRICE and FLUKER 1978; PINES et al. 1980; FRIEDRICH et al. 1980). Cefuroxime is less active against *S. aureus* than the first-generation cephalosporins; it is not recommended for severe staphylococcal and streptococcal infections.

VIII. Ceforanide

This cephalosporin has a microbiological spectrum of activity similar to cefamandole. It is presently under clinical investigation. The chemical structure is shown below.

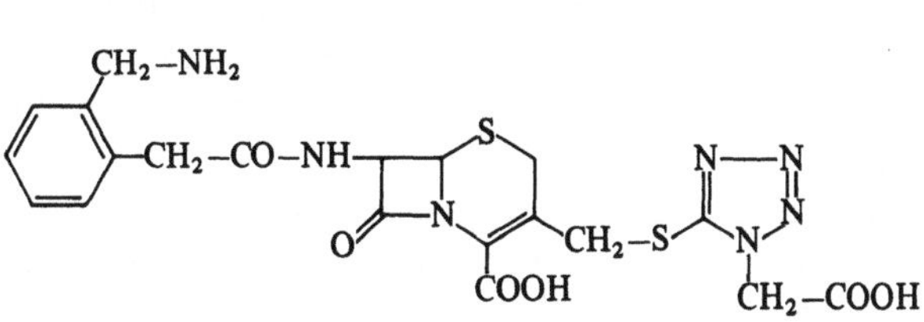

Ceforanide

Its advantage over cefamandole is its somewhat longer half-life (3.1 h) in man, allowing for twice-daily parenteral dosing. It was found efficacious and safe when administered in doses of 0.5, 1 or 2 g intramuscularly or intravenously every 12 h for 6–28 days. It was well tolerated and effective in the treatment of infections caused by sensitive organisms (BURCH et al. 1979; MUSHER et al. 1980; RAWSON et al. 1980). In healthy volunteers probenecid did not increase its plasma concentration or its urinary excretion. This may mean that the two drugs interact in the secretion or that ceforanide is mainly eliminated by glomerular filtration (JOVANOVICH 1981).

IX. Cefonicid

Cefonicid, of which the structure is shown below, resulted from a search designed to uncover long-acting cephalosporins.

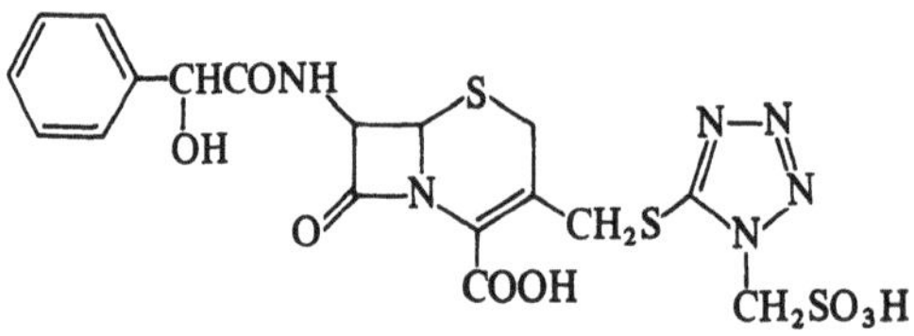

Cefonicid

It is currently under clinical investigation. It has a broad antibacterial spectrum that includes gram-positive and gram-negative bacteria (ACTOR et al. 1978). It produces high and prolonged serum levels in man and is excreted unchanged in the urine (PITKIN et al. 1980). Despite high serum binding (98%) it penetrates well into body fluids and tissues. The half-life after intravenous administration to man is approximately doubled (8 h) following oral administration of 1 g probenecid. Clinical reports show this cephalosporin to be efficacious in a once-daily regimen administered either intramuscularly or intravenously. This cephalosporin should be the drug of choice in surgical prophylaxis and as an outpatient treatment of such chronic infection as osteomyelitis.

X. Third-Generation Cephalosporins

Cefotaxime is the first, cefsulodin the second, and moxalactam the third marketed members of the so-called third-generation cephalosporins with great prospects in the therapy of a wide-range of infectious diseases. The other third-generation cephalosporins are under clinical evaluation. They are: ceftizoxime, cefoperazone (now approved), ceftazidime, cefmenoxime, cefotiam, and ceftriaxon. These newer compounds may significantly alter our approach to the treatment of serious bacterial infections.

The general characteristics of the third-generation cephalosporins include:

1) Extremely broad in vitro antibacterial activity including *P. aeruginosa.* They combine the favorable characteristics of the first and second generation cephalosporins with activity against a much broader range of bacteria including *Enterobacter* spp., *Serratia marcescens*, *Proteus mirabilis*, indole-positive *Proteus* spp., *H. influenzae*, *N. gonorrhoeae* and *B. fragilis*. Cefotiam inhibits almost all of the above bacteria but not *P. aeruginosa*, while cefsulodin has very good antipseudomonal activity with negligible effects against the other bacteria.

2) Potent in vitro activities against the gram-negative bacteria with MIC values usually well below 1.0 μg/ml. Their antistaphylococcal and antistreptococcal activities are usually less than those of the first-generation cephalosporins.

3) Increased resistance to both plasmid- and chromosomally-mediated β-lactamases. Therefore, these agents are being used for the treatment of infections caused by bacteria resistant to penicillin, ampicillin, cephalothin and cefazolin.

4) Retention of the excellent pharmacokinetic properties of the older cephalosporins. Some have been reported to penetrate into the CNS.

1. Cefotaxime

Third–generation cephalosporins

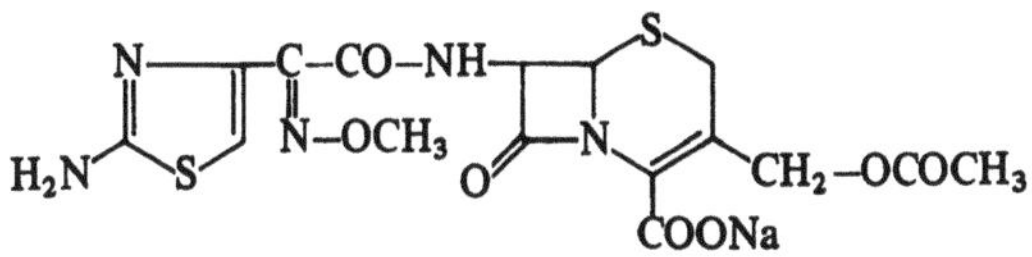

Cefotaxime

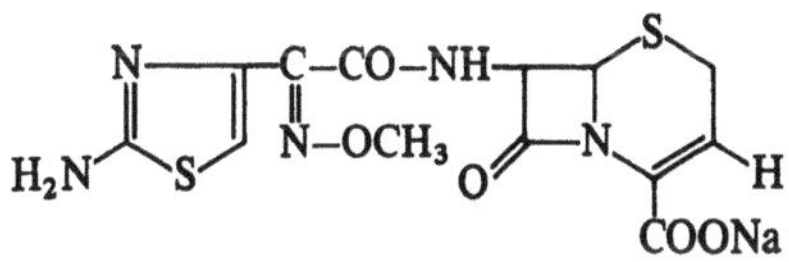

Ceftizoxime

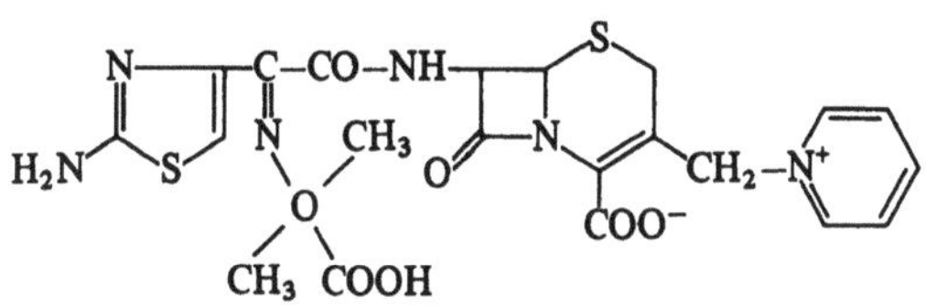

Ceftazidime

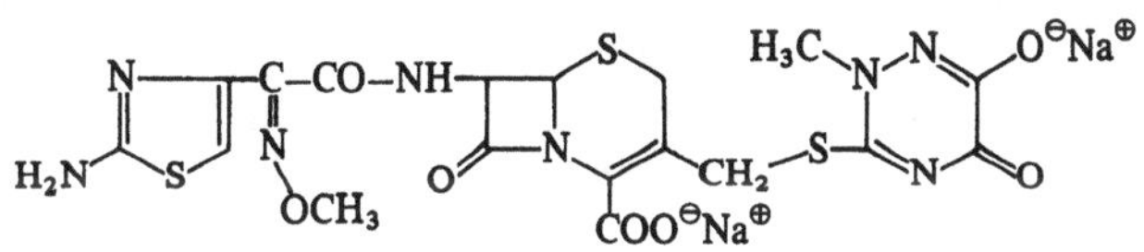

Ceftriaxon

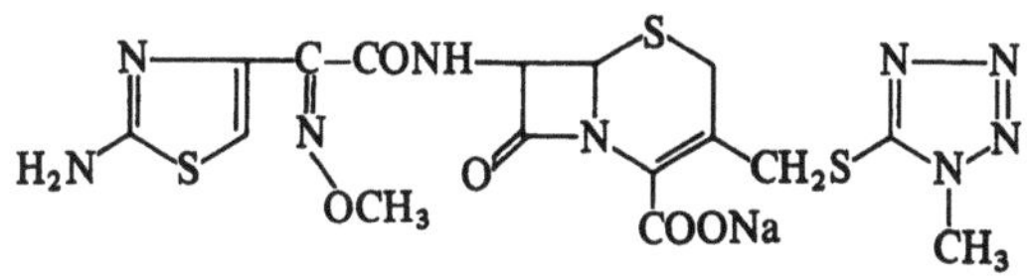

Cefmenoxime

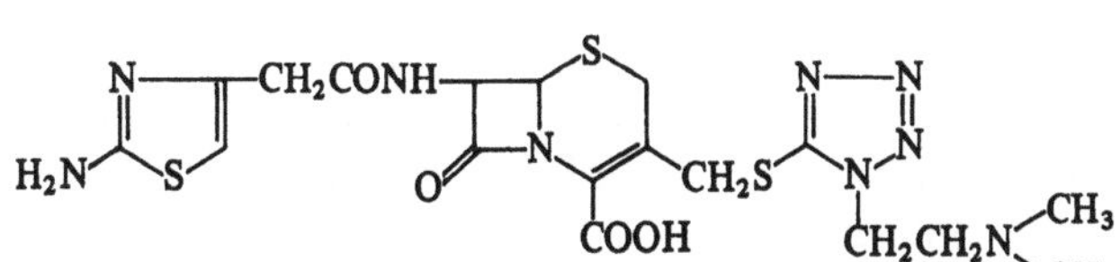

Cefotiam

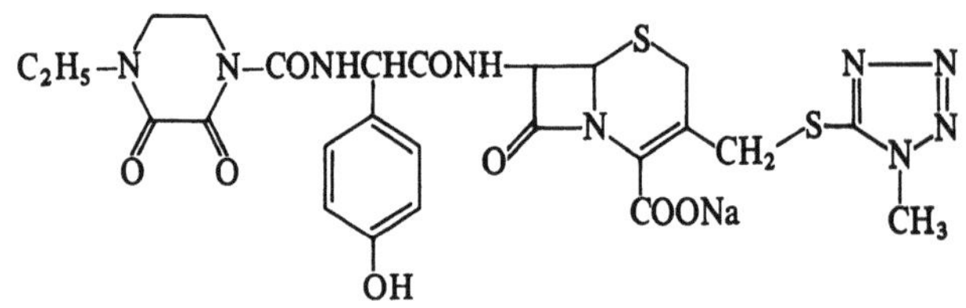

Cefoperazone

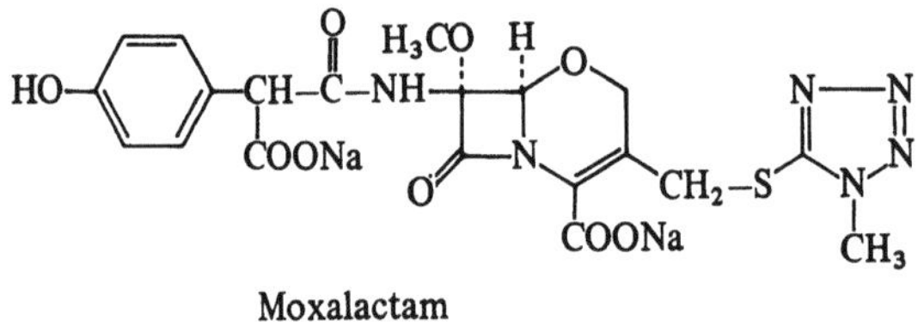

Moxalactam

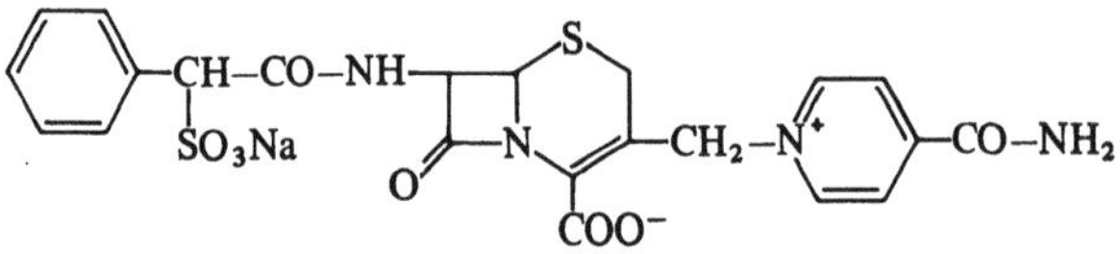

Cefsulodin

Cefotaxime (HR756) was first described by BUCOURT et al. (1977 and 1978); OCHIAI et al. (1977); NUMATA et al. (1977); CHABBERT and LUTZ (1978); HEYMÈS et al. (1979). The first preclinical study was published by HEYMÈS et al. (1977). Additional reports on its therapeutic results can be found in the manufacturer's (HOECHST 1980), pamphlet, "CLAFORAN – cefotaxime." We have drawn extensively on the following selected clinical papers related to adults: SHAH et al. (1979); SACK et al. (1978); NINANE (1979); CLUMECK et al. (1979); BROWN and FALLON (1979); SLACK et al. (1980); MCKENDRICK et al. (1980); NEWSON et al. (1980); RIMMER (1980); WRIGHT and WISE (1980); and these related to infants and children: REYNOLDS et al. (1979); BELOHRADSKY et al. (1980); HELWIG (1980) and KAFETZIS et al. (1980).

The therapeutic results of clinical trials basically reflect the microbiologic data. Adequate serum levels with about a 1 h half-life, good absorption after intramuscular injection, and good distribution into almost all body tissues and fluids have been reported. Cefotaxime is eliminated predominantly by renal excretion (glomerular filtration and tubular secretion), in a ratio of 60% unchanged and 20% the microbiologically less active desacetyl metabolite in the urine. The renal clearance was found to be about 120 ml/min per 1.73 m^2. In patients with kidney impairment, the dose should be reduced as dictated by the decrease in creatinine clearance.

Cefotaxime has been reported highly effective with very good cure rates in treatment of the following infections of adults and children: gastrointestinal, genito-urinary and respiratory tract infections, septicemia and infections of the ear, nose and throat. High cure rate was obtained in patients who were previously unsuccessfully treated with other antibiotics. Cefotaxime can also be used for the treatment of (often mixed) infections caused by sensitive microbes in obstetrics and gynecology, abdominal infections and those of bone, skin, joints and soft tissues as well as infected wounds and burns. Gonorrhoea caused even by penicillinase-producing strains was found to be cured by a single 1 g intramuscular dose of cefotaxime (sometimes with concomitant probenecid). Tests for syphilis prior to treatment should be instituted. Therapeutic usefulness was demonstrated in the treatment of newborn and childhood meningitides after failure with ampicillin or chloramphenicol, even in patients with compromised defense mechanisms (BELOHRADSKY et al. 1980). The response to treatment of *P. aeruginosa* infections is variable.

Cefotaxime is available in vials containing 0.25, 0.5, and 1.0 g of the sodium salt for intravenous or intramuscular injection. The recommended adult dose is 1 g every 8–12 h. In severe infections the dose should be increased to 2 g 2–3 times a day or 2 g can be injected every 6 h. As much as 12 g cefotaxime has been given per day without adverse effects. The regular pediatric doses are 50–100 mg/kg per day (in severe cases 150–200 mg/kg per day) in equally divided doses every 6–12 h. Premature babies should not be given more than 50 mg/kg/day.

2. Ceftizoxime

Ceftizoxime (FK749) was first described by KAMIMURA et al. (1979). Its broad antibacterial activity includes pseudomonal species and *A. calcoaceticus* (GOTOH et al. 1980) and β-lactamase stability. Pharmacokinetics and clinical pharmacology have been reported (NAKASHIMA 1980). Against many bacterial species it is 2–4 times more active and also more lytic than is cefotaxime (GREENWOOD et al. 1980). *Serratia* spp. are exceptionally sensitive to it as is *Bacteroides fragilis*. Ceftizoxime is not metabolized and is excreted in the urine as the active parent compound. It penetrates well into tissues and body fluids and produces high and prolonged serum levels permitting twice-daily dosing for most indications (NEU and SRINIVASAN 1981). In clinical trials in Japan it was administered to more than 1,500 patients with excellent results and low side effects. The results of these extensive clinical evaluations, along with numerous laboratory studies, were published in Chemotherapy (Tokyo) in 1980 (vol 28, pp 1–900) and those in USA in J Antimicrob Chemother (1982) Suppl. C, pp 1–355. Ceftizoxime is usually administered either intramuscularly or intravenously in doses of 0.5–2.0 g twice a day. In severe infections increased doses can be given more frequently, up to 12 g per day.

3. Moxalactam

Moxalactam (6059-S; LY127935) is an oxacephamycin, the first member of this class evaluated in man. Like other third-generation compounds, it possesses a broad spectrum of antibacterial activity, high level of potency and stability to many β-lactamases. Moxalactam is produced by synthesis starting from penicillin G.

Moxalactam is most active against Enterobacteriaceae, usually with MICs less than 1 μg/ml (JORGENSEN et al. 1980; YOSHIDA et al. 1980). It was found to be markedly bactericidal to *E. coli*, both β-lactamase-producing and nonproducing strains. Its activity against *S. aureus* and other gram-positive bacteria is much weaker (about 10 μg/ml).

Moxalactam has a favorable pharmacokinetic profile in man. The time course of plasma level was found to be similar to that of cefazolin. After a 1 g intravenous infusion the mean peak serum level was about 72 µg/ml, and after a 1 g intramuscular injection about 52 µg/ml. The serum half-life is approximately 2.5 h. It is eliminated mainly by the kidney with high urine concentrations. About 70%–80% of the dose can be recovered in the urine within 24 h. It is primarily eliminated by glomerular filtration since probenecid did not alter in healthy volunteers the following parameters: plasma levels and urinary concentrations, apparent volume of distribution, elimination half-life and rate constant, plasma and renal clearances (DESANTE et al. 1982).

In clinical trials it was found to be a very effective and useful antibiotic in the treatment of infections of the respiratory and urinary tracts, meningitis, sepsis and cholecystitis. Superinfection with resistant *P. aeruginosa* or *S. faecalis* may complicate the cure rate (MATSUMOTO et al. 1980a). Because of its activity against *B. fragilis*, it is expected to be useful in mixed infections where anaerobic strains are also involved. It was evaluated in patients with puerperal and postabortal genital infections with an initial daily dose of 6 g for a minimum of 5 days with favorable cure rate (GIBBS et al. 1980).

In these studies moxalactam was well tolerated with minimal hepatic, renal or hematologic abnormalities. Local irritation was observed. An "Antabuse" type reaction was observed with moxalactam similar to that of cefoperazone in patients who received 2 g moxalactam intravenously every 8 h and had a drink later (NEU and PRINCE 1980). This disulfiram-like reaction is not observed if the drug is given after alcohol consumption, allowing Emergency Room administration. It was found to be related to the methyltetrazolethiol side-chain at the 3 position (BUENING et al. 1981) and the accumulation of acetaldehyde in the blood.

4. Cefoperazone

Cefoperazone (T-1551), in addition to its broad and potent antibacterial spectrum, shows good activity against *P. aeruginosa* (≦8 µg/ml). The most susceptible organisms are: *H. influenzae*, *N. gonorrhoeae* and *meningitidis* (including β-lactamase producing strains), *Salmonella* spp. and viridans streptococci. Against *S. aureus* it is less active than the older cephalosporins. *Acinetobacter*, *B. fragilis* and some *Serratia* spp. are resistant to it. It is stable to many β-lactamases, but less so than other third-generation compounds (NEU et al. 1979).

Intravenous infusion of 2 g gives mean serum peak concentrations of 134–143 µg/ml. Half-life is 1.7 h and serum binding is high (90%). Cefoperazone is mainly excreted via the bile, with only 25% recovered in the urine (ALLAZ et al. 1979). It is administered twice-daily intravenously or intramuscularly. It has been found safe in the usual therapeutic doses of 2–4 g per day in intravenous drip. The daily dose may be increased up to 9 g. Pediatric dose is 25–100 mg/kg every 12 h. "Antabuse" type effects were observed in volunteers who consumed alcoholic beverages up to 36 h after a dose of 1 or 2 g cefoperazone similar to those with moxalactam, cefamandole and most probably cefmenoxime (KEMMERICH and LODE 1981). The marked incidence of lower gastrointestinal side effects, sometimes with diarrhea, may be the consequence of the high (60%) biliary excretion (REEVES and DAVIES 1980).

The clinical data are in agreement with the laboratory results. Good therapeutic results were obtained in respiratory and urinary tract as well as gynecologic and intra-abdominal infections and bacteremia on the basis of the evaluation of more than 2,500 patients treated worldwide (UEDA et al. 1980; MATSUDA et al. 1980; MATSUMOTO et al. 1980b). Its long half-life makes administration every 12 h an appropriate dosage. If further clinical studies prove its anti-*Pseudomonas* efficacy valid, it should be a significant cephalosporin. A special issue deals with cefoperazone sodium in Clinical Therapeutics (vol 3S, pp. 1–208, 1980).

5. Ceftriaxon

Ceftriaxon (Ro 13-9904) possesses, in general, all the attributes of the parenteral third-generation cephalosporins with the added unique property of an 8-h plasma half-life in man and strong experimental prophylactic efficacy (REINER et al. 1980; HINKLE and BODEY 1980; ANGEHRN et al. 1980). The extremely long half-life may be related to its high serum protein binding (95%). It penetrates well and rapidly into artificially produced blister fluid. Against gram-negative bacteria (*H. influenzae*, *N. gonorrhoeae*, *E. coli*, *Shigella*, and *Salmonella* spp.) isolated from pediatric patients ceftriaxon was found to be more active than cefotaxime, moxalactam, and cefoperazone. While it is stable to most β-lactamases, enzymes of *B. fragilis*, *E. cloacae* and indole-positive *Proteus* spp. hydrolyze it. It is presently under clinical trial [ANGEHRN et al. 1980; Reports on ceftriaxon (Rocephin) 1981].

6. Cefmenoxime

Cefmenoxime (SCE 1365) is a typical representative of the methoxyimino-aminothiazolyl cephalosporins both chemically and biologically. In addition to its broad-spectrum antibacterial activity it has a relatively high biliary excretion (about 15%–30%), but is mainly excreted in the urine, by both glomerular filtration and tubular secretion (OCHIAI et al. 1977; TANAYAMA et al. 1980; GOTO et al. 1980). Recent studies show that the tubular secretion predominates (GRANNEMAN et al. 1982). It was selected for further clinical studies as a compound with improved antibacterial spectrum, high degree of β-lactamase stability and other pharmacokinetic properties in animals. Basically it has similar characteristics and antimicrobial activity to cefotaxime with a longer duration of action. It is in early phase of clinical trial. Since it contains the methyltetrazolethiol side chain at the 3-position like cefamandole, moxalactam and cefoperazone, it is prone to produce the disulfiram-like reaction.

7. Ceftazidime

Ceftazidime (GR 20263) has perhaps the broadest spectrum and most potent activity against gram-negative bacteria of the third-generation cephalosporins. In addition to the general characteristics of the third-generation cephalosporins, it is as active as gentamicin against strains of *P. aeruginosa*. It has very low binding to serum proteins with a serum half-life of about 1.8 h. Ceftazidime has the potential to be used alone as a nontoxic alternative to the aminoglycoside antibiotics for the therapy of *Pseudomonas* infections (O'CALLAGHAN et al. 1980; ACRED et al. 1980).

Against *S. aureus* strains it appears to be very inferior to cefotaxime. *B. fragilis* and *S. faecalis* are not sensitive to it. Its human pharmacokinetics are promising and clinical trials are going on an 8-h dose interval.

8. Cefotiam

Cefotiam (SCE-963) is a broad-spectrum aminothiazolyl cephalosporin, without antipseudomonal activity. Its antibacterial spectrum includes *Enterobacter* spp., *Citrobacter* and indole-positive *Proteus* spp. (NUMATA et al. 1978). It was found to be superior to cefazolin in the treatment of postoperative and urinary tract infections (ISHIGAMI et al. 1980; SHIRAHA et al. 1980). It showed superior activity to cefamandole, cefuroxime, and cefazolin. *H. influenzae* and *N. gonorrhoeae*, including β-lactamase-producing strains are 100% inhibited by cefotiam. It is presently under clinical trial (YAMAMOTO et al. 1979).

9. Cefsulodin

Cefsulodin (SCE 129; CGP-7174/E) is an injectable antipseudomonal cephalosporin. It is unique among the β-lactams because it has activity only against *P. aeruginosa* and certain other pseudomonads, as well as some gram-positive cocci but not against any other gram-negative bacteria (TSUCHIYA et al. 1978). It has significant β-lactamase stability (KING et al. 1980).

Cefsulodin has good pharmacokinetic properties. Tissue penetration is good and reaches significant levels at the site of infection after 1–2 g intravenous injection. A regular dose should be 2 g 3 times daily. Intramuscular injection may be painful (WITTKE and ADAM 1980). About 90% of the dose is excreted unchanged in the urine over 24 h.

The clinical trials included infections caused by *P. aeruginosa*, such as pyelonephritis, septicemia, chronic bronchitis, burns, and soft tissue infections. The best therapeutic results were obtained in cases of chronic pyelonephritis (GUIBERT et al. 1980; GRANINGER et al. 1980; NAKATOMI et al. 1980). Further clinical trials are needed to establish its therapeutic indications and uses as an alternate to the aminoglycosides in the treatment of *Pseudomonas* infections, even after its marketing.

It is expected that the broader spectrum, enhanced potency, greatly improved β-lactamase stability, excellent pharmacokinetics and relative lack of toxicity of the third-generation cephalosporins will be translated into better and improved therapeutic usefulness (NEUMAN 1980). Undoubtedly many of the third-generation cephalosporins will be drug(s) of first choice in the treatment of infections where other drugs were placed earlier (Table 1). The initiation of clinical evaluation of two newer members of the 2-aminothiazolyl cephalosporins (cefodizime and 42980 RP) was reported recently (Personal Communication 1982).

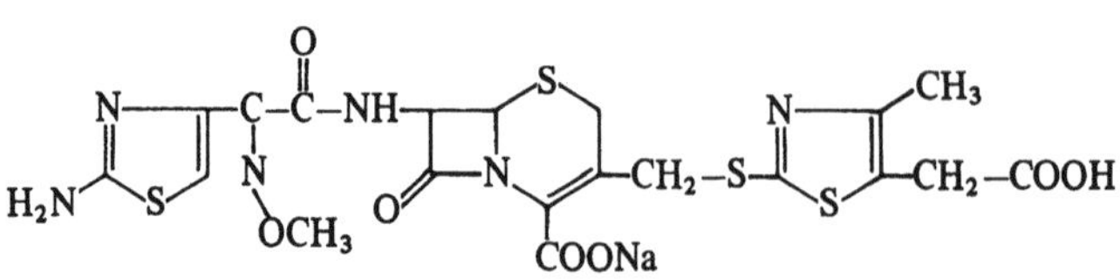

Cefodizime (HR 221)

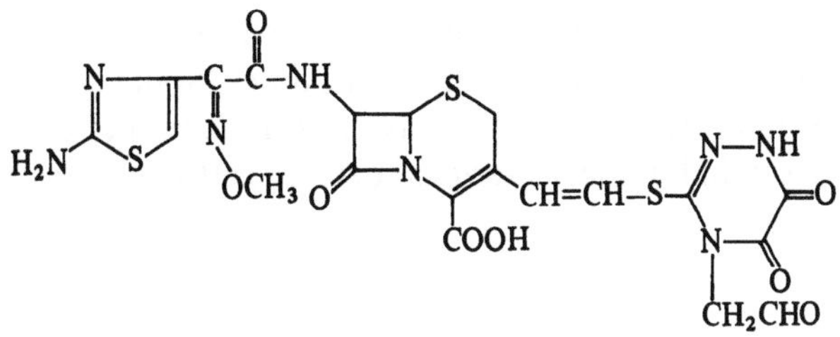

42980 RP

XI. The Oral Cephalosporins

All of the oral cephalosporins show a general similarity in their basic chemistry and profile of antimicrobial activity, although some of the newer compounds (cefatrizine and cefaclor) have extended the spectrum of activity slightly.

Oral cephalosporins

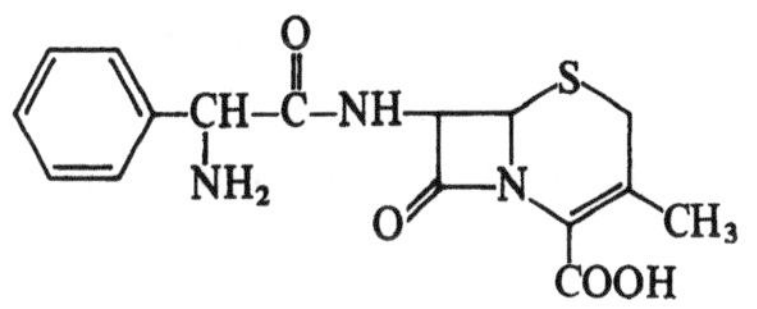

Cephalexin

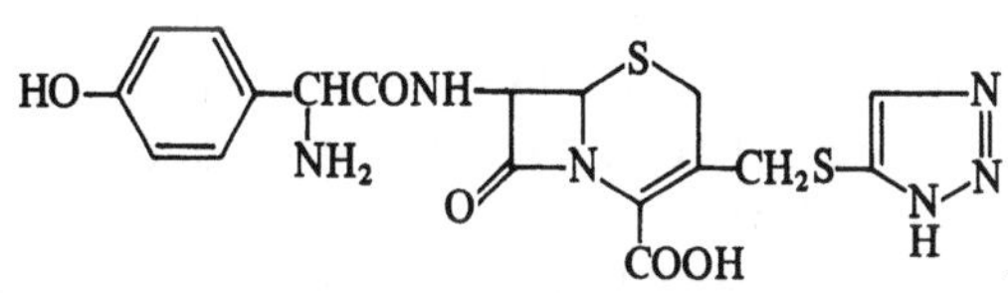

Cefatrizine

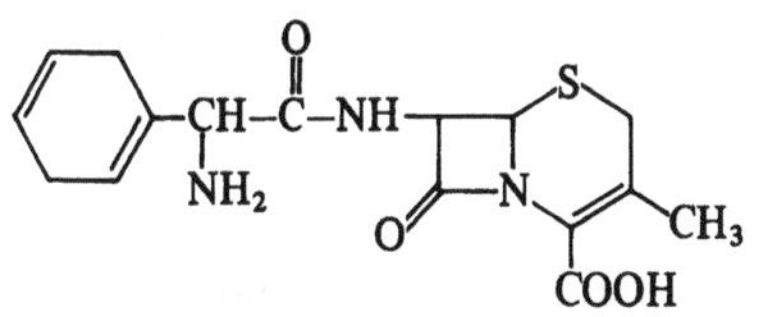

Cephradine

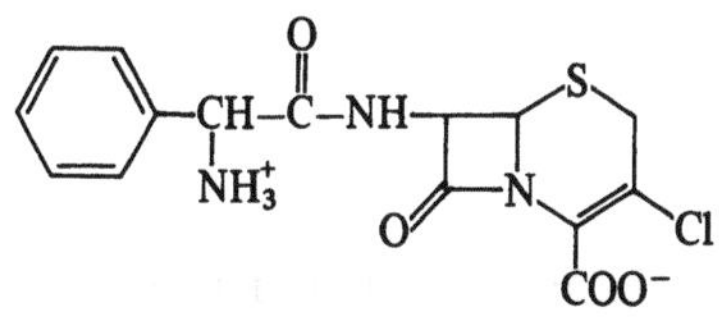

Cefaclor

1. Cephalexin

Cephalexin is the most frequently used oral cephalosporin. It is well absorbed from the gastrointestinal tract. Its antibacterial spectrum is similar to that of the first generation parenteral cephalosporins (cephalothin, cefazolin, etc.). It is less active than the parenteral preparations, especially against staphylococci. It was introduced in 1971, after the first phenylglycine-type oral cephalosporin, cephaloglycin (in 1970) showed poor oral absorption, although it was found to be acid stable.

Cephalexin therapy is indicated when oral administration is judged appropriate, such as mild infections caused by streptococci or pneumococci or if the patient has a history of hypersensitivity to oral penicillins. Urinary tract infections due to sensitive *E. coli* and *P. mirabilis* strains may be treated with this more convenient oral cephalosporin (KUNIN and FINKELBERG 1970).

Cephalexin is absorbed better from an empty stomach. The average serum peak level is about 18 µg/ml after 0.5 g orally. It is excreted by tubular secretion and probenecid increases and prolongs serum concentrations.

Cephalexin is available in capsules (250 and 500 mg), pediatric drops (100 mg/ml) and oral suspension (125 or 250 mg/5 ml). The usual adult dose is 250 or

500 mg 4 times a day. The dose for children ranges from 25 to 50 mg/kg/day, divided into 4 portions. For serious infections, the doses should be increased. It may cause gastrointestinal disturbances such as nausea, vomiting, diarrhea, and abdominal cramps. Cephalexin lacks serious toxic side effects (SPEIGHT et al. 1972).

2. Cephradine

Cephradine has the same clinical application as cephalexin, namely the treatment of moderate infections caused by sensitive gram-positive and gram-negative bacteria. Its indication and dosage are basically the same as for cephalexin (PERJÉS 1974), and they can be used interchangeably.

Cephradine is rapidly absorbed from the gastrointestinal tract and excreted unchanged in the urine. It is the first (and presently the only) semisynthetic cephalosporin which is available both in oral and parenteral forms. Intramuscular injection may be painful, therefore the intravenous injection is preferable. Some authorities prefer to use cephradine because they can start the treatment with parenteral injection and continue with oral administration of the same drug (SELWYN 1976a, b; REEVES 1976; BRUMFITT and HAMILTON-MILLER 1976; PHILLIPS and EYKYN 1976).

It is available in capsules (250 and 500 mg) and also as oral suspension (125 or 250 mg/5 ml). For intramuscular or intravenous uses the vials contain 250, 500, or 1,000 mg. Its oral dosage schedule is the same as for cephalexin. The usual parenteral adult dose is 0.5 to 1 g 6-hourly. The pediatric dose is 25 to 100 mg/kg/day in divided doses. No side effects were reported even when higher doses were taken.

3. Cefatrizine

Cefatrizine, sold only in Japan, has the same antibacterial spectrum as cephalexin but with 4- to 8-fold greater activity, in addition to inhibitory effects against *Enterobacter* spp. at clinically achievable concentrations (ACTOR et al. 1975; JONES et al. 1979). It has a somewhat broader spectrum than the first generation cephalosporins. In healthy human subjects after 0.5 g oral or intramuscular administration the peak serum level is lower than that of cephalexin but the area under the curve is similar (ACTOR et al. 1976). Although it can be injected intramuscularly, it is administered almost exclusively orally to adults in doses of 0.5–1 g 3 times daily or in serious infections in 1–3 g 2 to 4 times daily. It was found effective in various infections caused by *S. pneumoniae*, *β*-hemolytic *Streptococcus*, *S. aureus*, *E. coli*, *P. mirabilis* and *Klebsiella* spp. (UEDA 1976). Good therapeutic results were obtained in the treatment of genitourinary tract infections inlcuding cystitis, pyelonephritis and gonococcal urethritis, respiratory tract infections, sinusitis and soft-tissue infections with an oral dosage regimen of 500 mg of cefatrizine three to four times daily for 7–10 days (RIBNER et al. 1978a). All clinical and basic aspects of cefatrizine have been published in one volume (Cefatrizine, 1976).

4. Cefaclor

Cefaclor is the newest member of the group of orally active cephalosporins to be marketed. It is somewhat more active than cephalexin against gram-positive cocci and *N. gonorrhoeae* and significantly more active against gram-negative bacilli. Cefaclor is active against ampicillin-resistant *H. influenzae* strains. Its enhanced in vitro activity is counterbalanced by its poorer oral absorption when compared with cephalexin. It is safe. It has been used in pediatric medicine for the treatment of children allergic to penicillin (GINSBURG and MCCRACKEN 1980).

The therapeutic indications of cefaclor are: otitis media, respiratory and urinary tract infections and those of skin and soft tissues (MASBERNARD and SALORD 1979; HÖFFLER 1979; FEDERSPIL and BACH 1979; KAMMER and SHORT 1979; CODY et al. 1979; MAFGAARD et al. 1979).

Cefaclor is available in 250 and 500 mg capsules and in oral suspension containing 125 and 250 mg/5 ml. The adult dose is 250–500 mg three to four times a day for 7–10 days depending on the severity of the infection. The recommended pediatric dose is 40 mg/kg per day.

5. Cefroxadine, Cefadroxil, and Cephaloglycin

Cefroxadine is claimed to have some stronger bactericidal action than cephalexin and its absorption may not be influenced by food intake (YASUDA et al. 1980; MASHIMO et al. 1980).

Cefadroxil is absorbed and excreted by tubular secretion at a slower rate than is cephalexin and thus has a sustained antimicrobial effect. It can be administered orally in a dose of 0.5 g every 8–12 h (SANTELLA and BERMAN 1978; GORDON 1978). It is an expensive alternative to cephalexin.

Cephaloglycin, the first of the oral cephalosporins, is prctically never used anymore.

Unfortunately, there have been no major advances in the field of oral cephalosporins since the introduction of cephalexin. Some of the newer compounds offer some borderline therapeutic advantages. Developments similar to the third-generation parenteral cephalosporins are expected.

D. Antibacterial Chemoprophylaxis with the β-Lactam Antibiotics

Although the role of antibiotic prophylaxis for many medical uses has been firmly established, it is still, in many cases, a subject of debate. Antibiotic prophylaxis has been applied more in medicine than in surgery. Attitudes toward chemoprophylaxis of antibacterial agents, especially with β-lactams, have changed during the past decade (KEIGHLEY 1978). However, the controversy centered around the use and overuse of prophylactic antibiotics still continues. In certain well-defined situations patients benefit from prophylaxis, but in other situations its value is not clear-cut (GOLDMAN and PETERSDORF 1979). In many cases prophylactic use of antibiotics may not be fully justified, especially if we consider the estimate that more than one-third of all antibiotic use is for this purpose (NEU 1979b). According to a recent survey, an estimated 72% of patients received appropriate antibiotics for treatment, whereas only 36% received the appropriate antibiotics for prophylaxis (JOGERST and DIPPE 1981). The definition of antimicrobial chemoprophylaxis as used in this text is a composite of the thinking of a number of authors, such as KRUPP and CHATTON (1980), MEYERS et al. (1980), BRACHMAN (1979), WATTEL

(1975), MARGET (1979), JAWETZ et al. (1980). A propyhlactic agent is used not only for the purpose of preventing the establishment of pathogenic microorganisms in the body, but also in a broader sense, for administration during or shortly after exposure to and acquisition of an infectious agent and prior to clear development of a disease syndrome.

General considerations of chemoprophylaxis should first be considered (GARROD 1975; SANFORD 1977, HIRSCHMANN 1981; HIRSCHMANN and INUI 1980; LORD 1979; NICHOLS and CONDON 1980; PAULSON et al. 1980). The expected value of antibiotic prophylaxis should be weighed against the eventual risks. Timing of antibiotic prophylaxis is as important as is the route of administration of the antibiotic chosen. This is very often based on the knowledge of the major microflora of the appropriate anatomic part of the body. The duration of use of prophylactic agents also is important. With the exception of a few indications where chronic prophylaxis is necessary, the antimicrobials should be employed for as short a period as possible. Prophylactic antibiotics should be of low toxic potential, with preferably bactericidal action. The cost factors can also be considered.

The β-lactam antibiotics are frequently the most ideal drugs for prophylaxis and are usually the drugs of choice. Situations where the β-lactams are indicated and justified are: extraction of a tooth (penicillin, cephalosporin); infective endocarditis (prolonged penicillin, cephalosporins); vaginal hysterectomy (cephalosporin, penicillin); total abdominal hysterectomy (cephalosporin); high-risk cesarian section (cephalosporin); cystoscopic examination (amoxicillin, cephalosporin); sigmoidoscopy (ampicillin, cephalosporin); vascular grafts of the abdominal aorta or lower extremity vasculature (cephalosporin); total hip replacement and valvular prosthesis (cephalosporin or penicillinase-resistant penicillin); head and neck cancer surgery (cephalosporin). Other antimicrobial agents used for chemoprophylaxis include doxycycline, rifampicin, erythromycin, neomycin, isoniazid, clindamycin, metronidazole, sulfonamides, trimethoprim-sulfamethoxazole, aminoglycosides alone or in combination with β-lactams. The term penicillin as used above usually refers to benzylpenicillin but many other members of the penicillin group may be justified depending on the route of administration and the sensitivity of the suspected bacteria. Cephalosporins may include any member of the group, in addition to the available third-generation cephalosporins.

The prophylactic uses of β-lactam antibiotics will be discussed under two headings, the medical uses and the surgical uses.

I. Prophylactic Uses in Medicine

There are many diseases or clinical settings where the β-lactams are highly recommended for prophylactic treatment. Among these situations, the prolonged, continuous use of penicillins in bacterial endocarditis and recurrent rheumatic fever is well established and highly indicated.

Rheumatic fever is an outstanding example of the application of chemoprophylaxis. Prevention of infections with *S. pyogenes* in patients with normal susceptibility can prevent the late complications, such as rheumatic fever and/or glomerulonephritis. After established infections or past history of rheumatic fever, protection against reinfection with any type of group A streptococci may prevent the development of heart disease. Prevention of reinfection is not indicated in nephritis since the number of nephritogenic strains is negligible and the development of type-specific postinfection immunity is common.

Since the causative agents, the streptococci, are extremely sensitive to penicillin G, it is used widely. In the case of primary infection the first choice of drug is benzathine penicillin G in a single dose of 1.2 million units intramuscularly. An alternative drug is penicillin V orally 250 mg 4 times a day for 10 days. In case of penicillin allergy, oral erythromycin is the drug of choice, 200 mg 4 times daily for 10 days. An oral cephalosporin may also be a second choice. For the prevention of recurrent episodes, again, benzathine penicillin G is the drug of first choice in a dose of 1.2 million units intramuscularly every month for years, often for life (the optimum duration of antistreptococcal prophylaxis has not been firmly established). Penicillin V, in 500 mg oral doses 4 times a day for years, or a sulfonamide 0.5–1 g a day, may be the alternate prophylactic agents. Dosage may be discontinued at age 40 if no recurrence is observed.

Prevention of bacterial endocarditis in patients with increased susceptibility to infections with viridans streptococci and other organisms is discussed in Sect. E. Here it is suffice to emphasize the conditions which can lead to increased susceptibility to infections. Conditions which predispose to bacterial endocarditis and frequently require prophylaxis are: patients with prosthetic valves; dental (oral) procedures; patients with congenital, rheumatic or mitral prolapse or valvular disease; following many genitourinary procedures; and cardiac catheterization.

The bactericidal penicillin G is usually the prophylactic drug of choice, in a single dose (Shanson 1978; Neu 1979b; Goldman and Petersdorf 1979; Garrod 1975; Paulson et al. 1980; Sipes et al. 1977; Kaye 1976; Meyers et al. 1980; Krupp and Chatton 1980; Parrillo et al. 1979). An extensive review, including β-lactam prophylaxis, on the prevention of heart disease in infants and children was published by Rao (1977). Despite the heroic prophylactic antibiotic measures, rheumatic fever and its consequences are still serious problems and it causes more deaths than would be expected (Lyon et al. 1979). More controlled trials are needed for the prospective evaluation of the effectiveness of the present treatment regimens and, if necessary, for their rational modification (Sipes et al. 1977).

Other medical prophylactic uses of β-lactams should be based on logic and analogies relating to other situations (Paulson et al. 1980). These problems can usually be handled by general practitioners, internists, and pediatricians. The physician has to decide what organism is expected to be involved and whether it is expected to be sensitive to the β-lactam intended to be administered. The problem of mixed infections as well as the immune status (compromised) of the patients should also be taken into account when considering the prophylactic use of a specific β-lactam. Only the most frequent additional medical situations will be discussed below.

Neonatal infections are acquired from vaginal source by group B streptococci during delivery. This can be prevented by injecting benzylpenicillin to the neonate to prevent colonization or giving ampicillin to the mother intrapartum to prevent transmission. Occasionally, group A streptococci can cause outbreaks of nursery-acquired infections, sometimes with devastating effects such as sepsis and meningitis. Immediate treatment and the prevention of spread to other infants is usually effected by intramuscular injection of 50,000 units/kg of benzathine penicillin G. Further administration of the same drug will depend on the umbilical and throat cultures of all the infants and personnel. Prophylactic treatment is applied to mothers after premature rupture of the fetal membranes for fear of infection of the infant with gram-negative species. The newer cephalosporins are effective in this indication.

Recurrent urinary tract infections in women are often a difficult therapeutic problem. Most infections are due to *E. coli* or *S. faecalis*, but mixed infections are very common. Large doses of ampicillin or amoxicillin can prevent recurrence. Other antimicrobial agents are also employed for this indication.

Meningitis in patients with frequent meningococcemia may be a severe problem in closed population groups such as military installations, where pathogenic meningococci are disseminated by carriers. Treatment or prevention of contact infection is achieved by administration of 20 million units of aqueous penicillin parenterally (ARTENSTEIN 1975).

Lower respiratory infections are treated especially in patients with anatomic abnormalities of the respiratory tract (emphysema, bronchiectasis), elderly patients; and states after abdominal surgery, coma or paralysis where bronchitis may develop recurrently. *H. influenzae*, pneumococci and *S. aureus* (mostly resistant) are the most common pathogens. Ampicillin, amoxicillin and cloxacillin are β-lactams most often used. Superinfection with *P. aeruginosa* or *Proteus* spp., often in hospital conditions, aggravates the situation especially in children with cystic fibrosis. In most cases carbenicillin, ticarcillin, piperacillin, azlocillin and some of the third generation cephalosporins, alone or more often in combination with an aminoglycoside, are mandatory.

Acquisition of gonorrhoea and syphilis can be prevented by chemoprophylaxis with penicillin G. In the case of gonorrhoea, procaine penicillin G and in the case of syphilis, benzathine penicillin G (2.5 million units intramuscularly) can prevent or abort infections. Attention must be given to eventual β-lactamase producing *N. gonorrhoeae* strains as well as to the possibility of masked clinical syphilis, therefore prolonged follow-up serologic tests are mandatory (SÖNNICHSEN and ENGEL 1978).

Recurrent otitis media, especially its purulent form, can be prevented by continuous administration of low doses of ampicillin or amoxicillin.

Opportunistic infections in compromised patients in whom the natural protective mechanisms are seriously impaired by disease and/or drug treatment (corticosteroids and immunosuppressive agents) with severe granulocytopenia (leukocyte counts less than 500) are treated prophylactically. The drug selection and treatment schedule may vary from center to center. The feared bacteria are *Listeria monocytogenes*, *P. aeruginosa*, *S. marcescens*, *E. coli*, *Klebsiella* spp., *Enterobacter* spp., *Proteus* spp., resistant *S. aureus* and anaerobes. (Viral, fungal and *Pneumocystis carinii* infections are also common.) For prophylaxis all the respective penicillins and cephalosporins can be used (depending on the expected pathogen) often in combination with an aminoglycoside and other antibiotics or chemotherapeutic agents. These patients are generally very ill and of high risk of infection, therefore the chemoprophylaxis is desperately needed (GILLETT et al. 1978). The picture may change with the introduction of the new broad-spectrum β-lactamase stable cephalosporins.

In postcoital cystitis, the exacerbation of symptoms in women can often be prevented by oral ampicillin taken soon after intercourse.

II. Prophylactic Uses in Surgery

Surgical applications of antibiotics are predominantly for prophylactic purposes, usually for well-established indications, but occasionally of questionable benefit.

There obviously is no antibiotic which would give prophylaxis against all types of possible postoperative infections. However, in special cases retrospective studies suggest that postoperative infections can be prevented by prophylaxis. Some general features of the subject should be considered prior to a discussion of specific surgical indications (GOLDMAN and PETERSDORF 1979; NICHOLS and CONDON 1980; KRUPP and CHATTON 1980; WEINER et al. 1980). In clean elective surgery, where no normal flora-bearing tissue is involved, routine antibiotic prophylaxis has no advantage. Whenever the expected rate of contamination exceeds 5%, like clean-contaminated operations, contaminated and dirty traumatic wounds, antibacterial prophylaxis is justified. In cardiovascular, prosthetic and orthopedic surgery where an eventual infection may have catastrophic consequences, prophylactic administration of antibiotic(s) is mandatory. It is essential that the antibiotic be present at a killing level in the tissue spaces of the site of operation. Usually the antibiotic is administered 2 h before surgery. If the operation lasts longer than 3 h, the dose should be repeated. It is customary to inject another dose before the patient leaves the operating room. This dosing schedule is based on the observation that antibiotics, including β-lactams, suppress infections most effectively within three hours following contamination. The amount of contaminating microbes as well as their level of virulence are important but not always predictable factors. If, in spite of the prophylactic measures, infection establishes itself, naturally, adequate treatment must be instituted immediately. The prophylactic administration of antibiotics should not last more than 1 to 3 days. Of the β-lactams, at present, the broad-spectrum and bactericidal cefazolin is used most often and is reported to have a high degree of protective value in cardiovascular and orthopedic surgery as well as gastrointestinal, gallbladder, and gynecologic operations. Cefazolin is given intramuscularly 1 g 2 h before surgery and again at 2, 10, and 18 h after operation. In the case of cardiovascular operations, the dosage should be continued for 2–3 additional days.

GOLDMAN and PETERSDORF (1979) summarized the surgical procedures which have a high risk of contamination. These situations are: excision or drainage of brain abscess; excision of lung abscess; pulmonary decortication with empyema; excision of tuberculous process; acute cholangitis, common duct stone, obstructive jaundice; perforated diverticulum; perforation of colon due to carcinoma; ruptured appendix; vaginal hysterectomy; cesarean section; surgical procedures involving implantation of foreign bodies – cardiac valves, orthopedic prostheses, vascular grafts; debridement of traumatic contaminated wounds and debridement of burn wounds. Many of the β-lactams are beneficially used alone or in combination in the "chemoprophylaxis" in most of these surgical procedures.

A short acount of the indications and recommended β-lactams for surgical prophylaxis is given below:

Prevention of gas gangrene caused by *Clostridium perfringens* (*welchii*) is very important, since it is one of the most dangerous of acute wound infections. The spores are introduced by contaminated soil or dirt following various forms of trauma. Large doses of penicillin G (500,000 units every 6 h) for several days are required for prevention. If surgical intervention is needed, the first dose should be given at the beginning of the operation.

A single dose of 1.5 g cefuroxime intravenously prior to induction of anesthesia can prevent post-operative adominal wound sepsis or septicemia (LAMBERT and MULLINGER 1980).

Cardiac, cardiovascular and orthopedic procedures utilizing prosthetic devices always need antibacterial prophylaxis because of the possible potential devastating consequences of infection. If infection is established, the mortality may be as high as 70%. The infecting agents are almost always staphylococci and/or streptococci, therefore any of the penicillinase-resistant penicillins (methicillin, nafcillin, the isoxazolylpenicillins (0.5–1.0–2.0 g every 4 h) and especially cefazolin (0.5–1.0 g every 6 h) intramuscularly or intravenously, or cephalothin (1.0–2.0 g) intravenously have been successfully used (EIGEL et al. 1978; PIEN et al. 1979; CLARK 1979). Against the coagulase-negative staphylococci the anti-staphylococcal penicillins are less active than the cephalosporins; therefore the latter are more indicated in prosthetic valve and orthopedic surgery and in vascular surgery where grafts are involved.

Many β-lactam antibiotics have useful roles in the prophylaxis of abdominal surgery. For the sake of brevity all forms of surgical intervention in the gastrointestinal tract are handled here together, including surgery on the esophagus, stomach, biliary tract, distal ileum, colon and rectum, as well as ruptured viscus. In the case of elective operations in the lower gastrointestinal tract, in addition to cleansing of the colon, topical antibiotic agents (neomycin, insoluble sulfonamides) are used customarily to partially and transiently suppress bowel flora. Since contamination is expected from the normal flora of the gastrointestinal tract, the prophylactic β-lactams or other antibiotics are selected accordingly (DELALANDE et al. 1981). Carbenicillin, cefamandole, cefoxitin, other β-lactams or combinations of aminoglycosides and clindamycin are used most often. They are injected at the beginning of surgery to obtain effective suppressive levels in the tissues of the operation site. They should not be given longer than 24–48 h after surgery. Additional detailed data can be found in the publications of HURLEY et al. 1979, THADEPALLI 1979; CONDON 1975; SLAMA et al. 1979; KEIGHLEY et al. 1979; BUSUTTIL et al. 1981; LINDHAGEN et al. 1981.

In selected cases of pelvic surgery, such as abdominal and vaginal hysterectomy (POLK et al. 1980; CHODAK and PLAUT 1978) and cesarean section (GALL 1979) prophylactic β-lactams can reduce the incidence of infection. Ampicillin, cefamandole, cefoxitin, cefazolin and cephalothin have been successfully used alone or with gentamicin metronidazole and clindamycin to cover both aerobic and anaerobic flora in frequently-occurring mixed flora infections, usually as a one-day therapy.

In genitourinary surgery the prophylactic use of amoxicillin, cephalexin, cefazolin and cephalothin, with or without an aminoglycoside can significantly reduce the incidence of postoperative urinary tract infections. They may also be of benefit in patients undergoing transurethral prostatic resection and in vaginal hysterectomies. Pivmecillinam and co-trimoxazole have been reported to reduce postoperative bacterial episodes and hospital stay following prostatectomy (BANNISTER et al. 1981). Cefotaxime and cefazolin were used with success for the antibiotic prophylaxis in genitourinary surgery (CHILDS et al. 1981).

Preoperative administration of various β-lactams, predominantly penicillin G, ampicillin, cephalothin and cefazolin have been found beneficial in musculoskeletal and soft-tissue surgery (head and neck, chest and other soft-tissue wounds). These are also employed in burns, in combination with other appropriate medical and surgical measures.

Despite the beneficial prophylactic effect of β-lactam and other antibiotics, it should be kept in mind that excellent surgical technique and rigorous asepsis are equally if not more important means of preventing surgical infections. With the introduction of newer, more potent β-lactams, the prophylactic use of antibiotics will change in the future. More detailed information is contained in the bibliography and in an objective review on "Antimicrobial prophylaxis for surgery" (The Medical Letter 21:73–76, 1979).

E. Use of β-Lactam Antibiotics in Dental Medicine

All of the general rules with respect to β-lactam therapy of infections apply to the use of β-lactam antibiotics in dental medicine. The oral infections and their treatment are grouped into three classes (LANGDON 1974; CAWSON and SPECTOR 1975; BLACK 1978): treatment of established infections; prevention of infections in the oral cavity of particularly vulnerable patients; and protection of patients from the development of bacterial endocarditis following dental (oral) manipulations. The last of these categories represents a special problem in dental medicine (surgery) and in application of β-lactam antibiotics (EVERETT and HIRSCHMANN 1977).

The cause and treatment of dental and oral cavity infections and the prevention of localized infections in the mouth following dental manipulations can be considered together. Infections in the oral cavity of otherwise healthy persons, in general, are not very frequent and they usually resolve rapidly on local measures. Treatment only rarely requires systemic antibiotic therapy. Uncomplicated simple dental extractions and other minor oral surgery usually do not require antibiotic treatment. Removal of impacted teeth or any bone removal may be followed by antibiotic dosage in order to reduce post-operative infections. This is at the discretion of the dental surgeon. The case is the same with pericoronitis around eruption or partially erupted teeth and periapical infections. They will resolve usually without specific antibiotic treatment, after extraction or drainage through the root canal. However, if the local treatment is late or inadequate, abscess may develop with systemic infection. When serious symptoms develop, like facial swelling, pain and restriction of opening the mouth, local inflammation with lymph node enlargement, fever and malaise, urgent adequate antibiotic treatment is mandatory. Simple soft tissue injury during small oral surgery usually does not require systemic antibiotic treatment. In contrast, osteomyelitis is an absolute indication for introduction of rigorous prolonged antibiotic therapy.

Of the acute spreading infections, in the case of cellulitis of the oral cavity and the face, the development of cavernous sinus thrombosis is a danger, requiring immediate antibiotic therapy. Ludwig's angina, with swelling of the neck as well as swelling of the floor of the mouth, may lead to respiratory obstruction which needs antibiotic treatment together with surgery. Acute ulcerative gingivitis and bacterial gingivostomatitis are extremely painful and when they are associated with fever, malaise, lymphadenitis of the neck, they require prompt antibiotic treatment.

Fractures of the jaw almost always are compound fractures into the oral cavity and are prone to infection with oral bacteria. Therefore, immediate antibiotic therapy is mandatory and should be continued for 7–10 days after immobilization of the fractures.

Various dental procedures and manipulations, of which dental extraction is the most frequent, are associated with bacteremia which may cause bacterial endocarditis, especially in patients with damaged or abnormal heart valves, congenital heart disease or rheumatic fever. Since it is impossible to predict who will and who will not acquire endocarditis in such situations, and since endocarditis cannot occur without bacteremia, prophylactic antibiotic treatment is highly recommended in the above situations.

In addition to dental extraction, the following oral conditions and dental manipulations are potential risk factors for bacteremia and bacterial endocarditis in susceptible subjects: periodontal disease with tooth mobility, periodontal surgery, gingivectomy, osteoplasty, denture ulceration (even without natural teeth), poor dental hygiene, scaling and flap operations, periapical infection and root canal treatment, and pericoronal infection. Basically, all dental manipulations, like routine professional cleaning with gingival bleeding, topical application of fluoride substances, daily tooth brushing, chewing hard candy or gum and oral irrigation device working under pressure of water for cleansing can produce bacteremia and subsequent endocarditis in patients at risk but the incidence is much lower than after major surgical procedures. Prophylactic antibiotic treatment should be instituted in many of these situations. If the manipulation procedures and instrumentation are planned, it is advisable that they should be carried out during the period of peak antibiotic concentration.

Since alpha-hemolytic streptococci (viridans streptococci) are the most commonly implicated bacteria following dental manipulations, antibiotic treatment and prophylaxis should be specifically directed toward them. In this case, penicillin G is the drug of first choice. Penicillin V and ampicillin are also effective. In penicillin allergy, erythromycin or some of the cephalosporins (cefazolin, cefamandole) can be selected. In addition to the alpha-hemolytic streptococci very few other bacteria are implicated as causes of bacteremia with dental extractions and other dental manipulations. These are diphteroides, *S. epidermidis*, occasionally *S. aureus* and strains of the anaerobic mouth flora. They may require different therapy to the viridans streptococci.

For the treatment of severe dental infections, benzylpenicillin (penicillin G) remains the antibiotic of choice. It should be given intramuscularly about 20–30 min before any dental manipulation in a dose fo 1–2 million units. The usual dose of procaine benzylpenicillin G is 600,000 units intramuscularly about 30 min before any procedure. The oral phenoxymethylpenicillin (penicillin V) can be substituted or follow the intramuscular benzylpenicillin treatment. Tablets containing 125 or 250 mg should be taken every 6 h for a few days.

Rarely, *S. aureus* is the infecting agent. It should always be suspected to be a penicillinase-producer (prior to sensitivity testing); therefore, any of the penicillinase-resistant penicillins, most usually the oral oxacillin, cloxacillin, dicloxacillin or flucloxacillin should be taken first in adequate doses. The oral cephalexin would be a more expensive alternative. The broad spectrum penicillins (ampicillin, amoxicillin) are rarely, if ever, indicated in dentistry. The periapical infections are usually mixed infections including anaerobic bacteria. If *B. fragilis* is involved, the penicillins are not effective. The cephamycin cefoxitin or perhaps third generation cephalosporins should be administered. Clindamycin and metronidazole are also very effective drugs. The adult dose range for cefoxitin may be 1–2 g every 6 or 8 h intramuscularly or preferably intravenously depending on the severity of infection and the patient tolerance.

As mentioned above, in the case of penicillin allergy, a corresponding cephalosporin may be tried cautiously. Erythromycin estolate is also a logical choice. It is given orally in a dose of 500 mg 2 h before the dental manipulation which is followed by 250 mg orally every 6 h for 2–4 days.

For the prevention of endocarditis following dental manipulations intramuscular penicillin in combination with streptomycin, or large doses of procaine penicillin G or penicillin G combined with benzathine penicillin, or vancomycin alone in 1 g intravenous dose are used successfully often in a single dose. Phenoxymethylpenicillin and cefazolin in multiple doses have also been found to be effective. For prophylactic purposes, erythromycin alone is barely satisfactory because it is not bactericidal in its mode of action. The two basic regimens (A and B) for chemoprophylaxis of bacterial endocarditis following dental procedures have been suggested by the American Heart Association (1977).

Despite parenteral prophylaxis, some patients still develop bacterial endocarditis. The American Heart Association is in the process of evaluating the situation and, if needed, will make new recommendations with the cooperation of practicing physicians and dentists.

F. Use of β-Lactam Antibiotics in Veterinary Practice

The β-lactam antibiotics can be used in veterinary practice for the same indications as they are used in the treatment of infectious diseases in man.

This section will be restricted to a discussion of those β-lactam sensitive bacteria which are characteristically involved in various animal infections. These infectious diseases can be found in considerable detail in the comprehensive book of JONES (1965) and their treatment with penicillins and certain cephalosporins in the chapter of HUBER (1977), and in the publications of CLARK (1976, 1977). The use of cephalosporins, other than mentioned in HUBER's chapter, but which have been used with success in veterinary medicine will be discussed later.

Benzylpenicillin (water soluble salts, procaine and benzathine preparations) is used most extensively. Penicillin G is administered intravenously (without significant thrombophlebitis) in divided doses or by continuous infusion. The intramuscular injection is always intermittent administration. It can also be injected subcutaneously. The topical application of penicillin (ointment, powder and solution) is discouraged to avoid eventual sensitization and allergic reactions, and the emergence of resistant strains.

In addition to the systemic treatment, penicillin is often used intramammarily in the treatment of acute and chronic bovine mastitis by infusion via the teat canal. It is a useful treatment because the causative bacteria, *Staphylococcus agalactiae* and *S. aureus; Streptococcus dysgalactiae* and *S. uberis* as well as *Corynebacterium pyogenes*, are very sensitive to benzyl- and phenoxymethylpenicillins. If the *S. aureus* is a β-lactamase-producing strain, some of the β-lactamase-resistant antistaphylococcal penicillins (methicillin, nafcillin or any of the isoxazolyl penicillins) must be used. The purpose of their administration is two-fold, the successful treatment of the cattle and also the prevention of the dissemination of the resistant strain(s) to other animals and to man. Animals harboring such β-lactamase-producing staphylococcus are a potential source of infection for attendants of veterinary hospitals who may disseminate the strains to a larger human population. Hospitalized dogs were also found to harbour a much higher percentage of resistant staphylococci.

Another public health problem connected with the intramammary infusion of penicillin for the treatment or prevention of bovine mastitis is that penicillin traces may remain in the milk or in milk products, resulting in possible sensitization. To prevent this allergic sequela, public health measures have been introduced (Food and Drug Administration). To prevent allergies, treated cattle should be removed from the milking line until the penicillin is eliminated from the milk (usually about 96 h after treatment). The time must be longer when long-acting depot penicillin preparations are used.

Tests for penicillin residue in milk are available. Of the biologic methods the disc-assay using *B. subtilis* as the test organism or the morphologic changes induced in *S. thermophilus* are recommended. The chemical test utilizing the color change of triphenyltetrazolium chloride after incubation with milk is also used. Recently a simple fermentation test to detect penicillin, streptomycin, dihydrostreptomycin, or chloramphenicol residues in milk has been published (JURDI and ASMAR 1981).

Penicillin residue may be present in the edible tissues (muscle, liver, kidney) of swine and calves treated for various infections, most often erysipelas and leptospirosis. Erysipelas caused by *Erysipelothrix insidiosa* in sheep, chicken and turkey may raise the same problem as the residual penicillin in edible tissues of large animals used for human consumption.

Other animal diseases that respond well to benzylpenicillin or ampicillin treatment are too numerous to list here. Some, however, will be mentioned because of their frequency. Calf diarrhea, swine dysentery and enteritis, feline enteritis, all digestive infections and peritonitis are ususally caused by gram-negative bacilli, often a *Salmonella* sp., therefore ampicillin or carbenicillin is the β-lactam of choice for treatment. Blackleg caused by *Clostridium chauvei* and other clostridial infections react well to penicillin therapy as does pyosepticemia following navel infections. The bovine, equine, porcine, and feline respiratory infections, including pneumonia, as well as the urinary tract infections are well treatable with benzylpenicillin or ampicillin. The newer broader spectrum penicillins as well as cephalosporins used in human therapy can be considered as useful drugs if they are available for veterinary practice at a reasonable price. Penicillin G is the drug most often used in treatment of wounds, either surgical or traumatic.

Although penicillin G is of low toxic potential, two toxic reactions which may occur in animals should be mentioned. As previously pointed out, fatal reactions of unknown etiology in guinea-pigs are observed. If for some reason penicillin G reaches the central nervous system of cats, dogs, monkeys (and man) it causes cortical stimulation, sometimes with serious convulsions which can be treated with intravenous barbiturates. The penicillin concentration in the cerebrospinal fluid to produce convulsions in dogs exceeds 300 units/ml. Another toxic sign which was reported in dogs and in dairy cows are acute allergic reactions similar to those observed in humans. The symptoms are salivation, labored breathing, edema of the head and perineal region, and in the dog, additionally, vomiting, shivering, and urticaria. These symptoms appear 15 min after parenteral dosing, and either subside spontaneously within 2–4 h or after parenteral injection of epinephrine.

Cephalosporins, like penicillins, are useful drugs in veterinary practice (CLARK 1977). Although the cephalosporins used in human therapy can also be used with great success in veterinary medicine, they are used less often because of cost. Cephaloridine, in spite of its nephrotoxic potential, is successful in various bacterial infections in dogs and cats in 10 mg/kg dose intramuscularly or intravenously. The oral cephalexin and cephaloglycin are used in the treatment of smaller animals.

To overcome the disadvantages of penicillin, two cephalosporins have been introduced for the treatment and prevention of bovine mastitis (HARRIS et al. 1976). Cephalonium and cephoxazole were selected for the purpose. Neither is used in human therapy. The cerate preparations are nonirritant and tolerated within the udder after infusion. Cephoxazole was found to potentiate the action of benzylpenicillin by protecting it from the destruction of penicillinases. Cephoxazole is highly stable to β-lactamases (BOULTON and ROSS 1977). The cephoxazole-penicillin preparation contains 200 mg cephoxazole and 250,000 units of procaine penicillin G in an oily base and is used as an intramammary cerate with quick release properties. Good clinical cure was observed when the pathogens were *S. aureus*, *S. agalactiae*, *S. dysgalactiae*, *S. uberis* and *E. coli*. The two antibiotics are excreted at similar rates and there was no residual antibiotic found (triphenyltetrazolium chloride test) 3 days after the last infusion. The efficacy of this cerate preparation in the primary treatment of clinical mastitis of varied etiology was found also in field conditions after infusion with 3 g cerate, after milking, for 3 consecutive days (HARRIS et al. 1977).

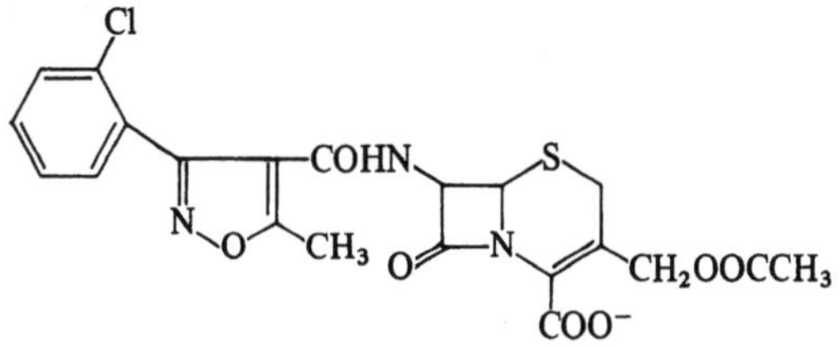

Cephoxazole

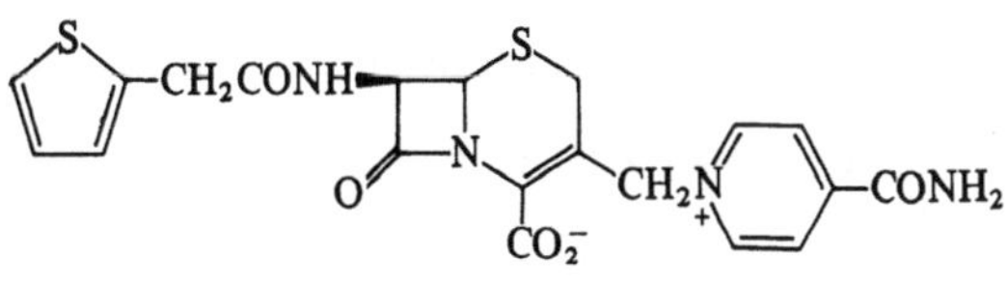

Cephalonium

Cephalonium is almost insoluble in water. The cerate containing 200 mg antibiotic is useful not only for the treatment of the existing mastitis but also for the prophylaxis of dry udder infections in dairy cattle. It is a long-acting intramammary cerate. The infusion of the cerate starts at the beginning of the dry period, and since the provision of prophylaxis covers for the dry period of about ten days, no clinical cases of mastitis were observed during this time (CURTIS et al. 1977). The cephalonium cerate is non-irritant and was found to be a very valuable β-lactam for routine prophylaxis of dry cow infections.

Other cephalosporins, such as cefazolin with its high blood levels and relatively long-lasting action may serve also a useful purpose not only in the treatment but also in the prophylaxis of parenteral therapy of mastitis and other veterinary infections caused by susceptible organisms. The third generation cephalosporins and newer penicillins with their uniquely broad antibacterial spectra and high degree of potency and stability to β-lactamases will be valuable antibiotics in veterinary practice when they become available for general use.

References

Acred P, Ryan DM, Harding SM, Muggleton PW (1980) In vivo properties of GR 20263 [ceftazidime]. In: Nelson JD, Grassi C (eds) Current chemotherapy and infectious disease, vol. I. American Society for Microbiology, Washington, DC, pp 271–273

Actor P, Uri JV, Phillips L, Sachs CS, Guarini JR, Zajac I, Berges DA, Dunn GL, Hoover JRE, Weisbach JA (1975) Laboratory studies with cefatrizine (SK & F 60771) a new broad-spectrum orally-active cephalosporin. J Antibiot 28:594–601

Actor P, Pitkin DH, Lucyszin G, Weisbach JA, Bran JL (1976) Cefatrizine (SK & F 60771), a new oral cephalosporin: serum levels and urinary recovery in humans after oral or intramuscular administration–comparative study with cephalexin and cefazolin. Antimicrob Agents Chemother 9:800–803

Actor P, Uri JV, Zajac I, Guarini JR, Phillips L, Pitkin DH, Berges DA, Dunn GL, Hoover JRE, Weisbach JA (1978) SK & F 75073 (cefonicid), a new parenteral broad-spectrum cephalosporin with high and prolonged serum levels. Antimicrob Agents Chemother 13:784–790

Alfthan O, Renkonen OV, Ohlsson H (1979) Treatment with azlocillin in complicated urinary tract infectons. Arzneim Forsch 29:1919–1981

Allaz AF, Dayer P, Fabre J, Rudhardt M, Balant M (1979) Pharmacocinétique d'une nouvelle céphalosporine, la céfopérazone. Schweiz Med Wochenschr 109:1999–2005

American Heart Association Committee on Rheumatic Fever and Bacterial Endocarditis: Prevention of Endocarditis. Circulation (1977) 56:139A

Almeida TR de, Prieto P, Calvalho JAM de, Trabulsi LR (1979) Mezlocillin in the treatment of urinary tract infections. Arzneim Forsch 29:1992–1994

Anderson JD (1977) Mecillinam resistance in clinical practice – a review. J Antimicrob Chemother 3:89–96

Anderson RJ, Gambertoglio JG, Schrier RW (1975) Clinical uses of drugs in renal failure. Thomas Springfield, p 33

Angehrn P, Probst PJ, Reiner R, Then RL (1980) Ro 13-9904 (ceftriaxon), a long-acting broad-spectrum cephalosporin: in vitro and in vivo studies. Antimicrob Agents Chemother 18:913–921

Anonymous (1980) Cefmetazole. Drugs Future 5:417–418 (editorial)

Artenstein MS (1975) Prophylaxis of meningococcal disease. JAMA 231:1035–1037

Asscher AW (1978) Use of antibiotics, management of frequency and dysuria. Br Med J 1:1531–1533

Baier R, Puppel H, Zelder O, Zehner R (1981) Piperacillin: Kinetische Studien über biliäre und renale Ausscheidung. Arzneim Forsch 31:857–861

Baisch C, Grimm H, Schmidt D, Suhayda A (1979) Klinische Erfahrungen mit Azlocillin. Med Welt 30:1735–1794

Ball AP, Gray JA, Murdoch JMcC (1978) Antibacterial drugs today. University Park Press, Baltimore, pp 6–29, 53–59

Bannister G, Arkell DG, Menday AP (1981) Prostatectomy and prophylaxis. J Antimicrob Chemother 7:209–210

Barriere SL, Gambertoglio JG, Lin ET, Conte JE (1982) Multiple dose pharmacokinetics of amdinocillin in healthy volunteers. Antimicrob Agents Chemother 21:54–57

Barza M, Miao PVW (1977) Antimicrobial spectrum, pharmacology and therapeutic use of antibiotics, part 3: cephalosporins. Am J Hosp Pharm 34:621–629

Basker MJ, Boon RJ, Hunter PA (1980) Comparative antibacterial properties in vitro of seven olivanic acid derivatives: MM 4550, MM 13902, MM 17880, MM 22380, MM 22381, MM 22382 and MM 22383. J Antibiot 33:878–884

Batchelor FR, Doyle FP, Nayler JHC, Rolinson GN (1959) Synthesis of penicillin: 6-aminopenicillanic acid in penicillin fermentation. Nature 183:257–258

Bax RN, White LO, Holt A, Bywater M, Reeves DS (1981) Metabolism of β-lactam antibiotics. N Engl J Med 304:734–735

Belli L, Gondolfo S, Varela M, Gennaro EA (1979) Local tolerance of I.M. mezlocillin injection. Arzneim Forsch 29:1985–1987

Belohradsky BH, Geiss D, Marget W, Bruch K, Kafetzis D, Peters G (1980) Intravenous cefotaxime in children with bacterial meningitis. Lancet 1:61–63

Bint AJ (1980) Esters of penicillins – are they hepatotoxic? J Antimicrob Chemother 6:697–699
Bint AJ, Reeves DS (1978) A guide to new antibiotics. Br J Hosp Med 19:335–342
Black CG (1978) Antibiotics in dentistry. NZ Med J 87:330–331
Botta GA, Park JT (1981) Evidence of involvement of penicillin binding protein 3 in murein synthesis during septation but not during cell elongation. J Bacteriol 145:333–340
Boulton MG, Ross GW (1977) Resistance of cephoxazole-benzyl-penicillin combinations to destruction by β-lactamases associated with bovine mastitis. J Comp Pathol 87:145–153
Brachman PS (1979) Principles of chemoprophylaxis and immunoprophylaxis. In: Mandell GL, Douglas RG, Bennett JE (eds) Principles and practice of infectious diseases. Wiley, New York, p 126
Brogden RN, Heel RC, Speight TM, Avery GS (1979a) Amoxycillin injectable: a review of its antibacterial spectrum, pharmacokinetics and therapeutic use. Drugs 18:169–184
Brogden RN, Heel RC, Speight TM, Avery GS (1979b) Cefoxitin: a review of its antibacterial activity, pharmacological properties and therapeutic use. Drugs 17:1–37
Brogden RN, Carmine A, Heel RC, Morley PA, Speight TM, Avery GS (1981) Amoxycillin/clavulanic acid; review of its antibacterial activity, pharmacokinetics and therapeutic use. Drugs 22:337–362
Brown AG (1981) New naturally occurring β-lactam antibiotics and related compounds. J Antimicrob Chemother 7:15–48
Brown WM, Fallon RJ (1979) Cefotaxime for bacterial meningitis. Lancet 1:1246
Brumfitt W, Hamilton-Miller J (1976) Rational choice of antibiotic. Lancet 2:900–901
Bucourt R, Heymès R, Lutz A, Pénasse L, Perronnet J (1977) Propriétés antibiotiques inattendues dans le domaine des céphalosporines. C R Acad Sci [D] (Paris) 284:1847–1849
Bucourt R, Heymès R, Lutz A, Pénasse L, Perronnet J (1978) Céphalosporines a chaine amino-2-thiazolyl-4 acétyles. Influence de la présence et de la configuration d'un groupe oxyimino sur l'activité antibactérienne. Tetrahedron 34:2233–2243
Buening MK, Wold JS, Israel KS, Kammer RB (1981) Disulfiram-like reaction to β-lactams. JAMA 245:2027–2028
Burch KH, Pohlod D, Saravolatz LD, Madhavan T, Kiani D, Quinn EL, Delbusto R, Cardenas J, Fisher EJ (1979) Ceforanide: in vitro and clinical evaluation. Antimicrob Agents Chemother 16:386–391
Busuttil RW, Davidson RK, Fine M, Tompkins RK (1981) Effect of prophylactic antibiotics in acute nonperforated appendicitis. Ann Surg 194:502–509
Carlone NA, Cuffini AM, Mastroviti S (1980) Cefuroxime: evaluation in vitro and in vivo. Drugs Exp Clin Res 6:437–448
Cawson RA, Spector RG (1975) Clinical pharmacology in dentistry. Churchill Livingstone, Edinbourgh
Cefatrizine (1976) Chemotherapy (Tokyo) 24:1661–1984
Chabert YA, Lutz AJ (1978) HR 756 (cefotaxime), the *syn* isomer of a new methoxyimino cephalosporin with unusual antibacterial activity. Antimicrob Agents Chemother 14:749–754
Childs SJ, Wood PD, Kosola JW (1981) Antibiotic prophylaxis in genitourinary surgery. Clin Ther 4:111–123
Chodak GW, Plaut M (1978) Wound infections and systemic antibiotic prophylaxis in gynecologic surgery. Obstet Gynecol 51:123–127
Clarke AM (1979) Prophylactic antibiotics for total hip arthroplasty–the significance of *Staphyloccus epidermidis*. J Antimicrob Chemother 5:493–502
Clark CH (1976a) Broad-spectrum penicillins. Mod Vet Pract 57:936–940
Clark CH (1976b) Penicillins in veterinary practice. Mod Vet Pract 57:1019–1023
Clark CH (1977) Cephalosporins in veterinary practice. Mod Vet Pract 58:47–50
Clumeck N, Vanhoof R, Vanlaetham Y, Butzler JP (1979) Cefotaxime and nephrotoxicity. Lancet 1:835
Cody CL, Spencer MJ, Millett VE (1979) Treatment of common pediatric infections with oral cefaclor. Curr Ther Res 26:133–140
Condon RE (1975) Rational use of prophylactic antibiotics in gastrointestinal surgery. Surg Clin North Am 55:1309–1318

Cosmidis J, Anifantis A, Stathakis CH, Mantopoulos K, Daikos GK (1980) Augmentin (amoxicillin plus sodium clavulinate, a β-lactamase inhibitor) is active in amoxicillin-resistant infections. In: Nelson JD, Grassi C (eds) Current Chemotherapy and Infectious Disease, vol I. American Society for Microbiology, Washington, DC, pp 330–331
Csáky TZ (1979) Cutting's handbook of pharmacology, 6th edn. Appleton-Century-Crofts, New York, pp 10–21
Curtis R, Hendy PG, Watson DJ, Harris AM, Devis AM, Marshall MJ (1977) A cerate containing cephalonium for the prophylaxis of dry udder infections in dairy cows. Vet Rec 100:557–560
Delalande JP, Perramant M, Colloc ML, Egreteau JP, Chastel C (1981) Infections post-opératoires à germes anaerobies en chirurgie abdominale. Sem Hôp Paris 57:1699–1703
DeSante KL, Israel KS, Brier GL, Wolny JD, Hatcher BL (1982) Effect of probenecid on the pharmacokinetics of moxalactam. Antimicrob Agents Chemother 21:58–61
Eigel P, Tschirkov A, Satter P, Knothe H (1978) Assays of cephalosporin antibiotics administered prophylactically in open-heart surgery. Infection 6:23–28
Ellis CJ, Geddes AM, Davey PG (1979) Mezlocillin and azlocillin: an evaluation of two new β-lactam antibiotics. J Antimicrob Chemother 5:517–525
Ernst JA, Lorian V (1980) Mecillinam in urinary tract infections. In: Nelson JD, Grassi C (eds) Current Chemotherapy and Infectious Disease, vol I. American Society for Microbiology, Washington, DC, pp 318–319
Everett ED, Hirschmann JV (1977) Transient bacteremia and endocarditis prophylaxis: a review. Medicine 56:61–77
Federspil P, Bach R (1979) Cefaclor in the treatment of infections of the ears, nose, and throat. Postgrad Med J 55:53–55
Finch R (1980) Immunomodulating effects of antimicrobial agents. J Antimicrob Chemother 6:691–694
Florey HW (1943–1944) Discussion on penicillin. Proc R Soc Med 37:104–105
Florey HW, Chain E, Heatley NG, Jennings MA, Sanders AG, Abraham EP, Florey ME (1949) Antibiotics, a survey of penicillin, streptomycin, and other antimicrobial substances from fungi, actinomycetes, bacteria, and plants, vol II. Oxford University Press, London, p 647
Fossati C (1978) Le Cephalosporine. Clin Ter 84:167–193
Fowler W, Khan MH (1979) Mezlocillin in gonorrhoea: a pilot study. Curr Med Res Opin 5:790–792
Fraser DG (1979) Drug therapy reviews: antimicrobial spectrum, pharmacology and therapeutic use of cefamandole and cefoxitin. Am J Hosp Pharm 36:1503–1508
Friedrich H, Haensel-Friedrich G, Langmaak H, Daschner FD (1980) Investigations of cefuroxime levels in the cerebrospinal fluid of patients with and without meningitis. Chemotherapy 26:91–97
Fu KP, Neu HC (1978) Azlocillin and mezlocillin – new ureido penicillins. Antimicrob Agents Chemother 13:930–938
Fujii R (1979) Ergebnisse multizentrischer klinischer Prüfungen mit Mezlocillin in Japan. Arzneim Forsch 29:2005–2008
Fujii R (1980) Clinical effects of cefmetazole in pediatric patients. In: Nelson JD, Grassi C (eds) Current Chemotherapy and Infectious Disease, vol I. American Society for Microbiology, Washington, DC, pp 240–242
Gall SA (1979) The efficacy of prophylactic antibiotics in cesarean section. Am J Obstet Gynecol 134:506–511
Gambertoglio JG, Barriere SL, Lin ET, Conte JE (1980) Pharmacokinetics of mecillinam in healthy subjects. Antimicrob Agents Chemother 18:952–956
Garrod LP (1974) Choice among penicillins and cephalosporins. Br Med J 2:96–100
Garrod LP (1975) Chemoprophylaxis. Br Med J 4:501–564
Geddes AM, Clarke PD (1977) The treatment of enteric fever with mecillinam. J Antimicrob Chemother [Suppl B] 3:101–102
Gibbs RS, Blanco JD, Castaneda YS, St. Clail PJ (1980) Therapy of obstetrical infections with moxalactam. Antimicrob Agents Chemother 17:1004–1007
Gillett AP, Wise R, Geddes AM (1978) Infection of the compromised host. Br Med J 2:335–337

Ginsburg CM, McCracken GH (1980) Cefaclor and cefadroxil: a commentary on their properties and possible indications for use in pediatrics. J Pediatr 96:340–342
Giron JA, Meyers BR, Hirschman SZ (1981a) Biliary concentrations of piperacillin in patients undergoing cholecystectomy. Antimicrob Agents Chemother 19:309–311
Giron JA, Meyers BR, Hirschman SZ, Srulevitch E (1981b) Pharmacokinetics of piperacillin in patients with moderate renal failure and in patients undergoing hemodialysis. Antimicrob Agents Chemother 19:279–283
Goldman PL, Petersdorf RG (1979) Prophylactic antibiotics: controversies give way to guidelines. Drug Therapy 9:57–77
Goldstein FW, Kitzis MD, Malhuret C, Bourquelot P, Acar JF (1980) Clinical evaluation of the formulation clavulanic acid plus amoxicillin in the treatment of urinary tract infections due to β-lactamase-producing bacteria. In: Nelson JD, Grassi C (eds) Current Chemotherapy and Infectious Disease, vol I. American Society for Microbiology, Washington, DC, pp 349–351
Gordon WE (1978) Efficacy and safety of cefadroxil. J K Med Assoc 76:121–123
Goto S, Tsuji A, Ogawa M, Kaneko Y, Miyazaki S, Kuwahara S (1980) Ceftizoxime. Chemotherapy (Tokyo) 28:7–23
Goto S, Ogawa M, Tsuji A, Kuwahara S, Tsuchiya K, Kondo M, Kida M (1980) SCE-1365, a new cephalosporin: in vitro antibacterial activities. In: Nelson JD, Grassi C (eds) Current Chemotherapy and Infectious Disease, vol I. American Society for Microbiology, Washington, DC, pp 264–266
Graninger W, Spitzy KH, Pichler H, Diem E, Slany J, Scherzer W, Gassner A, Breyer S (1980) Cefsulodin (CGP 7174/E) in the treatment of *Pseudomonas* infections in intensive-care patients. In: Nelson JD, Grassi C (eds) Current Chemotherapy and Infectious Disease, vol I. American Society for Microbiology, Washington, DC, pp 200–202
Granneman GR, Sennello LT, Steinberg FJ, Sonders RC (1982) Intramuscular and intravenous pharmacokinetics of cefmenoxime, a new broad-spectrum cephalosporin, in healthy subjects. Antimicrob Agents Chemother 21:141–145
Greenwood D, Pearson N, Eley A, O'Grady F (1980) Comparative in vitro activities of cefotaxime and ceftizoxime (FK749): new cephalosporins with exceptional potency. Antimicrob Agents Chemother 17:397–401
Griffith RS (1974) Ten years of cephalosporins. Adv Clin Pharmacol 8:6–17
Guibert J, Kitzis MD, Acar JF (1980) Clinical evaluation of cefsoludin (CGP 7174/E) in urinary tract infections caused by *Pseudomonas aeruginosa*. In: Nelson JD, Grassi C (eds) Current Chemotherapy and Infectious Disease, vol I. American Society for Microbiology, Washington, DC, pp 199–200
Hamilton-Miller JMT, Smith JT (1979) β-Lactamases. Academic, London
Harris AM, Davies AM, Marshall MJ, Evans JM, Hendy PG, Watson DJ (1977) The treatment of clinical mastitis with cephoxazole and penicillin. Vet Rec 101:4–7
Harris AM, Marshall MJ, Curtis R, Evans JM, Watson DJ (1976) Cephalosporins in the prevention and treatment of mastitis. Vet Rec 99:128–129
Helwig HF (1980) Cefotaxime in pediatrics. In: Nelson JD, Grassi C (eds) Current Chemotherapy and Infectious Disease, vol I. American Society for Microbiology, Washington, DC, pp 128–129
Heymès R, Lutz A, Schrinner E (1977) Experimental evaluation of HR 756 (cefotaxime), a new cephalosporin derivative: pre-clinical study. Infection 5:259–260
Heymès R, Bucourt R, Lutz A, Pénase L, Perronnet J (1979) Considerable magnification of the antibacterial activity of cephalosporin derivatives with 2-amino-4-thiazolyl acetyl side chain by introduction of a *syn*-alkoxyimino group (HR 756; cefotaxime). Drugs Exp Clin Res 5:23–30
Hinkle AM, Bodey GP (1980) In vitro evaluation of Ro 13-9904 (ceftriaxon). Antimicrob Agents Chemother 18:574–578
Hirschmann JV (1981) Rational antibiotic prophylaxis. Hosp Pract Nov 1981:105–123
Hirschmann JV, Inui TS (1980) Antimicrobial prophylaxis: a critique of recent trials. Rev Infect Dis 2:1–23
Hoechst (1980) Claforan (Cefotaxime) An inf Document Hoechst AG, Frankfurt/Main, 1–88
Hoeprich PD (1968) The penicillins, old and new. Med Prog 109:301–308

Höffler D (1979) Cefaclor – ein neues, orales Cephalosporin, MMW 121:229–230
Höffler D, Palmer WR (1976) Neuere Antibiotika – eine Übersicht. Aktuell Urol 7:89–99
Huber WG (1977) Penicillins. In: Jones LM, Booth NH, McDonald LE (eds) Veterinary pharmacology and therapeutics, 4th edn. Iowa State University Press, Ames, pp 912–928
Humbert G, Guibert J, Rogez JP (1979) Principales propriétés antibactériennes et pharmacologiques des pénicillines. Rev Med 6:263–272
Hurley DL, Howard P Jr, Hahn HH (1979) Perioperative prophylactic antibiotics in abdominal surgery. Surg Clin North Am 59:919–933
Imada A, Kitano K, Kintaka K, Muroi M, Asai M (1981) Sulfazecin and isosulfazecin, novel β-lactam antibiotics of bacterial origin. Nature 289:590–591
Ishigami J, Mita T, Momose S, Kumazawa J (1980) Clinical evaluation of cefotiam in complicated urinary tract infections: a comparative study with cefazolin by a randomized double-blind method. In: Nelson JD, Grassi C (eds) Current Chemotherapy and Infectious Disease, vol I. American Society for Microbiology, Washington, DC, pp 218–219
Jawetz E, Melnick JL, Adelberg EA (1980) Review of medical microbiology, 14th edn. Lange Medical, Los Altos, pp 127–131
Jogerst GJ, Dippe SE (1981) Antibiotic use among medical specialties in a community hospital. JAMA 245:842–846
Jones LM (1965) Veterinary pharmacology and therapeutics, 3rd edn. Iowa State University Press, Ames
Jones RN, Fuchs PC, Thornsberry C, Barry AL, Gavan TL, Gerlach EH (1979) Cefaclor and cefatrizine: new investigational orally administered cephalosporins. Am J Clin Pathol 72:578–585
Jonsson M, Tunevall G (1975) FL1039 (mecillinam): a new β-lactam derivative for the treatment of infections with gram-negative bacteria. Infection 3:31–36
Jovanovich JF, Saravolatz LD, Burch K, Pohlod DJ (1981) Failure of probenecid to alter the pharmacokinetics of ceforanide. Antimicrob Agents Chemother 20:530–532
Jurdi DA, Asmar JA (1981) Use of a simple fermentation test to detect antibiotic residues in milk. J Food Prot 44:674–676
Jorgensen JH, Crawford SA, Alexander GA (1980) In vitro activities of moxalactam and cefotaxime against aerobic gram-negative bacilli. Antimicrob Agents Chemother 17:937–942
Kafetzis DA, Kanarios J, Sinaniotis CA, Papadatos CJ (1980) Clinical and pharmacokinetic study of cefotaxime (HR 756) in infants and children. In: Nelson JD, Grassi C (eds) Current Chemotherapy and Infectious Disease, vol I. American Society for Microbiology, Washington, DC, pp 134–137
Kamimura T, Matsumoto Y, Okada N, Mini Y, Nishida M, Goto S, Kuwahara S (1979) Ceftizoxime (FK 749), a new parenteral cephalosporin: in vitro and in vivo antibacterial activities. Antimicrob Agents Chemother 16:540–548
Kammer RB, Short LJ (1979) Cefaclor: summary of clinical experience. Infection [Suppl] 7:631–635
Kaye D (1976) Infective endocarditis. University Park Press, Baltimore
Keighley MRB (1978) Use of antibiotics: surgical infections. Br Med J 1:1603–1606
Keighley MRB, Arabi Y, Alexander-Williams J, Youngs D, Burdon DW (1979) Comparison between systemic and oral antimicrobial prophylaxis in colorectal surgery. Lancet 1:894–897
Kemmerich B, Lode H (1981) Cefoperazone – another cephalosporin with a disulfiram type alcohol incompatibility. Infection 9:110
Kesado T, Hashizume T, Asahi Y (1980) Antibacterial activities of a new stabilized thienamycin, N-formimidoylthienamycin, in comparison with other antibiotics. Antimicrob Agents Chemother 17:912–917
King A, Shannon K, Phillips I (1980) In vitro antibacterial activity and susceptibility of cefsulodin, an antipseudomonal cephalosporin, to β-lactamases. Antimicrob Agents Chemother 17:165–169
König HB, Metzger KG, Mürmann RP, Offe HA, Schacht P, Schröck W (1977) Azlocillin – ein neues Penicillin gegen *Pseudomonas aeruginosa* und andere gramnegative Bakteria. Infection 5:170–182

Kropp H, Sundelof JG, Hajdu R, Kahan FM (1980a) Metabolism of thienamycin and related carbapenem antibiotics by the renal dipeptidase: dehydropeptidase I. 20th Intersci Conf Antimicrob Agents Chemother. New Orleans, Abstract No 2722

Kropp H, Sundelof JG, Bohn DL, Kahan FM (1980b) Improved urinary-tract bioavailability of MK0787 (N-formimidoylthienamycin) when coadministered with inhibitors of renal dehydropeptidase I. 20th Intersci Conf Antimicrob Agents Chemother. New Orleans, Abstract No 270

Kropp H, Sundelof JG, Kahan JS, Kahan FM, Birnbaum J (1980c) MK0787 (N-formimidoylthienamycin): evaluation of in vitro and in vivo activities. Antimicrob Agents Chemother 17:993–1000

Krupp MA, Chatton MJ (1980) Current medical diagnosis and treatment. Lange Medical, Los Altos, pp 943–945

Kucers A, Bennett N McK (1977) The use of antibiotics, a comprehensive review with clinical emphasis. Heinemann Medical, London, pp 3–172

Kunin CM, Finkelberg Z (1970) Oral cephalexin and ampicillin: antimicrobial activity, recovery in urine, and persistence of uremic patients. Ann Intern Med 72:349–356

Lambert WG, Mullinger BM (1980) Single-dose cefuroxime in the prophylaxis of abdominal wound sepsis. Curr Med Res Opin 6:404–406

Langdon JD (1974) Antibiotics in general dental practice. Br Dent J 136:309–316

Lassus A, Renkonen OV (1979) Mezlocillin in the treatment of gonorrhoea. Br J Vener Dis 55:191–193

Leigh DA, Bradnock K (1980) Amoxicillin/clavulanic acid (augmentin) therapy in complicated urinary tract infection. In: Nelson JD, Grassi C (eds) Current Chemotherapy and Infectious Disease, vol I. American Society for Microbiology, Washington, DC, pp 332–334

Leisinger T, Margraff R (1979) Secondary metabolites of the fluorescent pseudomonads. Microbiol Rev 43:422–442

Lernestedt JO, Pring BG, Westerlund D (1980) Comparative clinical pharmacology of bacmecillinam alone or in combination with bacampicillin and of pivmecillinam. In: Nelson JD, Grassi C (eds) Current Chemotherapy and Infectious Disease, vol I. American Society for Microbiology, Washington, DC, pp 314–316

Lindhagen J, Hadziomerović A, Nordland S, Zbornik J (1981) Comparison of systemic prophylaxis with metronidazole-fosfomycin and metronidazole-cephalothin in elective colorectal surgery. Acta Chir Scand 147:277–283

Linglöf TO, Cars O, Nordbring F (1980) Piperacillin in the treatment of severe infections: clinical evaluation and pharmacokinetics in serum, wound fluid, and subcutaneous tissue. In: Nelson JD, Grassi C (eds) Current Chemotherapy and Infectious Disease, vol I. American Society for Microbiology, Washington, DC, pp 285–287

Little PJ, Peddie BA, Pearson S (1979) Clinical use of cefamandole: a new cephalosporin. Med J Aust 1:97–99

Llorens-Terol J, Lobato A, Adam D (1979) Treatment of childhood meningitis with mezlocillin. Arzneim Forsch 29:2001–2002

Lode H, Baruch B, Koeppe P, Lehmann-Brauns S (1978) Neue Entwicklungen bei den Cephalosporin-Antibiotika. Infection 6 [Suppl] 2:197–202

Lord JW (1979) Prevent disaster-take a history. JAMA 242:153

Lyon JA, Thompson ME, Pazin GJ (1979) Prophylaxis for antibiotic endocarditis. Am Pharm 19:37–38

Maigaard S, Frimodt-Möller N, Madsen PO (1979) Treatment of complicated urinary tract infections with cefaclor: a comparison of twice daily and three times daily dosage forms. Clin Ther 2:252–257

Mandell GL (1979) Cephalosporins. In: Mandell GL, Douglas RG, Bennett JE (eds) Principles and practice of infectious diseases. Wiley, New York, pp 238–248

Mandell GL, Sande MA (1980) Penicillins and cephalosporins. In: Gilman AG, Goodman LS, Gilman A (eds) The pharmacologic basis of therapeutics, 6th edn. Macmillan, New York, pp 1126–1161

Marget W (1979) Präventive und therapeutische Anwendungsmöglichkeiten neurer Antibiotika. MMW 121:1133–1136

Masbernard A, Salord JC (1979) Therapy with cefaclor: analysis of infections in 189 French patients. Postgrad Med J 55:72–76
Mashimo K (1980) Clinical experiences with cefmetazole in Japan. In: Nelson JD, Grassi C (eds) Current Chemotherapy and Infectious Disease, vol I. American Society for Microbiology, Washington, DC, pp 238–240
Mashimo K, Kunii O, Ishigami J, Matsumoto K (1980) Clinical experience with CGP 9000 (cefroxadine) in Japan. In: Nelson JD, Grassi C (eds) Current Chemotherapy and Infectious Disease, vol I. American Society for Microbiology, Washington, DC, pp 206–207
Matsuda S, Tanno M, Kashiwagura T, Furuya H (1980) Placental transfer of cefoperazone (T-1551) and a clinical study of its use in obstetric and gynecological infections. In: Nelson JD, Grassi C (eds) Current Chemotherapy and Infectious Disease, vol I. American Society for Microbiology, Washington, DC, pp 167–168
Matsumoto K, Uzuka Y, Nagatake T, Shishido H (1980a) Clinical evaluation of 6059-S (moxalactam), a new active oxacephem. In: Nelson JD, Grassi C (eds) Current Chemotherapy and Infectious Disease, vol I. American Society for Microbiology, Washington, DC, pp 112–113
Matsumoto K, Uzuka Y, Shishido H, Nagatake T, Suzuki H (1980b) Clinical and laboratory evaluation of cefoperazone (T-1551) in respiratory infections. In: Nelson JD, Grassi C (eds) Current Chemotherapy and Infectious Disease, vol I. American Society for Microbiology, Washington, DC, pp 169–170
McKendrick MW, Geddes AM, Wise R (1980) Clinical experience with cefotaxime (HR 756). In: Nelson JD, Grassi C (eds) Current Chemotherapy and Infectious Disease, vol I. American Society for Microbiology, Washington, DC, pp 123–125
Meyers FH, Jawetz E, Goldfien A (1980) Review of medical pharmacology, 7th edn. Lange Medical, Los Altos, pp 542–550, 603–607
Michalsen H, Bergan T (1980) Azlocillin in respiratory tract infections with *Pseudomonas aeuruginosa* in children with cystic fibrosis. Chemotherapy 26:135–140
Mine Y, Nonoyama S, Kojo H, Fukada S, Nishida M (1977) Nocardicin A, a new monocyclic β-lactam antibiotic, VI, Absorption, excretion and tissue distribution in animals. J Antibiot 30:938–944
Moellering RC, Swartz MN (1976) The newer cephalosporins. N Engl J Med 294:24–28
Mogabgab WJ, Alvarez S, Beville RB (1978) Clinical experience with cefoxitin sodium in extensive trials. J Antimicrob Chemother [Suppl B] 4:215–218
Münnich D, Uri J, Valu G (1964b) Die kombinierte langfristig-hochdosierte Ampicillin- und Probenecid-Behandlung der Typhus-Bacterien-Dauerausscheider. Chemotherapy 8:226–240
Münnich D, Valu G, Uri J (1964a) Treatment of typhoid carriers with ampicillin (in Hungarian). Orvosi Hetilap (Medical Weekly) 105:205–208
Musher DM, Fainstein V, Young EJ (1980) Treatment of cellulitis with ceforanide. Antimicrob Agents Chemother 17:254–257
Nakashima M (1980) Clinical pharmacokinetics and safety of FK 749 (ceftizoxime) in healthy volunteers. In: Nelson JD, Grassi C (eds) Current Chemotherapy and Infectious Disease, vol I. American Society for Microbiology, Washington, DC, pp 254–255
Nakatomi M, Nasu M, Nagasawa T, Shigeno Y, Saito A, Hara K (1980) Cefsulodin in treatment of chronic bronchitis due to *Pseudomonas aeruginosa*. In: Nelson JD, Grassi C (eds) Current Chemotherapy and Infectious Disease, vol I. American Society for Microbiology, Washington, DC, pp 204–205
Najjar S, Messihi J, Smith LG (1980) Mecillinam, a new amidino-penicillin derivative in the treatment of serious gram-negative infections. In: Nelson JD, Grassi C (eds) Current Chemotherapy and Infectious Disease, vol I. American Society for Microbiology, Washington, DC, pp 316–318
Neu HC (1975) Aminopenicillins – clinical pharmacology and use in disease state. Int J Clin Pharmacol 11:132–144
Neu HC (1977) The penicillins, overview of pharmacology, toxicology, and clinical use. NY State J Med 962–967
Neu HC (1979a) Prophylaxis – has it at last come of age? J Antimicrob Chemother 5:331–333

Neu HC (1979b) Penicillins. In: Mandell GL, Douglas RG, Bennett JE (eds) Principles and practice of infectious diseases. Wiley, New York, pp 218–238
Neu HC (1980) The cephalosporins: a group of drugs in search of definite indications. Infect Dis 4:1–19
Neu HC, Prince AS (1980) Interaction between moxalactam and alcohol. Lancet 1:1422
Neu HC, Srinivasan S (1981) Pharmacology of ceftizoxime compared with that of cefamandole. Antimicrob Agents Chemother 20:366–369
Neu HC, Fu KP, Aswapokee N, Aswapokee P, Kung K (1979) Comparative activity and β-lactamase stability of cefoperazone, a piperazine cephalosporin. Antimicrob Agents Chemother 15:150–157
Neuman M (1980) Future perspectives in the field of β-lactam antibiotics. Drugs Exp Clin Res 6:491–513
Newsom SWB, Matthews J, Connellan SJ, Pearce VR (1980) Clinical studies with cefotaxime. In: Nelson JD, Grassi C (eds) Current Chemotherapy and Infectious Disease, vol I. American Society for Microbiology, Washington, DC, pp 125–126
Nichols RL, Condon RE (1980) Prophylactic antibiotics in surgery. In: Kagan BM (ed) Antimicrobial therapy, 3rd edn. Saunders, Philadelphia, pp 350–360
Ninane G (1979) Cefotaxime (HR 756) and nephrotoxicity. Lancet 1:332
Norrby R (1978) Newer cephalosporins and cephamycins – a review. Scand J Infect Dis [Suppl] 13:83–87
Numata M, Minamida I, Tsushima S, Nishimura T, Yamaoka M, Matsumoto N (1977) Synthesis of new cephalosporins with potent antibacterial activities. Chem Pharm Bull 25:3117–3119
Numata M, Minamida I, Yamaoka M, Shiraishi M, Miyawaki T, Akimoto H, Naito K, Kida M (1978) A new cephalosporin: SCE-963 (cefotiam), chemistry and structure-activity relationship. J Antibiot 31:1262–1271
O'Callaghan CH (1975) Classification of cephalosporins by their antibacterial activity and pharmacokinetic properties. J Antimicrob Chemother [Suppl] 1:1–12
O'Callaghan CH (1979) Description and classification of the newer cephalosporins and their relationships with the established compounds. J Antimicrob Chemother 5:635–671
O'Callaghan CH, Acred P, Harper PB, Ryan DM, Kirby SM, Harding SM (1980) GR 20263 (ceftazidime), a new broad-spectrum cephalosporin with anti-pseudomonal activity. Antimicrob Agents Chemother 17:876–883
Ochiai M, Aki O, Morimoto A, Okada T, Matsushita Y (1977) New cephalosporin derivatives with high antibacterial activities. Chem Pharm Bull 25:3115–3117
O'Grady FW (1982) Twenty-one years of beating β-lactamases. Br Med J 1:369–370
Ohkoshi M, Kimura S, Okada K, Kawamura N (1980) Clinical use of cefmetazole in urinary tract infections not responding to initial treatment with β-lactam antibiotics. In: Nelson JD, Grassi C (eds) Current Chemotherapy and Infectious Disease, vol I. American Society for Microbiology, Washington, DC, pp 232–234
Owens DR, Luscombe DK, Russel AD, Nicholls PJ (1975) The cephalosporin group of antibiotics. Adv Pharmacol Chemother 13:83–172
Pancoast SJ, Jahre JA, Neu HC (1979) Mezlocillin in the therapy of serious infections. Am J Med 67:747–752
Pancoast SJ, Francke EL, Neu HC (1980) Treatment of systemic infections with mecillinam alone or combined with other β-lactam antibiotics. In: Nelson JD, Grassi C (eds) Current Chemotherapy and Infectious Disease, vol I. American Society for Microbiology, Washington, DC, pp 320–322
Parrillo JE, Borst GC, Mazur MH, Iannini P, Klempner MS, Moellering RC Jr, Anderson SE (1979) Endocarditis due to resistant viridans streptococci during oral penicillin chemoprophylaxis. N Engl J Med 300:296–300
Paulson JA, Gordon IB, Mortimer EA (1980) Prophylactic antibiotics. In: Kagan BM (ed) Antimicrobial therapy, 3rd edn. Saunders, Philadelphia, pp 468–480
Perjés OC (1974) Klinische Untersuchung des neuen Cefalosporinderivates Cefradin. Med Welt 25:1564–1568
Phillips I, Eykyn S (1976) Rational choice of antibiotic. Lancet 2:900

Pien FD, Michael NL, Mamiya R, Takaki H, Slavish S, Bruce A, Moreno-Cabral RJ (1979) Comparative study of prophylactic antibiotics in cardiac surgery. J Thorac Cardiovasc Surg 77:908–913

Pines A, Raafat H, Kennedy MRK, Mullinger BM (1980) Experience with cefuroxime in 190 patients with severe respiratory infections. Chemotherapy 26:212–217

Pitkin DH, Actor P, Alexander F, Dubb J, Stote R, Weisbach JA (1980) Cefonicid (SK&F 75073) serum levels and urinary recovery after intramuscular and intravenous administration. In: Nelson JD, Grassi C (eds) Current Chemotherapy and Infectious Disease, vol I. American Society for Microbiology, Washington, DC, pp 252–254

Plempel M, Otten H (1969) Walter/Heilmeyer Antibiotika-Fibel, 3rd edn. Thieme, Stuttgart, pp 147–241

Polk BF, Tager IB, Shapiro M, Goren-White B, Goldstein P, Schoenbaum SC (1980) Randomized clinical trial of perioperative cefazolin in preventing infection after hysterectomy. Lancet 1:437–440

Popa G, Nuri M, Peters HJ (1979) Behandlung chronischer Harnwegsinfektion mit Mezlocillin. Med Welt 20:441–444

Price JD, Fluker JL (1978) The efficacy of cefuroxime for the treatment of acute gonorrhoea in men. Br J Vener Dis 54:165–167

Prince AS, Pancoast SJ, Neu HC (1980) Efficacy of piperacillin in the therapy of serious infections. In: Nelson JD, Grassi C (eds) Current Chemotherapy and Infectious Disease, vol I. American Society for Microbiology, Washington, DC, pp 295–296

Quintiliani R, Nightingale CH (1978) Cefazolin – diagnosis and treatment. Ann Intern Med 138:915–917

Rao PS (1977) Prevention of heart disease in infants and children. Curr Probl Pediatr 7/7, pp 1–48

Rawson D, Jones DS, Crain D, Perlino CA (1980) Comparison of ceforanide and cefazolin treatment of bacterial pneumonia. In: Nelson JD, Grassi C (eds) Current Chemotherapy and Infectious Disease, vol I. American Society for Microbiology, Washington, DC, pp 450–451

Reeves DS (1976) Rational choice of antibiotic. Lancet 2:900

Reeves DS, Bullock DW (1979) The aminopenicillins: development and comparative properties. Infection [Suppl 5] 7:425–433

Reeves DS, Davies AJ (1980) "Antabuse" effect with cephalosporins. Lancet 2:540

Regamey C (1975) Die Cephalosporine aus der Sicht des Klinikers. Int J Clin Pharmacol 11:93–102

Reports on ceftriaxon (Rocephin) (1981) Chemotherapy (Basel) [Suppl 1] 27:1–103

Retsema JA, Schelkly WU, Girard AE, English AR (1981) Beta-lactamase inhibitor CP-45,899 (sulbactam), mode of action against type III β-lactamase and synergy effect with cephalosporins. Drugs Exp Clin Res 7:255–261

Ribner BS, Billiard BS, Freimer EH (1978a) Clinical evaluation of cefatrizine in 101 patients. Curr Ther Res 24:614–621

Ribner BS, Freimer EH, Billiard BS (1978b) Clinical experience with cefoxitin sodium. J Antimicrob Chemother [Suppl B] 4:209–210

Richmond MH (1978) β-Lactamase insensitive or inhibitory β-lactams: two approaches to the challenge of ampicillin-resistant *E. coli*. Scand J Infect Dis [Suppl] 13:11–15

Rimmer DMD (1980) Cefotaxime in the treatment of septicemia. In: Nelson JD, Grassi C (eds) Current Chemotherapy and Infectious Disease, vol I. American Society for Microbiology, Washington, DC, pp 132–133

Reiner R, Weiss U, Brombacher U, Lanz P, Montavon M, Furlenmeier A, Angern P, Pobst PJ (1980) Ro 13-9904 (ceftriaxon) a novel potent and long-acting parenteral cephalosporin. J Antibiot 33:783–786

Reynolds V, Oates JK, Newsom SWB (1979) Prepubertal gonococcal vulvovaginitis: a penicillin-resistant infection treated with cefotaxime. Lancet 2:206–207

Rolinson GN (1979) 6-APA and the development of the β-lactam antibiotics. J Antimicrob Chemother 5:7–14

Rosett W, Hodges GR, Harms J, Gerjarusek P, Dworzak D, Hinthorn DR, Liu C (1977) Clinical evaluation of cefamandole nafate. Am J Med Sci 274:153–161

Sabath LD, Wallace SJ (1971) Factors influencing methicillin resistance in staphylococci. Ann NY Acad Sci 182:258–266
Sack K, Lepére A, Schwieder G (1978) Nierenverträglichkeit von Cephalosporinantibiotika: Cefoxitin und HR 756 (Cefotaxim). Med Welt 29:1233–1236
Sander S, Bergan T, Fossberg E (1980) Piperacillin in the treatment of urinary tract infections. Chemotherapy 26:141–144
Sanford JP (1977) Prophylactic use of antibiotics: basic considerations. South Med J 70:2–3
Santella PJ, Berman E (1978) Cefadroxil: sustained antimicrobial effect in bacterial infections, a review of clinical studies. Curr Ther Res 23:148–158
Schacht P (1978) Neue Entwicklungen und theoretische Grundlagen bei Penizillinen. Med Welt 29:696–700
Schacht P, Tettenborn D, Hullmann R, Bruck H (1979) Ergebnisse der klinischen Prüfung von Azlocillin. Arzneim Forsch 29:1981–1985
Schoutens E, Potvliege C, Yourassowsky E (1979) Intramuscular piperacillin sodium in uncomplicated lower urinary tract infections: evaluation of safety, clinical and bacteriological responses and blood levels. Curr Ther Res 26:848–855
Selwyn S (1976a) Rational choice of penicillins and cephalosporins based on parallel in vitro and in vivo tests. Lancet 2:616–618
Selwyn S (1976b) Rational choice of antibiotic. Lancet 2:901–902
Selwyn S (1980) The β-lactam antibiotics: penicillins and cephalosporins in perspective. Hodder and Stoughton, London
Shah PM, Helm EB, Stille W (1979) Klinische Erfahrungen mit Cefotaxim, einem neuen Cephalosporin-Derivat. Med Welt 30:298–301
Shanson DC (1978) The prophylaxis of infective endocarditis. J Antimicrob Chemother 4:2–4
Shiraha Y, Kawabata N, Yura J (1980) Double-blind comparison of cefotiam (SCE-963) and cefazolin in post-operative infections. In: Nelson JD, Grassi C (eds) Current Chemotherapy and Infectious Disease, vol I. American Society for Microbiology, Washington, DC, pp 220–221
Sipes JN, Thompson RL, Hook EW (1977) Prophylaxis of infective endocarditis: a reevaluation. Annu Rev Med 28:371–391
Slack MPE (1981) Antipseudomonal β-lactams. J Antimicrob Chemother 8:165–170
Slack RCB, Bittiner JB, Finch R (1980) Treatment of gonorrhoea caused by β-lactamase producing strains of *Neisseria gonorrhoeae* with cefotaxime. Lancet 1:431–432
Slama TG, Carey LC, Fass RJ (1979) Comparative efficacy of prophylactic cephalothin and cefamandole in elective colon sugery. Am J Surg 137:593–596
Slocombe B, Basker MJ, Bentley PH et al. (1981) BRL-17421 (Temocillin), a novel β-lactam antibiotic, highly resistant to β-lactamases, giving high and prolonged serum levels in humans. Antimicrob Agents Chemother 20:38–46
Smith H (1977) Antibiotics in clinical practice, 3rd edn. University Park Press, Baltimore, pp 25–55
Sönnichsen N, Engel S (1978) Zur Problematik der prophylaktischen Behandlung bei Kontaktpersonen von Syphilitikern und Gonorrhoikern. Dtsch Gesundheitswes 33:2296–2299
Speight TM, Brogden RN, Avery GS (1972) Cephalexin: a review of its antibacterial, pharmacological and therapeutic properties. Drugs 3:9–78
Spicehandler TR, Bernhardt L, Simberkoff MS, Rahal JJ (1980) Mezlocillin and piperacillin: a comparative clinical evaluation. In: Nelson JD, Grassi C (eds) Current Chemotherapy and Infectious Disease, vol I. American Society for Microbiology, Washington, DC, pp 293–294
Spitzy KH (1978) Neuere Preparata zur antibacteriellen Chemotherapie in der Inneren Medizin. Med Welt 29:705–707
Spratt BG (1977) The mechanism of action of mecillinam. J Antimicrob Chemother 3:13–19
Stoney DW (1979) Cefuroxime in post-operative chest infections. Curr Med Res Opin 6:209–212
Swabb EA, Leitz MA, Pilkiewicz FG, Sugerman AA (1981) Pharmacokinetics of the monobactam SQ 26,776 [Azthreonam] after single intravenous doses in healthy subjects. J Antimicrob Chemother 85:131–140

Sykes RB, Cimarusti CM, Bonner DP, Bush K, Floyd DM, Georgopapadakou NH, Koster WH et al. (1981) Monocyclic β-lactam antibiotics produced by bacteria. Nature 291:289–291
Sykes RB, Bonner DP, Bush K, Georgopapadakou NH (1982) Azthreonam (SQ 26,776), a synthetic monobactam specifically active against aerobic gram-negative bacteria. Antimicrob Agents Chemother 21:85–92
Tanayama S, Yoshida K, Adachi K, Kondo T (1980) Metabolic fate of SCE-1365, a new broad-spectrum cephalosporin, after parenteral administration to rats and dogs. Antimicrob Agents Chemother 18:511–518
Tanphaichitra D, Bussayanond A, Christensen O (1981) The combination of pivmecillinam and pivampicillin in the treatment of acute enteric fever. J Antimicrob Chemother 8:23–28
Tettenborn D, Schacht P, Hullmann R, Bruck H (1979) Ergebnisse der klinischen Prüfung von Mezlocillin. Arzneim Forsch 29:2009–2014
Thadepalli H (1979) Principles and practice of antibiotic therapy for post-traumatic abdominal injuries. Surg Gynecol Obstet 148:937–950
Thadepalli H, Rao B (1979) Clinical evaluation of mezlocillin. Antimicrob Agents Chemother 16:605–610
Thompson MIB, Ruso ME, Matsen JM, Atkin-Thor E (1981) Piperacillin pharmacokinetics in subjects with chronic renal failure. Antimicrob Agents Chemother 19:450–453
Thrupp LD (1974) Newer cephalosporins and "expanded-spectrum" penicillins. Annu Rev Pharmacol 15:435–467
Tjandramaga TB, Mullie A, Verbesselt R, De Schepper PJ, Verbist L (1978) Piperacillin: human pharmacokinetics after intravenous and intramuscular administration. Antimicrob Agents Chemother 14:829–837
Tsuchiya K, Kondo M, Nagatomo H (1978) SCE-129 (cefsulodin), Antipseudomonal cephalosporin: in vitro and in vivo antibacterial activities. Antimicrob Agents Chemother 13:137–145
Ueda Y (1976) Clinical and experimental studies on cefatriazone. Chemotherapy (Tokyo) 9:1661–1984
Ueda Y, Saito A, Ohmori M, Siba K (1980) Clinical studies on cefoperazone (T-1551) in the field of internal medicine. In: Nelson JD, Grassi C (eds) Current Chemotherapy and Infectious Disease, vol I. American Society for Microbiology, Washington, DC, pp 165–166
Uri J (1963) Die Cephalosporine als Sonderarten von Penicillinen. Pharmazie 18:254–261
Uri J (1964a) Über neue Ergebnisse und Möglichkeiten der Penicillinforschung und Therapie. Pharmazie 19:85–103
Uri J (1964b) Neuere Ergebnisse der Cephalosporinforschung. Pharmazie 19:14–17
Uri J (1964c) 6-Aminopenicillanic acid research. II. Conferentia hungarica pro therapia et investigatione in pharmacologia. Akadémiai Kiadó, Budapest, pp 364–368
Uri J (1966) Semisynthetic penicillins. Proceedings of the 4th congress of the Hungarian Association of Microbiologists. Akadémiai Kiadó, Budapest, pp 43–46
Uri J, Valu G (1963) "The therapeutic map" of the penicillins (in Hungarian). Orvosi Hetilap (Medical Weekly) 104:1729–1736
Uri J, Guarini J, Phillips L, Actor P (1972) Cefazolin: in vitro and in vivo laboratory studies. 12th Intersci Conf Antimicrob Agents Chemother, Atlantic City. Abstract 139
Váczi L, Uri J (1954) Studies on the enzyme penicillinase. Acta Microbiol Acad Sci Hung 2:167–177
Vent J (1979) Mezlocillin-Konzentrationen im menschlichen Knochen. Arzneim Forsch 29:1969–1971
Verbist L (1979) Comparison of the activities of the new ureidopenicillins piperacillin, mezlocillin, azlocillin and Bay K 4999 (furazlocillin) against gram-negative organisms. Antimicrob Agents Chemother 16:115–119
Warren GH (1976) Cyclacillin: microbiological and pharmacological properties and use in chemotherapy of infection – a critical appraisal. Chemotherapy 22:154–182
Wattel F (1975) L'antibiothérapie préventive en réanimation médicale. Lille Med 20:921–922

Webb D, Thadepalli H, Bach V, Roy I (1979) Clinical and experimental evaluation of cefoxitin therapy. Chemotherapy 25:233–242
Weiner JP, Gibson G, Munster AM (1980) Use of prophylactic antibiotics in surgical procedures: peer review guidelines as a method for quality assurance. Am J Surg 139:348–351
Weinstein AJ (1976) Newer antibiotics – guidelines for use. Postgrad Med 60:75–80
Weinstein AJ (1980) The cephalosporins: activity and clinical use. Curr Ther 8:117–139
Weippl G (1979) Therapie der Pneumonien im Kindesalter mit Mezlocillin. Arzneim Forsch 29:2003–2004
Williams JD (1978) Which cephalosporin? J Antimicrob Chemother 4:109–111
Winston DJ, Young LS (1980) Cephalosporins. In: Kagan BM (ed) Antimicrobial therapy, 3rd edn. Saunders, Philadelphia, pp 35–55
Wise R (1978a) Use of antibiotics, penicillins. Br Med J 1:1679–1681
Wise R (1978b) Use of antibiotics: cephalosporins. Br Med J 2:40–42
Wise R, Reeves DS (1974) Clinical and laboratory investigations on ticarcillin, an anti-pseudomonal antibiotic. Chemotherapy 20:45–51
Wittke RR, Adam D (1980) Diffusion of cefsulodin (CGP 7174/E) into human tissues. In: Nelson JD, Grassi C (eds) Current Chemotherapy and Infectious Disease, vol I. American Society for Microbiology, Washington, DC, pp 197–198
World Health Organization (1979) Biological substances, international standards, reference preparations, and reference reagents. WHO, Geneva, pp 74–75
Wright N, Wise R (1980) Cefotaxime elimination in patients with renal and liver dysfunction. In: Nelson JD, Grassi C (eds) Current Chemotherapy and Infectious Disease, vol I. American Society for Microbiology, Washington, DC, pp 133–134
Yamamoto T, Kuwahara I, Adachi Y, Yamaguchi N (1979) Phase 1 clinical studies on cefotiam (SCE-963). Chemotherapy (Tokyo) 27:172–180
Yasuda K, Kurashige S, Mitsuhashi S (1980) Cefroxadine (CGP-9000), an orally active cephalosporin. Antimicrob Agents Chemother 18:105–110
Yoshida T, Matsuura S, Mayama M, Kameda Y, Kuwahara S (1980) Moxalactam (6059S), a novel 1-oxa-β-lactam with an expanded antibacterial spectrum: laboratory evaluation. Antimicrob Agents Chemother 17:302–312

Subject Index

Handbook of Experimental Pharmacology

Continuation of "Handbuch der experimentellen Pharmakologie"

Springer-Verlag
Berlin
Heidelberg
New York

Handbook of Experimental Pharmacology

Continuation of "Handbuch der experimentellen Pharmakologie"

Springer-Verlag
Berlin
Heidelberg
New York

Volume 44
Heme and Hemoproteins

Volume 45: Part 1
Drug Addiction I

Part 2
Drug Addiction II

Volume 46
Fibrinolytics and Antifibrinolytics

Volume 47
Kinetics of Drug Action

Volume 48
Arthropod Venoms

Volume 49
Ergot Alkaloids and Related Compounds

Volume 50: Part 1
Inflammation

Part 2
Anti-Inflammatory Drugs

Volume 51
Uric Acid

Volume 52
Snake Venoms

Volume 53
Pharmacology of Ganglionic Transmission

Volume 54: Part 1
Adrenergic Activators and Inhibitors I

Part 2
Adrenergic Activators and Inhibitors II

Volume 55
Psychotropic Agents

Part 1
Antipsychotics and Antidepressants I

Part 2
Anxiolytis, Gerontopsychopharmacological Agents and Psychomotor Stimulants

Part 3
Alcohol and Psychotomimetics, Psychotropic Effects of Central Acting Drugs

Volume 56, Part 1 + 2
Cardiac Glycosides

Volume 57
Tissue Growth Factors

Volume 58
Cyclic Nucleotides
Part 1: **Biochemistry**
Part 2: **Physiology and Pharmacology**

Volume 59
Mediators and Drugs in Gastrointestinal Motility
Part 1: **Morphological Basis and Neurophysiological Control**
Part 2: **Endogenis and Exogenous Agents**

Volume 60
Pyretics and Antipyretics

Volume 61
Chemotherapy of Viral Infections

Volume 62
Aminoglycosides

Volume 64
Inhibition of Folate Metabolism in Chemotherapy

Volume 65
Teratogenesis and Reproductive Toxicology